Third Edition

Atlas of Ultrasound-Guided Regional Anesthesia

Andrew T. Gray, MD, PhD

Professor of Clinical Anesthesia
Department of Anesthesia and Perioperative Care
School of Medicine
University of California, San Francisco
Staff Anesthesiologist
San Francisco General Hospital
San Francisco, California

ELSEVIER

ELSEVIER

1600 John F. Kennedy Blvd.
Ste 1800
Philadelphia, PA 19103-2899

ATLAS OF ULTRASOUND-GUIDED REGIONAL ANESTHESIA,
THIRD EDITION   ISBN: 978-0-323-50951-0

Copyright © 2019 by Elsevier, Inc. All rights reserved.

No part of this publication may be reproduced or transmitted in any form or by any means, electronic or mechanical, including photocopying, recording, or any information storage and retrieval system, without permission in writing from the publisher. Details on how to seek permission, further information about the Publisher's permissions policies and our arrangements with organizations such as the Copyright Clearance Center and the Copyright Licensing Agency, can be found at our website: www.elsevier.com/permissions.

This book and the individual contributions contained in it are protected under copyright by the Publisher (other than as may be noted herein).

Notices

Knowledge and best practice in this field are constantly changing. As new research and experience broaden our understanding, changes in research methods, professional practices, or medical treatment may become necessary.

Practitioners and researchers must always rely on their own experience and knowledge in evaluating and using any information, methods, compounds, or experiments described herein. In using such information or methods they should be mindful of their own safety and the safety of others, including parties for whom they have a professional responsibility.

With respect to any drug or pharmaceutical products identified, readers are advised to check the most current information provided (i) on procedures featured or (ii) by the manufacturer of each product to be administered, to verify the recommended dose or formula, the method and duration of administration, and contraindications. It is the responsibility of practitioners, relying on their own experience and knowledge of their patients, to make diagnoses, to determine dosages and the best treatment for each individual patient, and to take all appropriate safety precautions.

To the fullest extent of the law, neither the Publisher nor the authors, contributors, or editors, assume any liability for any injury and/or damage to persons or property as a matter of products liability, negligence or otherwise, or from any use or operation of any methods, products, instructions, or ideas contained in the material herein.

Previous editions copyright © 2013, 2010.

Library of Congress Cataloging-in-Publication Data

Names: Gray, Andrew T., author.
Title: Atlas of ultrasound-guided regional anesthesia / Andrew T. Gray.
Description: Third edition. | Philadelphia, PA : Elsevier, Inc., [2019] | Includes bibliographical references and index.
Identifiers: LCCN 2017056978 | ISBN 9780323509510 (hardcover : alk. paper)
Subjects: | MESH: Anesthesia, Conduction | Ultrasonography, Interventional | Atlases
Classification: LCC RD84 | NLM WO 517 | DDC 617.9/640222–dc23
LC record available at https://lccn.loc.gov/2017056978

Publisher: Dolores Meloni
Senior Content Development Specialist: Anne Snyder
Publishing Services Manager: Catherine Jackson
Project Manager: Kate Mannix
Design Direction: Patrick Ferguson
Illustrations Manager: Lesley Frazier

Printed in China

Last digit is the print number: 9 8 7 6 5 4 3 2 1

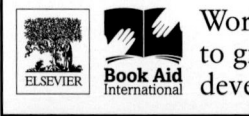

To my family of writers: Mary, Sarah, Alex, and Anna.

Preface

The third edition of *Atlas of Ultrasound-Guided Regional Anesthesia* marks a change in format. There are now many new chapters by contributing authors that vastly improve and expand the section of topics from what would be possible with a single-author text. A wide variety of newly described techniques are presented in this edition, and chapters from the previous editions underwent extensive editing and updating. The new chapters are mostly dedicated to blocks in the trunk and head and neck regions. The emphasis on safety continues, with a detailed contributed chapter that reviews large studies of rare events. Also included is a chapter on limited resources that discusses techniques and alternatives in different clinical settings.

We have tried to present clear and concise summaries of suggested techniques so that readers will have the confidence and background they need to begin using the interventional procedures. Wide fields of view, long axis views, three-dimensional imaging, and step-by-step instruction are all used to improve the educational format and illustrate anatomic structures that lie near or outside the conventional two-dimensional field of imaging. Where appropriate, chapters have additional sonograms that illustrate variations of normal anatomy that one may encounter in clinical practice. New videos show the dynamics of interventional acute pain medicine in stunning detail. All the chapters highlight recent advances and techniques in the rapidly changing field of ultrasound-guided regional anesthesia.

Very special thanks to Allegra Greher (artwork), Tin-na Kan (sciatic nerve blocks), David Mai (catheters), Ed Mathews (information technology), Stefan Simon (intercostal nerve blocks), Robin Stackhouse and Susan Yoo (figures and media production), and Ranier Litz and Tim Maecken (organizing the USRA Symposia at which much of this educational material was presented and discussed). We are grateful to the anesthesiologists, CRNAs, anesthesia technicians, and perioperative nurses at Kaiser Permanente hospitals in Oakland, Richmond, and San Francisco, California for their help with the catheter sonograms and video clips.

Andrew T. Gray, MD, PhD

Contributors

Michael J. Barrington, MBBS, FANZCA, PhD
Associate Professor
Faculty of Medicine, Dentistry and Health Sciences
University of Melbourne Medical School
Parkville, Victoria, Australia;
Department of Anaesthesia and Acute Pain Medicine
St. Vincent's Hospital Melbourne
Fitzroy, Victoria, Australia.
Chapter 74: Safety: Practical Techniques to Prevent Complications During Ultrasound-Guided Nerve Blocks

Gerald Dubowitz, MD
Associate Professor
Department of Anesthesia and Perioperative Care
University of California, San Francisco
San Francisco, California
Chapter 75: Regional Anesthesia in Resource-Constrained Environments

Urs Eichenberger, MD
Balgrist University Hospital
Chair, Department of Anaesthesia
Zürich, Switzerland
Chapter 58: Ilioinguinal and Iliohypogastric Nerve Blocks

Hesham Elsharkawy, MD, MBA, MSc
Staff Departments of General Anesthesia and Pain Management, Outcomes Research
Assistant Professor of Anesthesiology
CCLCM of Case Western Reserve University
Cleveland, Ohio
Chapter 60: Quadratus Lumborum Blocks

Jeffrey Ghassemi, MD, MPH
Assistant Clinical Professor
Department of Anesthesia and Perioperative Care
University of California, San Francisco
San Francisco, California;
Chief of Anesthesia
Diablo Service Area
The Permanente Medical Group
Kaiser Petrmanente
Walnut Creek, California
Chapter 42: The Adductor Canal Block

Andrew T. Gray, MD, PhD
Professor of Clinical Anesthesia
Department of Anesthesia and Perioperative Care
School of Medicine
University of California, San Francisco;
Staff Anesthesiologist
San Francisco General Hospital
San Francisco, California

Manfred Greher, MD, MBA
Hospital of the Sacred Heart of Jesus
Vienna, Austria
Chapter 69: Greater Occipital Nerve Block

Peter Hebbard, MD
Department of Anesthesia
University of Melbourne
Wangaratta, Austalia
Chapter 59: Transversus Abdominis Plane Blocks

Jens Kessler, MD
Department of Anesthesiology
University Hospital Heidelberg
Heidelberg, Germany
Chapter 73: Stellate Ganglion Block

Manoj Kumar Karmakar, MD, FRCA, DA (UK), FHKCA, FHKAM
Professor, Consultant Anaesthesiologist and Director of Paediatric Anaesthesia
Department of Anaesthesia and Intensive care
The Chinese University of Hong Kong
Prince of Wales Hospital
Shatin, Hong Kong, China
Chapter 61: Thoracic Paravertebral Block

Bradley Lee, MD
Department of Anesthesia and Perioperative Care
University of California, San Francisco
San Francisco, California
Chapter 47: Posterior Femoral Cutaneous Nerve Block

Michael S. Lipnick, MD
Assistant Professor
Department of Anesthesia and Perioperative Care
University of California, San Francisco
San Francisco, California
Chapter 75: Regional Anesthesia in Resource-Constrained Environments

L. Stephen Long, MD
Pediatric Anesthesiologist
Children's Anesthesia Medical Group
UCSF Benioff Children's Hospital Oakland
Oakland, California
Chapter 62: Pudendal Nerve Block in Children

Daniel A. Nahrwold, MD
Assistant Professor
Department of Anesthesia and Perioperative Care
University of California, San Francisco
San Francisco, California
Chapter 14: Ultrasound-Guided Continuous Peripheral Nerve Blocks

Contributors

Ronald Seidel, MD
Department of Anaesthesiology and Intensive Care Medicine
HELIOS Medical Center Schwerin
Schwerin, Germany
Chapter 72: Cervical Plexus Block

Agnes Wabule, MMED
Head of Department
Department of Anesthesia and Critical Care
Mulago Hospital
Kampala, Uganda
Chapter 75: Regional Anesthesia in Resource-Constrained Environments

Daniel M. Wong, MBBS, FANZCA
Honorary Clinical Senior Fellow
University of Melbourne Medical School
Parkville, Victoria, Australia;
Department of Anaesthesia and Acute Pain Medicine
St. Vincent's Hospital Melbourne
Fitzroy, Victoria, Australia
Chapter 74: Safety: Practical Techniques to Prevent Complications During Ultrasound-Guided Nerve Blocks

Contents

SECTION 1 Introduction to Ultrasound Imaging

1. Ultrasound — 2
2. Speed of Sound — 3
3. Attenuation — 5
4. Reflection — 7
5. Beam Width (Slice Thickness) — 11
6. Anisotropy — 13
7. Spatial Compound Imaging — 15
8. Doppler Imaging — 19
9. Ultrasound Transducers — 21
10. Transducer Manipulation — 22
11. Needle Imaging — 24
12. Approach and Techniques — 28
13. Sonographic Signs of Successful Injections — 32
14. Ultrasound-Guided Continuous Peripheral Nerve Blocks — 34
    Daniel A. Nahrwold
15. Three-Dimensional Ultrasound — 42

SECTION 2 Structures

16. Anatomic Structures — 46
17. Skin and Subcutaneous Tissue — 47
18. Peripheral Nerves — 48
19. Muscle — 53
20. Tendons and Ligaments — 56
21. Arteries — 60
22. Veins — 64
23. Bone — 66
24. Pleura — 67
25. Peritoneum — 68
26. Lymph Nodes — 69

SECTION 3 Upper Extremity Blocks

27. Supraclavicular Nerve Block (of the Cervical Plexus) — 72
28. Interscalene and Supraclavicular Blocks (of the Brachial Plexus) — 74
29. Phrenic Nerve Imaging — 84
30. Dorsal Scapular Nerve Imaging — 87
31. Suprascapular Nerve Block (Anterior Approach above the Clavicle) — 89
32. Infraclavicular Block — 93
33. Axillary Block — 104
34. Musculocutaneous Nerve Block — 117
35. Forearm Blocks — 125
36. Radial Nerve Block — 126
37. Median Nerve Block — 132
38. Ulnar Nerve Block — 138

SECTION 4 Lower Extremity Blocks

39. Lateral Femoral Cutaneous Nerve Block — 144
40. Fascia Iliaca Block — 150
41. Femoral Nerve Block — 156
42. Adductor Canal Block — 169
    Jeffrey Ghassemi
43. Obturator Nerve Block — 174
44. Sciatic Nerve Block — 179
45. Anterior Sciatic Nerve Block — 189
46. Popliteal Block — 193
47. Posterior Femoral Cutaneous Nerve Block — 200
    Bradley Lee
48. Ankle Block — 204
49. Saphenous Nerve Block in the Leg — 205
50. Deep Peroneal Nerve Block — 208
51. Superficial Peroneal Nerve Block — 214
52. Sural Nerve Block — 221
53. Tibial Nerve Block — 227

SECTION 5 Trunk Blocks

54. Intercostal Nerve Block — 234
55. Pectoral Nerve Block (the Pecs Block) — 239
56. Transversus Thoracis Muscular Plane Block — 244
57. Rectus Sheath Block — 249
58. Ilioinguinal and Iliohypogastric Nerve Blocks — 259
    Urs Eichenberger
59. Transversus Abdominis Plane Blocks — 267
    Peter Hebbard
60. Quadratus Lumborum Blocks — 277
    Hesham Elsharkawy
61. Thoracic Paravertebral Block — 286
    Manoj Kumar Karmakar
62. Pudendal Nerve Block in Children — 316
    L. Stephen Long
63. Neuraxial Block — 319
64. Caudal Epidural Block — 328

SECTION 6 Head and Neck Blocks

65. Supraorbital Nerve Block — 337
66. Mental Nerve Block — 342
67. Superior Laryngeal Nerve Block — 347
68. Transtracheal Block — 353
69. Greater Occipital Nerve Block — 357
    Manfred Greher
70. Lesser Occipital Nerve Block — 363
71. Great Auricular Nerve Block — 366
72. Cervical Plexus Block — 372
    Ronald Seidel
73. Stellate Ganglion Block (Cervicothoracic Sympathetic Ganglion Block) — 381
    Jens Kessler

Contents

SECTION 7 **Safety Issues**

74 Safety: Practical Techniques to Prevent Complications During Ultrasound-Guided Nerve Blocks 389
Michael J. Barrington and Daniel M. Wong

75 Regional Anesthesia in Resource-Constrained Environments 405
Michael S Lipnick, Gerald Dubowitz, and Agnes Wabule

Available on ExpertConsult.com
Appendix 1. Self-Assessment Questions: Text
Appendix 2. Self-Assessment Questions: Images
Appendix 3. Advanced Self-Assessment Questions: Text
Appendix 4. Advanced Self-Assessment Questions: Images

Index 413

Video Contents

INTRODUCTION TO ULTRASOUND IMAGING
Chapters 1-15
Video 1.1 — Introduction to Ultrasound Imaging
Chapter 14
Video 14.1 — Ultrasound-Guided Continuous Peripheral Nerve Blocks

UPPER EXTREMITY BLOCKS
Chapter 28
Video 28.1 — Interscalene and Supraclavicular Blocks
Chapter 32
Video 32.1 — Infraclavicular Blocks
Chapter 33
Video 33.1 — Axillary Block
Chapter 35
Video 35.1 — Forearm Blocks

LOWER EXTREMITY BLOCKS
Chapter 40
Video 40.1 — Fascia iliaca Block
Chapter 41
Video 41.1 — Femoral Nerve Block
Chapter 42
Video 42.1 — Adductor Canal Block
Chapter 43
Video 43.1 — Obturator Nerve Block
Chapter 44
Video 44.1 — Sciatic Nerve Block
Chapter 46
Video 46.1 — Popliteal Nerve Block
Chapter 48
Video 48.1 — Ankle Block
Chapter 49
Video 49.1 — Saphenous Nerve Block

TRUNK BLOCKS
Chapters 57 and 58
Video 57.1 — Truncal Blocks
Chapter 59
Video 59.1 — Transversus Abdominis Plane (TAP) Block
Chapter 61
Video 61.1 — Paravertebral Block
Chapter 63
Video 63.1 — Neuraxial Block

HEAD AND NECK BLOCKS
Chapter 72
Video 72.1 — Cervical Plexus Block

SAFETY ISSUES
Chapter 74
Video 74.1 — Ultrasound Safety Issues

SECTION 1

Introduction to Ultrasound Imaging

CHAPTER 1

Ultrasound

 See Video 1.1 on ExpertConsult.com.

Ultrasound waves are high-frequency sound waves generated in specific frequency ranges and sent through tissues.[1] How sound waves penetrate a tissue depends on the range of the frequency produced. Lower frequencies penetrate deeper than high frequencies do. The frequencies for clinical imaging (1 to 70 MHz) are well above the upper limit of normal human hearing (15 to 20 KHz). Wave motion transports energy and momentum from one point in space to another without transport of matter. In mechanical waves (e.g., water waves, waves on a string, and sound waves), energy and momentum are transported by means of disturbance in the medium because the medium has elastic properties. Any wave in which the disturbance is parallel to the direction of propagation is referred to as a longitudinal wave. Sound waves are longitudinal waves of compression and rarefaction of a medium such as air or soft tissue. *Compression* refers to high-pressure zones, and *rarefaction* refers to low-pressure zones (these zones alternate in position).

As the sound passes through tissues, it is absorbed, reflected, or allowed to pass through, depending on the echodensity of the tissue. Substances with high water content (e.g., blood, cerebrospinal fluid) conduct sound very well and reflect very poorly and thus are termed *echolucent*. Because they reflect very little of the sound, they appear as dark areas (hypoechoic). Substances low in water content or high in materials that are poor sound conductors (e.g., air, bone) reflect almost all the sound and appear very bright (hyperechoic). Substances with sound conduction properties between these extremes appear darker to lighter, depending on the amount of wave energy they reflect.

Audible sounds spread out in all directions, whereas ultrasound beams are well collimated. The frequency of sound does not change with propagation unless the wave strikes a moving object, in which case the changes are small. The product of the frequency and wavelength of sound waves is the wave speed. Because the speed of sound in soft tissue is nearly constant, higher-frequency sound waves have shorter wavelengths. Two adjacent structures cannot be identified as separate entities on an ultrasound scan if they are less than one wavelength apart. Therefore sound wave frequency is one of the main determinants of spatial resolution of ultrasound scans.

Reference

1. Aldrich JE. Basic physics of ultrasound imaging. *Crit Care Med*. 2007;35:S131–S137.

Speed of Sound

CHAPTER 2

See Video 1.1 on ExpertConsult.com.

The speed of sound is determined by properties of the medium in which it propagates. The sound velocity equals $\sqrt{(B/rho)}$, where *B* equals the bulk modulus and *rho* equals density. The bulk modulus is proportional to stiffness. Thus stiffness (change in shape) and wave speed are related. Density (weight per unit volume) and wave speed are inversely related. The speed of sound in a given medium is essentially independent of frequency.

Because the velocity of sound in soft tissue is 1540 m/s, 13 microseconds elapse for each centimeter of tissue the sound wave must travel (the back-and-forth time of flight). Speed-of-sound artifacts relate to both time-of-flight considerations and refraction that occurs at the interface of tissues with different speeds of sound.[1-3]

References

1. Scanlan KA. Sonographic artifacts and their origins. *AJR Am J Roentgenol*. 1991;156:1267–1272.
2. Fornage BD. Sonographically guided core-needle biopsy of breast masses: the "bayonet artifact". *AJR Am J Roentgenol*. 1995;164:1022–1023.
3. Gray AT, Schafhalter-Zoppoth I. "Bayonet artifact" during ultrasound-guided transarterial axillary block. *Anesthesiology*. 2005;102:1291–1292.

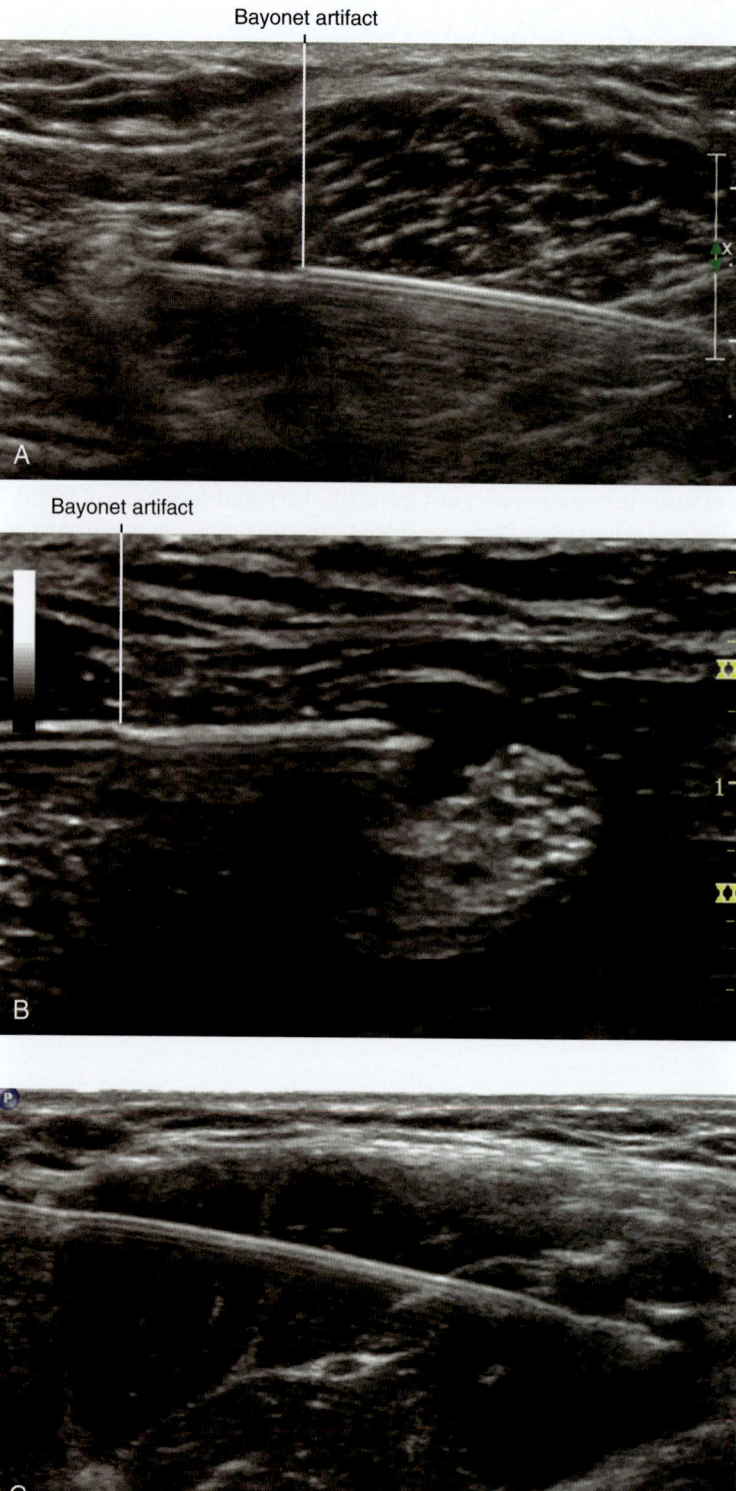

FIGURE 2.1 Bayonet artifacts during popliteal block (A and B). Because the speed of sound is not necessarily homogeneous in soft tissue, the needle can sometimes appear to bend, similar to a bayonet. Actual mechanical bending of the needle typically appears as gentle bowing of the needle (C).

CHAPTER 3

Attenuation

See Video 1.1 on ExpertConsult.com.

Attenuation is a decrease in wave amplitude as it travels through a medium. The attenuation of ultrasound in soft tissue is approximately 0.5 to 0.75 dB/(MHz-cm), indicating that the extent of attenuation depends on the distance traveled and the frequency of insonation. The units of the attenuation coefficient directly show the greater attenuation of high-frequency ultrasound beams. In soft tissue, 80% or more of the total attenuation is caused by absorption of the ultrasound wave, thereby generating heat.

Time gain compensation (TGC) adjusts for attenuation of an ultrasound beam as a function of depth. When TGC is properly adjusted, images of similar reflectors appear the same regardless of depth.

An acoustic shadow is said to exist when a localized object reflects or attenuates sound to impede transmission. Bone is a strong absorber of ultrasound waves. Therefore shadowing occurs deep to bony structures ("bone shadow").

When a nonattenuating fluid (e.g., blood or injected local anesthetic) lies within an attenuating sound field (e.g., soft tissue), enhancement of echoes deep to the fluid occurs. This phenomenon, originally described as posterior acoustic enhancement (also called increased through-transmission), is due to lack of absorption of the sound waves by the fluid.[1] This attenuation artifact is a potential source of problems, especially during regional blocks where nerves are situated close to blood vessels.

Clinical Pearls

- In general, the highest frequency capable of adequate penetration to the depth of interest should be used for imaging.
- Decibels (dB) are a relative logarithmic measure of sound wave intensity.

Reference

1. Filly RA, Sommer FG, Minton MJ. Characterization of biological fluids by ultrasound and computed tomography. *Radiology*. 1980;134:167–171.

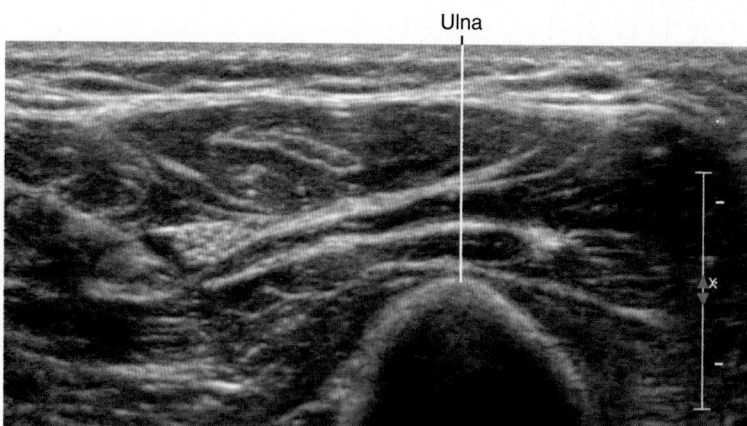

FIGURE 3.1 Acoustic shadowing by bone. In this sonogram from the forearm, the acoustic shadowing by the ulna is evident. The bright cortical line of the surface of the bone is followed by extinction of the sound wave below.

Reflection

CHAPTER 4

See Video 1.1 on ExpertConsult.com.

Ultrasonography measures the amplitude of the return echo as a function of time.[1] Sound waves are reflected at the interface of tissues with different acoustic impedances. The acoustic impedance ($kg/[m^2\text{-}s]$) is the product of the density (kg/m^3) and velocity (m/sec). The extent of reflection is governed by the reflection coefficient: $R = (Z1 - Z2)/(Z1 + Z2)$. If $Z1 = Z2$, there is no reflected wave.[2] Ultrasound characteristics of biologic tissue and interventional materials are summarized in Table 4.1.

Reflections off a smooth surface are called *specular*. If two specular reflectors are close to each other, reverberation within the sound field can result, displayed as parallel, equally spaced lines deep to the reflectors. Csomet-tail artifact, which is a form of reverberation artifact, is caused by multiple internal reflections from a small, highly reflective interface.[3,4]

Clinical Pearls

- The normal pleural line is thin and smooth, which generates a few comet-tail artifacts (between one and three artifacts per intercostal space scan). In the presence of parenchymal lung disease, the pleural line is irregular and thickened, generating many more comet-tail artifacts.[5]
- No comet-tail artifact is observed from the lung when pneumothorax is present.
- Hyperechoic reverberation artifacts are seen with metallic foreign bodies such as block needles.

TABLE 4.1 Ultrasound Characteristics of Biologic Tissue and Interventional Materials

Substance	Velocity (m/s)	Attenuation (dB/[MHz-cm])	Impedance (mrayls × 10^{-6})
Air	330	7.5	0.0001
Water	1480	0.0022	1.5
Soft tissue	1540	0.75	1.7
Blood	1575	0.15	1.6
Bone	4080	15	8
Stainless steel	5790	0.2	47

Data from Ziskin MC. Fundamental physics of ultrasound and its propagation in tissue. *Radiographics*. 1993;13:705–709; Ziskin MC, Thickman DI, Goldenberg NJ, Lapayowker MS, Becker JM. The comet tail artifact. *J Ultrasound Med*. 1982;1:1–7; Gawdzinska K. Investigation into the propagation of acoustic waves in metal. *Metalurgija*. 2005;44:125–128; Smith SW, Booi RC, Light ED, Merdes CL, Wolf PD. Guidance of cardiac pacemaker leads using real time 3D ultrasound: feasibility studies. *Ultrason Imaging*. 2002;24:119–128.

References

1. Ziskin MC. Fundamental physics of ultrasound and its propagation in tissue. *Radiographics*. 1993;13:705–709.
2. Ziskin MC. Equation governing the transmission of ultrasound. *J Clin Ultrasound*. 1982;10:A21.
3. Ziskin MC, Thickman DI, Goldenberg NJ, Lapayowker MS, Becker JM. The comet tail artifact. *J Ultrasound Med*. 1982;1:1–7.
4. Thickman DI, Ziskin MC, Goldenberg NJ, Linder BE. Clinical manifestations of the comet tail artifact. *J Ultrasound Med*. 1983;2:225–230.
5. Reissig A, Kroegel C. Transthoracic sonography of diffuse parenchymal lung disease: the role of comet tail artifacts. *J Ultrasound Med*. 2003;22:173–180.

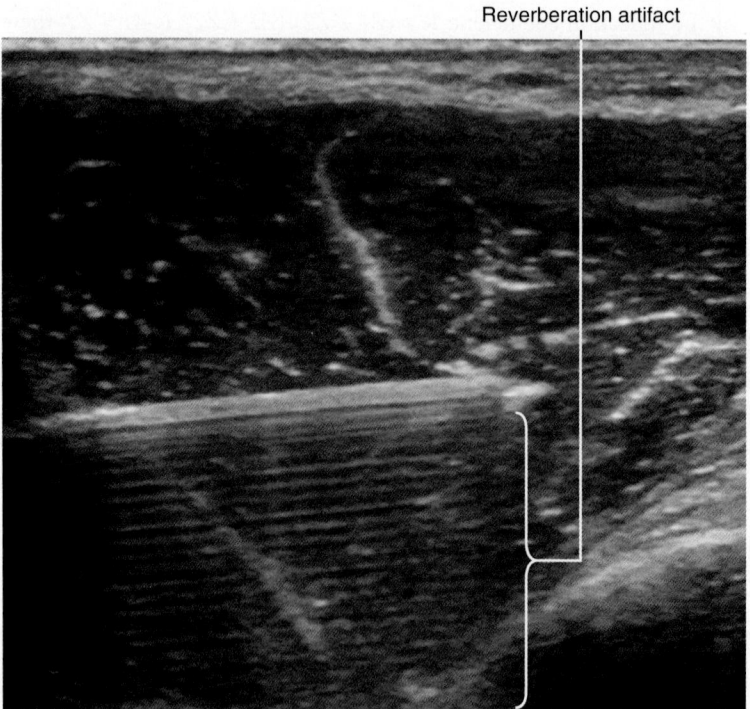

FIGURE 4.1 Reverberation artifact from a block needle placed nearly parallel to the active face of the transducer.

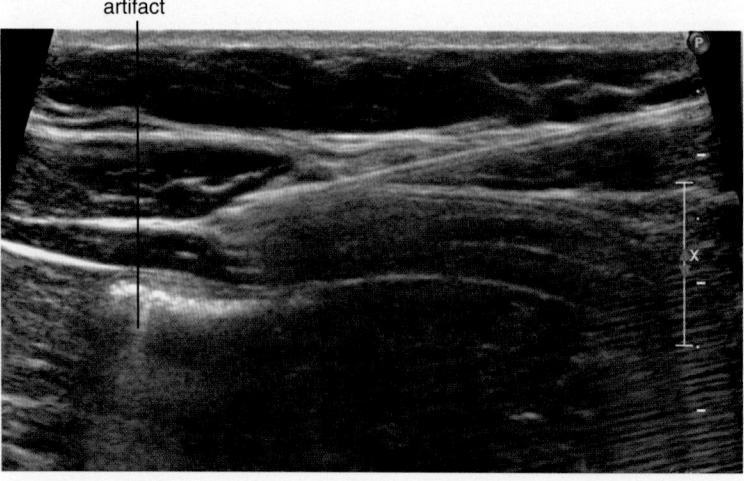

FIGURE 4.2 Comet-tail artifact from the peritoneum during rectus sheath block. The peritoneum and pleura have similar appearances on ultrasound scans.

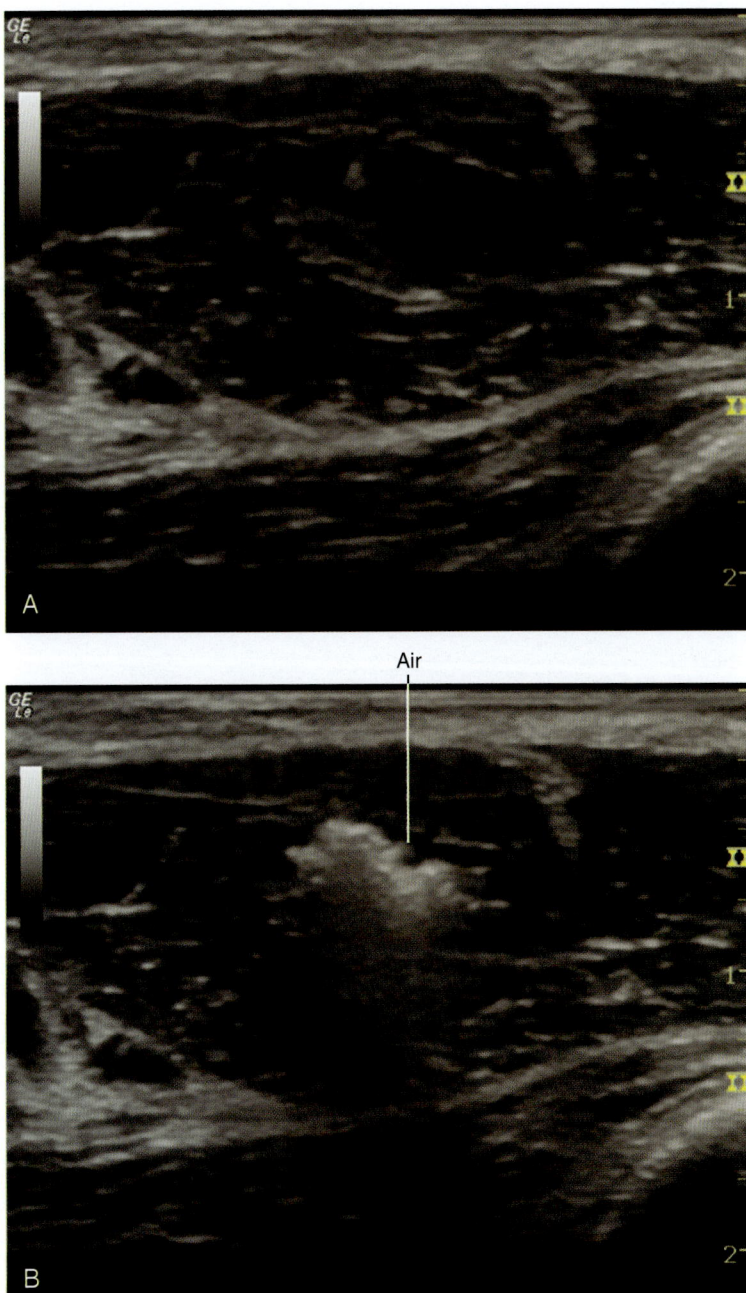

FIGURE 4.3 A strong echo and acoustic shadowing are observed when air is inadvertently injected during musculocutaneous nerve block in the axilla. Sonograms before injection (A) and after injection (B) are shown.

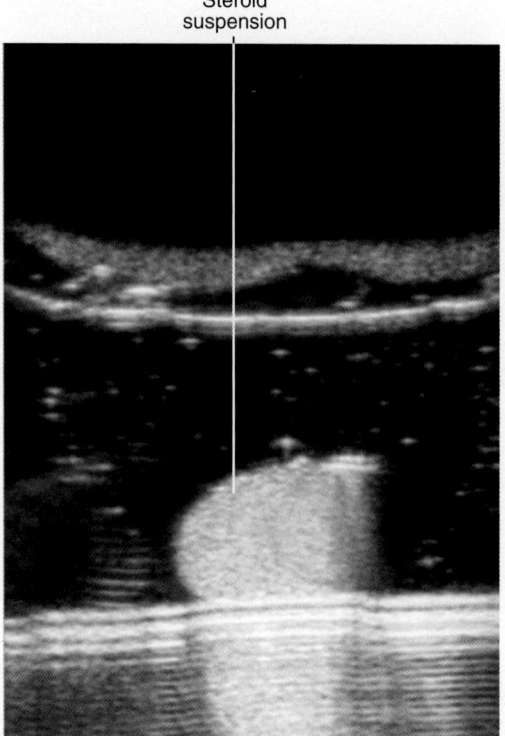

FIGURE 4.4 Acoustic properties of a steroid suspension. Although the local anesthetic injected for most regional blocks is anechoic, the particles of this steroid suspension are sufficiently large to produce a strong echo.

Beam Width (Slice Thickness)

CHAPTER 5

See Video 1.1 on ExpertConsult.com.

Ultrasound systems assume all reflectors lie directly along the main axis of the ultrasound beam (i.e., the acoustic axis or central ray)[1]; however, ultrasound beams have a finite size. The out-of-plane beam width (slice thickness) can be measured with a diffuse scattering plane.[2] The plane is oriented at a 45-degree angle so that the displayed echoes are equal to the out-of-plane echoes. Ultrasound beams can be focused to reduce the out-of-plane beam width and thereby improve image quality.

References

1. Goldstein A, Madrazo BL. Slice-thickness artifacts in gray-scale ultrasound. *J Clin Ultrasound*. 1981;9:365–375.
2. Goldstein A. Slice thickness measurements. *J Ultrasound Med*. 1988;7:487–498.

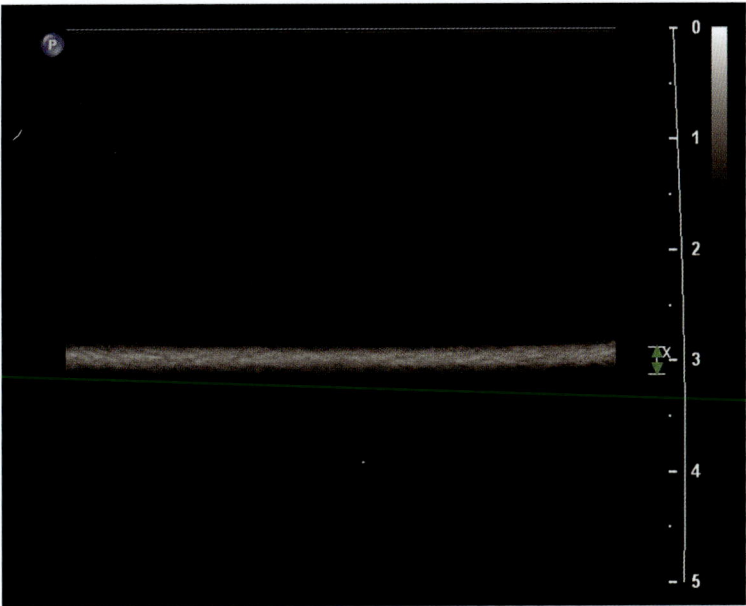

FIGURE 5.1 Out-of-plane slice thickness. Ultrasound scan of a diffuse scattering plane (a sheet of sandpaper).

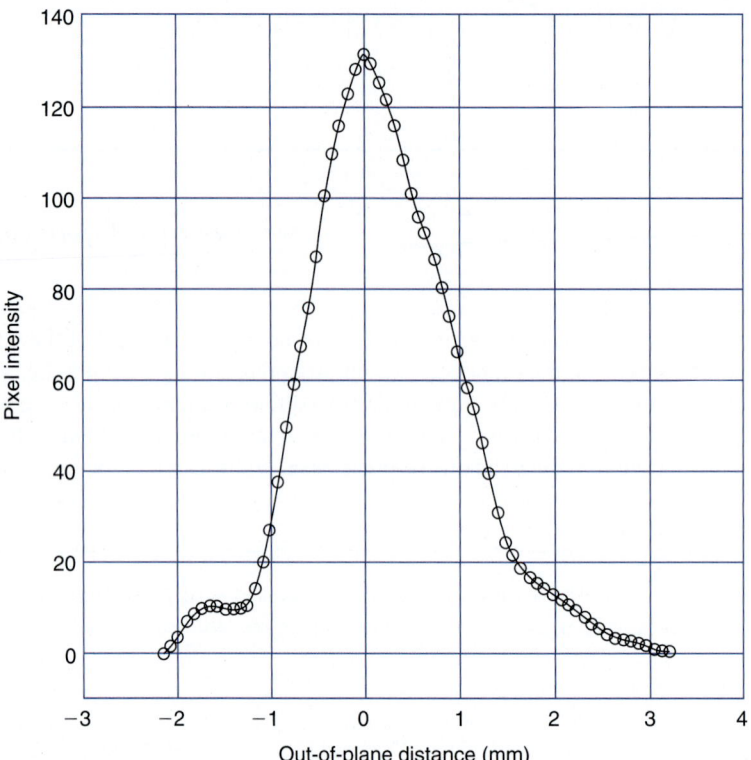

FIGURE 5.2 The beam profile is shown as a function of the distance from the central ray. Because needle diameters are substantially less than those of the slice plane, a strong relationship between needle diameter and visibility is expected.

Anisotropy

CHAPTER 6

See Video 1.1 on ExpertConsult.com.

Isotropic means equal in all directions. Anisotropic implies angle dependence. The latter term has been used to indicate the change in amplitude of received echoes from a structure when the angle of insonation is changed. Anisotropy is a discriminating feature between nerves and tendons. Tendons are more anisotropic than nerves are, meaning that smaller changes in angle (approximately 2 degrees) alter the echoes from tendons than the changes in angle (approximately 10 degrees) that alter the echoes from nerves. The anisotropy of nerves also is important because during interventions it can be challenging to maintain nerve visibility while manipulating the transducer to image the block needle.[1] With training, practitioners learn to naturally manipulate the transducer to fill in the received echoes from nerves. The amplitude of the received echoes from peripheral nerves is usually largest when the sound beam is perpendicular to the nerve path. Other structures, such as muscle, also exhibit anisotropy.[2]

Clinical Pearls

- Anisotropy means that the backscatter echoes from a specimen depend on the directional orientation within the sound field.
- Anisotropy can be quantified by specifying the transducer frequency and the decibel change in backscatter echoes with perpendicular and parallel orientation of the specimen.
- Nerves, tendons, and muscle all exhibit anisotropy. Of these structures, tendon echoes are the most sensitive to transducer manipulation.

References

1. Soong J, Schafhalter-Zoppoth I, Gray AT. The importance of transducer angle to ultrasound visibility of the femoral nerve. *Reg Anesth Pain Med.* 2005;30:505.
2. Rubin JM, Carson PL, Meyer CR. Anisotropic ultrasonic backscatter from the renal cortex. *Ultrasound Med Biol.* 1988;14:507–511.

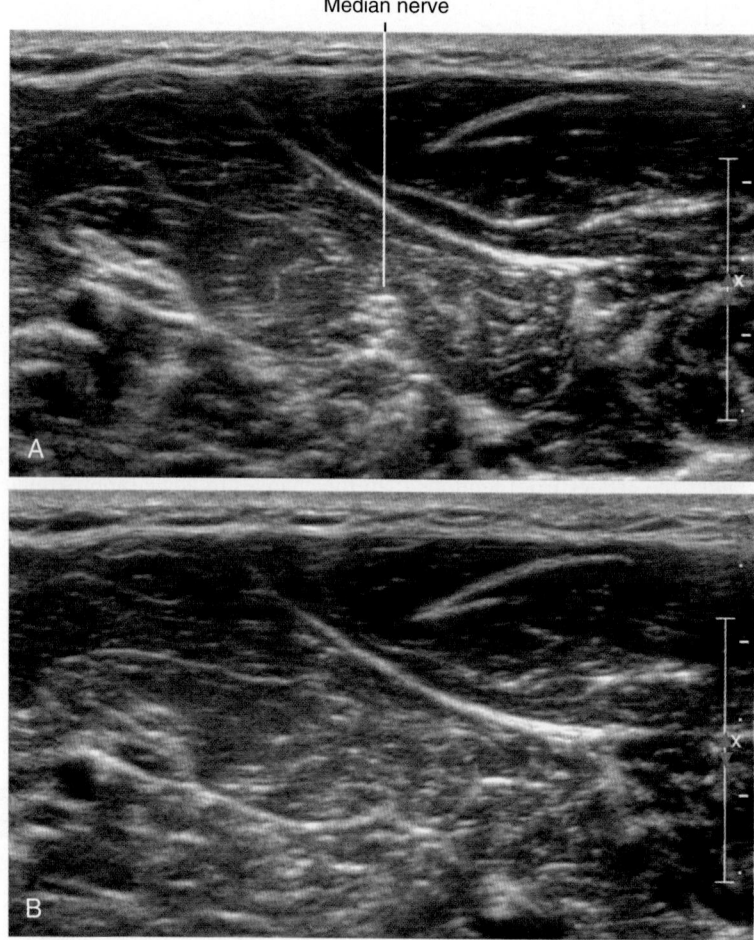

FIGURE 6.1 Anisotropy of the median nerve (A and B). With inclination of the transducer (tilting), the received echoes from the median nerve disappear.

Spatial Compound Imaging

CHAPTER 7

See Video 1.1 on ExpertConsult.com.

In conventional sonography, tissue is insonated from a single direction. Spatial compound imaging combines multiple lines of sight to form a single composite image at real-time frame rates. The ultrasound beam is steered by a different set of predetermined angles, typically within 20 degrees from the perpendicular.

One benefit of the use of spatial compound imaging is the reduction of angle-dependent artifacts (Table 7.1). *Speckle* is the granular appearance of a sonographic image that results from scattering of the ultrasound beam from small tissue reflectors. This speckle artifact results in the grainy appearance observed on sonograms, representing noise in the image. Improved image quality may be obtained by using spatial compound imaging, which can reduce speckle noise.

There is a central triangular region of overlap within the field of view where all angles mesh together for full compounding. The corners of the image receive only a subset of all the lines of sight; therefore not all the benefits of spatial compounding are manifest. Some machines allow the stray lines of sight (those off the rectangular field of view) to form a trapezoidal image format. This is sometimes useful to view the approaching needle with in-plane technique.

Spatial compound imaging was first designed to eliminate angle-dependent artifacts.[1] This can be accomplished with a narrow range of beam angles. The larger the range of angles subtended by spatial compounding, the smaller the region within the field of imaging that will receive all the lines of sight (i.e., the region of full compounding).

Ultrasound imaging near bone may be improved by spatial compound imaging. This has relevance to imaging for some blocks (e.g., neuraxial, paravertebral, lumbar plexus, intercostals, sacroiliac joint). Although ultrasound waves cannot penetrate mature bone (even with low-frequency ultrasound), spatial compound imaging allows better definition of the bone surface.

Linear test tool images can be used to reveal the number of lines of sight used in spatial compound imaging. These images are generated with a smooth metal surface, such as that of a paper clip, solid metal stylet, or a US nickel. Metal is used because it is relatively nonattenuating,

TABLE 7.1 Advantages and Disadvantages of Spatial Compound Imaging

Advantages	Disadvantages
Reduction of angle-dependent artifacts (e.g., posterior acoustic enhancement and speckle)	Frame averaging (persistence or motion blur effect)
Needle tip imaging	Limited range of angles (typically <20 degrees)
Nerve border definition	
Fascia contours	
Imaging around bone	
Wider field of view with stray lines of sight	

yet produces an echo. Smooth metal is used so that the test tool does not damage the transducer. For these measurements, high receiver gain and a single focal zone near the surface are used. As long as the test tool contact is less than the receiver aperture, the width of the displayed echoes will not change.

> **Clinical Pearls**
>
> - The use of spatial compound imaging can improve imaging of nerve borders and the block needle tip.
> - One potential disadvantage of compound imaging is that needle reverberations occur over a broader range of angles and can prevent imaging of deeper structures.
> - Compound imaging is being developed for both linear and curved arrays.
> - Sliding the transducer along the known course of the nerve is a well-established technique to improve small nerve imaging. However, frame rate reduction that occurs with spatial compound imaging can cause problems with this technique.
> - If compound imaging is not an advantage for a particular imaging situation, it can be turned off.

Reference

1. Baad M, Lu ZF, Reiser I, Paushter D. Clinical significance of US artifacts. *Radiographics*. 2017;37:1408–1423.

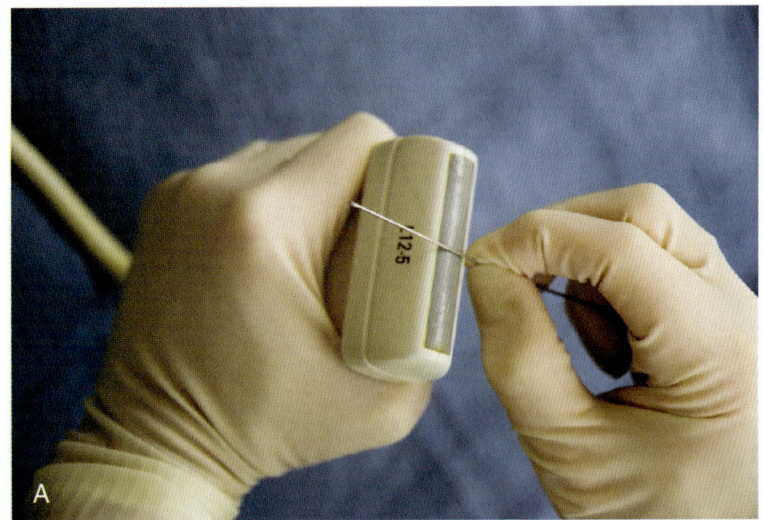
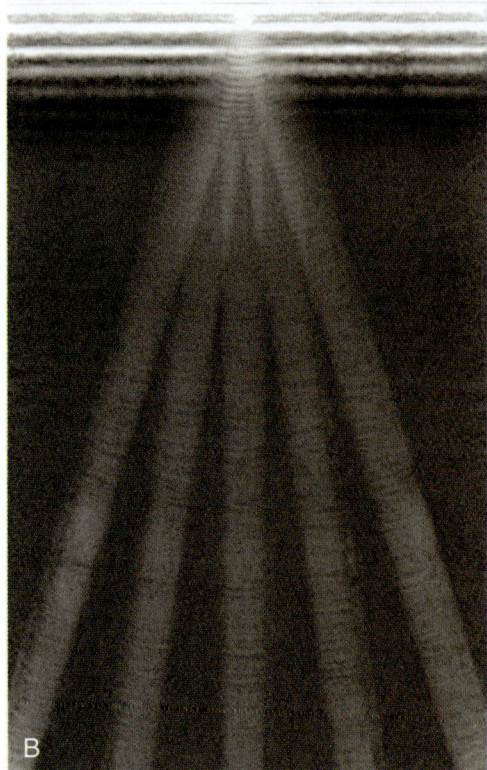

FIGURE 7.1 Spatial compound imaging. Some forms of ultrasound imaging use multiple lines of sight by electronically steering the beam to different angles. This sonogram was obtained by placing a linear array test tool (the solid metal stylet of a 17-gauge epidural needle) over the active face of the transducer to isolate a single element (A and B). The displayed test tool image consists of the receiver apertures of the transducer. In this case, five lines of sight are used to form a compound image.

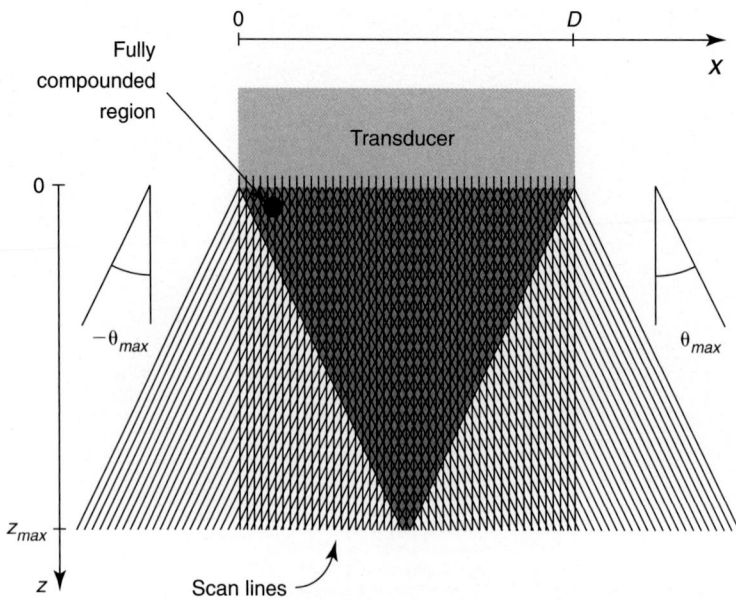

FIGURE 7.2 Conceptual illustration of transducer and associated scan lines for recording of three single-angle images. (Adapted from Jespersen SK, Wilhjelm JE, Sillesen H. In vitro spatial compound scanning for improved visualization of atherosclerosis. *Ultrasound Med Biol*. 2000;26:1357–1362.)

Doppler Imaging

CHAPTER 8

See Video 1.1 on ExpertConsult.com.

The Doppler shift is the change in frequency of sound when the sound wave strikes a moving object. This means the frequencies of the transmitted and reflected sound waves are not the same. Doppler shifts in clinical imaging are in the audible range (±10 KHz). Red blood cells are the primary reflectors that produce Doppler shifts. Ultrasound machines can color-encode the mean velocity (color Doppler), variance within the sample volume (variance Doppler), and power spectrum of the frequency shift (power Doppler).[1]

The optimal spectral Doppler angle is 30 to 60 degrees. Doppler angles greater than 60 degrees result in small Doppler shifts. Doppler angles less than 30 degrees result in loss of signal due to refraction.

Aliasing (incorrect or ambiguous estimation of the velocity) occurs when the velocity scale is set too small relative to the actual velocities. Wraparound transition between positive and negative velocity on spectral Doppler tracings indicates aliasing; therefore the peak velocities are off scale and not accurately estimated. This occurs because the pulse repetition frequency is insufficiently low relative to the frequency of the Doppler signal (a consequence of the sampling or Nyquist theorem).

Color Doppler is traditionally shown with the Nyquist velocity limits. Color aliasing is displayed as reversed flow within laminar flow areas, with no intervening black stripe between them. With true flow reversal, the transition has an intervening black stripe, indicating no flow estimation. This narrow colorless area occurs because of the absence of a Doppler shift where flow is perpendicular to the angle of insonation.

Clinical Pearls

- Blood has a low ultrasound attenuation coefficient. Red blood cells are the primary reflectors within blood.
- In power Doppler the gain threshold can be adjusted to the level at which there is no observed signal in bone.[2]
- In low-flow states (e.g., heart failure or atrial arrhythmias), aggregates of red blood cells can cause spontaneous echo contrast within blood vessels.

References

1. Bude RO, Rubin JM. Power Doppler sonography. *Radiology*. 1996;200:21–23.
2. Rubin JM. Musculoskeletal power Doppler. *Eur Radiol*. 1999;9(suppl 3):S403–S406.

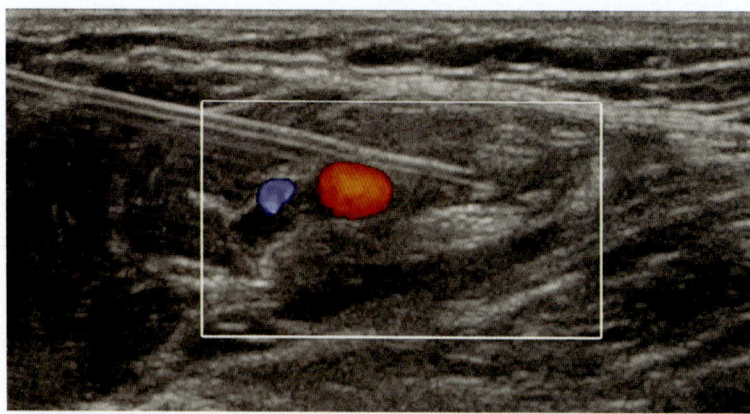

FIGURE 8.1 An example of color Doppler imaging during axillary block. A short-axis view of the neurovascular bundle is displayed.

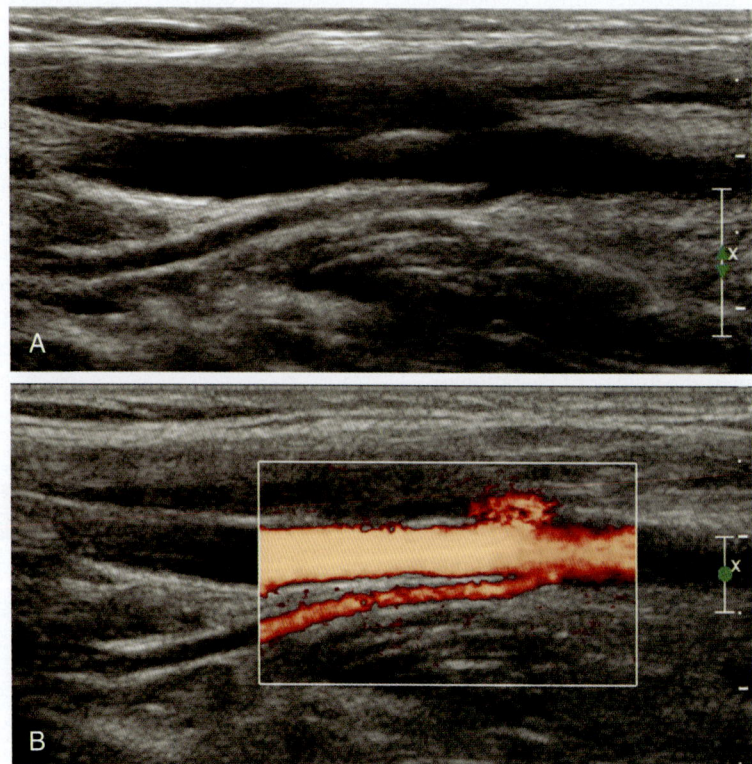

FIGURE 8.2 Long-axis view of the axillary artery and its profunda branch in conventional B-mode imaging (A) and with power Doppler (B).

Ultrasound Transducers

CHAPTER 9

See Video 1.1 on ExpertConsult.com.

Ultrasound transducers consist of arrays of piezoelectric crystals that produce high-frequency sound waves in response to an electrical signal. These crystals interconvert electrical and mechanical energy, allowing for both transmission and reception of sound waves. The piezoelectric element vibrates to produce ultrasound. Piezoelectric crystals change shape under the influence of an electric field. The thickness of the crystal and the propagation speed within determine the frequency. With some transducers, the sonographer can select different crystals within the assembly to produce a different frequency.

The first ultrasound transducers were made using natural piezoelectric crystals (quartz, Rochelle salts, tourmaline). Modern transducers use synthetic crystals, such as PZT (lead zirconate titanate), that have high density, velocity, and acoustic impedance.[1]

Linear arrays typically produce a rectangular image format. The piezoelectric crystals are arranged in a straight line. Curvilinear arrays produce images in sector format (that do not originate from a single point). The range of angles with curved arrays (typically, 0 to 60 degrees) is much larger than with beam steering for spatial compound imaging (typically, 0 to 20 degrees).

Most regional blocks are performed with linear transducers because the high scan line density produces the resolution necessary for direct nerve imaging. Small curved probes are useful for infraclavicular and suprascapular nerve blocks because working room is limited. With curved probes, inaccurate estimation of needle tip location can occur despite complete line-up due to the different angles at which the ultrasound beam hits the needle.

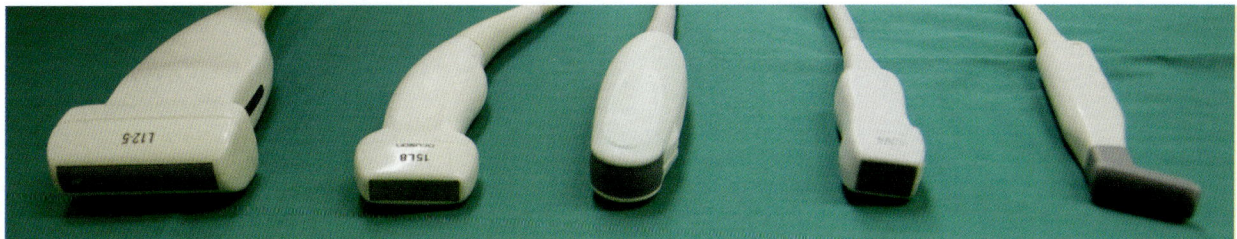

FIGURE 9.1 Ultrasound transducers for regional blocks. The photograph includes *(left to right)* broad linear, small footprint linear, curved, sector, and hockey stick transducers.

Reference

1. Szabo TL, Lewin PA. Ultrasound transducer selection in clinical imaging practice. *J Ultrasound Med.* 2013;32:573–582.

CHAPTER 10
Transducer Manipulation

 See Video 1.1 on ExpertConsult.com.

Nomenclature for transducer manipulation has been previously established.[1,2] Note that this nomenclature does not include specification of direction (e.g., rock back, rotate clockwise, tilt proximal). To control the transducer for interventions, the hands of the operator must be very close to the skin surface. The ulnar aspect of the transducer hand should rest on the skin of the patient.

References

1. AIUM technical bulletin. Transducer manipulation. American Institute of Ultrasound in Medicine. *J Ultrasound Med.* 1999;18:169–175.
2. Bahner DP, Blickendorf JM, Bockbrader M, et al. Language of transducer manipulation: codifying terms for effective teaching. *J Ultrasound Med.* 2016;35:183–188.

TRANSDUCER MANIPULATION 23

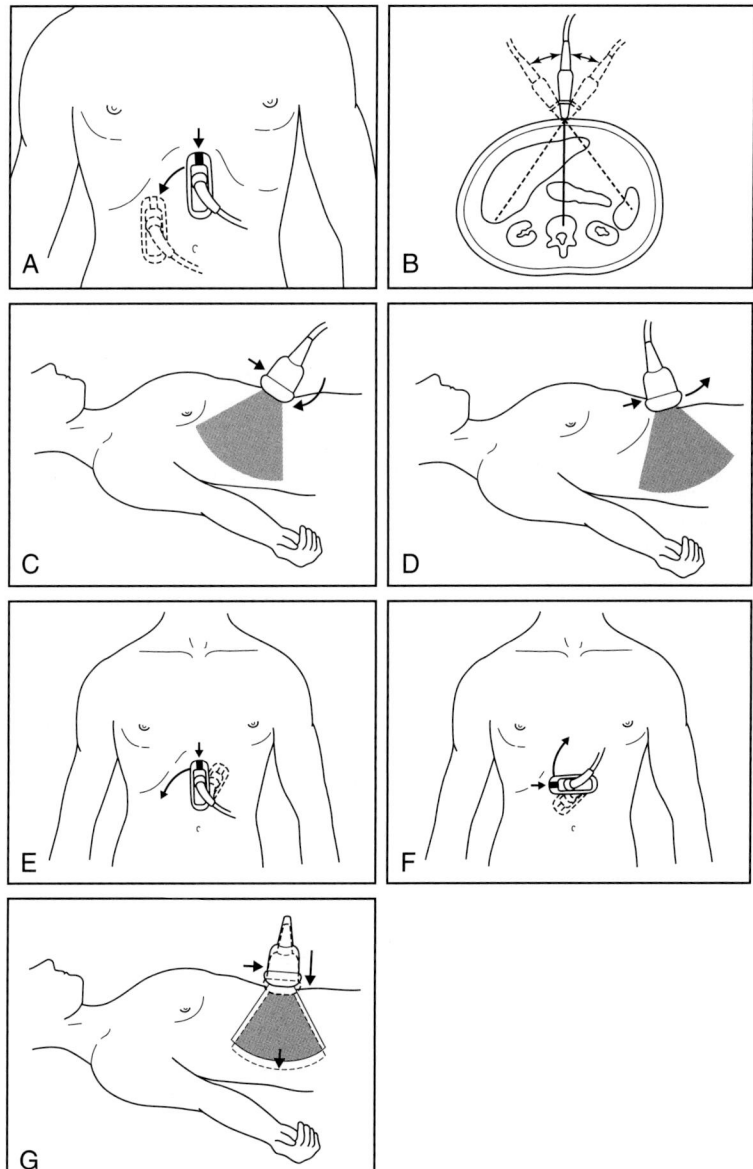

FIGURE 10.1 To optimally display anatomy for image presentation, the transducer must be manipulated. Transducer manipulation can be broken down into five basic movements: sliding (A), tilting (B), rocking (C and D), rotating (E and F), and compressing (G). Combining these movements allows for smooth scanning motion and anatomy visualization. (Adapted from AIUM technical bulletin. Transducer manipulation. American Institute of Ultrasound in Medicine. *J Ultrasound Med*. 1999;18:169–175.)

CHAPTER 11

Needle Imaging

 See Video 1.1 on ExpertConsult.com.

Needle tip visibility is critical to the success and safety of regional block interventions. It is imperative to identify the needle tip before advancing the needle. The cut on the bevel is the best identifier of the needle tip for a beveled needle. Partial line-ups (so that the needle tip is not within the plane of imaging but some of the needle shaft is) are a source of false reassurance with in-plane technique. A number of factors have been reported to influence needle tip visualization under clinical imaging conditions (Table 11.1).

INSERTION ANGLE (ANGLE OF INSONATION)

Needle tip imaging is optimal when the needle is parallel to the active face of the transducer. The cleanest needle echo is from a conventional needle at or near parallel. One study found a linear correlation between angle of incidence (measured from 0 to 75 degrees) and the mean needle tip brightness.[1]

NEEDLE GAUGE

There are multiple advantages to using a large needle for regional block. Needles as large as 17 gauge have been used to improve needle tip visibility for regional blocks.[2] Alignment of a large needle is faster with in-plane technique. An additional advantage of a large needle is the ability to redirect the needle within the scan plane. A large needle tip can be used to displace structures (e.g., arteries or nerves) before advancing. The disadvantages of the large needle are patient discomfort and the consequences of unintended puncture (e.g., of vessels, nerves), which are typically worse. In addition, the soft tissue properties (tent and recoil) are more noticeable with large needles. With finer needle tips, the hand motion and needle tip motion are more closely matched, and it is easier to place a fine needle tip within a thin fascial plane.

BEVEL ORIENTATION

Needle bevel orientation is important for needle tip visibility (Table 11.2).[3] The bevel should be facing the transducer to enhance needle tip imaging.

TABLE 11.1 Factors Reported to Influence Needle Tip Visibility
Angle of insonation
Needle gauge
Bevel orientation
Receiver gain
Needle motion and test injections
Echogenic modifications
Spatial compound imaging

TABLE 11.2 Influence of Bevel Orientation on Needle Tip Visibility

Angle (Degrees)	Poor	Fair	Good
0	0.14	0.45	0.41
90	0.33	0.51	0.17
180	0.14	0.45	0.41
270	0.25	0.52	0.23

From Hopkins RE, Bradley M. In-vitro visualization of biopsy needles with ultrasound: a comparative study of standard and echogenic needles using an ultrasound phantom. *Clin Radiol*. 2001;56:499–502.

RECEIVER GAIN

The overall two-dimensional receiver gain should be reduced to improve visibility of the needle tip. However, a competing consideration is the visibility of other structures, such as the local anesthetic injection and blood vessels.

NEEDLE MOTION AND TEST INJECTIONS

Some clinicians move the needle slightly or use small-volume test injections of fluid (<1 mL) to improve the needle tip visibility.[4] Because regional anesthesia interventions are performed near reactive structures, if needle motion is used, it should be small and slow (avoid rapid jabbing motions, which may cause puncture or paresthesia).

ECHOGENIC MODIFICATIONS

McGahan roughened up the surface of needles with a No. 11 surgical blade to improve the needle tip visibility.[5] Historically, this was one of the first echogenic needle designs. When the angle of approach is more the 30 degrees, an echogenic needle is of benefit because the roughened surface sends echoes back to the transducer.[6]

SPATIAL COMPOUND IMAGING

With an increasing angle of incidence, the decrease in needle visibility is more pronounced for single-line ultrasound than for compound imaging. However, at angles of incidence of more than 30 degrees, the needle was barely visible with either method of imaging.[7]

Clinical Pearls

- Among specialized needles used for regional blocks, Hustead needle tips tend to have better ultrasound visibility.
- Side-port needles for regional block do not appear to exhibit isotropic diffraction, which has been reported to enhance the ultrasound visibility of similar needles.[8]
- Large-bore needles can be used as nerve retractors, pushing or pulling nerves out of the way of the advancing needle.
- Bevel orientation should be toward the nerve (so that the needle will pass the nerve rather than puncture it).
- When navigating the block needle between two nerves, the bevel should be rotated to face the closer of the two. This helps the block needle shoot the intervening gap and makes the closer nerve roll to the side as the needle is advanced. The same bevel orientation strategy can be used when placing the block needle between a nerve and an artery.

References

1. Bondestam S, Kreula J. Needle tip echogenicity: a study with real-time ultrasound. *Invest Radiol.* 1989;24:555–560.
2. Sandhu NS, Capan LM. Ultrasound-guided infraclavicular brachial plexus block. *Br J Anaesth.* 2002;89:254–259.
3. Hopkins RE, Bradley M. In-vitro visualization of biopsy needles with ultrasound: a comparative study of standard and echogenic needles using an ultrasound phantom. *Clin Radiol.* 2001;56:499–502.
4. Feller-Kopman D. Ultrasound-guided internal jugular access: a proposed standardized approach and implications for training and practice. *Chest.* 2007;132:302–309.
5. McGahan JP. Laboratory assessment of ultrasonic needle and catheter visualization. *J Ultrasound Med.* 1986;5:373–377.
6. Deam RK, Kluger R, Barrington MJ, et al. Investigation of a new echogenic needle for use with ultrasound peripheral nerve blocks. *Anaesth Intensive Care.* 2007;35:582–586.
7. Cohnen M, Saleh A, Luthen R, et al. Improvement of sonographic needle visibility in cirrhotic livers during transjugular intrahepatic portosystemic stent-shunt procedures with use of real-time compound imaging. *J Vasc Interv Radiol.* 2003;14:103–106.
8. Hurwitz SR, Nageotte MP. Amniocentesis needle with improved sonographic visibility. *Radiology.* 1989;171:576–577.

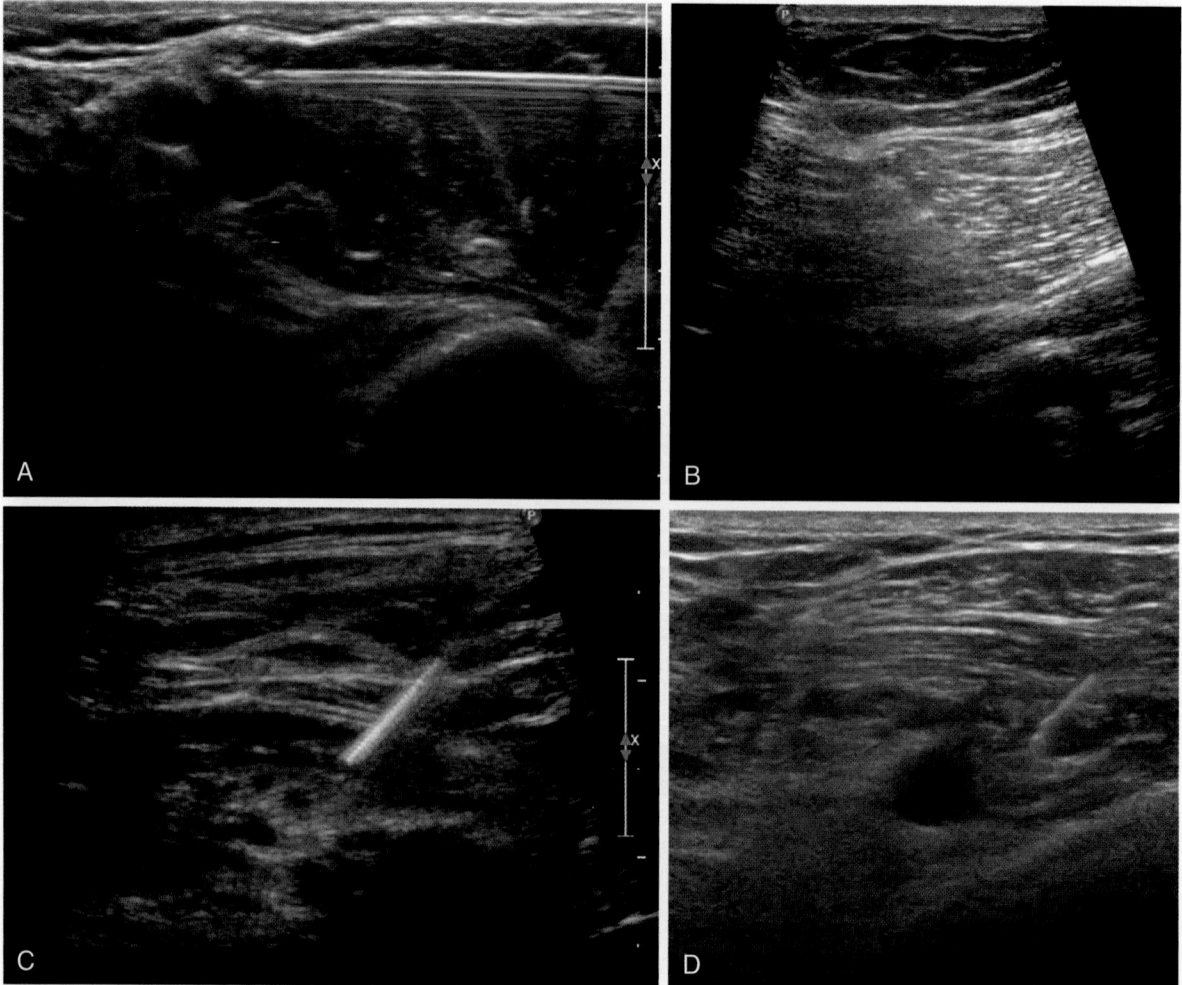

FIGURE 11.1 Influence of angle of insonation on needle tip visibility. When the needle is nearly parallel, the tip is easily identified (A). When the needle is at an angle, needle tip visibility is difficult (B). Echogenic needles can help improve needle tip visibility at steep angles under some clinical imaging conditions (C and D).

NEEDLE IMAGING   27

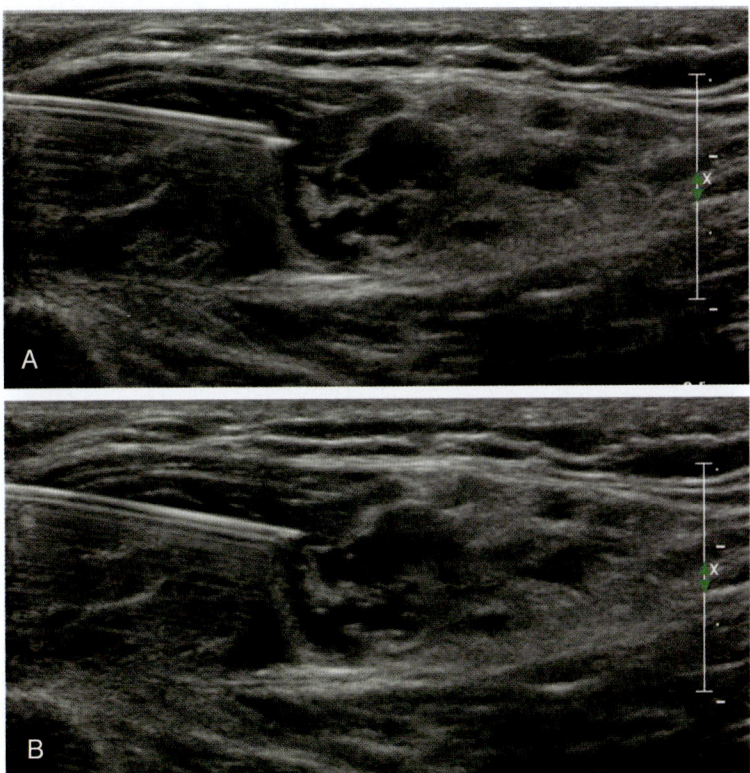

FIGURE 11.2 Influence of bevel orientation on needle tip visibility: bevel up (A) and bevel down (B).

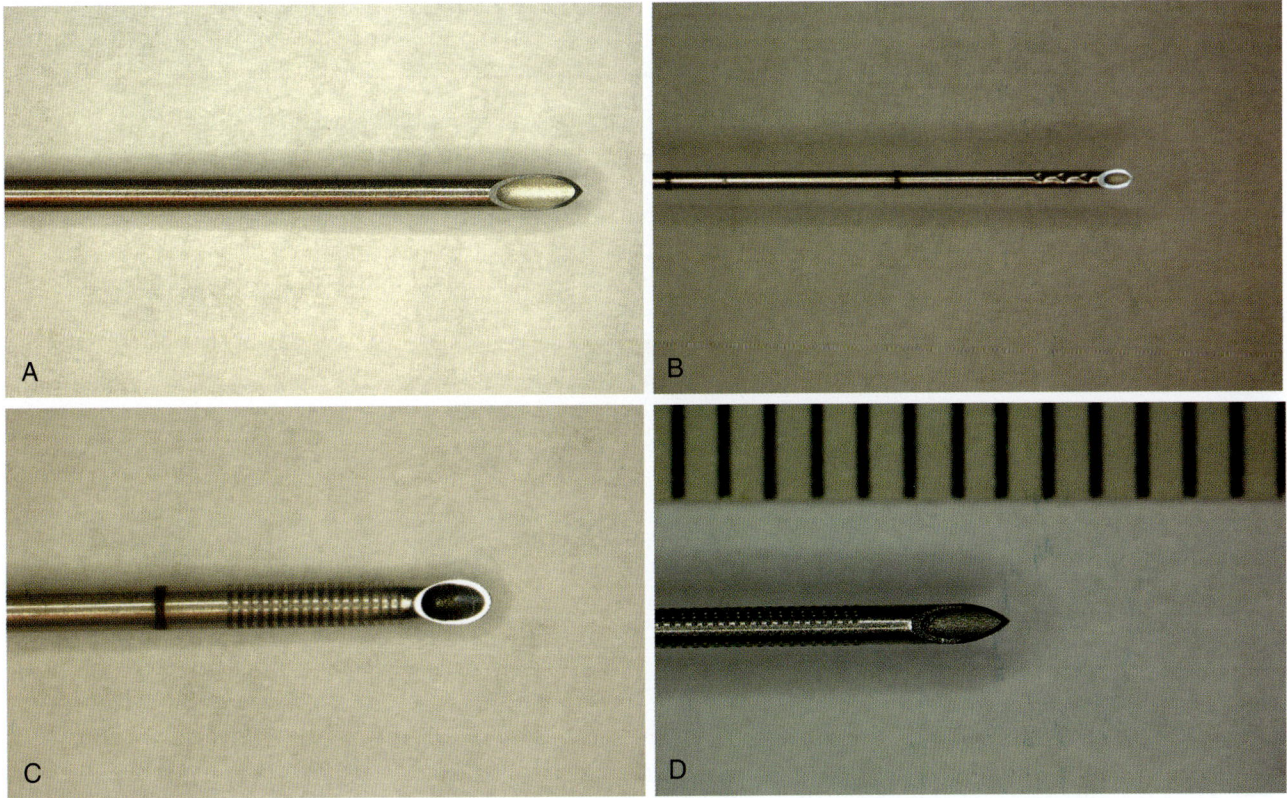

FIGURE 11.3 Photomicrographs of needles used for regional block. A plain conventional needle (A) and echogenic designs (B, C, and D) are shown. A smooth needle may not generate a recordable echo because its rounded shaft reflects most incident sound away from the source. A variety of textured surfaces are manufactured and marketed to improve needle tip detection on acquired sonograms.

CHAPTER 12

Approach and Techniques

 See Video 1.1 on ExpertConsult.com.

OFFLINE MARKINGS

Offline techniques involve external skin markings from ultrasound scans without imaging during needle placement.[1] Changes in patient position, mobility of the skin, and dynamic changes with needle placement and injection limit the utility of this approach, but this approach can be used for neuraxial blocks. The skin adjacent to the sides of the transducer can be marked. Alternatively, a paper clip or solid metal stylet (preferably with dull ends) can be used to create artifact within the field to mark the position of the object. For this technique, spatial compound imaging can be turned off to enhance the artifact.[2] The M-mode center line can be used to facilitate offline markings in the center of the field.

ONLINE GUIDANCE

There are two basic approaches to online ultrasound guidance (imaging during the intervention). With the out-of-plane technique, the needle tip crosses the plane of imaging as an echogenic dot. With the in-plane approach, the entire tip and shaft of the advancing needle are visible.

OUT-OF-PLANE APPROACH

There are several advantages to the out-of-plane approach to regional block (Table 12.1). This approach is most similar to traditional approaches to regional block guided by nerve stimulation or palpation. Therefore the out-of-plane approach provides a natural transition from one form of guidance to another. The out-of-plane approach uses a shorter needle path than do in-plane approaches. If short-axis views of the nerve are used, an out-of-plane approach results in catheter placement that is guided along the path of the nerve. One disadvantage of the out-of-plane

TABLE 12.1 Comparison of Out-of-Plane and In-Plane Approaches

Approach	Advantages	Disadvantages
Out-of-plane (OOP)	Most similar to other approaches to regional block (nerve stimulation or palpation)	Unimaged needle path, crossing the plane of imaging without recognition
	Shorter needle path than with in-plane approaches	
	Along the nerve path (catheters)	
In-plane (IP)	Most direct visualization	Partial line-ups (creating a false sense of security when the needle tip is not correctly identified)
		Some unimaged needle path occurs with IP approach, but typically less than with OOP approach
		Longer paths and therefore more structures to cross with the block needle

approach is the extent of the unimaged needle path (structures that may lie short of or beyond the scan plane). If the needle tip crosses the scan plane without recognition, it can be advanced beyond the scan plane into undesired tissue.

IN-PLANE APPROACH

There are several advantages to the in-plane approach. It provides the most direct visualization of the needle tip and injection. The amount of unimaged needle path is typically small. The needle tip is visualized before advancement. One disadvantage is the long needle path, which results in more tissue for the needle to cross. Large-bore needles are often used with this approach to facilitate alignment. Partial line-ups (visualization of the needle shaft without visualization of the needle tip in the scan plane) create a false sense of security and therefore compromise safety of the technique.

External marks on the transducer can be used to initially guide needle placement for in-plane technique. However, the mechanical axis of the transducer and its acoustic axis are not always precisely aligned.[3] The traditional teaching is that watching your hands during ultrasound-guided regional anesthesia is a quality-compromising behavior. However, recent evidence suggests that initial visual guidance can improve the speed of subsequent sonographic guidance for regional anesthesia interventions.[4] Furthermore, in-plane lineups of novices are typically better when the visual axis and needle path are aligned.[5]

NEEDLE REDIRECTION DURING IN-PLANE TECHNIQUE

The traditional teaching is that it is difficult to redirect the needle after it is placed within muscle and that it is necessary to pull it back to the subcutaneous tissue to effectively change the needle trajectory. However, there are some maneuvers that will influence the needle path when the needle is deep within soft tissue. Rotating the needle will change the bevel orientation and have a small effect on the trajectory. Quincke tip needles deflect away from the bevel surface.[6,7] Controlling the amount of transducer compression can alter the needle path, with more compression forcing a slightly steeper approach.[8] In some cases, injecting fluid can create a more favorable needle path if unintended (and displaceable) targets lie in the path.

Hand-on-needle hub provides better needle control for in-plane technique. This is important for blocks above the clavicle where the injection hand is stabilized. Hand-on-syringe provides the ability to control needle movement and injection by a single operator.

Skill is more important than approach alone. There will probably never be a good study comparing the two approaches (out-of-plane versus in-plane) because of strong institutional biases and effort dependence regarding how to perform regional blocks.

By musculoskeletal convention, the long-axis images are shown with the proximal side on the left and the distal side on the right. Long-axis views are useful for demonstrating longitudinal distribution of local anesthetic along the nerve path in one image. However, in clinical practice, it is usually easier to view the nerve in short axis and slide along the nerve path in a proximal-distal fashion to assess the longitudinal distribution.

References

1. Manickam BP, McDonald A. Surface marking technique to locate needle insertion point of ultrasound-guided neuraxial block. *Br J Anaesth.* 2016;116(4):568–569.
2. Gabriel H, Shulman L, Marko J, et al. Compound versus fundamental imaging in the detection of subdermal contraceptive implants. *J Ultrasound Med.* 2007;26:355–359.
3. Goldstein A, Parks JA, Osborne B. Visualization of B-scan transducer transverse cross-sectional beam patterns. *J Ultrasound Med.* 1982;1:23–35.
4. Lam NC, Fishburn SJ, Hammer AR, et al. A randomized controlled trial evaluating the see, tilt, align, and rotate (STAR) maneuver on skill acquisition for simulated ultrasound-guided interventional procedures. *J Ultrasound Med.* 2015;34(6):1019–1026.

5. Speer M, McLennan N, Nixon C. Novice learner in-plane ultrasound imaging: which visualization technique? *Reg Anesth Pain Med.* 2013;38(4):350–352.
6. Drummond GB, Scott DH. Deflection of spinal needles by the bevel. *Anaesthesia.* 1980;35(9):854–857.
7. Sitzman BT, Uncles DR. The effects of needle type, gauge, and tip bend on spinal needle deflection. *Anesth Analg.* 1996;82:297–301.
8. Hebbard PD, Barrington MJ, Vasey C. Ultrasound-guided continuous oblique subcostal transversus abdominis plane blockade: description of anatomy and clinical technique. *Reg Anesth Pain Med.* 2010;35(5):436–441.

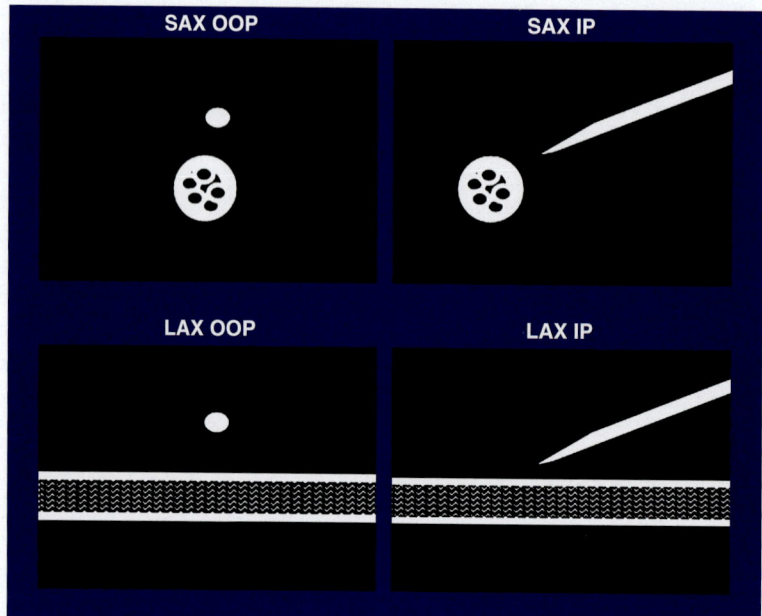

FIGURE 12.1 Schematic drawing of the short-axis (SAX) and long-axis (LAX) out-of-plane (OOP) imaging *(left panels)*, and SAX and LAX in-plane (IP) imaging *(right panels)*. (Adapted from Gray AT. Ultrasound-guided regional anesthesia: current state of the art. *Anesthesiology.* 2006;104:368–373.)

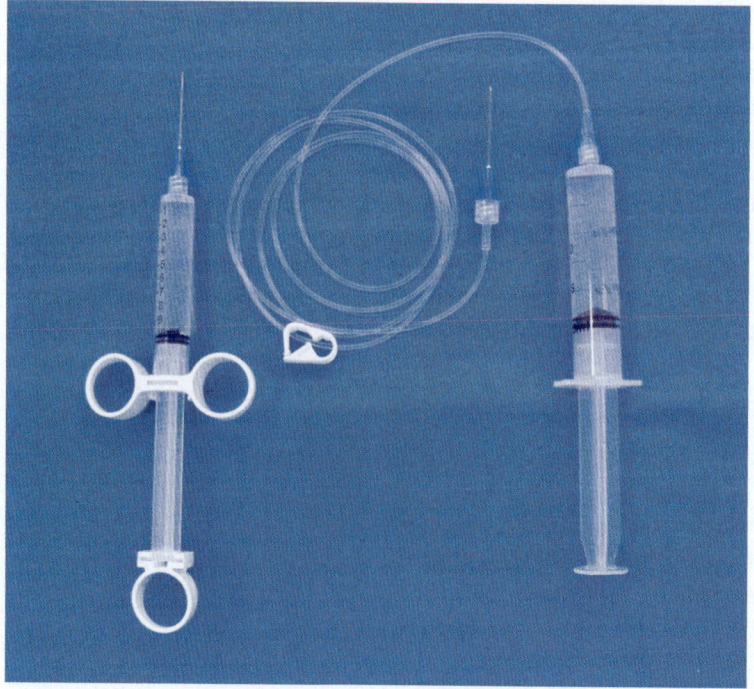

FIGURE 12.2 Setup for regional block with hand-on-syringe or hand-on-needle approaches.

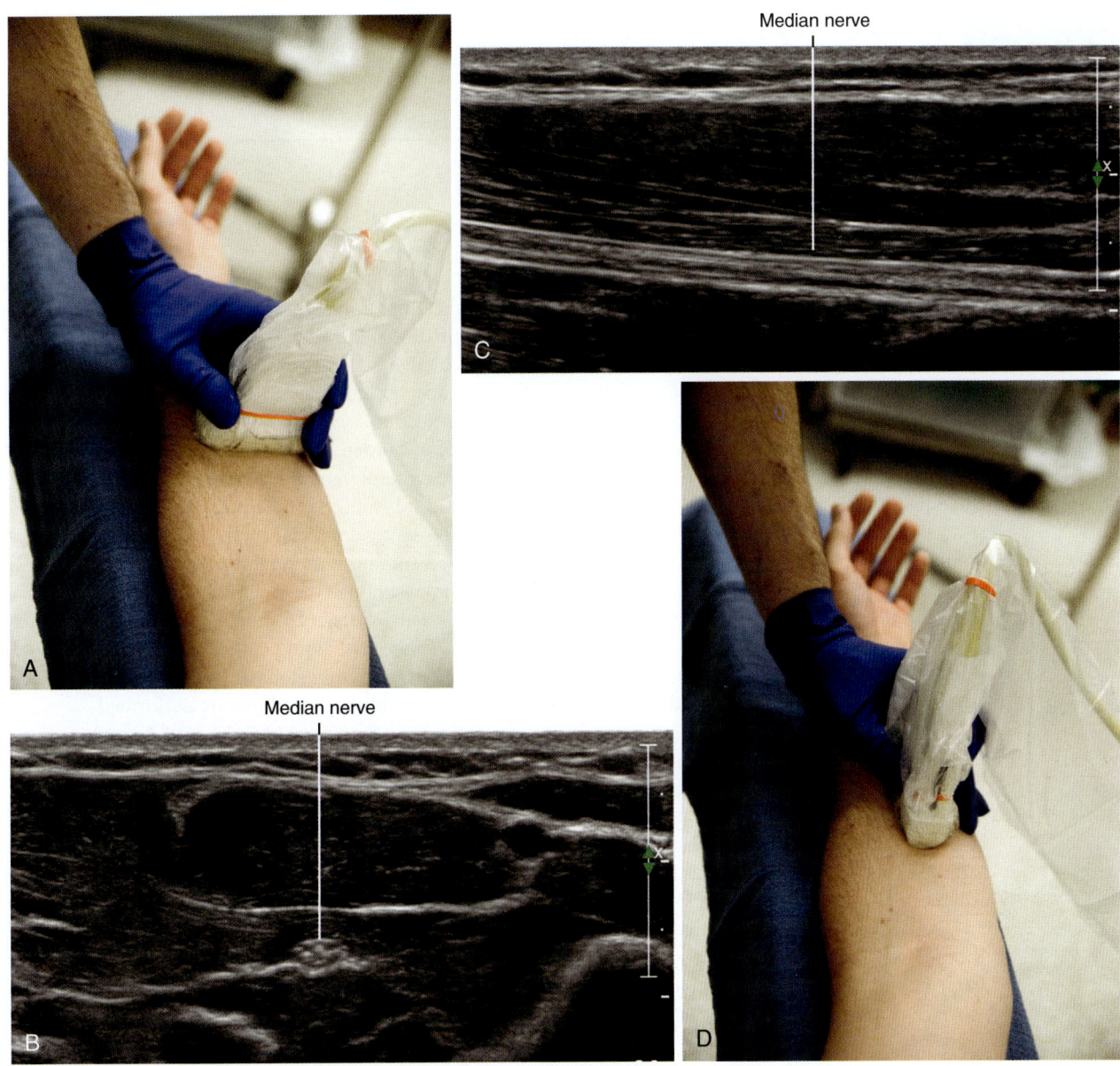

FIGURE 12.3 Median nerve viewed in short axis (A and B) and in long axis (C and D).

CHAPTER 13
Sonographic Signs of Successful Injections

 See Video 1.1 on ExpertConsult.com.

It seems simple enough to state that successful drug injections for regional blockade should surround the peripheral nerve. However, studies have reported that the doughnut sign, previously considered the gold standard for success, has a positive predictive value of only 90% for producing surgical anesthesia.[1] It is therefore important to carefully consider multiple factors that constitute sonographic signs for success that can be evaluated after injection.

First, successful drug injections should clarify the nerve border. Most regional blocks are performed with nerves viewed in short axis to evaluate the circumferential distribution. If more than half of the nerve border is contacted by local anesthetic, it is unlikely there is an intervening fascial plane that will serve as a barrier to diffusion. Therefore it is important that the injection round the corner of the nerve so that there is demonstrated curvature of the injection.

Second, successful drug injections will track along the nerve. Although the longitudinal distribution can be imaged with the nerve viewed in long axis, it is usually easier to slide the transducer along the nerve path with the nerve viewed in short axis (short-axis sliding assessment). If the local anesthetic truly tracks along the nerve, it will track along nerve divisions as well. This sign is especially useful for femoral and popliteal blocks because these block procedures are performed near points of nerve branching.

Third, peripheral nerves are often connected to adjacent structures, such as arteries or other peripheral nerves. Because they are covered in common connective tissue, successful injections should separate the connected structures. This is why practitioners often perform infraclavicular blocks or axillary blocks by placing the block needle tip between the axillary artery and the adjacent nerves. Understanding these connective tissue layers can provide a means of keeping the needle tip at a distance from the peripheral nerves.

Fourth, peripheral nerves are often more echogenic after injection of local anesthetic. This is because anechoic fluid has been injected into an attenuating sound field. This is not a perfect sign of success because anechoic fluid introduced anywhere between the nerve and the skin surface can cause this same effect.

Reference

1. Perlas A, Brull R, Chan VW, McCartney CJ, Nuica A, Abbas S. Ultrasound guidance improves the success of sciatic nerve block at the popliteal fossa. *Reg Anesth Pain Med.* 2008;33:259–265.

SONOGRAPHIC SIGNS OF SUCCESSFUL INJECTIONS

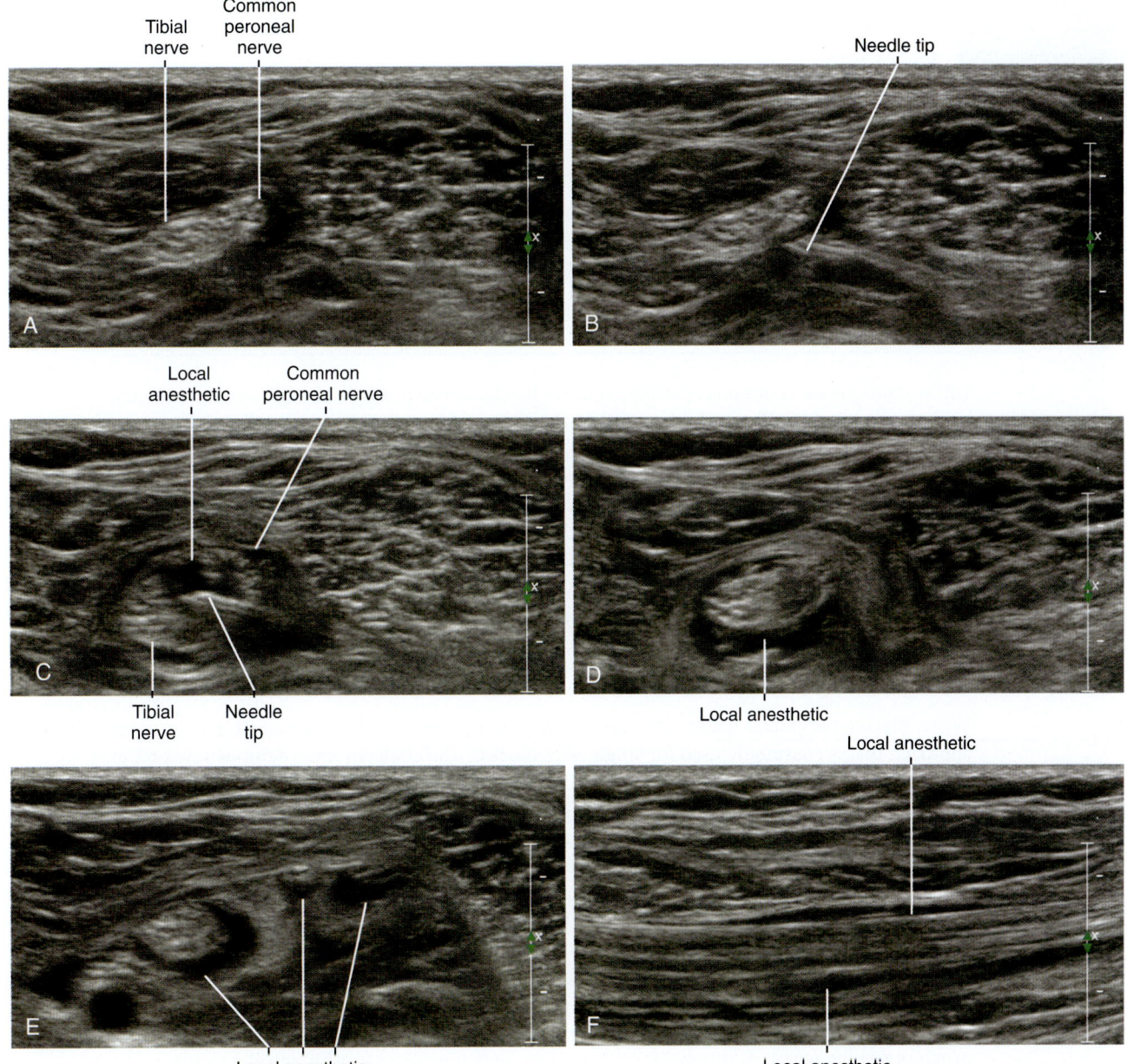

FIGURE 13.1 Image sequence showing successful sciatic nerve block in the popliteal fossa. The tibial and common peroneal contributions of the sciatic nerve are viewed in short axis before injection (A). An in-plane approach is demonstrated where the needle tip is placed between the tibial and common peroneal nerves (B). Local anesthetic is injected between the nerves (C). After injection, local anesthetic is distributed around the nerves (D) and tracks along nerve branches (E). A long-axis view also verifies the local anesthetic distribution along the sciatic nerve (F).

CHAPTER 14

Ultrasound-Guided Continuous Peripheral Nerve Blocks

Daniel A. Nahrwold

 See Video 1.1 and Video 14.1 on ExpertConsult.com.

INTRODUCTION

Ultrasound-guided continuous peripheral nerve blocks can be placed with high success rates and low complication profiles in both adults and children.[1,2] Peripheral nerve catheters are more beneficial than traditional opioid-based analgesia and also are associated with improved pain control, lower opioid requirements, less nausea, and greater patient satisfaction when compared with single-shot blocks.[3-5] Catheters are commonly placed at the interscalene, supraclavicular, infraclavicular, sciatic, femoral, adductor canal, and popliteal sites. A short-axis in-plane approach to peripheral nerve catheter insertion is popular, although out-of-plane techniques and long-axis approaches also have been described.[6]

SUGGESTED TECHNIQUE

When placing peripheral nerve catheters, many practitioners use the same short-axis in-plane approach that is commonly used for single-shot blocks.[7] The clinician must demonstrate proper hand hygiene and maintain sterile technique throughout the entire procedure.

After ultrasound imaging of the needle tip in close relation to the nerve has been obtained, the proceduralist typically injects 10 to 20 mL of local anesthetic or saline to create space into which the catheter can be advanced. The catheter is threaded through and then beyond the needle tip, leaving the catheter either alongside or around the peripheral nerve. Catheter advancement is usually accomplished without ultrasound guidance, although advances in ultrasound needle guidance systems can allow for catheter advancement with real-time ultrasound assistance.[8]

The needle is now withdrawn over the catheter. The catheter is then viewed using ultrasound, and tip placement can be confirmed by injecting 1 mL of air through the catheter.[9] Based on ultrasound interrogation, the catheter may be slightly withdrawn to an optimal location in close proximity to the nerve. Additional local anesthetic may now be given through the catheter. The catheter is then secured with a skin adhesive followed by transparent sterile dressing placement.[10]

A long-axis in-plane approach to continuous peripheral nerve blocks has been described.[11] In this approach, the peripheral nerve, needle shaft, and catheter tubing can all be viewed in the same ultrasound image. However, it can be difficult to manipulate the transducer to maintain all three structures within the plane of imaging. One study found that the onset of sensory anesthesia was faster only to be negated by a slower procedure time when using a long-axis in-plane approach to femoral nerve catheter placement.[6] No other advantages were described, and the complication profile was similar to catheters placed with the short-axis in-plane technique. Subgluteal sciatic nerve catheters seem particularly amenable to the long-axis in-plane approach when the patient is placed in the prone position.

DISCUSSION

Placing peripheral nerve catheters with ultrasound guidance alone is faster, causes less procedure-related pain, is more cost effective, and provides equivalent anesthesia when compared with catheters placed with stimulating needles and stimulating catheters both with and without ultrasound guidance.[12–15] When injecting local anesthetic, similar times to sensory and motor anesthesia can be achieved by injecting through the needle or the catheter.[16,17] Catheter-insertion distance past the needle does not appear to affect the quality of analgesia, and many practitioners aim to thread the catheter 1 to 5 cm beyond the needle tip.[18]

A relatively new method for placing peripheral nerve catheters is known as the catheter-over-needle (CON) technique. As its name suggests, the catheter is already loaded onto the block needle, and once the needle/catheter unit is in proper location adjacent to the nerve, the practitioner removes the needle as the catheter remains in place. As compared with the catheter-through-needle (CTN) technique, the CON approach may cause less fluid leakage at the skin insertion site and less catheter dislodgement. Further studies are in progress to evaluate these and other potential differences between the techniques.

Catheter orifice configuration may influence the quality of nerve blockade, with multiorifice catheters providing superior analgesia when compared with end-hole catheters.[19] Finally, complications related to continuous peripheral nerve blocks, such as bleeding, infection, neurologic injury, and local anesthetic toxicity, have been studied and remain relatively low.[1,20]

Clinical Pearls

- A successful peripheral nerve catheter program requires trust and collaboration between the anesthesia team and clinicians from other medical and surgical specialties.
- Customized peripheral nerve catheter kits that bundle high-quality and validated supplies may allow for greater efficiency and better results.
- In the short-axis in-plane approach to continuous peripheral nerve blocks, rotating the bevel of the needle 90 degrees may allow the catheter to be positioned alongside the nerve rather than above or below it. A styletted catheter is often easier to advance past the needle and into the tissue adjacent to the nerve. After injecting local anesthetic or saline through the block needle, withdrawing the needle slightly may allow the catheter to thread with more ease.
- Careful attention to ergonomics can lead to less fatigue and more success when placing peripheral nerve catheters. Keep the ultrasound screen at eye level directly across from where the block is being placed. Hold the ultrasound probe near its end, with the hand braced against the patient's skin. Be conscious of bed and procedure table height. Posture is particularly important, and sitting may aid placement of some continuous blocks, especially popliteal catheters.
- Dilute solutions of local anesthetics can be safely administered through peripheral nerve catheters using commercially available delivery systems both in the hospital and at home. Patient education including succinct written instructions must be provided to patients who will be managing and removing their catheters at home.[4]

References

1. Borgeat A, Blumenthal S, Lambert M, Theodorou P, Vienne P. The feasibility and complications of the continuous popliteal nerve block: a 1001-case survey. *Anesth Analg.* 2006;103(1):229–233.
2. Gurnaney H, Kraemer FW, Maxwell L, Muhly WT, Schleelein L, Ganesh A. Ambulatory continuous peripheral nerve blocks in children and adolescents: a longitudinal 8-year single center study. *Anesth Analg.* 2014;118(3):621–627.
3. Williams BA, Kentor ML, Vogt MT, et al. Reduction of verbal pain scores after anterior cruciate ligament reconstruction with 2-day continuous femoral nerve block: a randomized clinical trial. *Anesthesiology.* 2006;104(2):315–327.
4. Swenson JD, Cheng GS, Axelrod DA, Davis JJ. Ambulatory anesthesia and regional catheters: when and how. *Anesthesiol Clin.* 2010;28(2):267–280.
5. Bingham AE, Fu R, Horn JL, Abrahams MS. Continuous peripheral nerve block compared with single-injection peripheral nerve block: a systematic review and meta-analysis of randomized controlled trials. *Reg Anesth Pain Med.* 2012;37(6):583–594.

6. Mariano ER, Kim TE, Funck N, et al. A randomized comparison of long-and short-axis imaging for in-plane ultrasound-guided femoral perineural catheter insertion. *J Ultrasound Med.* 2013;32(1):149–156.
7. Ilfeld BM, Fredrickson MJ, Mariano ER. Ultrasound-guided perineural catheter insertion: three approaches but few illuminating data. *Reg Anesth Pain Med.* 2010;35(2):123–126.
8. Swenson JD, Klingler KR, Pace NL, Davis JJ, Loose EC. Evaluation of a new needle guidance system for ultrasound: results of a prospective, randomized, blinded study. *Reg Anesth Pain Med.* 2016;41(3):356–361.
9. Kan JM, Harrison TK, Kim TE, Howard SK, Kou A, Mariano ER. An in vitro study to evaluate the utility of the "air test" to infer perineural catheter tip location. *J Ultrasound Med.* 2013;32(3):529–533.
10. Gurnaney H, Kraemer FW, Ganesh A. Dermabond decreases pericatheter local anesthetic leakage after continuous perineural infusions. *Anesth Analg.* 2011;113(1):206.
11. Koscielniak-nielsen ZJ, Rasmussen H. Hesselbjerg L. Long-axis ultrasound imaging of the nerves and advancement of perineural catheters under direct vision: a preliminary report of four cases. *Reg Anesth Pain Med.* 2008;33(5):477–482.
12. Fredrickson MJ, Ball CM, Dalgleish AJ, Stewart AW, Short TG. A prospective randomized comparison of ultrasound and neurostimulation as needle end points for interscalene catheter placement. *Anesth Analg.* 2009;108(5):1695–1700.
13. Mariano ER, Loland VJ, Sandhu NS, et al. Ultrasound guidance versus electrical stimulation for femoral perineural catheter insertion. *J Ultrasound Med.* 2009;28(11):1453–1460.
14. Mariano ER, Loland VJ, Sandhu NS, et al. A trainee-based randomized comparison of stimulating interscalene perineural catheters with a new technique using ultrasound guidance alone. *J Ultrasound Med.* 2010;29(3):329–336.
15. Farag E, Atim A, Ghosh R, et al. Comparison of three techniques for ultrasound-guided femoral nerve catheter insertion: a randomized, blinded trial. *Anesthesiology.* 2014;121(2):239–248.
16. Slater ME, Williams SR, Harris P, et al. Preliminary evaluation of infraclavicular catheters inserted using ultrasound guidance: through-the-catheter anesthesia is not inferior to through-the-needle blocks. *Reg Anesth Pain Med.* 2007;32(4):296–302.
17. Harrison TK, Kim TE, Howard SK, et al. Comparative effectiveness of infraclavicular and supraclavicular perineural catheters for ultrasound-guided through-the-catheter bolus anesthesia. *J Ultrasound Med.* 2015;34(2):333–340.
18. Ilfeld BM, Sandhu NS, Loland VJ, et al. Ultrasound-guided (needle-in-plane) perineural catheter insertion: the effect of catheter-insertion distance on postoperative analgesia. *Reg Anesth Pain Med.* 2011;36(3):261–265.
19. Fredrickson MJ, Ball CM, Dalgleish AJ. Catheter orifice configuration influences the effectiveness of continuous peripheral nerve blockade. *Reg Anesth Pain Med.* 2011;36(5):470–475.
20. Capdevila X, Pirat P, Bringuier S, et al. Continuous peripheral nerve blocks in hospital wards after orthopedic surgery: a multicenter prospective analysis of the quality of postoperative analgesia and complications in 1,416 patients. *Anesthesiology.* 2005;103(5):1035–1045.

ULTRASOUND-GUIDED CONTINUOUS PERIPHERAL NERVE BLOCKS

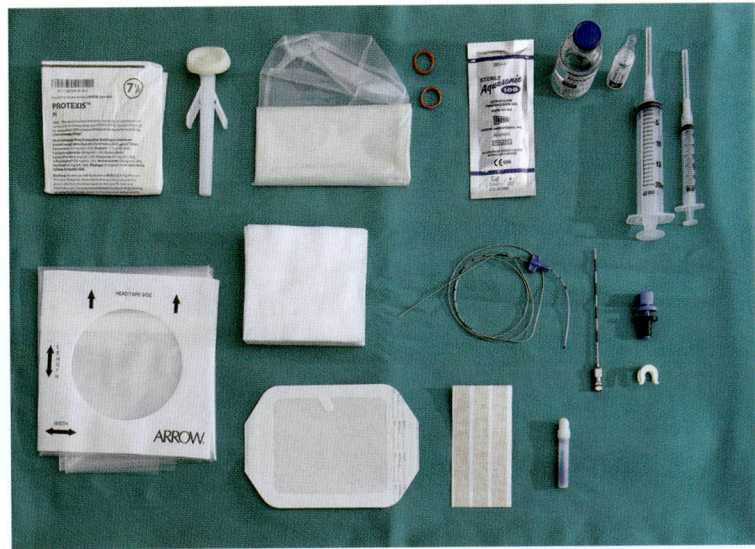

FIGURE 14.1 The equipment necessary for ultrasound-guided peripheral nerve catheter placement.

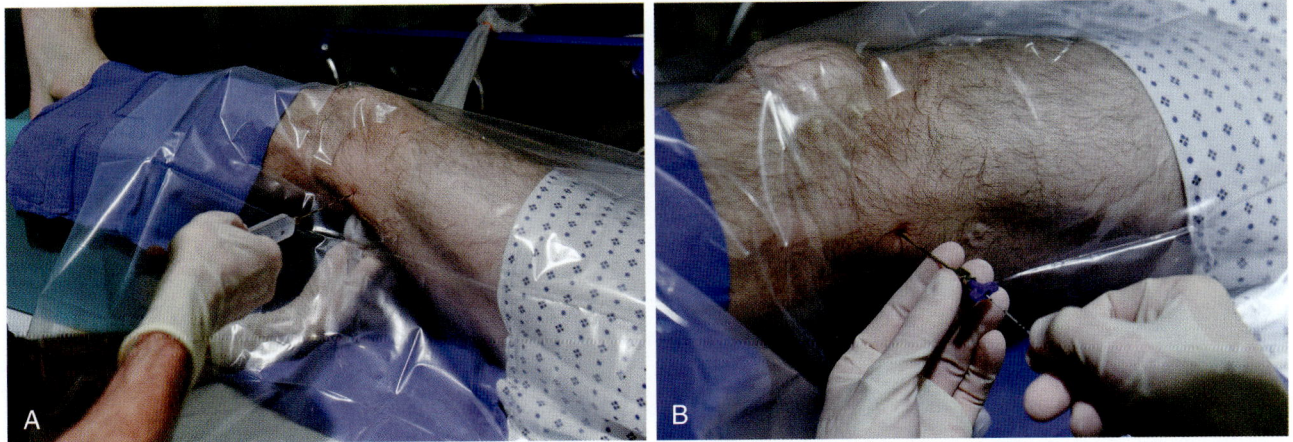

FIGURE 14.2 External photographs showing the approach to popliteal catheter placement. The proceduralist shown connects a 20-mL syringe directly to the Tuohy needle and advances into the popliteal fossa with ultrasound guidance (A). The catheter is then threaded into and past the Tuohy needle (B). Catheter placement is confirmed by sonographic assessment.

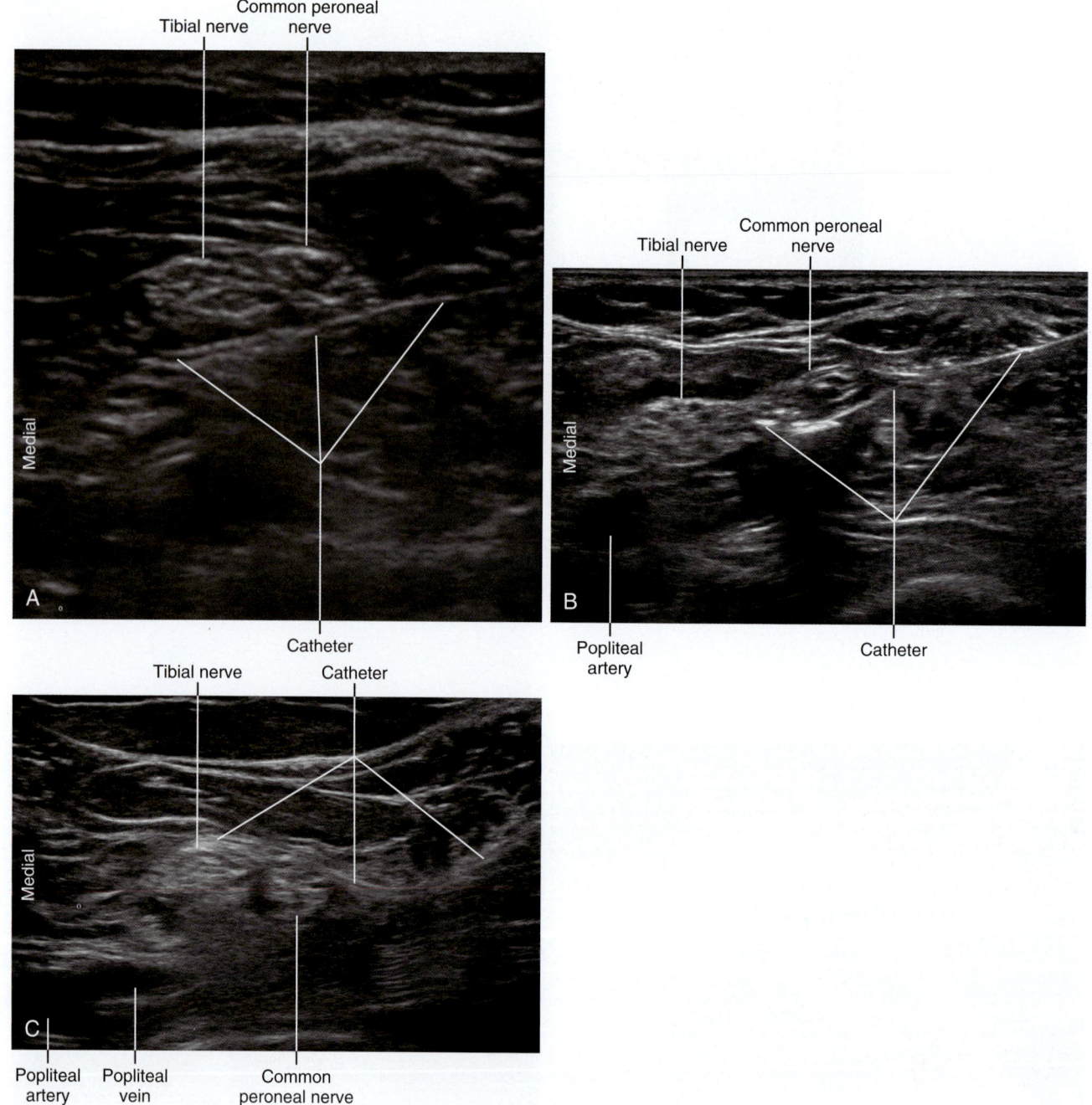

FIGURE 14.3 Ultrasound imaging of a peripheral nerve catheter in the popliteal fossa. The catheter is placed below (A), between (B), or above (C) the common peroneal and tibial branches of the sciatic nerve. All catheters were functional.

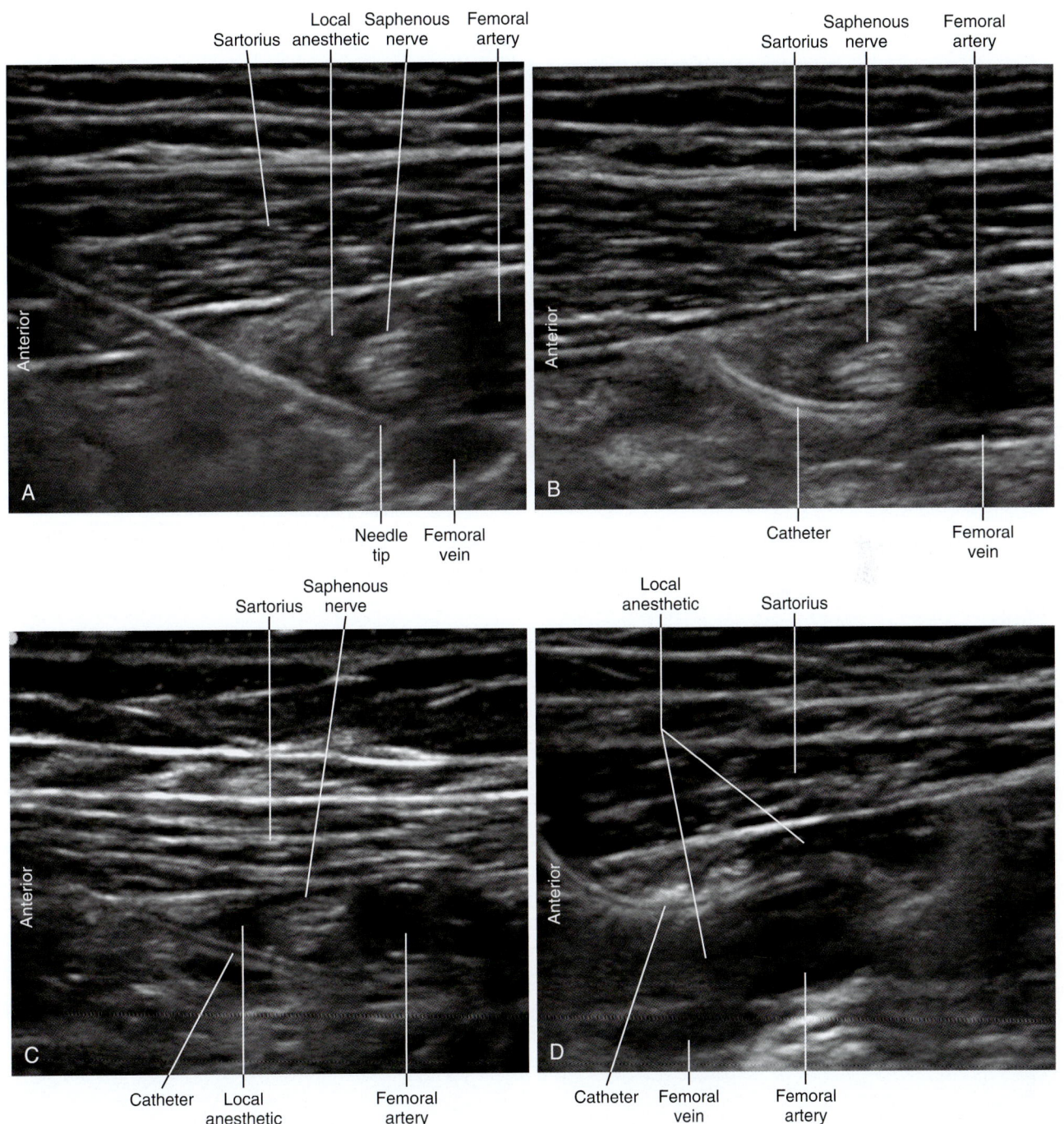

FIGURE 14.4 Sonographic assessment of a peripheral nerve catheter in the adductor canal. The space is dilated with an injection of local anesthetic or saline through the needle (A). The catheter is then advanced and typically tracks adjacent to (B and C) or above (D) the femoral artery.

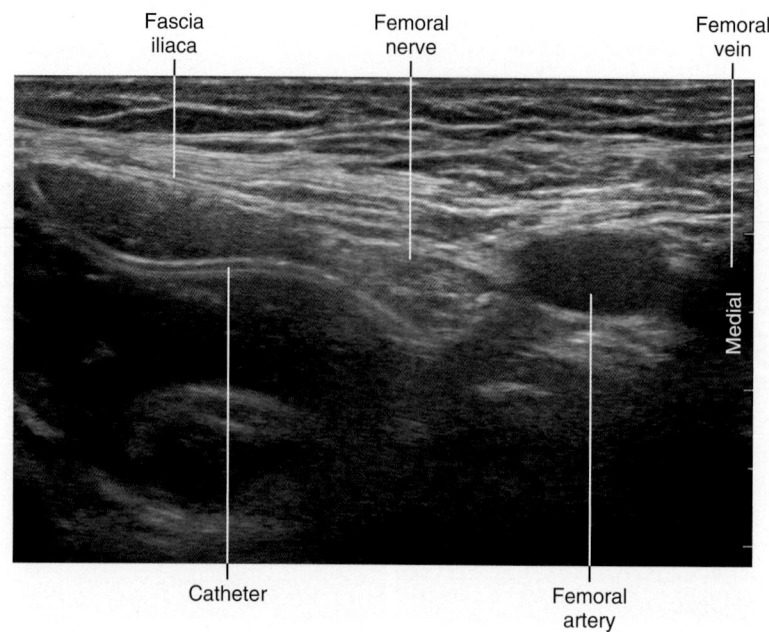

FIGURE 14.5 Advancement of a peripheral nerve catheter for continuous femoral nerve block. Note the triangular appearance of the femoral nerve and the catheter tracking below it.

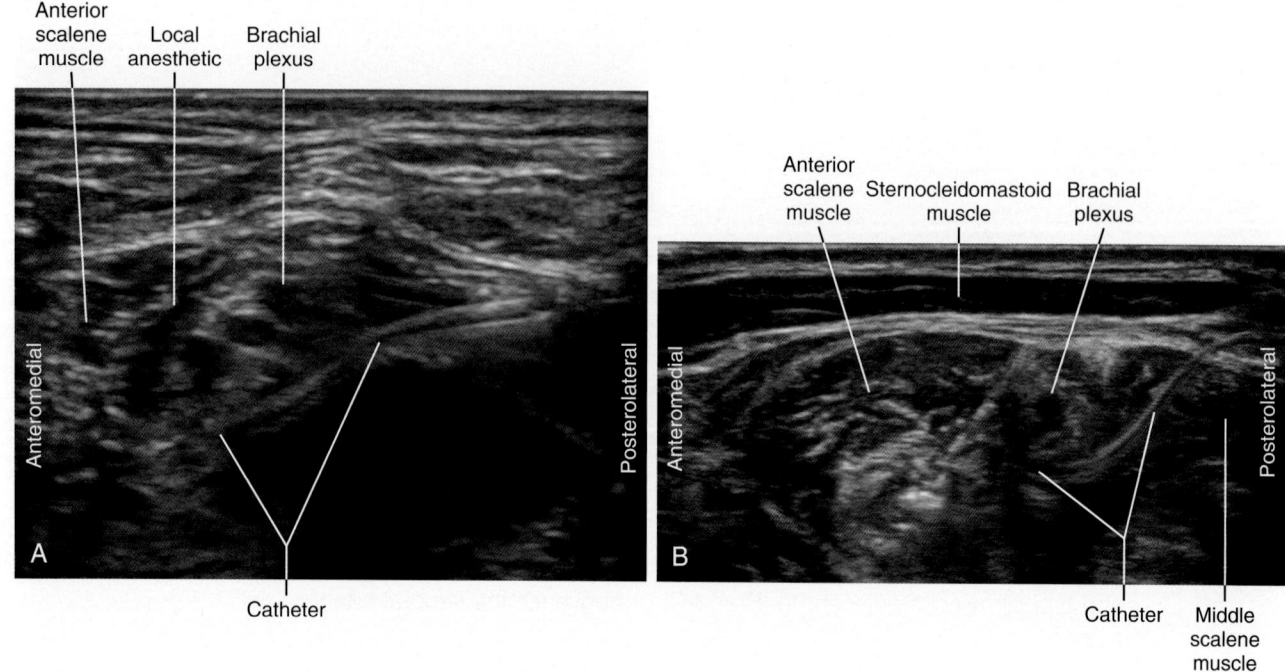

FIGURE 14.6 Ultrasound imaging of a peripheral nerve catheter in the interscalene groove (A and B). If the catheter is placed within the groove, it does not matter on which side of the brachial plexus the catheter is positioned for adequate nerve blockade to occur.

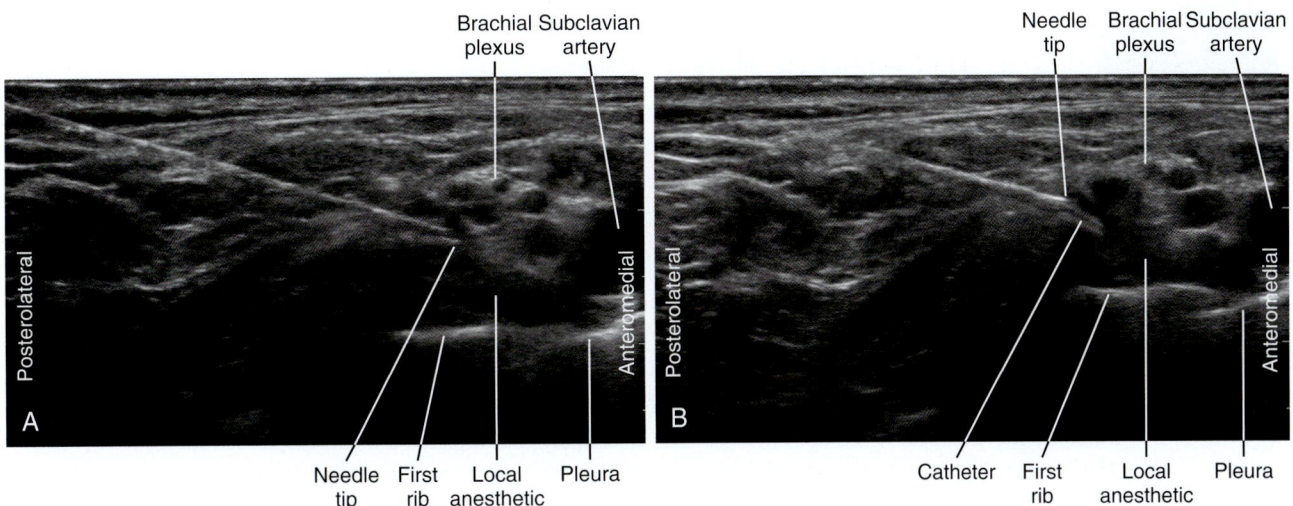

FIGURE 14.7 Image sequence showing continuous supraclavicular nerve block. The needle tip is advanced toward the subclavian artery. Local anesthetic or saline is then injected in close proximity to the divisions of the brachial plexus (A), creating a space for threading the peripheral nerve catheter (B).

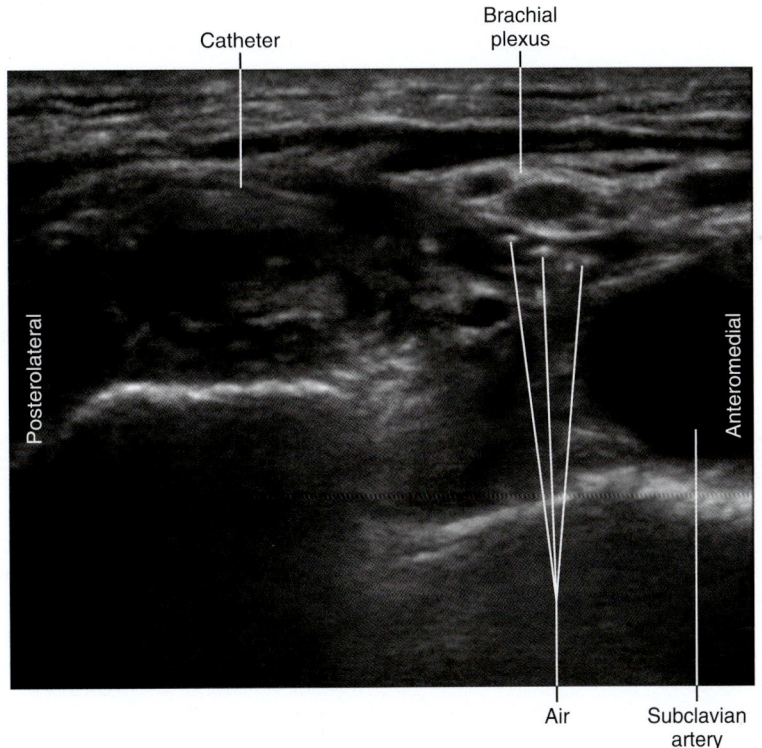

FIGURE 14.8 Sonogram showing an air test to confirm catheter placement for continuous supraclavicular nerve block. Ultrasound imaging of the peripheral nerve catheter often proves difficult to obtain. Injecting 0.5 to 1 mL of air through the catheter can help identify catheter tip location.

CHAPTER 15: Three-Dimensional Ultrasound

 See Video 1.1 on ExpertConsult.com.

There are several reports of the use of three- or four-dimensional imaging to image nerves and guide regional blocks.[1-3] Furthermore, higher-dimensional imaging may be useful for detecting focal nerve pathology.[4] The complexity of the surrounding echoes in musculoskeletal tissue can make rendering clear three-dimensional images challenging. Injected anechoic fluid can improve the interface for three-dimensional imaging of the nerve surface. Rendered volumes are often shown with sepia coloring to improve contrast resolution.

One potential advantage of three-dimensional imaging is to avoid partial line-ups of the block needle that can occur with two-dimensional in-plane technique. Because line-up is not necessary, performance time and accuracy of the procedure would benefit. One study found that the use of higher-dimensional imaging improved needle tip identification.[5] However, another study found that multiplanar reformatted displays improved needle conspicuity compared with volume-rendered displays.[6] Serious considerations for this developing technology balance obtaining more useful information with unnecessary distraction. Interventional procedure times tend to be longer with this technology.[7]

Manual acquisition of images by sliding the transducer at a constant velocity is difficult. Subsequent rendering of three-dimensional images is then done offline. Another problem is that some probes used for three-dimensional imaging using automated sweeps of acquisition are large and bulky. The biggest benefit of three-dimensional imaging may be the detection of injections that would be out of plane with two-dimensional imaging (whether it is within a vessel or along a nerve). One of the newer three-dimensional imaging display formats is "niche" format in which all three orthogonal imaging planes are shown in the single image. This format has been reported to improve imaging of the proximal sciatic nerve.[8]

Live four-dimensional imaging with matrix arrays may reduce probe manipulation during interventions and improve detection of catheter tips. However, this technology has low frame.

Clinical Pearls

- Three-dimensional ultrasound has the same artifacts as does two-dimensional imaging. Additional artifacts can arise from acquisition and rendering of three-dimensional images. As a rule, three-dimensional imaging is more subject to shadowing artifacts than two-dimensional imaging is.
- Three-dimensional ultrasound may be useful for imaging the local anesthetic distribution or catheter when it tracks out of the plane with two-dimensional imaging.

References

1. Karmakar MK, Li X, Li J, Hadzic A. Volumetric three-dimensional ultrasound imaging of the anatomy relevant for thoracic paravertebral block. *Anesth Analg.* 2012;115(5):1246–1250.
2. Clendenen SR, Pirris S, Robards CB, Leone B, Nottmeier EW. Symptomatic postlaminectomy cerebrospinal fluid leak treated with 4-dimensional ultrasound-guided epidural blood patch. *J Neurosurg Anesthesiol.* 2012;24(3):222–225.

3. Clendenen NJ, Robards CB, Clendenen SR. A standardized method for 4D ultrasound-guided peripheral nerve blockade and catheter placement. *Biomed Res Int*. 2014;2014:920538.
4. Pelz JO, Busch M, Weinreich A, Saur D, Weise D. Evaluation of freehand high-resolution 3D ultrasound of the median nerve. *Muscle Nerve*. 2017;12:e0167500. doi:10.1002/mus.25241.
5. Won HJ, Han JK, Do KH, et al. Value of four-dimensional ultrasonography in ultrasonographically guided biopsy of hepatic masses. *J Ultrasound Med*. 2003;22:215–220.
6. Rose SC, Nelson TR, Deutsch R. Display of 3-dimensional ultrasonographic images for interventional procedures: volume-rendered versus multiplanar display. *J Ultrasound Med*. 2004;23:1465–1473.
7. Tonni G, Centini G, Rosignoli L, Argento C, Centini G. 4D vs 2D ultrasound-guided amniocentesis. *J Clin Ultrasound*. 2009;37:431–435.
8. Karmakar M, Li X, Li J, Sala-Blanch X, Hadzic A, Gin T. Three-dimensional/four-dimensional volumetric ultrasound imaging of the sciatic nerve. *Reg Anesth Pain Med*. 2012;37(1):60–66.

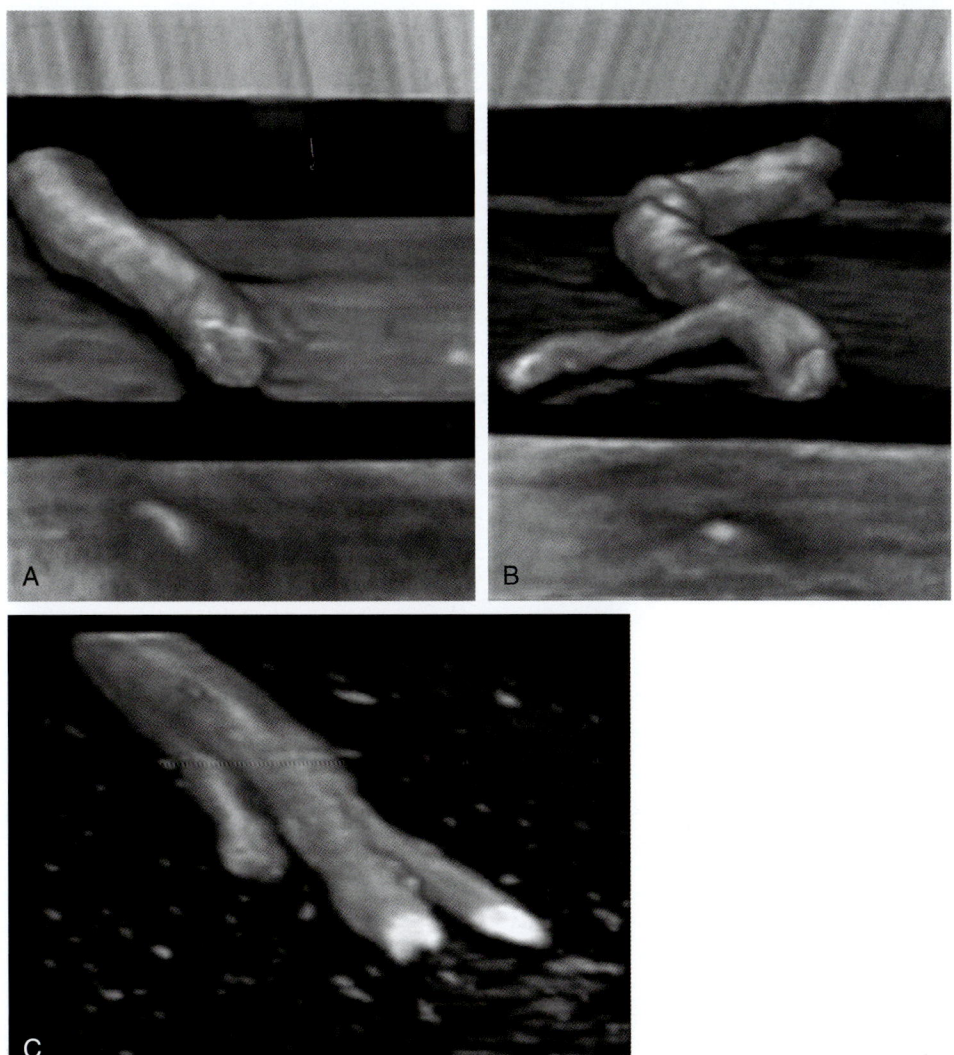

FIGURE 15.1 Excised ex vivo nerve specimen embedded in anechoic acoustic medium for three-dimensional imaging. A single nerve (A) and nerves with branching patterns (B and C) are displayed, demonstrating the echotexture of the nerve surface.

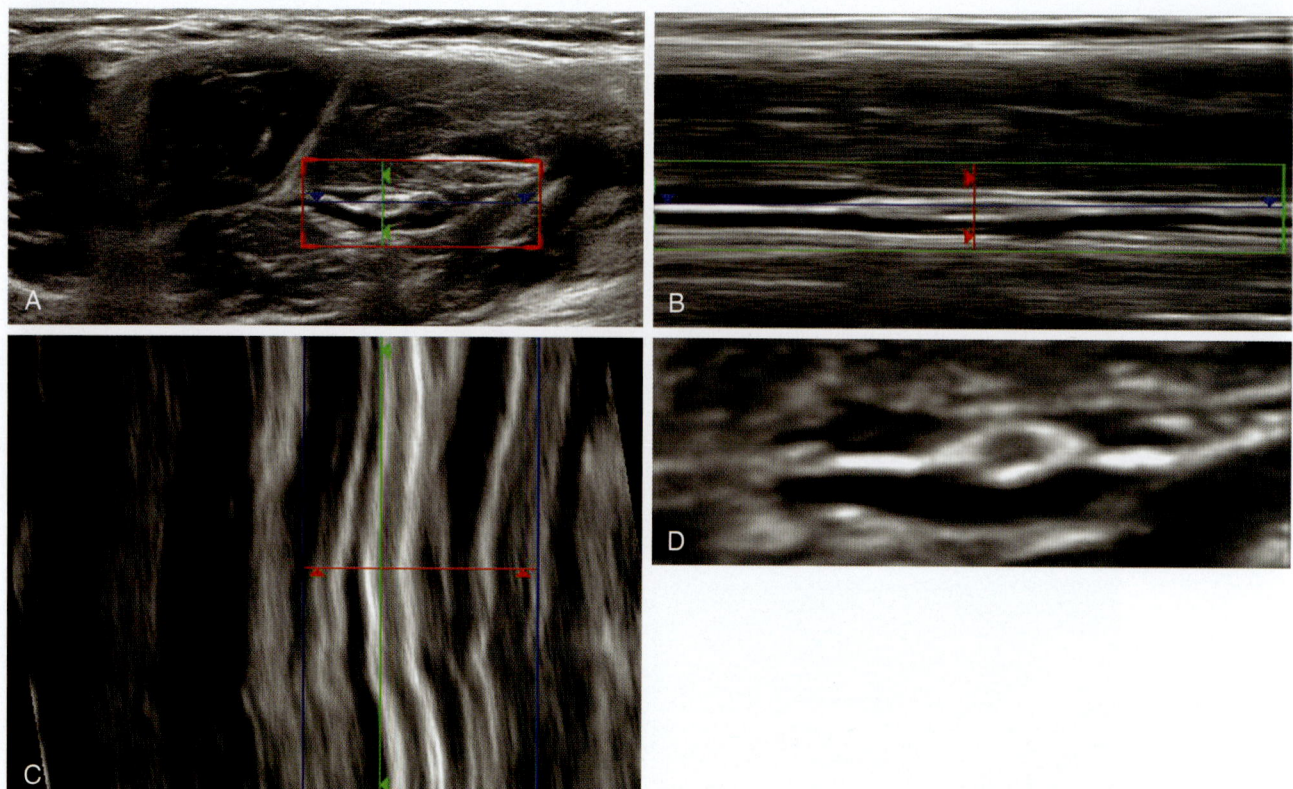

FIGURE 15.2 Clinical three-dimensional imaging of the musculocutaneous nerve and injection of local anesthetic. The nerve is seen in short-axis view (A), two long-axis views (B and C), and volume-rendered view (D).

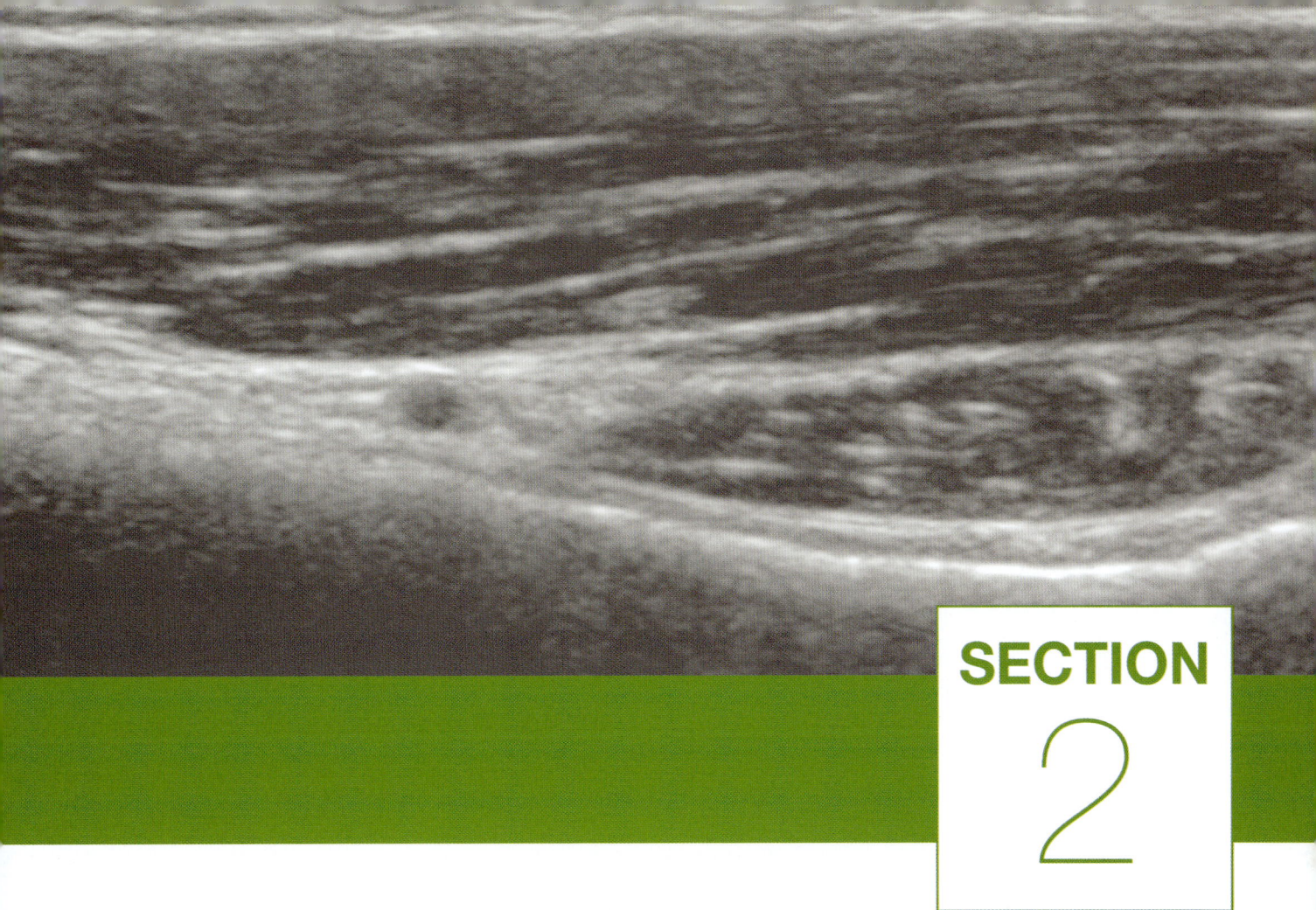

SECTION 2

Structures

CHAPTER 16

Anatomic Structures

Direct ultrasound visualization significantly improves the outcome of most techniques in regional anesthesia.[1] With the help of high-resolution ultrasonography, the anesthesiologist can directly visualize relevant structures for upper and lower extremity nerve blocks at all levels. Such direct visualization can improve the quality of nerve blocks and avoid complications. The benefits of directly visualizing targeted structures and monitoring the distribution of local anesthetic are significant. This ultrasound monitoring allows the anesthesiologist to reposition the block needle in the event of maldistribution of injected local anesthetic.

This section contains a brief overview of musculoskeletal imaging with ultrasound. Several structures are commonly imaged during regional blocks. Precise identification of these anatomic structures often involves tracking their course from start to end with ultrasound imaging.

Reference

1. Marhofer P, Greher M, Kapral S. Ultrasound guidance in regional anaesthesia. *Br J Anaesth*. 2005;94:7–17.

Skin and Subcutaneous Tissue

CHAPTER 17

Normal skin (epidermis and dermis) varies in thickness from 1 to 5 mm throughout the body and is uniformly hyperechoic.[1] The attenuation of ultrasound by skin (>1 dB/[MHz-cm]) is more than other soft tissues (0.5 to 0.75 dB/[MHz-cm]).[2,3] This is particularly important for thoracic paravertebral blocks in the upper back region where the skin is thick. Subcutaneous tissue is hypoechoic with connective septa visible as streaks parallel or nearly parallel to the skin surface.

References

1. Fornage BD, Deshayes JL. Ultrasound of normal skin. *J Clin Ultrasound*. 1986;14(8):619–622.
2. Moran CM, Bush NL, Bamber JC. Ultrasonic propagation properties of excised human skin. *Ultrasound Med Biol*. 1995;21(9):1177–1190.
3. Lebertre M, Ossant F, Vaillant L, Diridollou S, Patat F. Spatial variation of acoustic parameters in human skin: an in vitro study between 22 and 45 MHz. *Ultrasound Med Biol*. 2002;28(5):599–615.

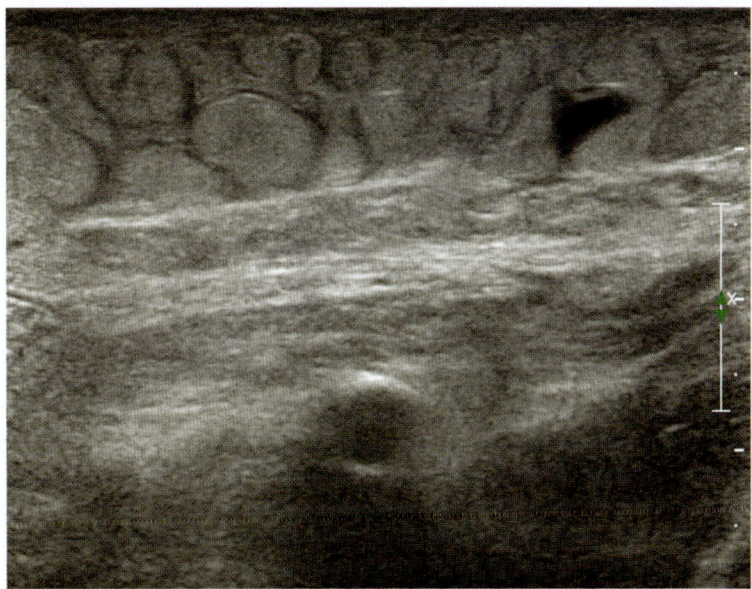

FIGURE 17.1 The dry river bed appearance to edema within subcutaneous tissue illustrating pathologic changes.

CHAPTER 18

Peripheral Nerves

Peripheral nerves have a fascicular or "honeycomb" echotexture. This consists of the mixture of nerve fiber (hypoechoic) and connective tissue (hyperechoic) content within the nerve. Because there is little connective tissue within more central nerves (e.g., the cervical ventral rami of the brachial plexus), these nerves have a monofascicular or oligofascicular appearance on ultrasound scans.[1] Nerves that are surrounded by hypoechoic muscle are usually easier to visualize than nerves that are surrounded by hyperechoic fat because the nerve borders are more evident.

Peripheral nerves have a complex architecture. Nerves are like a plexus within themselves, with fascicles combining and recombining internally along the nerve path. Because of this intertwined network, the fascicle count varies along the nerve path. Nerve sections taken 2 mm apart can have different fascicular patterns.[2] The connective tissue content and fascicle count of peripheral nerves vary directly. That is, the amount of connective tissue is more abundant in multifascicular nerves.[3] The connective tissue within nerves protects the fascicles from injury. Therefore monofascicular nerves are more vulnerable to damage.

Identification of nerve fascicles is the basis of peripheral nerve imaging. With ultrasound, only a small subset of the total number of fascicles is imaged. In one study of ex vivo nerve specimens, only approximately one-third the number of fascicles visible on light microscopy were visible on ultrasound scans.[4] It is difficult for imaging technologies to resolve thin collagenous boundaries between adjacent fascicles. For these reasons, fascicular discrimination is a standard by which to judge nerve imaging quality.

Nerves can be round, oval, or triangular and can change in shape along the nerve path. Heavy compression with the transducer can redistribute fascicles within a nerve to change its shape (the nerve shape flattens). Nerve fascicles are always round, and therefore monofascicular nerves are normally round and will not change shape with probe compression. Despite changes in shape that may occur, nerves have a relatively constant cross-sectional area along their path.

High ultrasound frequencies (10 to 15 MHz) provide better resolution of nerve fascicles.[5] However, at lower frequencies (7 to 10 MHz), peripheral nerves are still visible as cordlike structures. Commercial nerve imaging presets of imaging quality controls have been developed that enhance detection of nerve fascicles.

Short-axis sliding (sliding the transducer along the known nerve path with the nerve viewed in short axis) is a powerful technique not only to identify small nerves with ultrasound but also to assess the longitudinal distribution of local anesthetic along the nerve. Acoustic coupling gel can be placed over the known course of the nerve path before sliding to image a peripheral nerve in short-axis view (a gel trail). This will maintain effective contact with the skin for tracing the course of the nerve and local anesthetic distribution.

Among morphometric variables, the best correlate of nerve diameter is body height.[6] The best correlate of nerve visibility on ultrasound scans is the extremity size.[7]

A variety of pathologic conditions can influence nerve echotexture and mechanical properties. For example, diabetes is known to reduce nerve mobility and increase nerve stiffness.[8,9]

Clinical Pearls

- When nerves cross a tight passage, they assume a more homogeneous hypoechoic appearance from tight packing of the nerve fascicles.[1]
- When scanning superficial nerves, it is best to apply a generous amount of acoustic coupling gel (as if applying toothpaste to a toothbrush) to provide some acoustic standoff.[10]
- Sliding along the known course of a peripheral nerve with the nerve viewed in short axis can be useful for determining the edges of the distribution.

> **Clinical Pearls—cont'd**
>
> - The easiest way to obtain a long-axis view of a peripheral nerve is to view it in short axis and rotate the probe while keeping the nerve in the center of the field of view.
> - The outer band of collagen does not always produce a distinct echogenic nerve border. This can make long-axis assessments of local anesthetic distribution difficult.

References

1. Martinoli C, Bianchi S, Santacroce E, Pugliese F, Graif M, Derchi LE. Brachial plexus sonography: a technique for assessing the root level. *AJR Am J Roentgenol*. 2002;179:699–702.
2. Sunderland S. The anatomy and physiology of nerve injury. *Muscle Nerve*. 1990;13:771–784.
3. Sunderland S, Bradley KC. The cross-sectional area of peripheral nerve trunks devoted to nerve fi bers. *Brain*. 1949;72:428–449.
4. Silvestri E, Martinoli C, Derchi LE, Bertolotto M, Chiaramondia M, Rosenberg I. Echotexture of peripheral nerves: correlation between US and histologic findings and criteria to differentiate tendons. *Radiology*. 1995;197:291–296.
5. Giovagnorio F, Martinoli C. Sonography of the cervical vagus nerve: normal appearance and abnormal findings. *AJR Am J Roentgenol*. 2001;176:745–749.
6. Heinemeyer O, Reimers CD. Ultrasound of radial, ulnar, median, and sciatic nerves in healthy subjects and patients with hereditary motor and sensory neuropathies. *Ultrasound Med Biol*. 1999;25:481–485.
7. Schwemmer U, Markus CK, Greim CA, Brederlau J, Kredel M, Roewer N. Sonographic imaging of the sciatic nerve division in the popliteal fossa. *Ultraschall Med*. 2005;26:496–500.
8. Boyd BS, Gray AT, Dilley A, Wanek L, Topp KS. The pattern of tibial nerve excursion with active ankle dorsiflexion is different in older people with diabetes mellitus. *Clin Biomech (Bristol, Avon)*. 2012;27(9):967–971.
9. Dikici AS, Ustabasioglu FE, Delil S, et al. Evaluation of the tibial nerve with shear-wave elastography: a potential sonographic method for the diagnosis of diabetic peripheral neuropathy. *Radiology*. 2017;282:494–501.
10. Thain LM, Downey DB. Sonography of peripheral nerves: technique, anatomy, and pathology. *Ultrasound Q*. 2002;18:225–245.

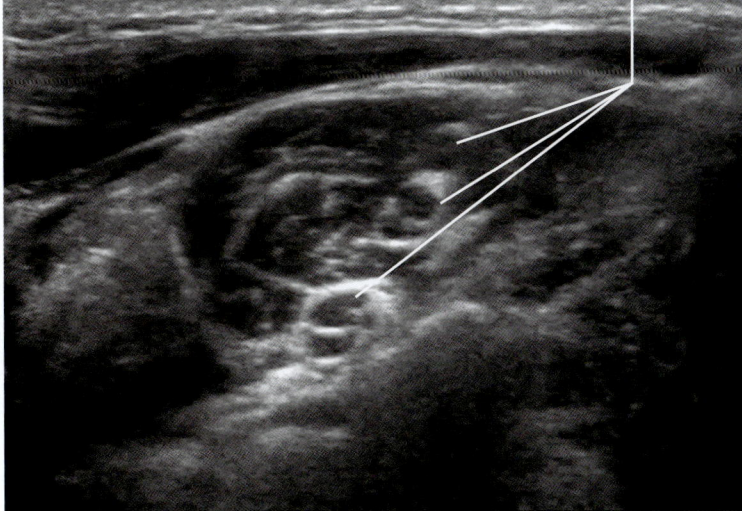

FIGURE 18.1 The cervical ventral rami of the brachial plexus viewed in short axis. This monofascicular echotexture is observed in more central nerves that contain little connective tissue.

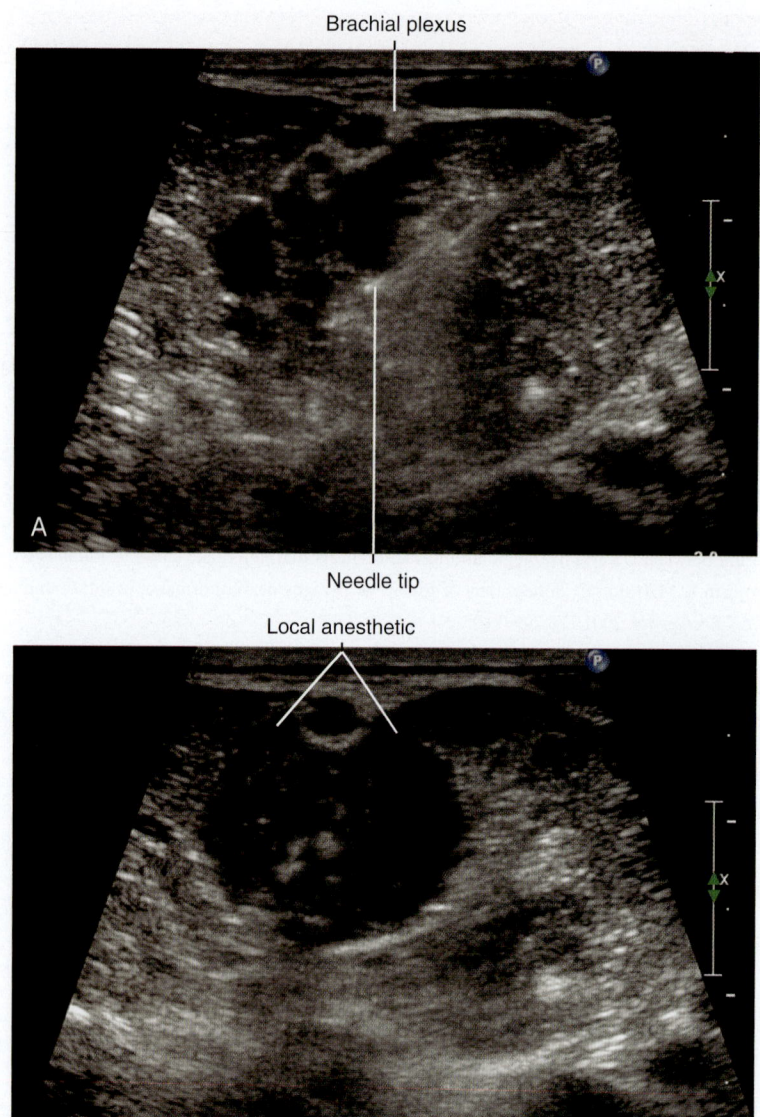

FIGURE 18.2 Interscalene block demonstrating monofascicular echotexture before (A) and after (B) injection of local anesthetic.

PERIPHERAL NERVES | 51

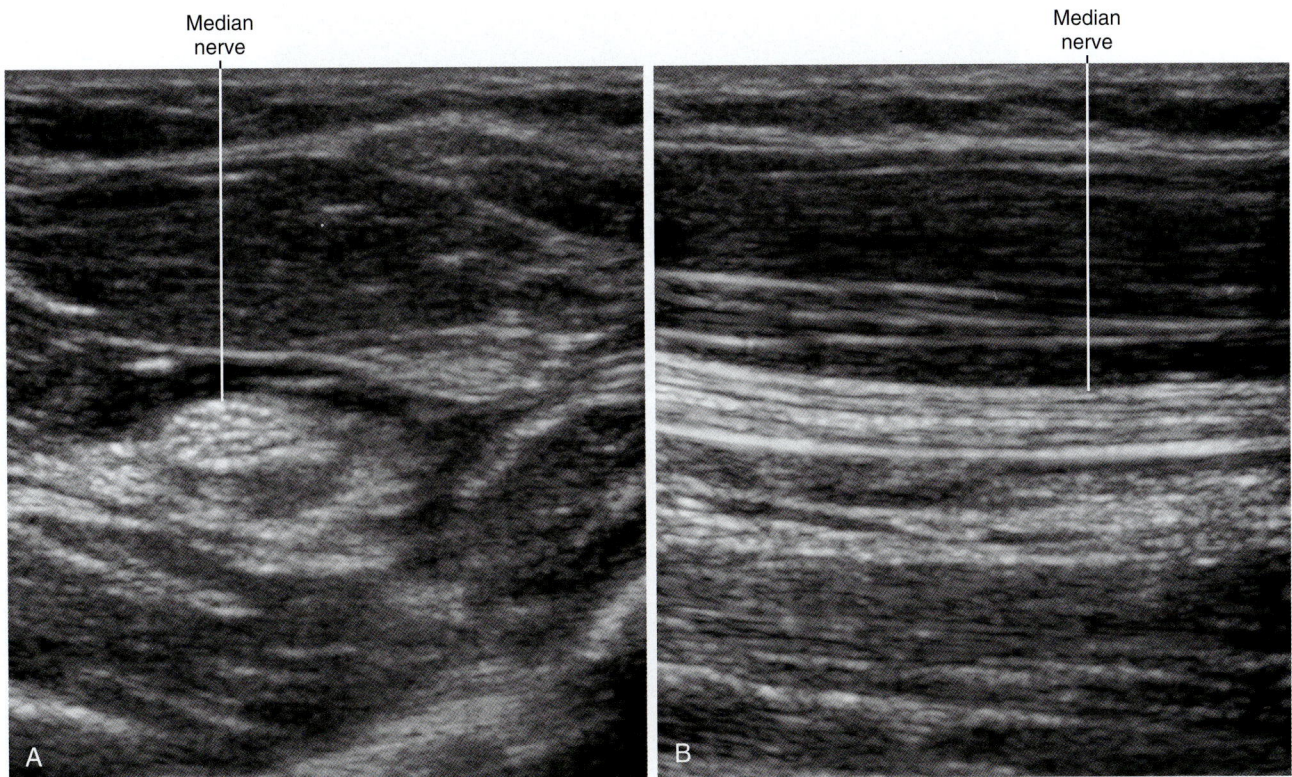

FIGURE 18.3 Median nerve in the forearm viewed in short axis (A) and long axis (B) demonstrating fascicular or honeycomb echotexture. These views were obtained after injection of local anesthetic around the nerve.

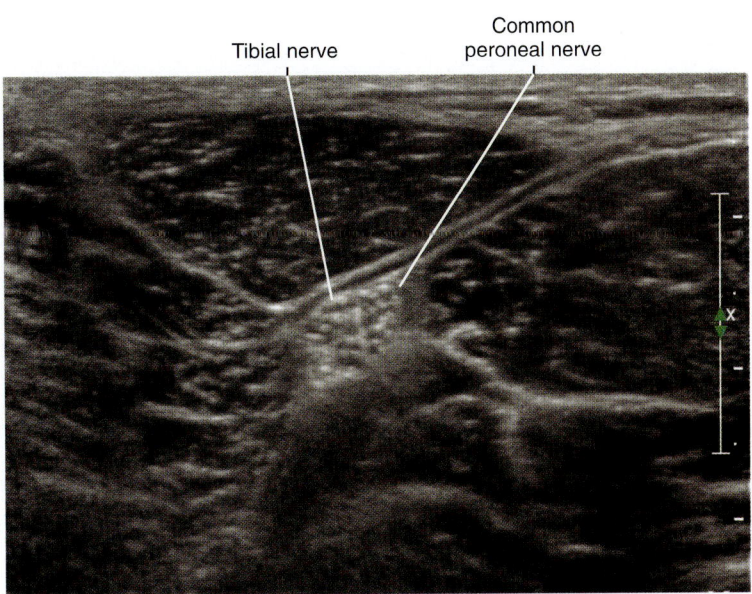

FIGURE 18.4 Sciatic nerve in the thigh demonstrating echobright connective tissue content and compartmentalization into its tibial and common peroneal nerve components.

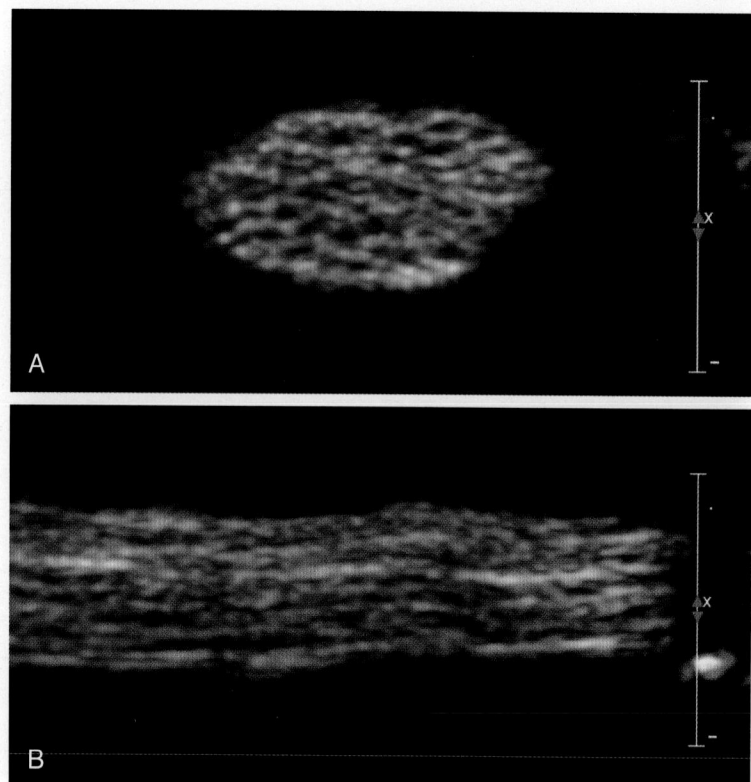

FIGURE 18.5 Excised ex vivo nerve specimen demonstrating fascicular echotexture in short-axis (A) and long-axis (B) views. Peripheral nerves viewed in long axis often exhibit parallel fascicles with coarse wavy echotexture.

Muscle

CHAPTER 19

Muscle consists of hypoechoic muscle bundles (fascicles) surrounded by linear hyperechoic streaks of fibroadipose connective tissue (perimysium). The overall echogenicity of muscle depends on the amount of intramuscular fat and (to less extent) fibroadipose tissue.[1] Healthy muscle becomes more echogenic with age due to age-related muscle replacement by fat and fibrous tissue.[2,3] The organization of fibroadipose septa within muscle can resemble peripheral nerves in some cases.

It is important to recognize muscle borders during regional blocks (Table 19.1). A thick fibrous layer surrounds the entire muscle (the epimysium or investing fascia). Adjacent muscles can often be distinguished by differences in their muscle fiber directions. When muscles are viewed in their long axis, the linear parallel arrangement of their fibers can be appreciated.[4]

Muscle exhibits anisotropy (the received echoes depend on the angle of insonation) but to less extent than tendons.[5]

Pennate muscles have a featherlike appearance from fiber insertions on a common aponeurosis. Tendons can lie in the center of muscle (central tendon of bipennate structure) or on the side of the muscle (eccentric tendon of unipennate structure).

Muscle contraction and motion can be used to improve definition of muscle borders. For example, external rotation of the leg can help define the borders of the piriformis muscle during sonography. Dynamic motion will improve the quality of scanning of the piriformis muscle because it will move independently of the adjacent muscles.

Anatomic variation is sometimes observed as accessory muscles (accessory soleus, peroneus quartus, scalenus minimus, cleidoatlanticus, etc.).

TABLE 19.1 Muscle Echogenicity (Echo Intensity) for Several Regional Blocks

Block	Hyperechoic	Hypoechoic	Reference
Transversus abdominis plane (TAP)	External oblique	Transversus abdominis	Hebbard et al.[a]
Quadratus lumborum	Psoas	Quadratus lumborum	Callen et al.[b]; King et al.[c]
Intercostal	External intercostal	Innermost intercostal and Diaphragm	Boon et al.[d]
Lateral femoral cutaneous nerve (LFCN)	Tensor Fascia Lata	Sartorius	Bass and Connell[e]

[a]Hebbard PD, Barrington MJ, Vasey C. Ultrasound-guided continuous oblique subcostal transversus abdominis plane blockade: description of anatomy and clinical technique. *Reg Anesth Pain Med*. 2010;35(5):436–441.
[b]Callen PW, Filly RA, Marks WM. The quadratus lumborum muscle: a possible source of confusion in sonographic of the retroperitoneum. *J Clin Ultrasound*. 1979;7(5):349–352.
[c]King AD, Hine AL, McDonald C, Abrahams P. The ultrasound appearance of the normal psoas muscle. *Clin Radiol*. 1993;48(5):316–318.
[d]Boon AJ, Harper CJ, Ghahfarokhi LS, Strommen JA, Watson JC, Sorenson EJ. Two-dimensional ultrasound imaging of the diaphragm: quantitative values in normal subjects. *Muscle Nerve*. 2013;47(6):884–889.
[e]Bass CJ, Connell DA. Sonographic findings of tensor fascia lata tendinopathy: another cause of anterior groin pain. *Skeletal Radiol*. 2002;31(3):143–148.

> **Clinical Pearls**
> - When muscles are viewed in their long axis, the echotexture consists of a set of parallel line segments from their fibers.
> - There is loose connective tissue between adjacent muscles to promote sliding.
> - One can often get a sense of the muscle borders/boundaries by the change in muscle fiber direction between adjacent muscles.
> - Pennate muscles have a featherlike appearance from fiber insertions on a common aponeurosis. Muscles can be unipennate or bipennate.

References

1. Reimers K, Reimers CD, Wagner S, Paetzke I, Pongratz DE. Skeletal muscle sonography: a correlative study of echogenicity and morphology. *J Ultrasound Med*. 1993;12(2):73–77.
2. Nijboer-Oosterveld J, Van Alfen N, Pillen S. New normal values for quantitative muscle ultrasound: obesity increases muscle echo intensity. *Muscle Nerve*. 2011;43(1):142–143.
3. Young HJ, Jenkins NT, Zhao Q, Mccully KK. Measurement of intramuscular fat by muscle echo intensity. *Muscle Nerve*. 2015;52(6):963–971.
4. Peetrons P. Ultrasound of muscles. *Eur Radiol*. 2002;12(1):35–43.
5. Ophir J, Maklad NF, Bigelow RH. Ultrasonic attenuation measurements of in vivo human muscle. *Ultrason Imaging*. 1982;4(3):290–295.

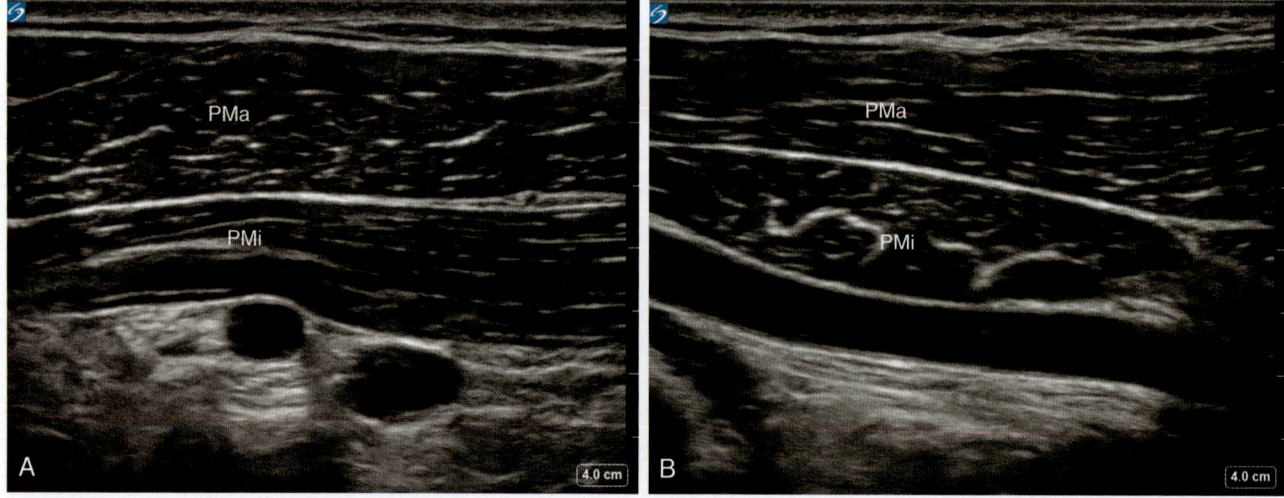

FIGURE 19.1 The pectoralis minor muscle is a key sonographic landmark for performing infraclavicular block. In this anatomic location the brachial plexus is relatively compact and surrounds the second part of the axillary artery. The muscle fibers of the pectoralis minor (PMi) muscle are easily distinguished from those of the pectoralis major (PMa) because they run in different directions. Short-axis (A) and long-axis (B) views of the axillary artery are shown to illustrate the different fiber directions of the pectoralis major and minor muscles.

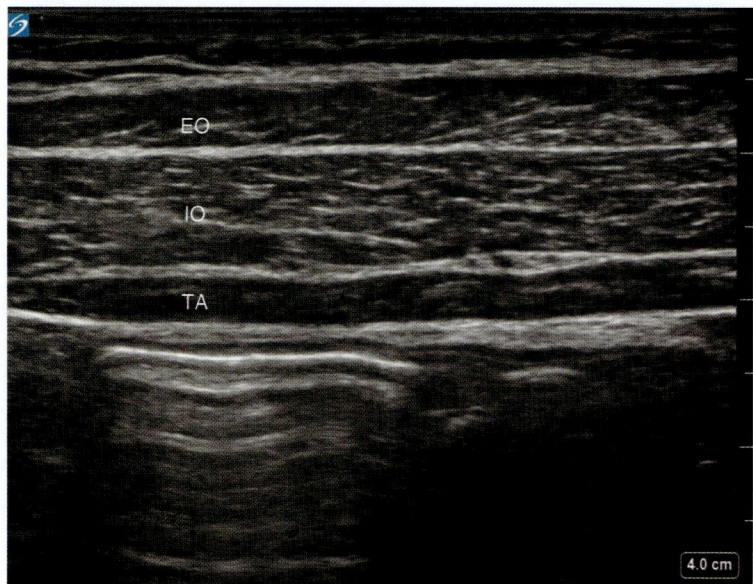

FIGURE 19.2 The transversus abdominis *(TA)* muscle is a hypoechoic muscle that lies deep to the external oblique (EO) and internal oblique (IO) in the abdominal wall. Other examples of hypoechoic muscles include the diaphragm and quadratus lumborum.

CHAPTER 20
Tendons and Ligaments

Tendons are the strong anatomic structures that connect muscle to bone. Their fibrillar echotexture (fiberlike, appearing as the fine hairs of a violin bow) results from parallel collagen bundles. Because of this ordered architecture, tendons are highly anisotropic, meaning that the received echoes are highly dependent on the angle of insonation.[1-3]

Tendons and nerves are both imaged during regional block procedures, and therefore some commentary regarding their discriminatory features is appropriate. Although the two structures can appear similar, tendons and nerves are primarily distinguished by tracing their course. Because tendons form only at the ends of muscle, changes in cross-sectional area along the course are substantial. For nerves, the cross-sectional area is relatively constant along the nerve path. In addition, the amplitudes of the received echoes from tendons are more sensitive to transducer inclination than nerves (tendons are more anisotropic than nerves). At high frequencies of insonation (≥10 MHz), the fibrillar echotexture of tendons can be distinguished from the fascicular echotexture of nerves (Table 20.1).[4]

Tendons can have central or eccentric location within muscle depending on whether the muscle is bipennate or unipennate, respectively. Multipennate muscles have more than one tendon. Normal tendons are avascular with no flow detectable either on color-flow or power Doppler examinations.[5] Direct injections into tendons have been associated with tendon rupture.[6]

Some tendons are valuable landmarks of nerve position. For example, the ulnar nerve lies between the flexor carpi ulnaris (FCU) tendon and the ulnar artery in the medial forearm. As another example, the common peroneal nerve lies posterior to the conjoint tendon of the biceps femoris in the distal thigh near the knee crease. In the axilla the neurovascular bundle lies anterior to the conjoint tendon of the latissimus dorsi and teres major.

Ligaments join adjacent osseous structures and are thickened at their ends (broad attachments forming a convex shape with "bowtie" appearance in long-axis view). Because ligaments are stabilizers that connect bone to bone, they are less mobile than tendons. Ligaments can be oval or triangular in short-axis view.[7] Most ligaments are 2 to 5 mm in thickness.

TABLE 20.1 Characteristics of Nerves and Tendons That Can Be Identified With Ultrasound Imaging

Characteristic	Nerve	Tendon
Echotexture	Fascicular	Fibrillar
Elemental composition	Fascicles (coarse, thick, wavy, less numerous)	Fibrils (fine, thin, straight, more numerous)
Internal architecture	Plexiform (combine and divide)	Parallel fibrils
Cross-sectional area	Constant along nerve path	Forms at the ends of muscle
Overall shape	Round, oval, or triangular Shape can change along path	Round, oval, or triangular; C or S Shape does not change along path
Branching	Yes	None
Anisotropy	Moderately sensitive	Highly sensitive
Adjacent vessels	Often	Infrequent
Border	Not as distinct	Distinct paratenon
Compressibility	More compressible	Less compressible

Both ligaments and tendons have fibrillar echotexture and exhibit marked anisotropy. However, ligaments have a more compact structure than tendons. Ligaments can serve as important sonographic landmarks for regional blocks (Table 20.2). For adequate imaging the angulation of the transducer must be adjusted for the ultrasound beam to be perpendicular to either ligaments or tendons.

TABLE 20.2 Examples of Regional Blocks and Ligaments as Sonographic Landmarks

Regional Block	Ligament
Suprascapular	Transverse scapular
Paravertebral	Superior costotransverse
Epidural	Ligamentum flavum
Spinal	Interspinous
Fascia iliaca	Inguinal
Pudendal	Sacrospinous, sacrotuberous
Caudal	Sacrococcygeal

Clinical Pearls

- The position of musculotendinous junctions is variable, making it difficult to identify tendons based on anatomic position alone.
- Tendons consist of a network of thin, parallel, and longitudinally oriented specular echoes that resemble fibrils. The septa consist of loose connective tissue with elastic fibers, vessels, and thin muscle fibers.
- Nerves typically have fewer and thicker echogenic lines than do tendons.

References

1. Fornage BD. The hypoechoic normal tendon: a pitfall. *J Ultrasound Med.* 1987;6:19–22.
2. Crass JR, van de Vegte GL, Harkavy LA. Tendon echogenicity: ex vivo study. *Radiology.* 1988;167:499–501.
3. Connolly DJ, Berman L, McNally EG. The use of beam angulation to overcome anisotropy when viewing human tendon with high-frequency linear array ultrasound. *Br J Radiol.* 2001;74:183–185.
4. Silvestri E, Martinoli C, Derchi LE, Bertolotto M, Chiaramondia M, Rosenberg I. Echotexture of peripheral nerves: correlation between US and histologic findings and criteria to differentiate tendons. *Radiology.* 1995;197:291–296.
5. O'Connor PJ, Grainger AJ, Morgan SR, Smith KL, Waterton JC, Nash AF. Ultrasound assessment of tendons in asymptomatic volunteers: a study of reproducibility. *Eur Radiol.* 2004;14:1968–1973.
6. Ford LT, DeBender J. Tendon rupture after local steroid injection. *South Med J.* 1979;72:827–830.
7. Ferreira FB, Fernandes ED, Silva FD, Vieira MC, Puchnick A, Fernandes AR. A sonographic technique to evaluate the anterior bundle of the ulnar collateral ligament of the elbow: imaging features and anatomic correlation. *J Ultrasound Med.* 2015;34(3):377–384.

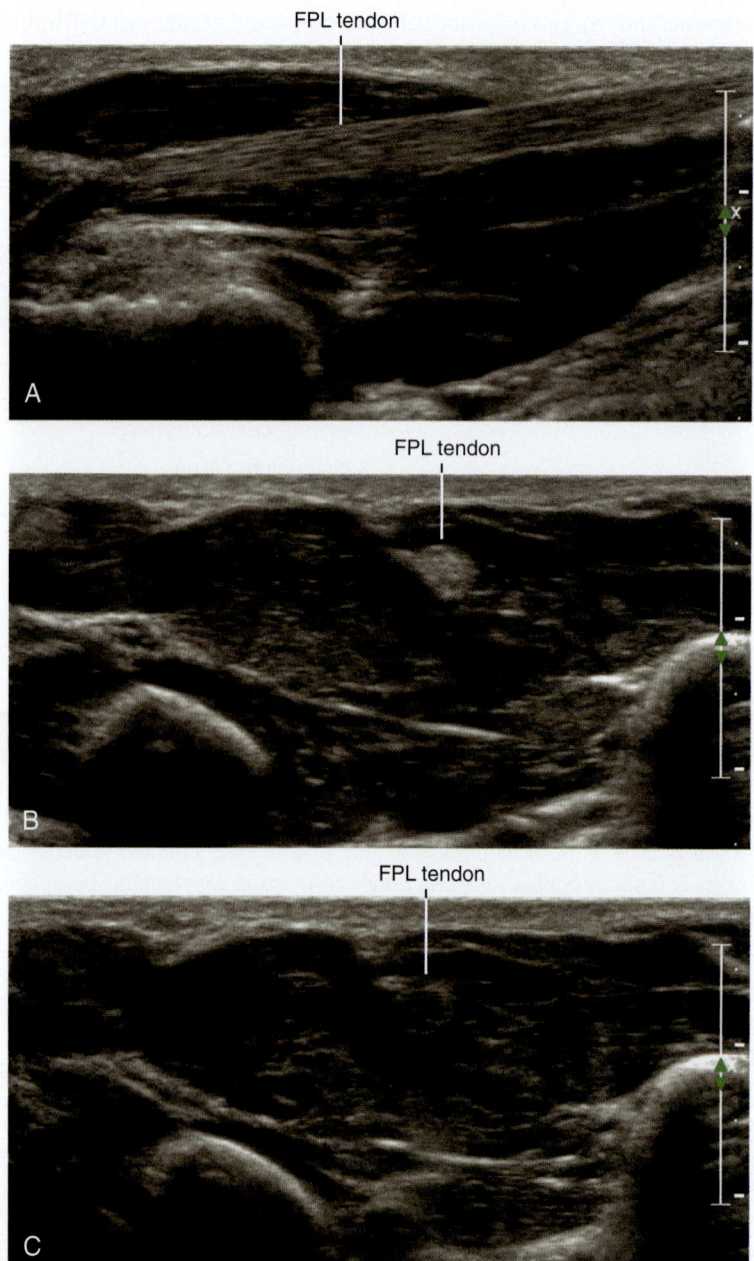

FIGURE 20.1 The flexor pollicis longus (FPL) tendon in long-axis view (A) and short-axis view (B). If the transducer is tilted slightly, echoes from the tendon will disappear, thereby demonstrating anisotropy (C).

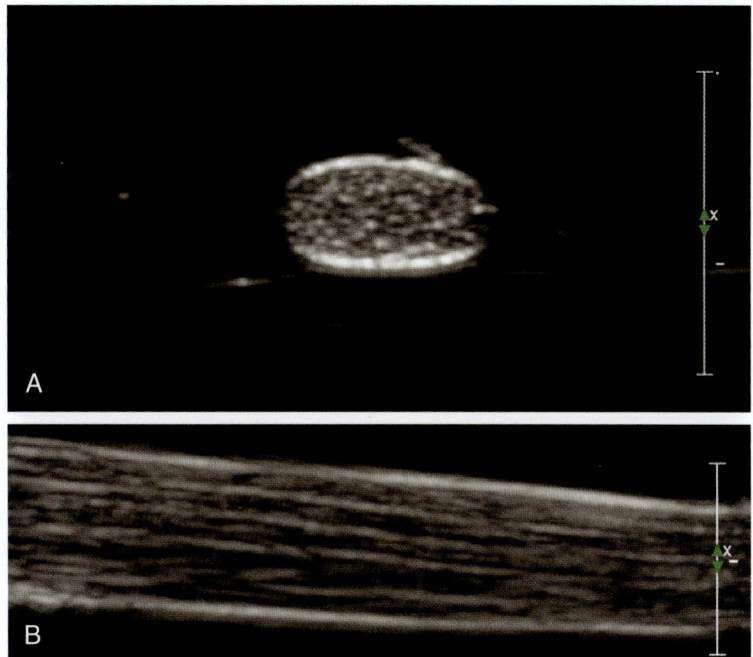

FIGURE 20.2 Excised ex vivo tendon specimen demonstrating fibrillar echotexture in short-axis (A) and long-axis (B) views.

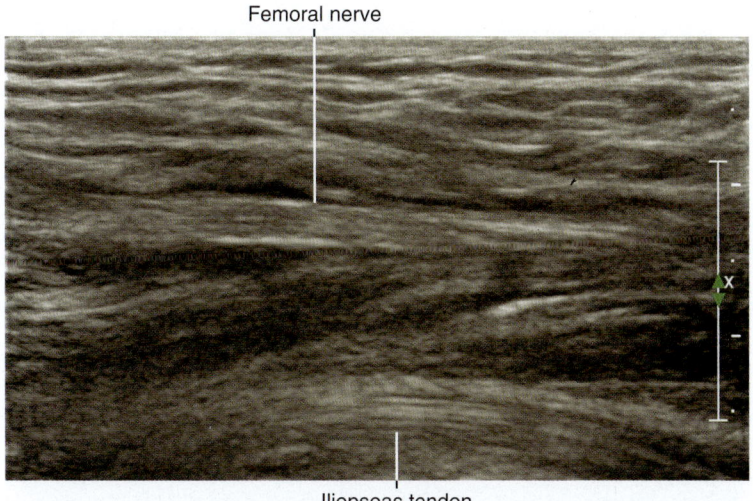

FIGURE 20.3 Comparison in echotexture of the femoral nerve and iliopsoas tendon in long-axis view after femoral nerve block. The sonogram illustrates the distinction between the fascicular and fibrillar patterns.

CHAPTER 21

Arteries

Visible pulsations from arteries are observed when compression is applied with the transducer to soft tissue. The amount of compression necessary for this depends on many variables, including the blood pressure, size and depth of the artery, and proximity of the artery to bone. Adjusting the amount of transducer compression to elicit visible pulsations is the fastest way to identify arteries. In some cases it is necessary to apply Doppler. Arteries have thicker walls than veins and do not have valves. Almost every peripheral nerve has a long running path with accompanying artery or vein.

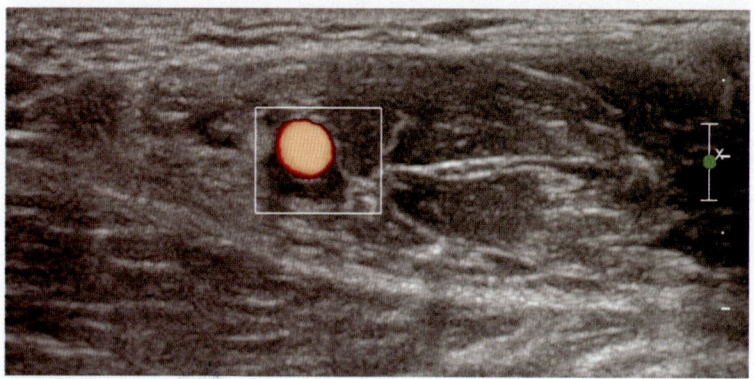

FIGURE 21.1 Short-axis view of the axillary artery in the axilla viewed with power Doppler.

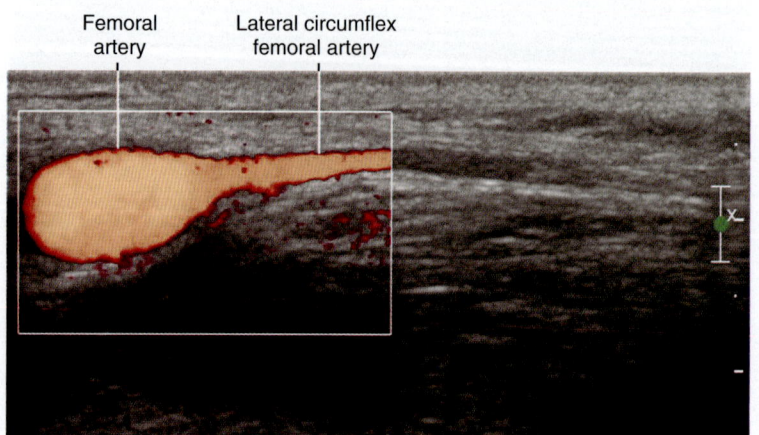

FIGURE 21.2 Power Doppler imaging of the femoral artery and lateral circumflex femoral artery. The lateral artery overlies the femoral nerve and is a potential site for bleeding complications.

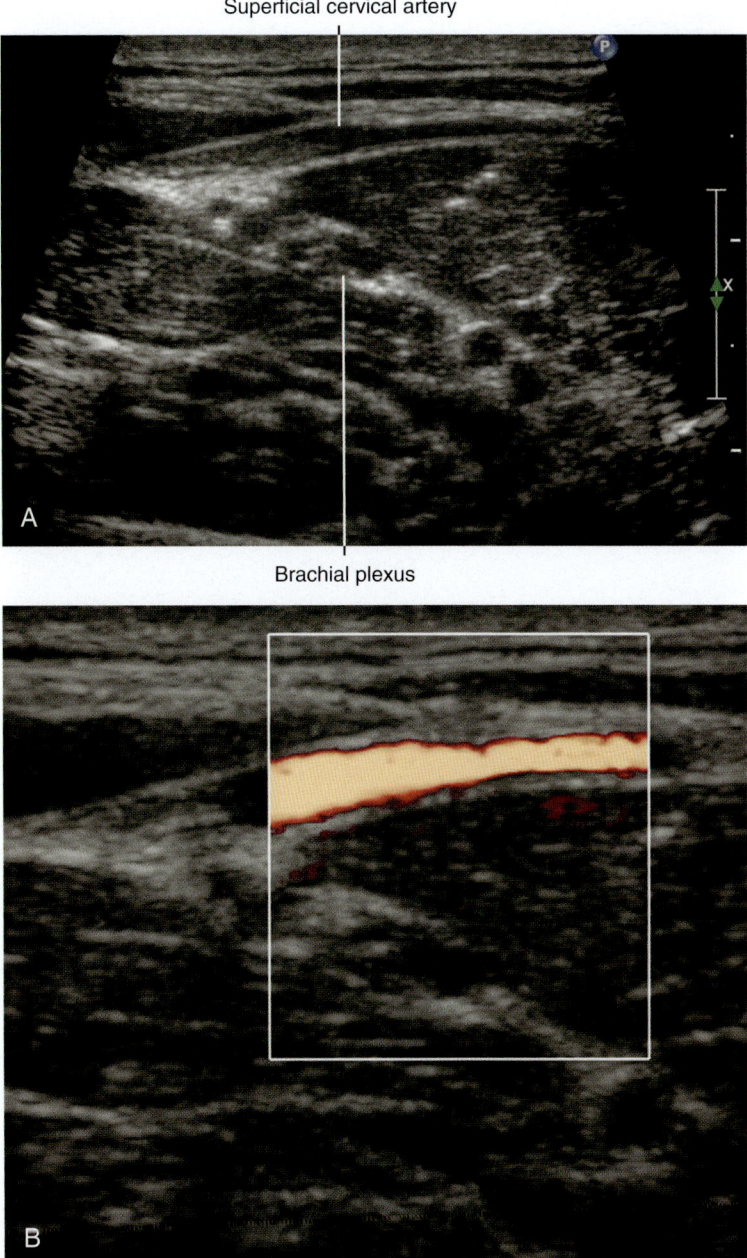

FIGURE 21.3 Superficial cervical artery is observed overlying the brachial plexus during interscalene block. (A) B-mode sonogram. (B) Power Doppler.

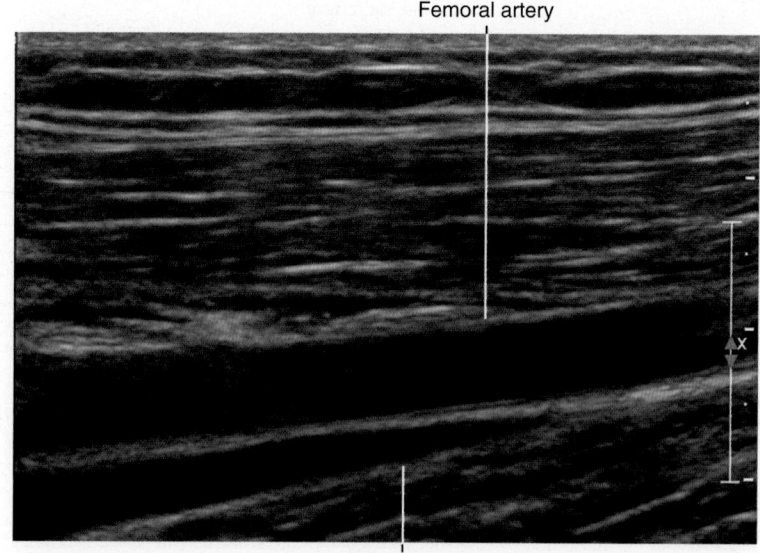

FIGURE 21.4 Long-axis view of femoral artery running under the sartorius muscle in the midthigh proximal to the adductor canal. The femoral vein also is seen in long-axis view. The femoral artery serves as a landmark for saphenous nerve block in the midthigh.

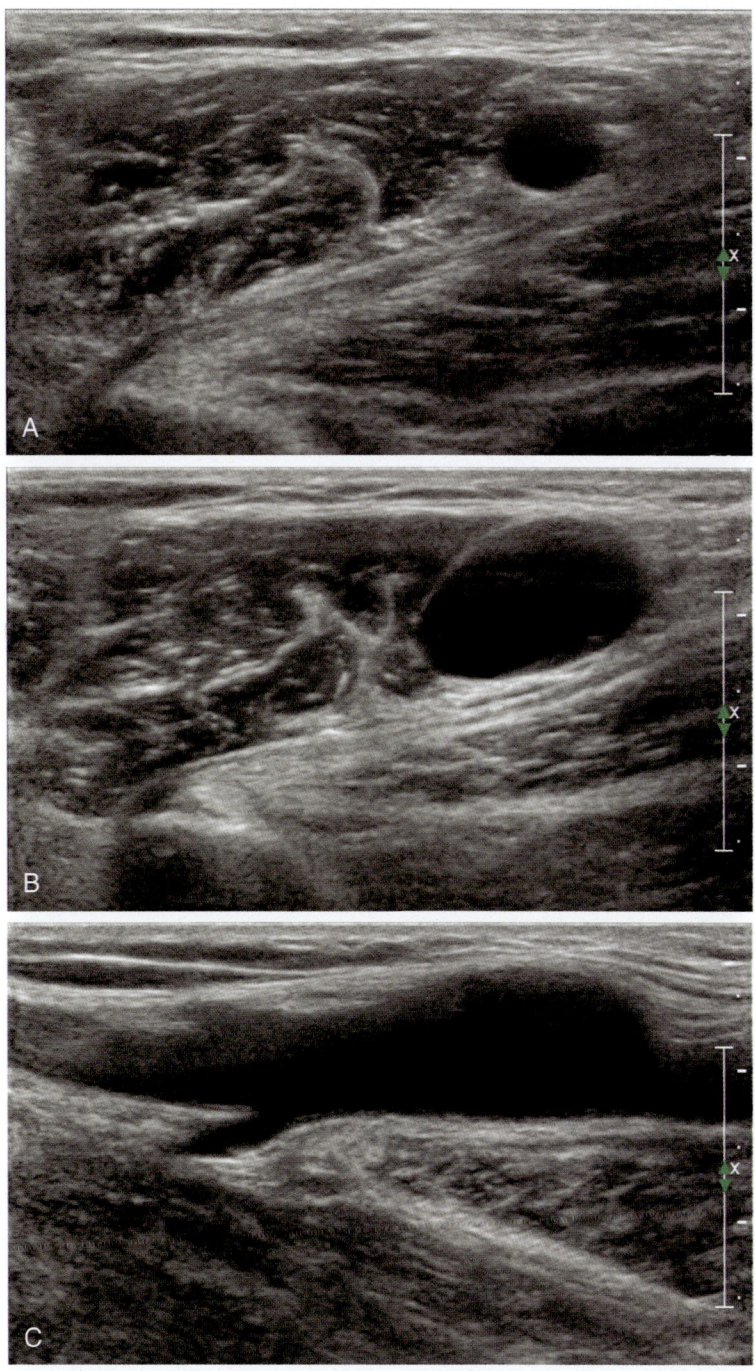

FIGURE 21.5 Arteries normally have a uniform caliber. In this case, aneurysmal dilatation of the axillary artery was detected. Short-axis views in the normal segment (A) and dilated segment (B) are shown, together with the long-axis view (C). Axillary block was performed away from this site where the artery appeared to be normal.

CHAPTER 22

Veins

Veins are easily compressed with the ultrasound transducer and have thin walls that are difficult to visualize. The vein shape is highly dependent on the amount of probe compression. Often, valves can be imaged inside the vein lumen. In contrast to the pulsatile flow of arteries, veins exhibit more continuous flow. Some degree of ACV waves (from **A**trial contraction, **C**ontraction of the ventricle, and **V**enous filling of the atrium) and respiratory variation in flow may be present, depending on how close the vein is to the thoracic cavity. Veins may have spontaneous echo contrast due to rouleaux formation of red blood cells in low flow states such as congestive heart failure.[1] At the usual amount of probe compression for nerve imaging, the veins are not visible in the field because the vein walls are coapted.

Some veins travel with peripheral nerves within the subcutaneous tissue. The saphenous vein travels with the saphenous nerve in the medial leg. The small saphenous vein travels with the sural nerve in the lateral leg.

Distal augmentation maneuvers can be used to help identify patent peripheral veins.[2] Squeezing the calf will distend the popliteal vein. A similar maneuver applied to the foot or lower calf will distend the posterior tibial veins.

References

1. Machi J, Sigel B, Beitler JC, Coelho JC, Justin JR. Relation of in vivo blood flow to ultrasound echogenicity. *J Clin Ultrasound*. 1983;11:3–10.
2. Polak JF, Culter SS, O'Leary DH. Deep veins of the calf: assessment with color Doppler flow imaging. *Radiology*. 1989;171(2):481–485.

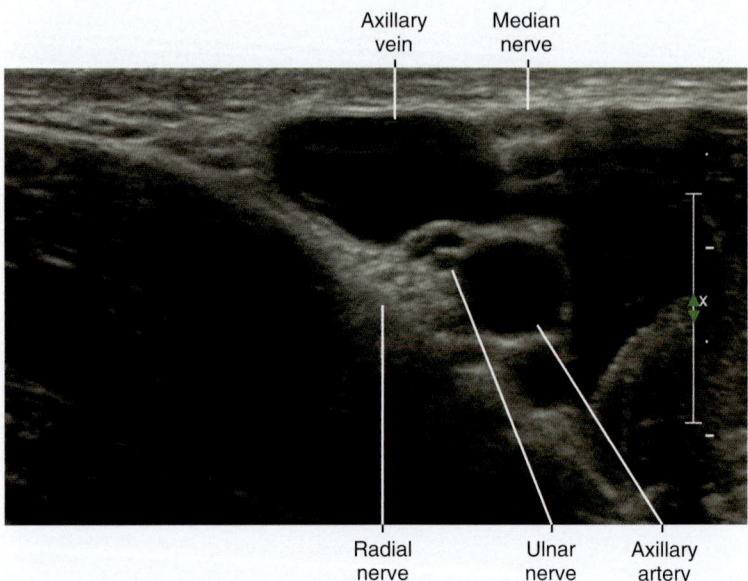

FIGURE 22.1 The axillary vein in the axilla. The ulnar nerve lies between the axillary artery and axillary vein in the axilla. The axillary vein can serve as an acoustic window for enhancing echoes from the ulnar nerve. In this sonogram, the ulnar nerve is shown in short-axis view deep to the axillary vein with light touch imaging (no compression by the ultrasound transducer).

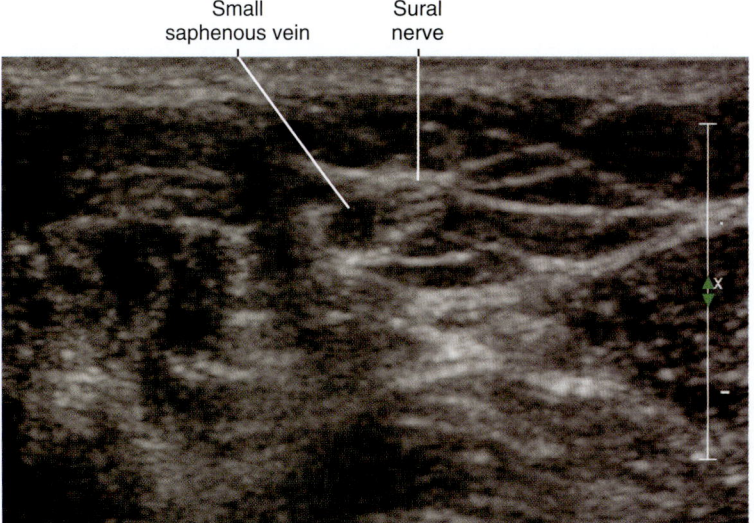

FIGURE 22.2 Short-axis view of the small saphenous vein and sural nerve within the subcutaneous tissue of the posterolateral calf. A calf tourniquet has been applied to distend the vein. Some veins serve as landmarks for nerve position.

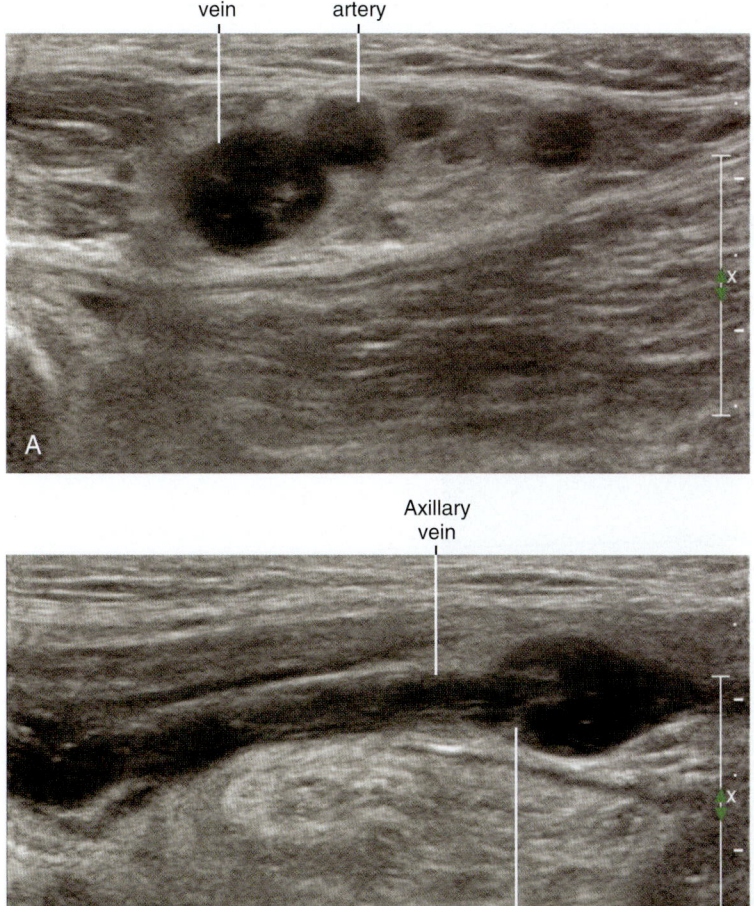

FIGURE 22.3 Thrombosed (uncompressible) axillary vein in the axilla viewed in short axis (A) and long axis (B). A valve is present in the long-axis view.

CHAPTER 23

Bone

The outer surface of cortical bone consists of dense fibrous connective tissue (the periosteum). There is a marked acoustic impedance mismatch between bone and soft tissue. This results in a bright line on ultrasound scans from reflection at the bone–soft tissue interface. Mature bone also is a strong absorber of sound waves.[1] Acoustic shadowing occurs deep to the interface because of extinction of the sound wave.

Clinical Pearls

- Neuraxial scans of pediatric patients are superior to those of adults, in part because skeletal maturity does not occur until approximately 2 years of age from an acoustic standpoint.
- The thermal index of bone is greater than thermal index of soft tissue because of the substantial absorption of ultrasound.

Reference

1. Han S, Medige J, Davis J, Fishkin Z, Mihalko W, Ziv I. Ultrasound velocity and broadband attenuation as predictors of load-bearing capacities of human calcanei. *Calcif Tissue Int.* 1997;60:21–25.

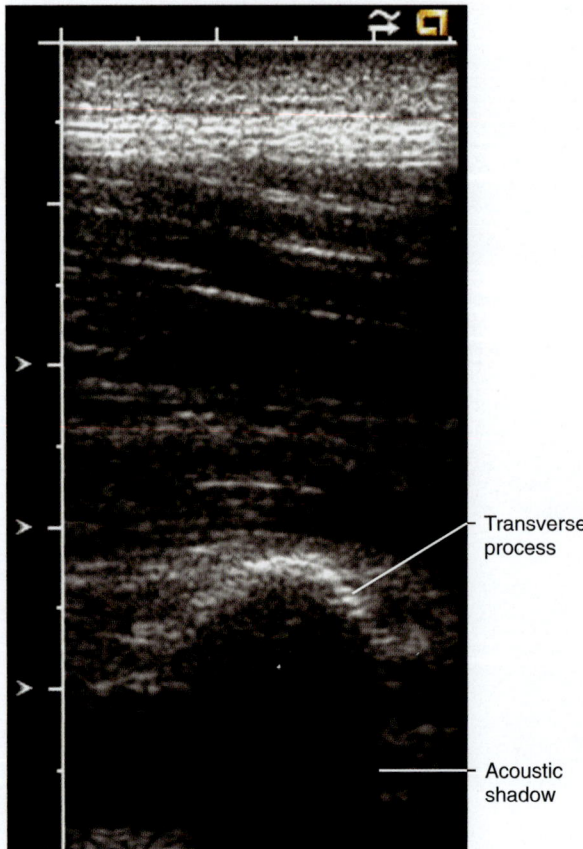

FIGURE 23.1 Ultrasound appearance of bone, demonstrating a bright cortical line and acoustic shadowing. In this sonogram, a short-axis view of a transverse process is shown.

Pleura

CHAPTER 24

The pleura is a strong reflector of ultrasound waves. Comet-tail artifact, indicating reverberation of sound waves, is observed deep to the pleural line on ultrasound scans.[1] Another characteristic feature of pleura with ultrasound imaging is "lung sliding."[2] The pleural line moves to and fro with ventilation. This motion is greatest at the base of the lung and least at the apex because most of the translational motion of the lung is generated by descent of the diaphragm. Both comet-tail artifact and lung sliding are eliminated when pneumothorax is present.[3]

References

1. Thickman DI, Ziskin MC, Goldenberg NJ, Linder BE. Clinical manifestations of the comet tail artifact. *J Ultrasound Med*. 1983;2:225–230.
2. Lichtenstein DA, Menu Y. A bedside ultrasound sign ruling out pneumothorax in the critically ill: lung sliding. *Chest*. 1995;108:1345–1348.
3. Lichtenstein D, Meziere G, Biderman P, Gepner A. The comet-tail artifact: an ultrasound sign ruling out pneumothorax. *Intensive Care Med*. 1999;25:383–388.

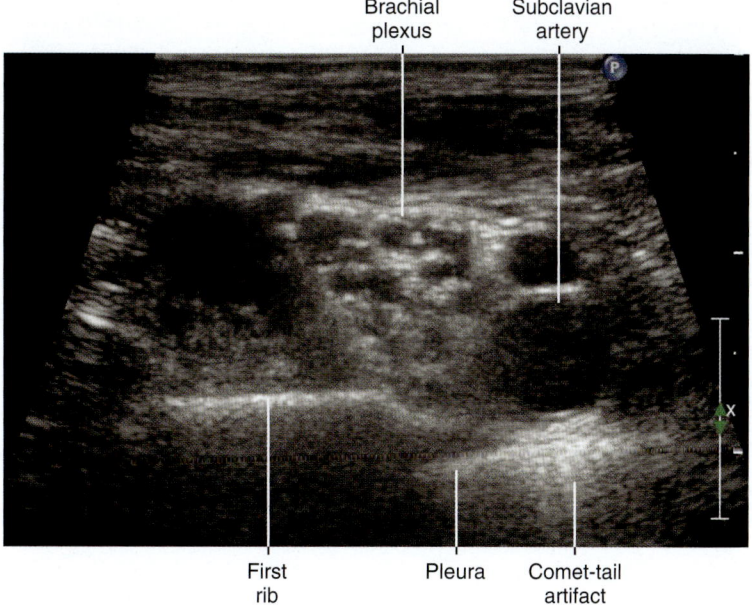

FIGURE 24.1 Comet-tail artifact observed deep to the pleural line during supraclavicular block of the brachial plexus.

CHAPTER 25

Peritoneum

The peritoneum appears as a discrete, thin, smooth, single echogenic line deep to the abdominal wall.[1] Like pleura, peritoneum can produce a type of reverberation artifact known as *comet-tail artifact*.[2] Motion of the peritoneum and abdominal cavity contents ("gut sliding") can sometimes be appreciated.

References

1. Hanbidge AE, Lynch D, Wilson SR. Ultrasound of the peritoneum. *Radiographics*. 2003;23:663–684.
2. Thickman DI, Ziskin MC, Goldenberg NJ, Linder BE. Clinical manifestations of the comet tail artifact. *J Ultrasound Med*. 1983;2:225–230.

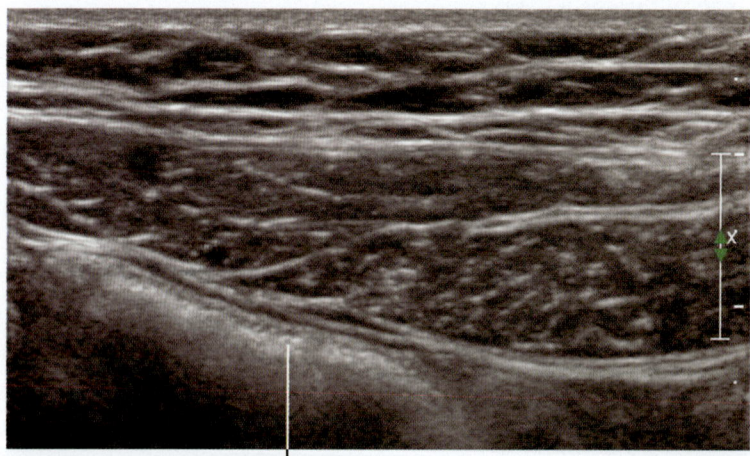

FIGURE 25.1 Peritoneum deep to the abdominal wall muscles observed during rectus sheath block.

Lymph Nodes

CHAPTER 26

Normal lymph nodes are well-defined, oval structures containing an echogenic hilum and hypoechoic rim. Central vascularity can be demonstrated on Doppler scans (a hilar pattern of blood flow). Inguinal lymph nodes are frequently encountered during femoral nerve blocks. Lymph nodes are more numerous in young patients, and nodes involute with aging. Normal lymph nodes are small with well-defined borders.

Clinical Pearls

- Reactive lymph nodes are sometimes identified during regional blocks.
- Lymph nodes are small, oval, or reniform (bean shaped).
- Lymphatic vessels resemble veins in structure, but valves are more numerous in lymphatic vessels. The lymphatic vessels primarily contain lymphocytes (not erythrocytes).

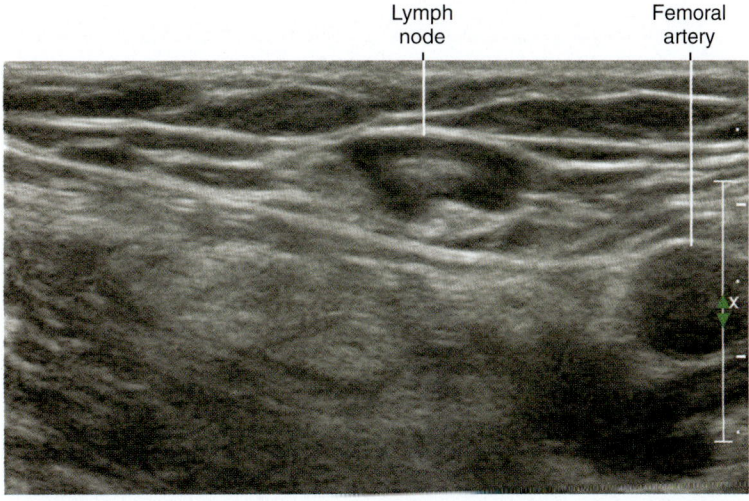

FIGURE 26.1 Ultrasound appearance of a lymph node in the inguinal region. This node was observed during femoral nerve block with ultrasound guidance.

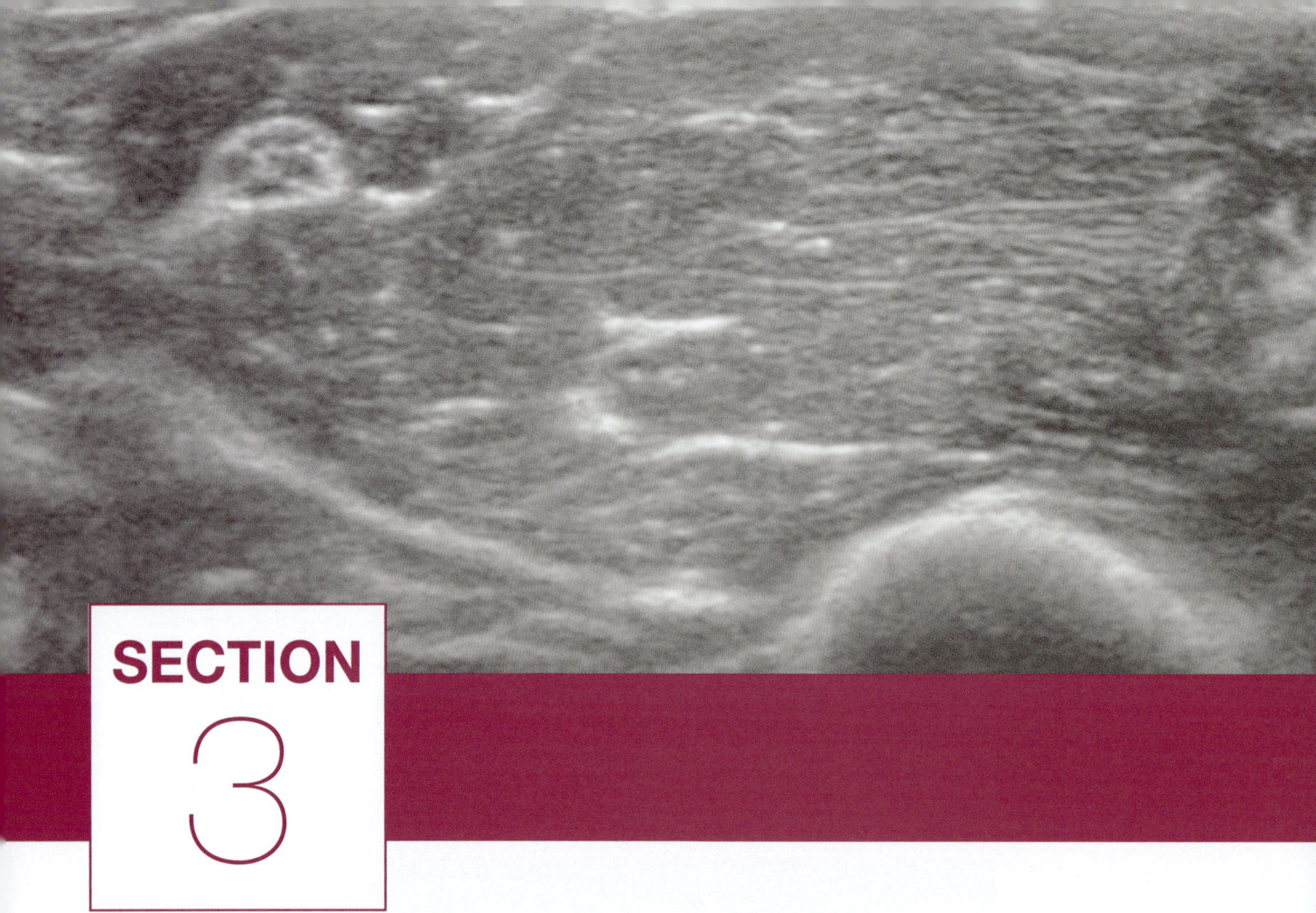

SECTION 3

Upper Extremity Blocks

Supraclavicular Nerve Block (of the Cervical Plexus)

CHAPTER 27

The supraclavicular nerve (SCN) is a branch of the superficial cervical plexus (see Fig. 72.1). It arises from the third and fourth cervical ventral rami and divides into three branches: medial, intermediate, and lateral. These branches are about 1 to 2 mm in diameter. The intermediate branch can in some cases be palpated over the midportion of the clavicle. The nerve has sensory fibers to the clavicle and shoulder, the chest wall to the level of the second rib, and the acromioclavicular and sternoclavicular joints. The supraclavicular branches usually pass over the clavicle but in some cases can actually travel through the clavicle. Block of the SCN is useful for pain relief from shoulder or clavicle surgery.[1,2]

SUGGESTED TECHNIQUE

The traditional supraclavicular block of the brachial plexus is not considered adequate for shoulder surgery.[3] Sensory blockade of the supraclavicular and axillary nerves has slower onset for the traditional supraclavicular technique compared with the interscalene technique of brachial plexus anesthesia. However, ultrasound-guided infiltration of local anesthetic for SCN block can augment low interscalene or supraclavicular blocks for shoulder surgery. The SCN is typically located over the prevertebral fascia and brachial plexus near the clavicle. SCN block is generally performed after the brachial plexus block.

Clinical Pearls

- The incidence of the SCN branches piercing the clavicle is 1% to 4%.[4] In some of these cases, the bony foramina are large enough to be visible on chest radiographs.
- Interscalene blocks often result in SCN block because the local anesthetic tracks to C4 within the interscalene groove.[3] This is less likely or has slower onset with supraclavicular blocks of the brachial plexus. SCN blocks can be assessed along the skin surface over the clavicle.
- The SCNs further divide before piercing the platysma.

SCN, Supraclavicular nerve.

References

1. Choi DS, Atchabahian A, Brown AR. Cervical plexus block provides postoperative analgesia after clavicle surgery. *Anesth Analg.* 2005;100:1542–1543.
2. Maybin J, Townsley P, Bedforth N, Allan A. Ultrasound guided supraclavicular nerve blockade: first technical description and the relevance for shoulder surgery under regional anaesthesia. *Anaesthesia.* 2011;66(11):1053–1055.
3. Lanz E, Theiss D, Jankovic D. The extent of blockade following various techniques of brachial plexus block. *Anesth Analg.* 1983;62:55–58.
4. Tubbs RS, Salter EG, Oakes WJ. Anomaly of the supraclavicular nerve: case report and review of the literature. *Clin Anat.* 2006;19:599–601.

72 UPPER EXTREMITY BLOCKS

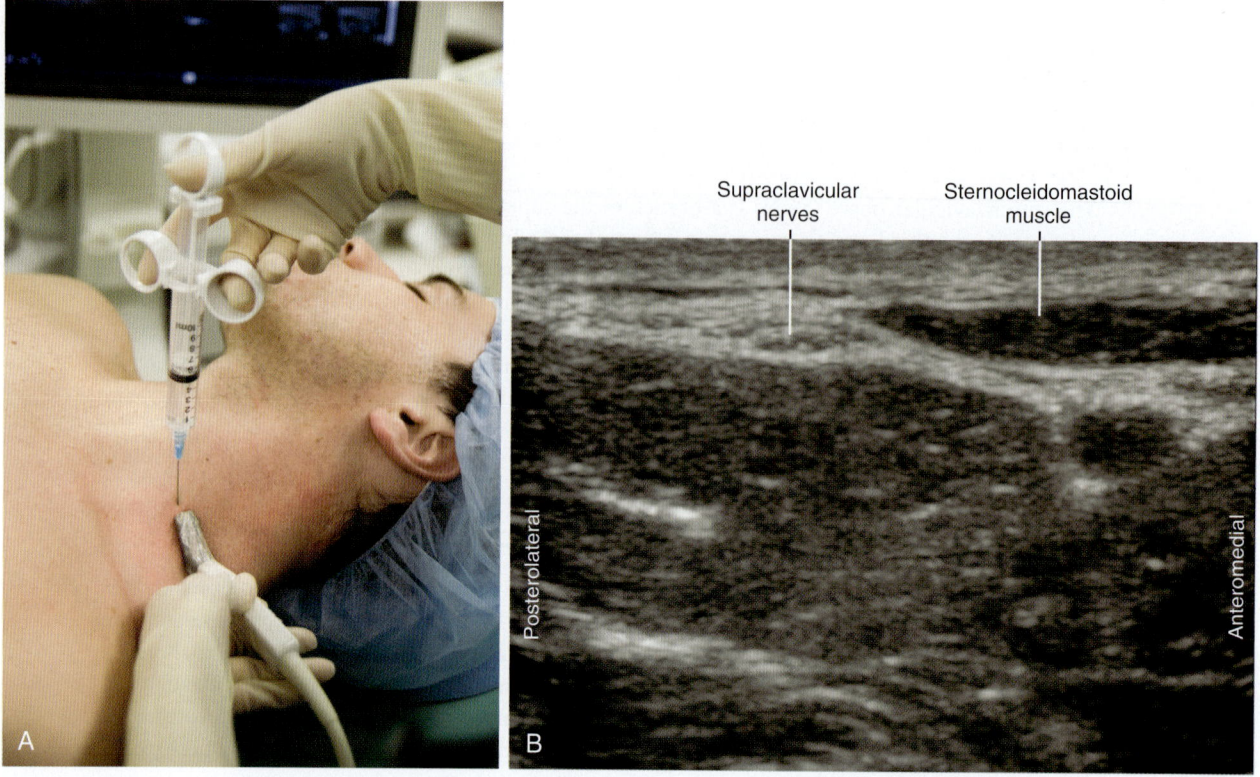

FIGURE 27.1 External photograph showing the approach to a supraclavicular nerve block in the cervical region (A) and corresponding sonogram (B).

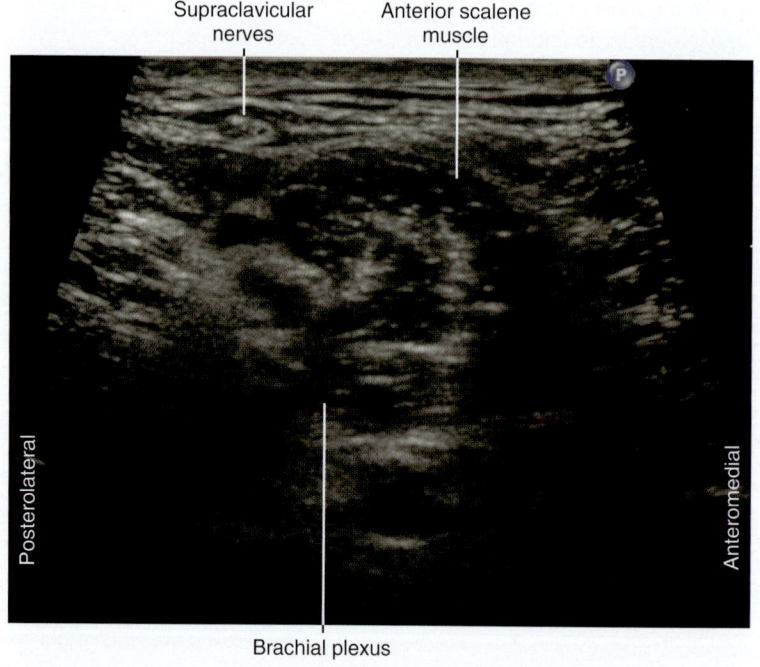

FIGURE 27.2 Short-axis view of the supraclavicular nerves before injection. The supraclavicular nerves are seen to lie superficial to the brachial plexus.

SUPRACLAVICULAR NERVE BLOCK

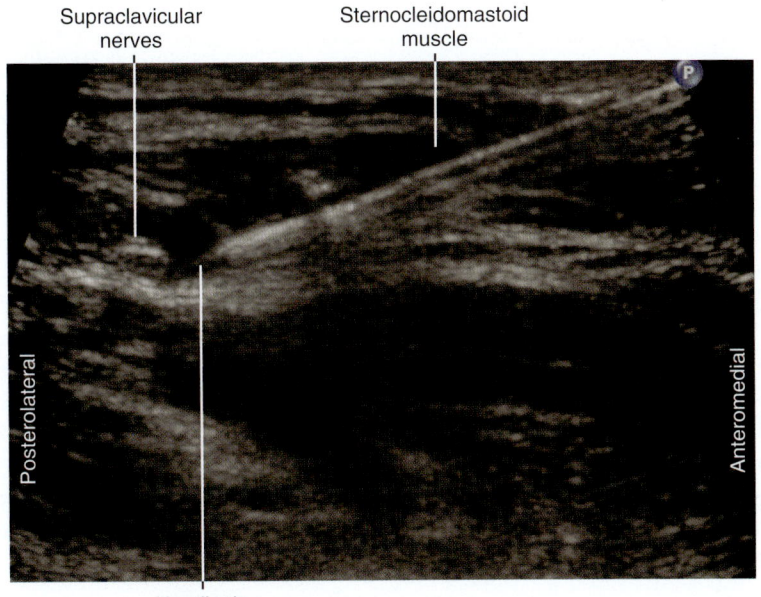

FIGURE 27.3 Short-axis in-plane approach to block of the supraclavicular nerves of the cervical plexus. The block needle tip approaches from the medial side through the sternocleidomastoid muscle.

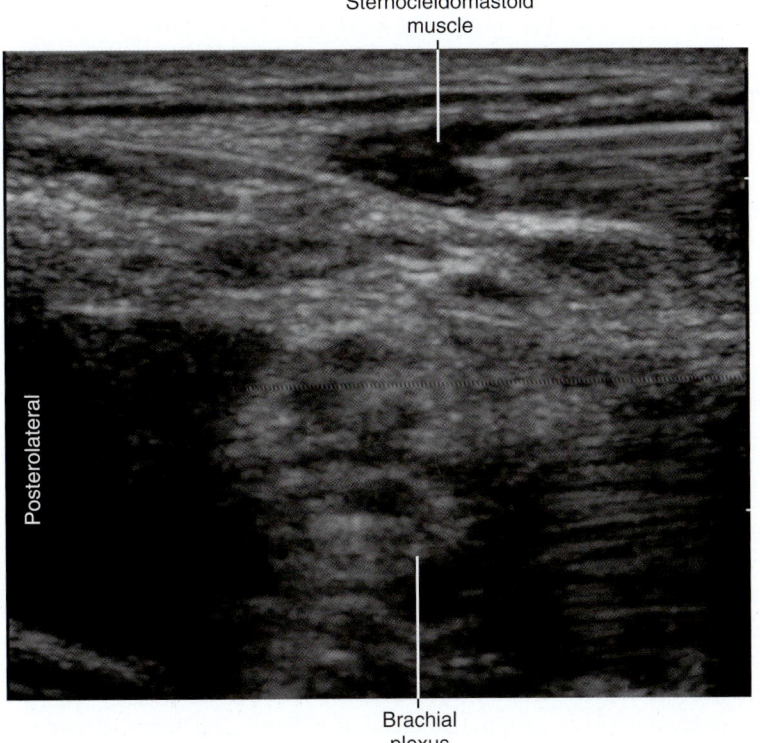

FIGURE 27.4 The proximity of the brachial plexus to the supraclavicular nerves is evident during this in-plane block through the sternocleidomastoid muscle. The brachial plexus is seen deep to the prevertebral fascia.

CHAPTER 28

Interscalene and Supraclavicular Blocks
(of the Brachial Plexus)

 See Video 28.1 on ExpertConsult.com.

The first reported use of ultrasound to guide regional block was for brachial plexus block above the clavicle.[1] These pioneers used an offline Doppler technique to mark the position of the subclavian artery as a surrogate landmark of the brachial plexus. Although today there may be many criticisms of this technique, their results were impressive: a 98% success rate with no complications.

Ultrasound imaging blurs the distinction between interscalene and supraclavicular blocks. If the brachial plexus is seen stacked between the anterior and middle scalene muscles, the block is generally referred to as an interscalene block. If the brachial plexus is seen as a compact group of nerves lying superior and lateral to the subclavian artery, the approach is generally referred to as a supraclavicular block. Because this distinction can be subtle, both blocks are treated together in this chapter.

SONOANATOMY OF THE POSTERIOR CERVICAL TRIANGLE

The brachial plexus typically forms from the ventral rami of C5, C6, C7, C8, and T1. The monofascicular ventral rami of the brachial plexus are hypoechoic and can sometimes be difficult to identify between the scalene muscles (the "stoplight sign").[2] The brachial plexus lies deep to the tapering posterolateral edge of the sternocleidomastoid in the neck. The ventral rami can be similar to blood vessels in their ultrasound appearance. The seventh cervical ventral ramus is usually the largest, with progressively smaller cephalad and caudad ventral rami.[3] These size differences tend to equalize the size of the three trunks that form from the ventral rami of the brachial plexus.

The anterior tubercle of C7 is rudimentary (the longus capitis and anterior scalene muscles do not insert on it, in contrast to the anterior tubercle of C6). This sonographic landmark can be used to trace the level of blocks in the posterior cervical triangle. The vertebral artery lies in close proximity to the ventral ramus of C7 as it emerges from the sulcus. The thoracic (T1) contributions rise to join the remainder of the brachial plexus over the first rib (ascending nerves of the brachial plexus). These contributions lie adjacent to the tendinous insertions of the middle scalene on the first rib.

ANATOMIC VARIATION

Variations in brachial plexus anatomy with respect to the scalene muscles are common. The cephalad components of the plexus (in particular, the C5 and C6 ventral rami) often pass over or through the anterior scalene muscle. This may pose a problem for nerve stimulation–based approaches to brachial plexus blocks above the clavicle. The incidence of scalene muscle anomalies is similar for sonography of volunteers and in cadaveric dissections, suggesting that ultrasound can accurately detect these anomalies.[4]

Cervical ribs are relatively uncommon, occurring in about 0.5% of the population. Most cervical ribs are partial (incomplete) and therefore do not pose a problem. However, if the cervical rib is sufficiently large, transducer manipulation can be difficult, and acoustic shadowing by the bone obscures imaging of the brachial plexus.

SUGGESTED TECHNIQUE

The best nerve visibility is usually near the first rib, because the brachial plexus is compact and lateral to the subclavian artery. The plexus contains more connective tissue moving from interscalene to supraclavicular views, resulting in more hyperechoic echotexture. To obtain a good supraclavicular view with the subclavian artery in true short axis, the imaging plane must face caudally at the brachial plexus (rather than posteriorly). Brachial plexus imaging in the supraclavicular region is most consistent and can be used to trace the plexus centrally to the interscalene groove. Perform the block where the imaging is most reliable.

The semi-sitting (beach-chair) position helps comfort the patient, lowers the arm and shoulder by gravity, and brings the plane of imaging closer to the plane of the display. The head-of-bed should be elevated about 45 degrees. The patient's head turns to the opposite side from the block, and the operator stands at the side of the bed.

Working room is limited above the clavicle; therefore, a compact transducer is favored. A small curved or small linear (20- to 25-mm footprint) transducer is generally preferred, and the compact transducer can be rocked back to improve needle tip visibility. Broad linear probes are more difficult to rock than narrow linear or curved transducers for this procedure but provide a larger field of view. The ulnar aspects of both hands of the operator are placed on the patient for the best control of the needle and transducer.

A short (50 mm), broad (21 gauge) echogenic needle is used for optimal control and visibility. Hand-on-needle hub (versus hand on syringe) is recommended for better needle control.

A medial to lateral in-plane needle path heads away from pleura, and a lateral to medial in-plane needle path is further from the phrenic nerve. Another approach is to place the needle so that it is advanced within the interscalene groove ("running the groove"). With this approach, the needle is placed in the space between the middle scalene muscle and brachial plexus, without the needle entering the muscle, advancing from lateral to medial down along the inclination of the interscalene groove. The advantage of this approach is that the needle runs along the side of the nerves of the brachial plexus rather than aiming at them. All approaches require some modification by multiple injections when brachial plexus pass-over or pass-through anatomic variation is identified.

Most authors recommend a multiple injection technique to ensure complete plexus anesthesia. With this approach, the initial aim of the needle is deep (under the more caudal elements of the brachial plexus) so that the brachial plexus rises closer to the skin surface with the injection of local anesthetic. This makes the subsequent needle manipulation easier to perform. The needle tip should be positioned adjacent to the components of the brachial plexus for injection within the interscalene groove.[5]

Inferior trunk sparing occurs less often with this multiple injection ultrasound technique compared with traditional nerve stimulation–based approaches to interscalene block.[6] The dorsal scapular artery can be used to help identify the inferior trunk, because this artery consistently divides the middle and the inferior trunks of the brachial plexus.[7] The inferior trunk can be blocked deep to the dorsal scapular artery near where it crosses over the first rib. A multiple injection technique is often used to assure complete brachial plexus anesthesia in this location.

Surprisingly, injections 8 mm from the brachial plexus result in effective interscalene block in half the cases with high-volume injections (20 mL).[8] Injections less than 10 mL are effective with minimal side effects if they are made immediately adjacent to the brachial plexus.[9]

The anatomy of the posterior triangle of the neck is complex. Nerves close to the brachial plexus, and therefore potentially in the needle path, include the phrenic nerve, dorsal scapular nerve, and spinal accessory nerve. The phrenic nerve lies medial to the brachial plexus and travels over the anterior scalene muscle toward the midline as it descends into the chest. The dorsal scapular nerve is a branch of the brachial plexus that is often observed lateral to the brachial plexus within the middle scalene muscle. The spinal accessory nerve is difficult to image but lies lateral to the brachial plexus within the posterior triangle of the neck. The suprascapular nerve takeoff from the brachial plexus can be seen deep to the omohyoid muscle.

The subclavian, dorsal scapular, and transverse cervical arteries are the primary vascular puncture risks of this procedure. Transverse cervical arteries are frequently observed running over the brachial plexus in the neck.[10]

Clinical Pearls

- The needle tip should be positioned adjacent to the ventral rami of C5, C6, and C7 to ensure complete plexus anesthesia with a multiple-injection technique.
- Arteries that traverse the interscalene brachial plexus can divide it into separate compartments. The deep cervical artery (the dorsal scapular artery) usually runs between the seventh and eighth cervical roots, and this artery continues between the middle and the lower trunks of the brachial plexus. Multiple injections may be necessary to obtain complete plexus anesthesia when this anatomy is present.
- The seventh cervical ventral ramus is usually the largest, with progressively smaller cephalad and caudad ventral rami. These size differences tend to equalize the size of the three trunks that form the brachial plexus.
- Both the medial to lateral and lateral to medial approaches to supraclavicular block have similar efficacy and safety profiles.[11]
- Low volumes of local anesthetic (10 mL or less) for interscalene block reduce the chance of concomitant phrenic nerve block.[12]
- Cervical ribs can obscure imaging during brachial plexus blocks above the clavicle.[13]

References

1. La Grange P, Foster PA, Pretorius LK. Application of the Doppler ultrasound bloodflow detector in supraclavicular brachial plexus block. *Br J Anaesth*. 1978;50:965–967.
2. Franco CD, Williams JM. Ultrasound-guided interscalene block: reevaluation of the "stoplight" sign and clinical implications. *Reg Anesth Pain Med*. 2016;41(4):452–459.
3. Haun DW, Cho JC, Kettner NW. Normative cross-sectional area of the C5-C8 nerve roots using ultrasonography. *Ultrasound Med Biol*. 2010;36(9):1422–1430.
4. Kessler J, Gray AT. Sonography of scalene muscle anomalies for brachial plexus block. *Reg Anesth Pain Med*. 2007;32:172–173.
5. Sinha SK, Abrams JH, Weller RS. Ultrasound-guided interscalene needle placement produces successful anesthesia regardless of motor stimulation above or below 0.5 mA. *Anesth Analg*. 2007;105:848–852.
6. Kapral S, Greher M, Huber G, et al. Ultrasonographic guidance improves the success rate of interscalene brachial plexus blockade. *Reg Anesth Pain Med*. 2008;33:253–258.
7. Demondion X, Boutry N, Drizenko A, et al. Thoracic outlet: anatomic correlation with MR imaging. *AJR Am J Roentgenol*. 2000;175(2):417–422.
8. Albrecht E, Kirkham KR, Taffé P, et al. The maximum effective needle-to-nerve distance for ultrasound-guided interscalene block: an exploratory study. *Reg Anesth Pain Med*. 2014;39(1):56–60.
9. Vandepitte C, Gautier P, Xu D, et al. Effective volume of ropivacaine 0.75% through a catheter required for interscalene brachial plexus blockade. *Anesthesiology*. 2013;118(4):863–867.
10. Weiglein AH, Moriggl B, Schalk C, et al. Arteries in the posterior cervical triangle in man. *Clin Anat*. 2005;18:553–557.
11. Subramanyam R, Vaishnav V, Chan VW, et al. Lateral versus medial needle approach for ultrasound-guided supraclavicular block: a randomized controlled trial. *Reg Anesth Pain Med*. 2011;36(4):387–392.
12. Gautier P, Vandepitte C, Schaub I, et al. The disposition of radiocontrast in the interscalene space in healthy volunteers. *Anesth Analg*. 2015;120:1138–1141.
13. Liu M, Peng P. Supraclavicular brachial plexus block in the presence of a cervical rib. *Anesthesiology*. 2017;126:979.

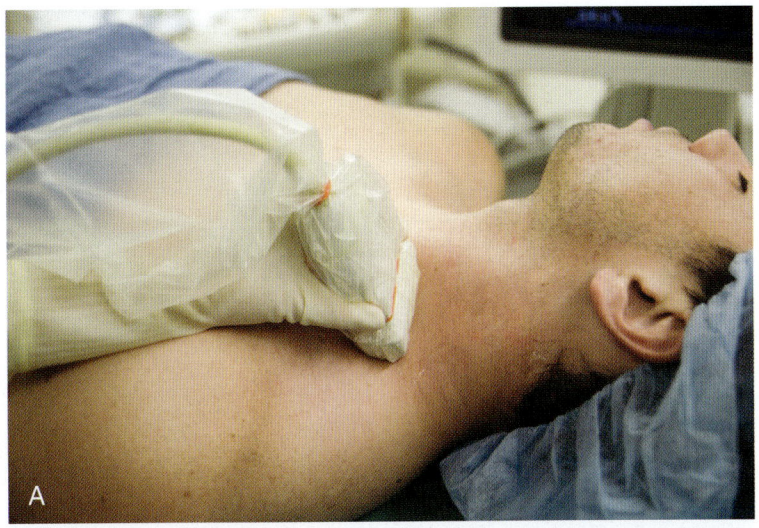
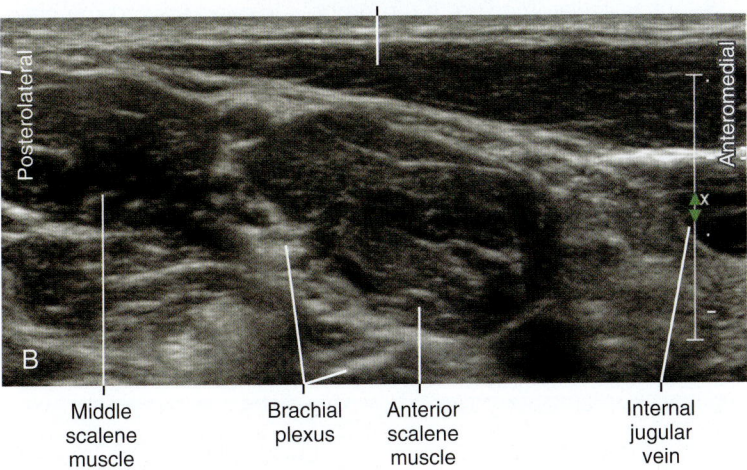

FIGURE 28.1 External photograph showing the transducer position for interscalene imaging (A) and corresponding sonogram (B). In this location, the components of the brachial plexus are stacked between the anterior and middle scalene muscles underneath the tapering anterolateral edge of the sternocleidomastoid muscle.

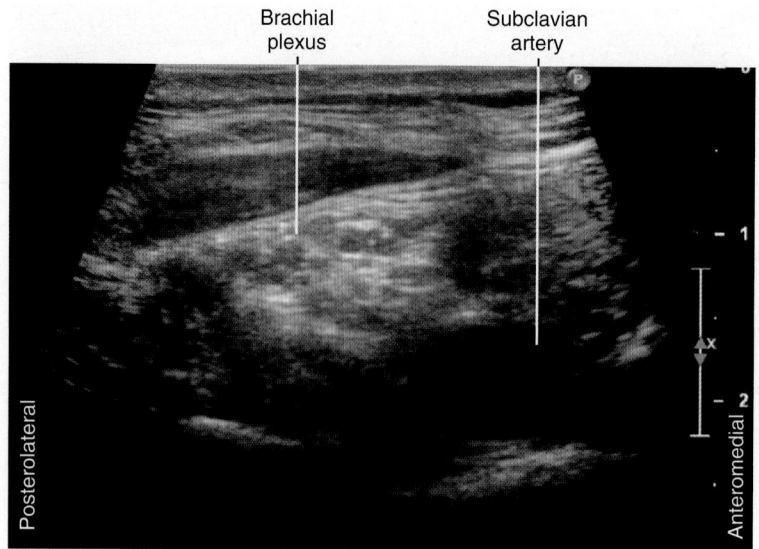

FIGURE 28.2 Supraclavicular imaging. If the probe is moved toward the clavicle and angled caudally, the brachial plexus is seen to bundle compactly in the superior and lateral positions with respect to the subclavian artery.

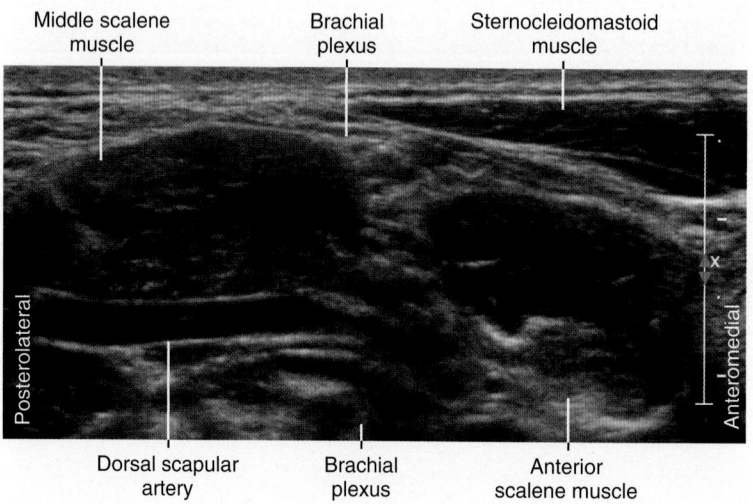

FIGURE 28.3 Interscalene imaging reveals a large artery passing through the middle scalene muscle in this subject. The deep cervical artery (the dorsal scapular artery) usually runs between the seventh and eighth cervical roots and can sometimes be identified dividing the middle and the lower trunks of the brachial plexus.

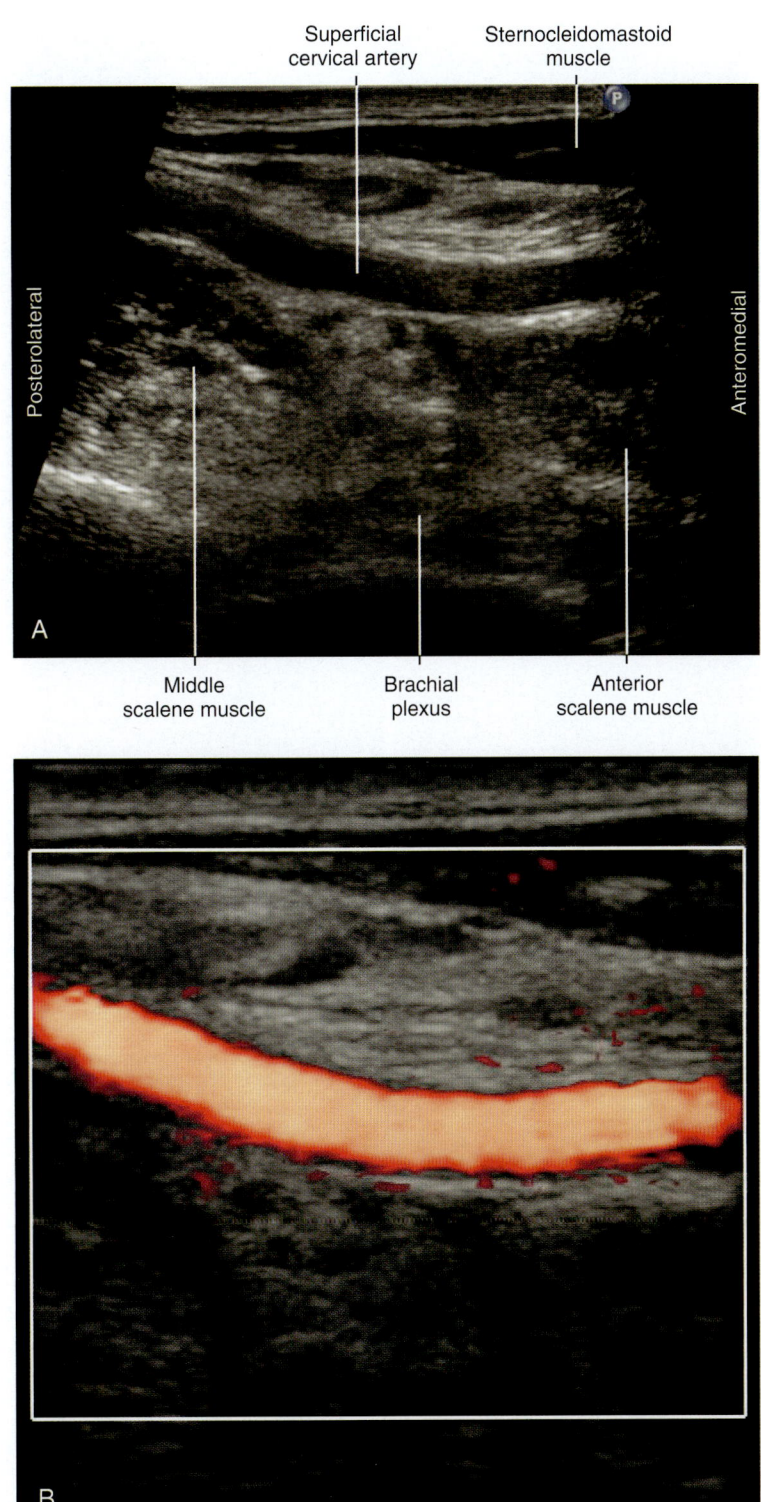

FIGURE 28.4 B-mode sonogram (A) and duplex power Doppler (B) identify a superficial cervical artery. The interscalene region is highly vascular. When these vessels are identified, the probe position for interscalene block is moved slightly cephalad or caudad.

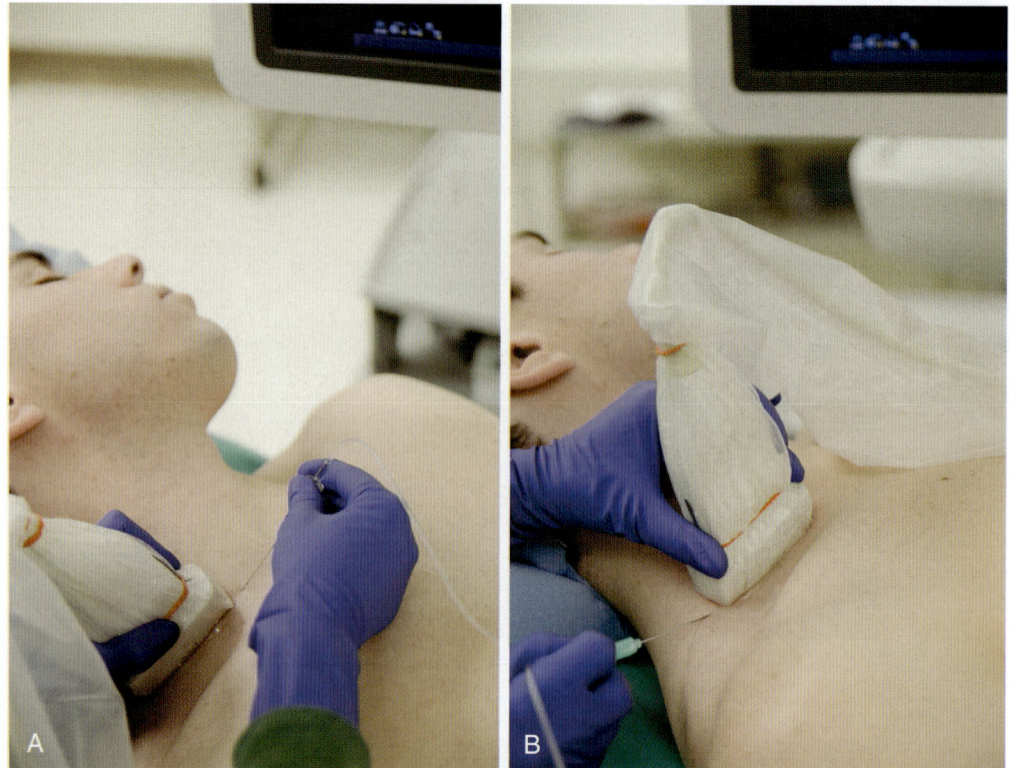

FIGURE 28.5 External photographs showing in-plane approaches to interscalene block. The medial to lateral approach (A) and the lateral to medial approach (B) are shown.

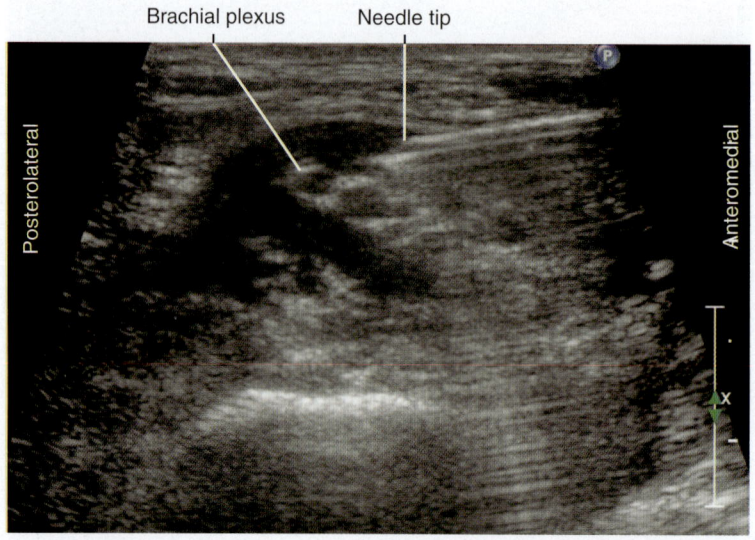

FIGURE 28.6 Short-axis view of the interscalene plexus during medial to lateral in-plane approach. Local anesthetic is seen to distribute around nerves of the brachial plexus.

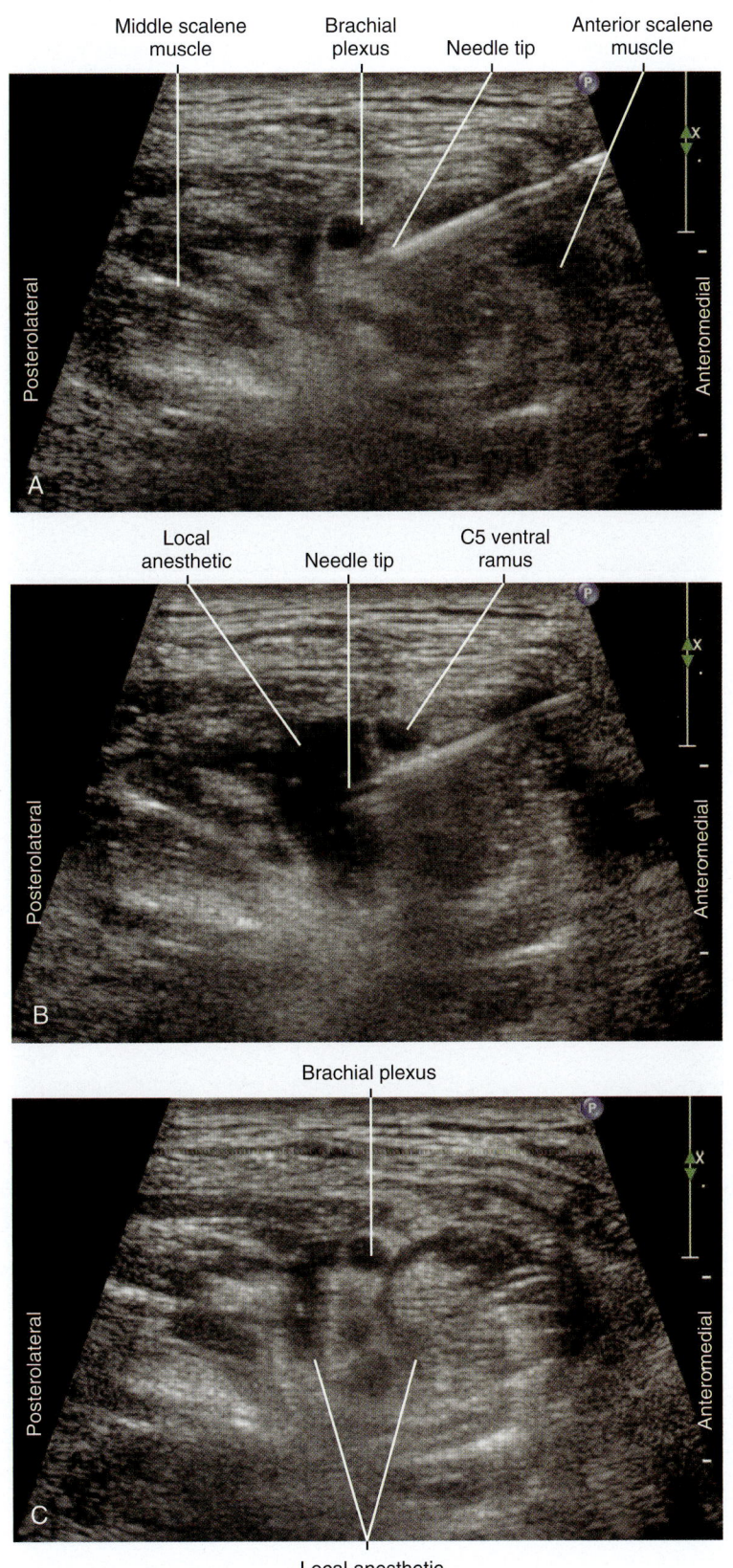

FIGURE 28.7 Image sequence showing interscalene block. A medial to lateral in-plane approach is demonstrated where the needle tip is carefully placed adjacent to the components of the plexus (A and B). After injection, local anesthetic is distributed around both sides of the brachial plexus (C).

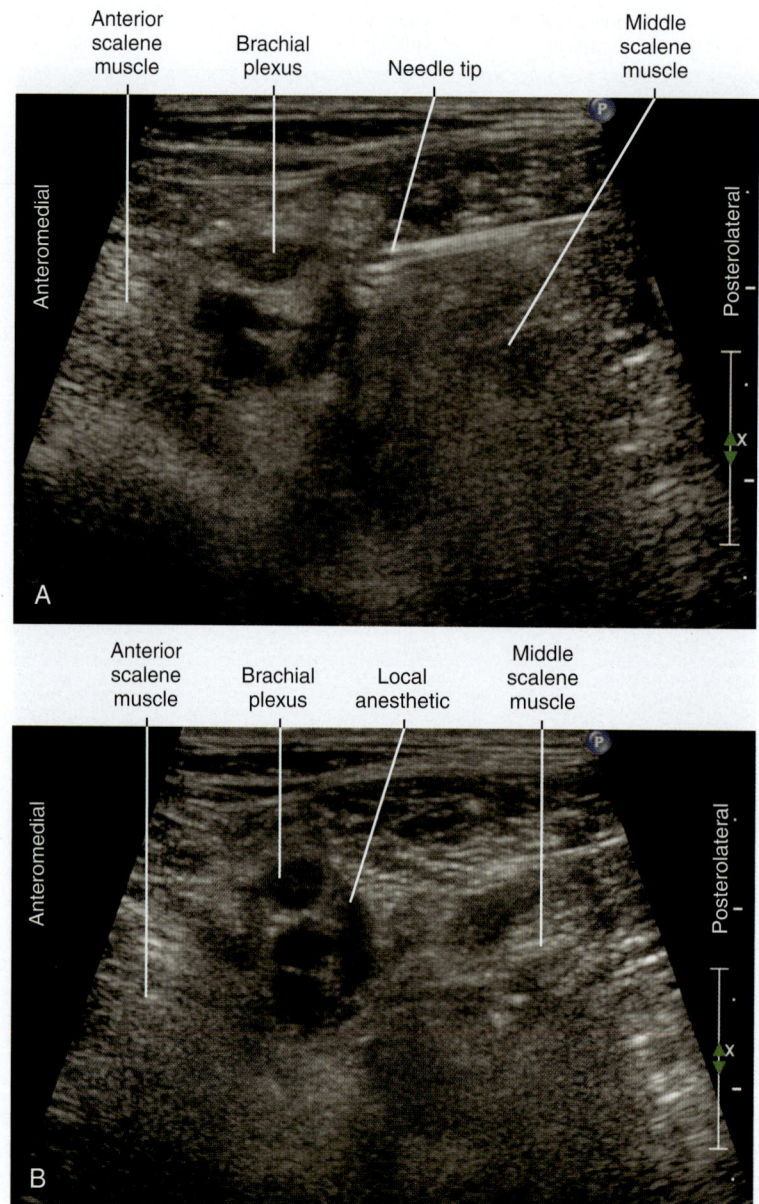

FIGURE 28.8 Image sequence showing interscalene block. A lateral to medial in-plane approach is demonstrated (A). After injection, local anesthetic is distributed around both sides of the brachial plexus (B).

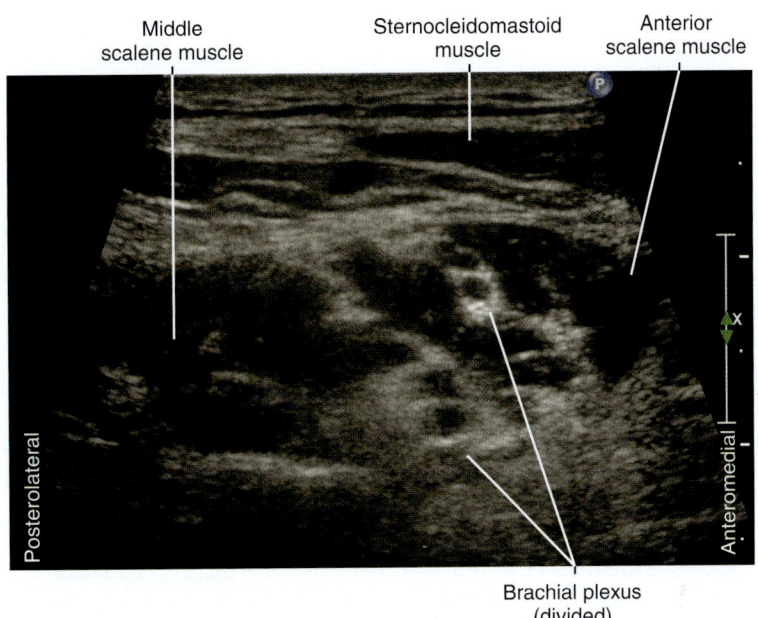

FIGURE 28.9 Pass-through brachial plexus. In this sonogram, cephalad elements of the brachial plexus are seen to pass through the anterior scalene muscle. This anatomic variation potentially divides the brachial plexus and has the potential for incomplete blocks.

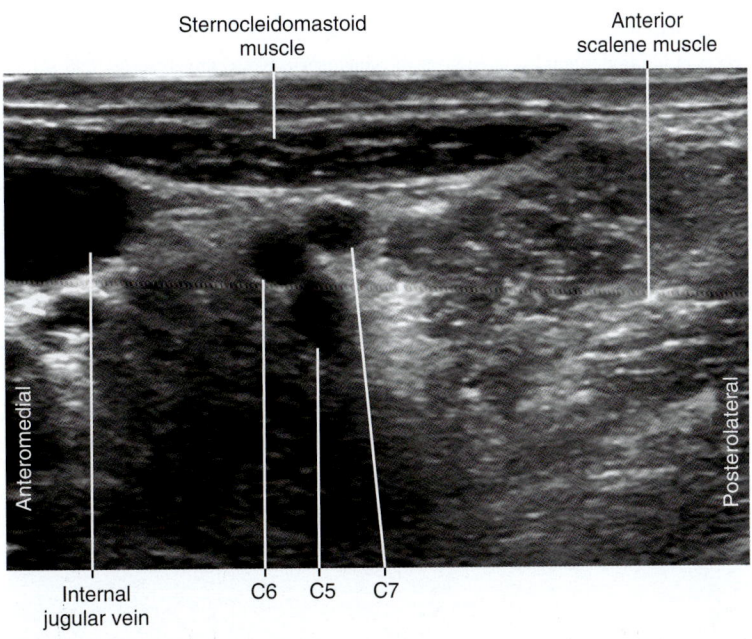

FIGURE 28.10 Pass-over brachial plexus. In this sonogram, three ventral rami (C5, C6, and C7) are seen to pass over the anterior scalene muscle. It is uncommon for three ventral rami to pass over the anterior scalene, although more commonly, C5 or both C5 and C6 can travel in this pathway.

CHAPTER 29

Phrenic Nerve Imaging

The phrenic nerve is a small (< 1 mm in diameter), monofascicular nerve that arises from the third, fourth, and fifth cervical ventral rami. The most consistent and largest contribution is from the fourth cervical ventral ramus. At the level of the cricoid cartilage, the phrenic nerve is essentially coincident with the C5 ventral ramus.[1] As the nerve descends the neck, it travels from lateral to medial over the surface of the anterior scalene muscle. The nerve usually enters the chest between the subclavian artery and vein. Accessory phrenic nerves are observed in 60% of specimens and often derive from the fifth cervical ventral ramus.[2]

Phrenic nerve imaging is important for several reasons. First, it may be possible to reduce the incidence of transient pulmonary complications related to phrenic nerve block using ultrasound. Low volumes of local anesthetic (5 to 10 mL) administered for interscalene block using ultrasound guidance appear to reduce the incidence of concomitant phrenic nerve block.[3] Ultrasound guidance allows more caudal approaches to brachial plexus block with an even lower chance of phrenic nerve block. Second, direct trauma to the nerve can potentially be avoided during regional anesthetic procedures in the cervical region. Third, ultrasound can be used to guide phrenic nerve blocks to treat intractable hiccups (singultus).[4]

References

1. Kessler J, Schafhalter-Zoppoth I, Gray AT. An ultrasound study of the phrenic nerve in the posterior cervical triangle: implications for the interscalene brachial plexus block. *Reg Anesth Pain Med*. 2008;33:545–550.
2. Loukas M, Kinsella CR Jr, Louis RG Jr, et al. Surgical anatomy of the accessory phrenic nerve. *Ann Thorac Surg*. 2006;82:1870–1875.
3. Riazi S, Carmichael N, Awad I, et al. Effect of local anaesthetic volume (20 vs 5 mL) on the efficacy and respiratory consequences of ultrasound-guided interscalene brachial plexus block. *Br J Anaesth*. 2008;101:549–556.
4. Kohse EK, Hollmann MW, Bardenheuer HJ, Kessler J. Chronic hiccups: an underestimated problem. Anesth Analg. 2017;125:1169–1183.

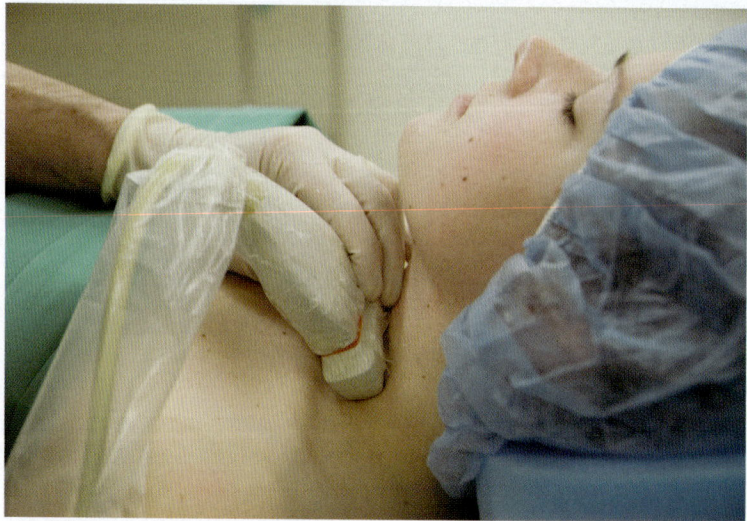

FIGURE 29.1 External photograph showing the approximate transducer position for phrenic nerve imaging in the cervical region.

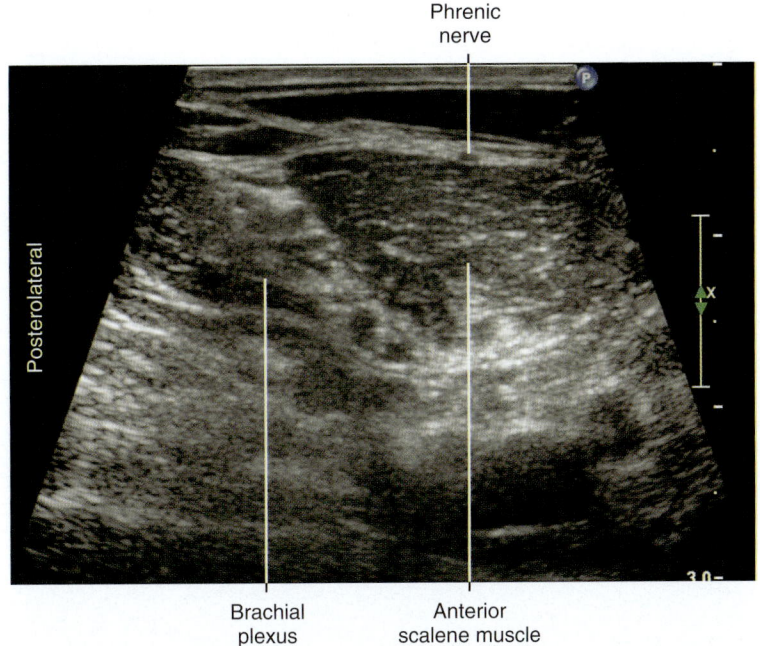

FIGURE 29.2 Phrenic nerve imaging with ultrasound. At the level of the cricoid cartilage, the phrenic nerve and C5 ventral ramus lie side by side. At more caudal positions in the neck, the phrenic nerve crosses medially over the surface of the anterior scalene muscle and appears monofascicular.

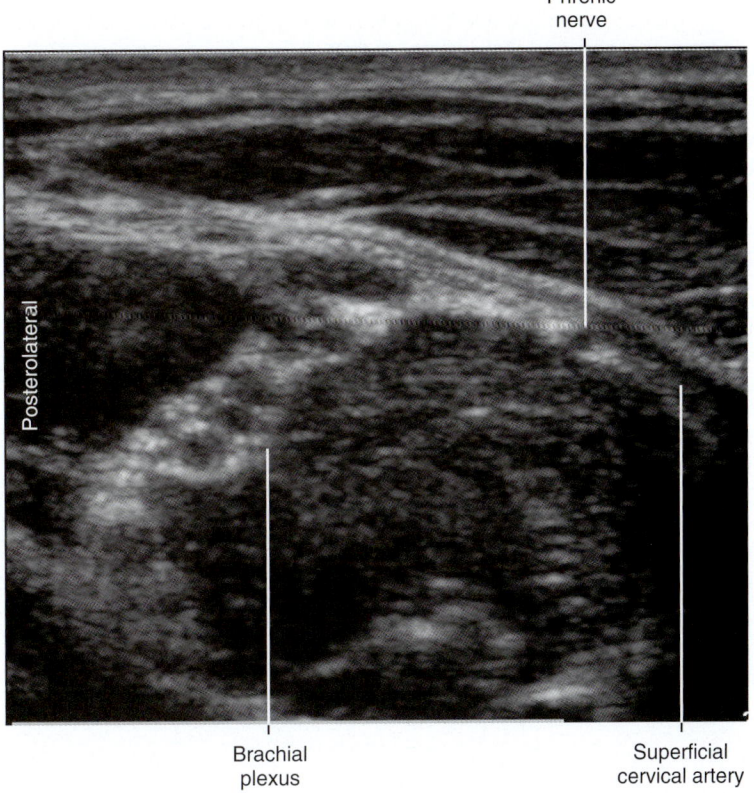

FIGURE 29.3 Sonogram showing the course of the phrenic nerve. The superficial (transverse) cervical artery lies superficial to the phrenic nerve in the midportion of the anterior scalene muscle.

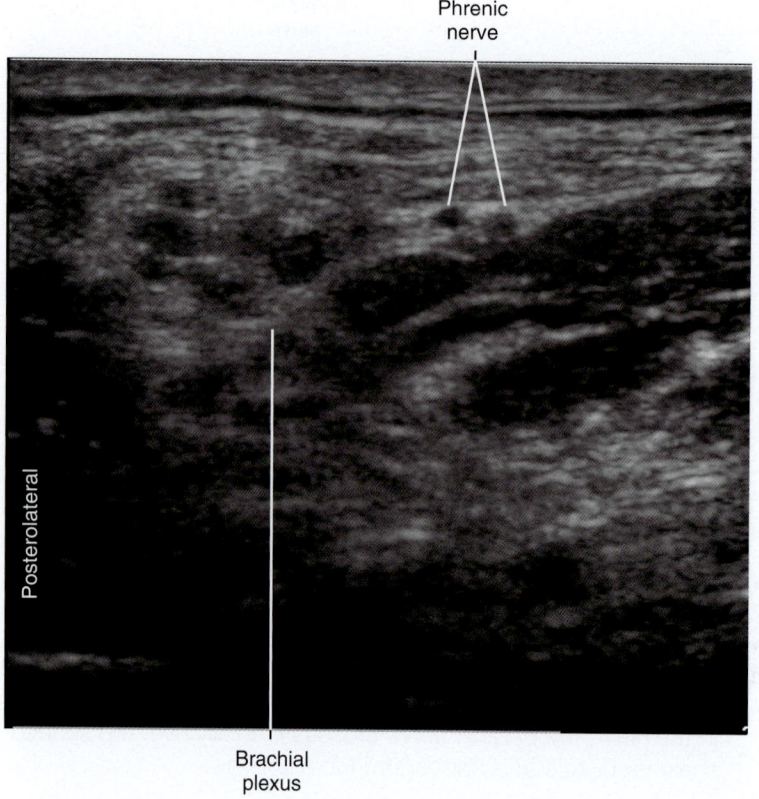

FIGURE 29.4 Echotexture of the phrenic nerve. On occasion, the phrenic nerve appears bifascicular on ultrasound scans, possibly from an accessory phrenic contribution from the fifth cervical ventral ramus.

Dorsal Scapular Nerve Imaging

CHAPTER 30

The dorsal scapular nerve (DSN) arises from the C5 ventral ramus and often contains contributions from C4.[1] The nerve is usually considered part of the brachial plexus. The DSN pierces the middle scalene muscle to innervate the rhomboid muscles and supplies some of the motor branches to the levator scapulae. The nerve joins the dorsal scapular artery that usually arises from the transverse cervical artery. There is no cutaneous innervation of the DSN.

It is important to recognize the DSN during interscalene blocks of the brachial plexus to avoid trauma to the nerve.[2] The nerve can often be visualized within the middle scalene muscle lateral to the brachial plexus.

Clinical Pearls

- The dorsal scapular nerve is a branch of the brachial plexus that can be identified during interscalene block.[3]
- Block of the dorsal scapular nerve may reduce pain following scapular surgery.[4]
- The DSN rounds in shape as it exits the middle scalene muscle, whereas it is flat within this muscle.
- The dorsal scapular artery courses between the inferior and middle trunks of the brachial plexus before joining the DSN.

References

1. Tubbs RS, Tyler-Kabara EC, Aikens AC, et al. Surgical anatomy of the dorsal scapular nerve. *J Neurosurg*. 2005;102:910–911.
2. Saporito A. Dorsal scapular nerve injury: a complication of ultrasound-guided interscalene block. *Br J Anaesth*. 2013;111:840–841.
3. Hanson NA, Auyong DB. Systematic ultrasound identification of the dorsal scapular and long thoracic nerves during interscalene block. *Reg Anesth Pain Med*. 2013;38:54–57.
4. Auyong DB, Cabbabe AA. Selective blockade of the dorsal scapular nerve for scapula surgery. *J Clin Anesth*. 2014;26:684–687.

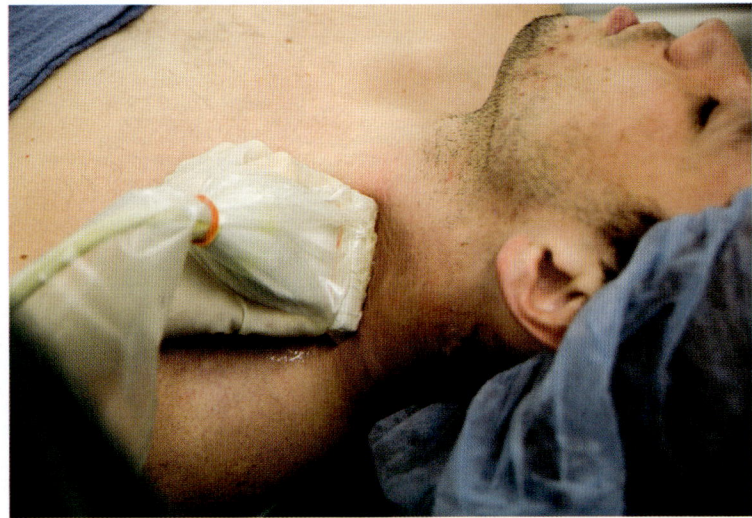

FIGURE 30.1 External photograph showing the transducer position for imaging the dorsal scapular nerve.

88 UPPER EXTREMITY BLOCKS

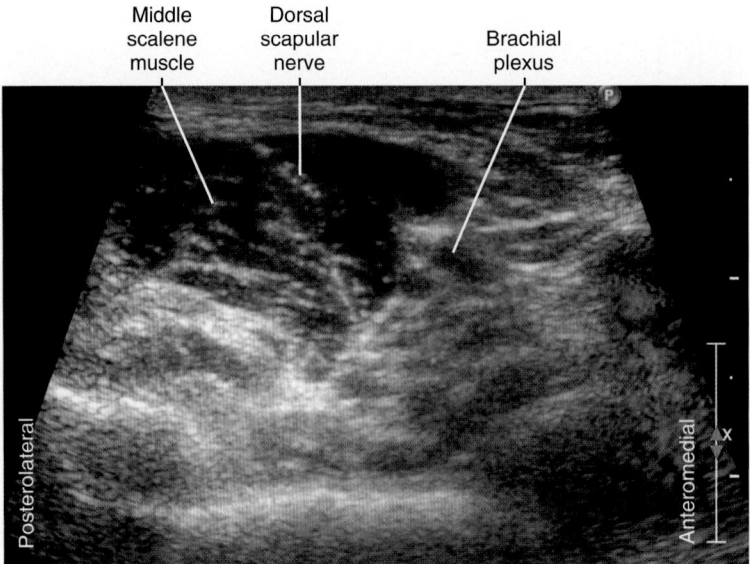

FIGURE 30.2 Short-axis view of the dorsal scapular nerve as it leaves the brachial plexus to travel through the middle scalene muscle.

Suprascapular Nerve Block
(Anterior Approach above the Clavicle)

CHAPTER 31

The suprascapular nerve (SSN) arises from the superior trunk of the brachial plexus, containing contributions from the C5 and C6 ventral rami. The SSN provides the majority of the sensory innervation of the shoulder joint (approximately 70% on anatomic dissections).[1] There also are articular fibers carried by the axillary nerve, lateral pectoral nerve, and the nerve to the subscapularis.[2] Isolated SSN block may be indicated in patients with severe pulmonary and compromise undergoing shoulder surgery or rehabilitation of adhesive capsulitis (frozen shoulder syndrome).[3,4]

Cutaneous innervation of the SSN is not common, being demonstrated in only about 10% to 15% of subjects.[5] When present, the cutaneous distribution is similar to the typical distribution for the axillary nerve. The SSN has motor branches to the supraspinatus and infraspinatus muscles.

The SSN diverges distally 2 cm from the junction of C5 and C6 into the superior trunk (range, 0 to 2.5 cm). Recognition of the takeoff of the SSN from the brachial plexus is an important consideration for complete brachial plexus blocks when performed low in the neck. Selective SSN block should not only spare the remainder of the brachial plexus but also the phrenic nerve.

LIMITATIONS TO TRADITIONAL APPROACH TO BLOCKS AT THE SUPRASCAPULAR NOTCH

Isolated SSN block is traditionally performed where the nerve crosses the suprascapular notch, because the nerve usually does not have major branches before this notch, and the bony landmark is useful. However, there are limitations to this traditional approach. The SSN lies deep to the trapezius and supraspinatus muscles within the suprascapular notch. While distal block of the SSN near the suprascapular notch is potentially more selective, the nerve and needle imaging for this procedure can be challenging.

The suprascapular notch, which is a landmark for the distal SSN block below the clavicle, is often absent (approximately 15% of scapulae).[6] The SSN always runs under the suprascapular ligament, while the position of the suprascapular artery and vein with respect to the ligament is variable. The suprascapular ligament is frequently ossified, thereby reducing image quality. In approximately 50% of cases, sensory branches already separate from the main stem before the main stem enters the suprascapular notch.[7] Injuries to the SSN after blocks performed near the suprascapular notch have been reported (blocks were performed near a site of nerve entrapment).

SUGGESTED TECHNIQUE

The semi-sitting (beach-chair) position helps comfort the patient, lowers the arm and shoulder by gravity, and brings the plane of imaging closer to the plane of the display. The head-of-bed should be elevated about 45 degrees. The patient's head turns to the opposite side from the block. The operator stands at the side of the bed.

A shoulder roll with arms at the side can improve exposure for the anterior approach to the SSN block (place a rolled towel longitudinally between the scapulae).

Working room is limited above the clavicle; therefore, a compact transducer is favored. A small to medium footprint linear (38-mm footprint) transducer is generally preferred. The compact transducer can be rocked back to improve needle tip visibility. Broad linear probes are more difficult to rock than narrow linear or curved transducers for this procedure, but they provide a larger field of view. The ulnar aspects of both hands of the operator are placed on the patient for the best control of the needle and transducer.

The inferior belly of the omohyoid muscle lies over the SSN in the posterior cervical triangle. The SSN obliquely travels underneath the omohyoid muscle from cranial to caudal. The depth of the SSN in this location is less than half the depth of the suprascapular notch. The expected nerve depth is approximately 10 mm in this anatomic location. The SSN is about 2 to 3 mm in diameter. The thickness of the omohyoid muscle is approximately 3 mm.[8]

The omohyoid muscle can be identified by its characteristic to-and-fro sliding motion with swallowing (the omohyoid muscle also moves with scapular movement). This motion is best identified when the muscle is viewed in long axis. Because the omohyoid muscle is the longest muscle of the infrahyoid muscles, the stretched force is comparatively large when swallowing.

The block can be approached in-plane (lateral to medial, or medial to lateral) with transducer held nearly parallel to the clavicle.[6] The needle tip is placed in the tissue plane deep to the omohyoid muscle. For the selective SSN block via anterior approach, inject through the distal part of the inferior belly of the omohyoid muscle (inject distal to the SSN rather than between SSN and brachial plexus).

SELECTIVITY

In this location, the SSN is separated from the remainder of brachial plexus (distance 9 mm on average, range 4 to 15 mm in one volunteer study).[6] Low volumes of local anesthetic can be used for selective block (<1 mL).

CLINICAL ASSESSMENT

The supraspinatus muscle abducts the upper arm (test with the arm at the side to avoid overlap with deltoid muscle function). The infraspinatus muscle externally rotates the upper arm at the shoulder. Block of the remainder of the brachial plexus block can be tested (dorsal scapular, axillary, and other brachial plexus nerves, both sensory and motor function).

Clinical Pearls

- The SSN is responsible for most of the sensory innervation to the shoulder joint.
- The SSN lies beneath the inferior belly of the omohyoid muscle and runs slightly oblique to its course. The SSN is accompanied by the suprascapular artery along the distal part of this course.
- Imaging the omohyoid muscle in long-axis view facilitates the visualization of the SSN above the clavicle.
- Selective SSN block can be performed prior to axillary block to improve mobility of the arm for positioning.

References

1. Vorster W, Lange CP, Briët RJ, et al. The sensory branch distribution of the suprascapular nerve: an anatomic study. *J Shoulder Elbow Surg*. 2008;17(3):500–502. PMID: 18262803.
2. Aszmann OC, Dellon AL, Birely BT, McFarland EG. Innervation of the human shoulder joint and its implications for surgery. *Clin Orthop Relat Res*. 1996;330:202–207. PMID: 8804294.
3. Neal JM, McDonald SB, Larkin KL, et al. Suprascapular nerve block prolongs analgesia after nonarthroscopic shoulder surgery but does not improve outcome. *Anesth Analg*. 2003;96:982–986.
4. Chang KV, Hung CY, Wang TG, Yang RS, Sun WZ, Lin CP. Ultrasound-guided proximal suprascapular nerve block with radiofrequency lesioning for patients with malignancy-associated recalcitrant shoulder pain. *J Ultrasound Med*. 2015;34(11):2099–2105. PMID: 26453125.
5. Ajmani ML. The cutaneous branch of the human suprascapular nerve. *J Anat*. 1994;185(Pt 2):439–442. PMID: 7961151.
6. Siegenthaler A, Moriggl B, Mlekusch S, et al. Ultrasound-guided suprascapular nerve block, description of a novel supraclavicular approach. *Reg Anesth Pain Med*. 2012;37(3):325–328. PMID: 22222688.
7. Rothe C, Steen-Hansen C, Lund J, Jenstrup MT, Lange KH. Ultrasound-guided block of the suprascapular nerve—a volunteer study of a new proximal approach. *Acta Anaesthesiol Scand*. 2014;58(10):1228–1232. PMID: 25186626.
8. Battaglia PJ, Haun DW, Dooley K, Kettner NW. Sonographic measurement of the normal suprascapular nerve and omohyoid muscle. *Man Ther*. 2014;19(2):165–168. PMID: 24412231.

SUPRASCAPULAR NERVE BLOCK (ANTERIOR APPROACH ABOVE THE CLAVICLE)

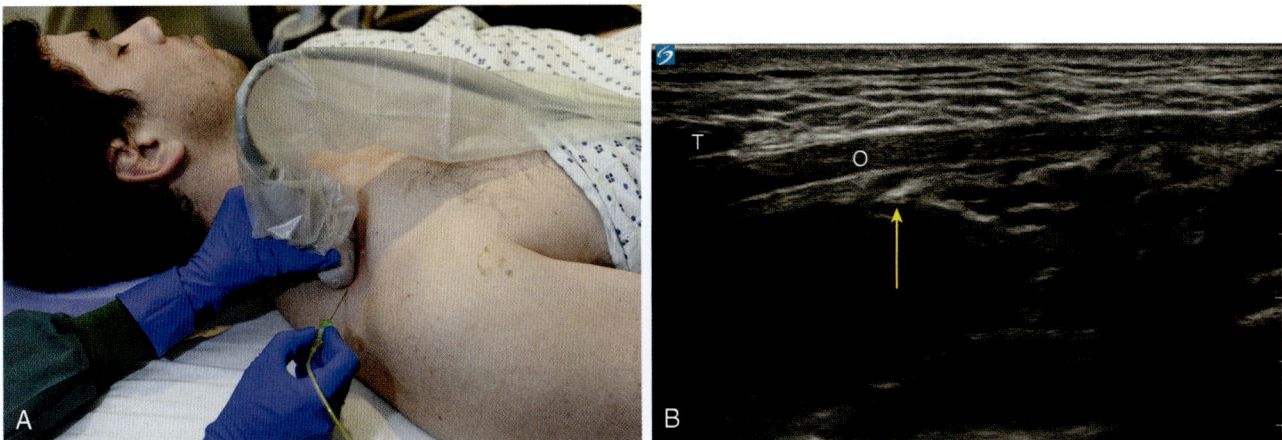

FIGURE 31.1 External photograph showing the probe position for suprascapular nerve (SSN) imaging at its takeoff from the brachial plexus (A). The lateral to medial in-plane approach to SSN block is shown with the transducer held nearly parallel to the clavicle. The corresponding sonogram is also shown (B). The SSN is responsible for most of the sensory innervation to the shoulder joint. The SSN *(yellow arrow)* lies deep to the inferior belly of the omohyoid muscle *(O)*, near the corner of the trapezius muscle *(T)*.

UPPER EXTREMITY BLOCKS

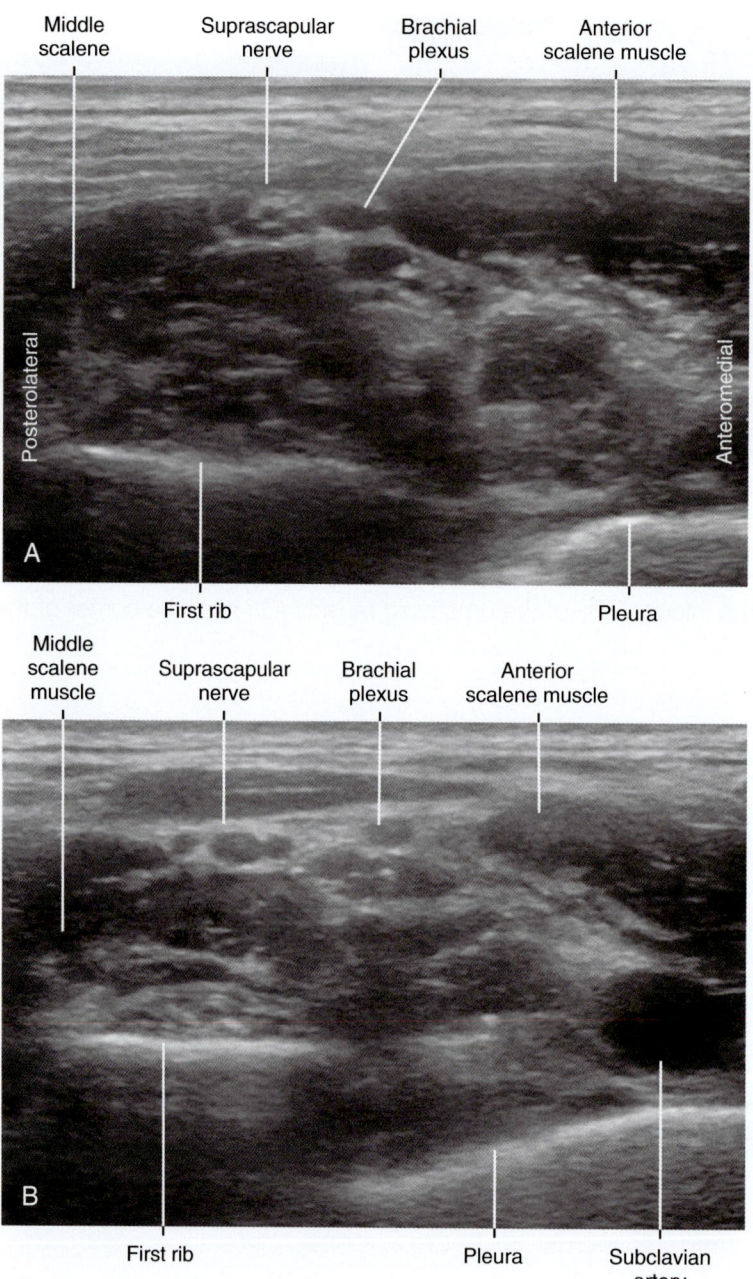

FIGURE 31.2 Short-axis views of the suprascapular nerve at the takeoff from the brachial plexus. The nerve diverges superior and lateral to the brachial plexus (A and B).

Infraclavicular Block

CHAPTER 32

See Video 32.1 on ExpertConsult.com.

Infraclavicular block of the brachial plexus was developed as a means to achieve complete brachial plexus anesthesia and was one of the first blocks to be described using ultrasound imaging.[1-3] This block is performed at the level of the pectoralis minor muscle. In this location, the brachial plexus consists of three cords that compactly hug the walls of the second part of the axillary artery.[4] The infraclavicular region has the advantage of being a secure place for a catheter that provides complete brachial plexus anesthesia. Another advantage is that anatomic variation is relatively uncommon in this region. In the infraclavicular region, the serratus anterior and subscapularis muscles form a margin of safety between the neurovascular bundle and the chest. Because proximal arm muscles are anesthetized (including the pectoralis and deltoid), infraclavicular blocks produce excellent tourniquet tolerance and conditions for upper extremity surgery.[5] The block can be performed with the arm abducted or at the patient's side (Table 32.1).

The major disadvantage of infraclavicular blocks is that the brachial plexus is deep, with the neurovascular bundle being covered by both the pectoralis major and pectoralis minor muscles. Therefore, medium-frequency, small, curved transducers are often favored. Although the block can be performed with the arm at the side, it is best to abduct the arm if possible to straighten the neurovascular bundle and retract the clavicle to provide more working room. Because the block is deep with a relatively steep angle of approach, an echogenic or large-bore needle is recommended (17 or 18 gauge) to improve needle tip visibility.

The three cords of the brachial plexus (medial, lateral, and posterior) are closely adherent to the second part of the axillary artery that lies beneath the pectoralis minor muscle. This arrangement of cords around the second part of the axillary artery resembles a "three-point star" or "tristar" configuration with the artery centered in the middle. The subscapularis muscle separates the infraclavicular brachial plexus from the lung, with a larger margin of safety laterally than medially. The pectoral nerves are sometimes visualized between the pectoralis major and pectoralis minor muscles. Refractile shadowing and posterior acoustic enhancement artifacts are often observed deep to the second part of the axillary artery.

Cord topography changes along the length of the axillary artery in the infraclavicular region. Proximally, the cords of the brachial plexus have more of a "supraclavicular" configuration in which all the cords are on the lateral side of the axillary artery. Following distally, the true "infraclavicular" configuration is when all cords surround the axillary artery before the takeoff of the axillary and musculocutaneous nerves. When the transducer is too proximal, the curved inclination of the ribs and pleura can be recognized (as well as the recurrent thoracoacromial branch of the axillary artery and the cephalic vein, as it joins the axillary vein). When the transducer is too distal, the coracobrachialis muscle and musculocutaneous nerve can be appreciated on the lateral side of artery.

TABLE 32.1 Clinical Considerations for Infraclavicular Block

Advantages	Disadvantages
Compact brachial plexus	Deeper block
Anatomic variation uncommon	Specialized equipment (small curved probe)
Stable location for catheters	
Arm positioning	
Tourniquet tolerance	

The axillary vein lies on the medial (caudal) side of the axillary artery. The medial cord is the only cord of the brachial plexus that lies medial to the axillary artery (between the axillary artery and vein).[4] Occasionally, a duplicate axillary vein is observed. The cephalic vein enters the axillary vein from the lateral side by traveling through the deltopectoral groove. The cephalic vein can lie over the axillary artery in the infraclavicular region and can be recognized by its "tadpole" shape. Otherwise, there are few veins within the field of imaging for infraclavicular block.

The artery refers to the second part of the axillary artery (deep to the pectoralis minor muscle). The axillary artery can appear transiently smaller (or elevation of the posterior wall) with small bolus injections for infraclavicular block.

The "white walls sign" indicates that local anesthetic surrounds the artery and that the wall-hugging cords have been separated from the artery.

The "dark stripe sign" indicates a layer of local anesthetic distributing along the posterior aspect of the axillary artery seen in long axis view. This layer separates the posterior or medial cord from the undersurface of the artery.

SUGGESTED TECHNIQUE

Infraclavicular block is performed in supine position with the arm abducted. The transducer is placed about halfway between the supraclavicular and axillary locations for brachial plexus block. A short-axis view of the axillary artery under the pectoralis minor muscle is obtained. The needle tip is usually placed in-plane between the lateral cord and artery to inject local anesthetic that results in a U-shaped distribution under the posterior aspect of the artery. Some retraction of the lateral cord with the needle may be necessary to pull this cord farther laterally away from the axillary artery.

The fascial layers under the pectoralis minor and over the subscapularis muscle are effective for containing local anesthetic. The injection(s) should ideally separate the cords from the artery by placing the needle tip between each of the three cords and the artery. The anatomic location immediately posterior to the axillary artery appears to result in the most consistent brachial plexus anesthesia for both single-shot injections and catheters.

If a U-shaped distribution is observed from a small test injection (with local anesthetic ascending on both medial and lateral sides of the artery), the majority of local anesthetic should be injected deep to the axillary artery (typically 20 to 30 mL for average sized adult patients). However, if this is not observed, then the needle tip should be repositioned as close as possible to the posterior aspect of the artery. If a medial or lateral J distribution is observed, the needle tip can be adjusted for a more complete U distribution. Local anesthetic can be deposited in small aliquots as the needle is withdrawn and redirected over the artery and along the medial wall to surround the artery.

It is possible to use a linear transducer for infraclavicular block. However, this can be difficult because the working room is limited by the location of the clavicle and the coracoid process. If a linear transducer is chosen, it is especially important to retract the clavicle away from the infraclavicular site by abducting the arm. Another difficulty with linear transducers is that it is difficult to rock the transducer back against the inclination of the chest wall.

COMMENTS

One advantage of infraclavicular block over axillary block is that the infraclavicular block of the brachial plexus can be achieved with a single injection and therefore better functionality of indwelling catheters.

With use of nerve stimulation, posterior cord stimulation tends to be the most predictive of complete brachial plexus anesthesia. This is consistent with the observation that the posterior cord lies between the medial and lateral cords. This also agrees with the sonographic observation that a U-shaped distribution under the second part of the arterial artery is predictive of infraclavicular block success (Table 32.2).

TABLE 32.2 Sonographic Signs of Infraclavicular Block Success

U-shaped distribution under the artery

Separation of cords and artery

"White walls" appearance of the artery

"Dark stripe" under the artery (long axis view)

Arterial compression or elevation during injection

A steep angle of approach between the lateral cord and artery together with loss-of-resistance technique as the needle is advanced can improve the chance of achieving a U-shaped distribution underneath the axillary artery.

Infraclavicular block does not cover the suprascapular nerve of the brachial plexus. This can be important when arm and shoulder manipulation is required during surgery.[6]

The optimal point for infraclavicular block appears to be where the brachial plexus cords form a true neurovascular bundle around the second part of the axillary artery. The benefit of more proximal approaches to infraclavicular block is under current investigation.[7]

KEY POINTS

Infraclavicular Block	The Essential Points
Anatomy	The PMi defines the second part of the AA. The cords of the BP hug the walls of the second part of the AA. The BP cords (lateral, posterior, and medial) are named with respect to the second part of the AA The cephalic vein ("tadpole sign") crosses over the AA to enter the AV.
Image orientation	The AV lies medial (caudad) to the AA.
Positioning	Supine, with arm abducted if possible A blue foam headrest provides working room.
Operator	Standing on the lateral (cephalad) side of the armboard (for laptop system) At the side of patient (for system with movable display)
Display	Across the armboard (for laptop system) Across the table (for system with movable display)
Transducer	Medium-frequency curved, small footprint Initial depth setting: 40–50 mm
Needle	20–21 gauge, 70–90 mm in length
Anatomic location	Begin by scanning halfway between supraclavicular region and axilla. Slide transducer to obtain SAX view of AA underneath PMa and PMi. Perform infraclavicular block at the level of the PMi. The CB (and therefore MCN takeoff) should not be in view.
Approach	SAX view of second part of AA (under PMi), in-plane. Place the needle tip between the cords and AA. A U-shaped distribution under the AA is desired.
Sonographic assessment	The injection should separate the cords of the BP from the AA. Duplicate axillary vein on lateral side of AA is common. "Supraclavicular" configuration to the BP cords is possible. This means all three cords of BP lie on the lateral side of the AA. If this condition is recognized, slide the probe more distally.

AA, Axillary artery; *AV*, axillary vein; *BP*, brachial plexus; *CB*, coracobrachialis muscle; *MCN*, musculocutaneous nerve; *PMa*, pectoralis major muscle; *PMi*, pectoralis minor muscle; *SAX*, short axis.

> **Clinical Pearls**
> - Infraclavicular block is best performed at the level of the pectoralis minor muscle.
> - The cords of the brachial plexus surround the second part of the axillary artery. If the coracobrachialis muscle is within the field of imaging, there is some potential for takeoff of the musculocutaneous nerve and therefore incomplete block.
> - Abducting the arm retracts the clavicle, thereby allowing more space to place the block needle. Furthermore, the neurovascular bundle is straightened, thereby making imaging easier. In this position, the brachial plexus lies closer to the skin surface and farther from the pleura compared with other arm positions.
> - In the infraclavicular region, the axillary artery and vein are separated when the medial cord of the brachial plexus lies between them. This gap can be identified on ultrasound imaging and indicates wall-hugging cords of the brachial plexus (rather than a bundle or cluster of cords that lie on the lateral side of the axillary artery). Performing an infraclavicular block where the cords surround the axillary artery is desired for complete brachial plexus anesthesia.
> - Although debate continues, most clinical studies have suggested that brachial plexus anesthesia can be achieved with a single injection of local anesthetic under the second part of the axillary artery for infraclavicular block.

References

1. Raj PP, Montgomery SJ, Nettles D, et al. Infraclavicular brachial plexus block: a new approach. *Anesth Analg.* 1973;52:897–904.
2. Ootaki C, Hayashi H, Amano M. Ultrasound-guided infraclavicular brachial plexus block: an alternative technique to anatomical landmark-guided approaches. *Reg Anesth Pain Med.* 2000;25(6):600–604.
3. Sandhu NS, Capan LM. Ultrasound-guided infraclavicular brachial plexus block. *Br J Anaesth.* 2002;89(2):254–259.
4. Sauter AR, Smith HJ, Stubhaug A, et al. Use of magnetic resonance imaging to define the anatomical location closest to all three cords of the infraclavicular brachial plexus. *Anesth Analg.* 2006;103:1574–1576.
5. Chin KJ, Singh M, Velayutham V, et al. Infraclavicular brachial plexus block for regional anaesthesia of the lower arm. *Anesth Analg.* 2010;111(4):1072.
6. Flohr-Madsen S, Ytrebø LM, Valen K, et al. A randomized placebo-controlled trial examining the effect on hand supination after the addition of a suprascapular nerve block to infraclavicular branch plexus blockade. *Anaesthesia.* 2016;71(8):938–947.
7. Sala-Blanch X, Reina MA, Pangthipampai P, Karmakar MK. Anatomic basis for brachial plexus block at the costoclavicular space: a cadaver anatomic study. *Reg Anesth Pain Med.* 2016;41(3):387–391.

INFRACLAVICULAR BLOCK

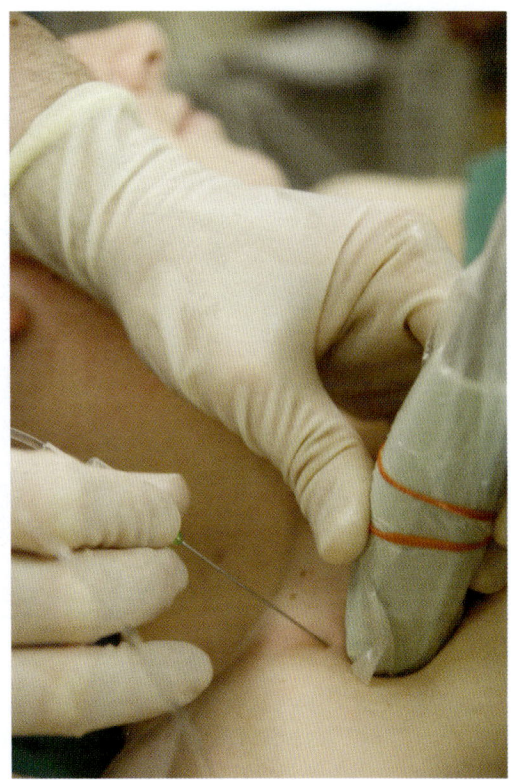

FIGURE 32.1 External photograph showing an in-plane approach to infraclavicular block. The operator can stand at the head or side of the table. A curved probe is usually chosen because of the working room limitation imposed by the clavicle. If possible, the arm should be abducted to straighten the neurovascular bundle for infraclavicular block.

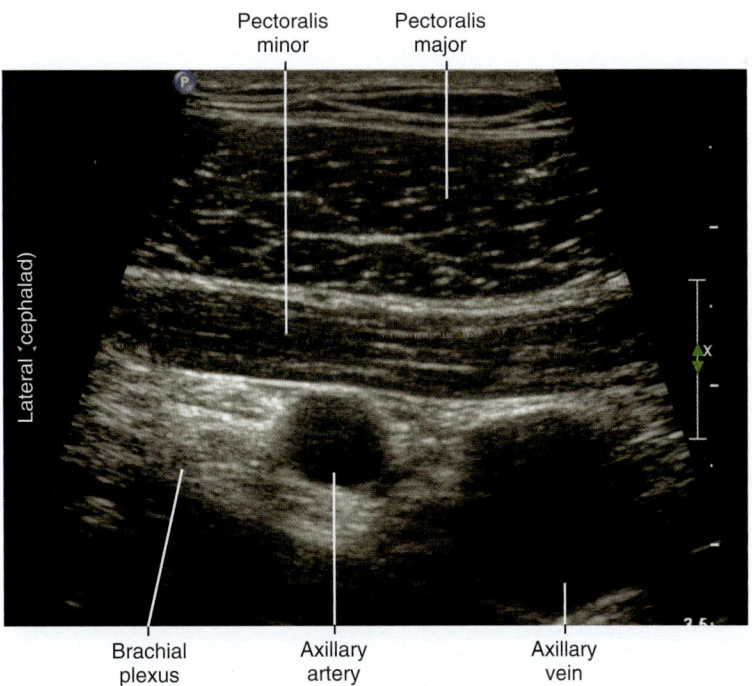

FIGURE 32.2 Short-axis view of the second part of the axillary artery under the pectoralis major and pectoralis minor muscles. The cords of the brachial plexus are named for their position with respect to the artery. The three cords of the brachial plexus have a triangular arrangement around the second part of the axillary artery, which lies underneath the pectoralis minor muscle. The clavipectoral fascia creates a favorable space for injection of local anesthetic and catheter placement in the infraclavicular region.

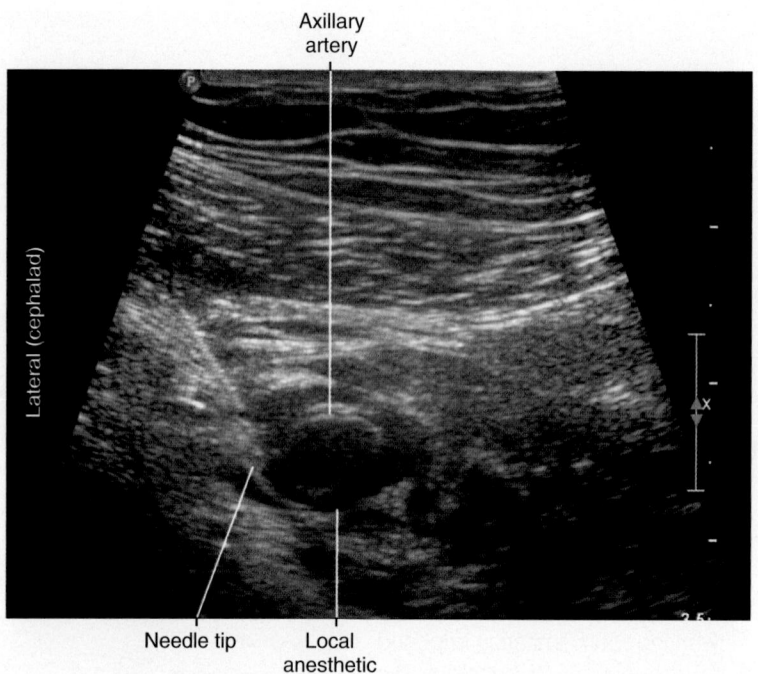

FIGURE 32.3 Sonogram showing in-plane approach to infraclavicular block. An echogenic needle has been used to place local anesthetic underneath the axillary artery deep to the pectoralis minor muscle.

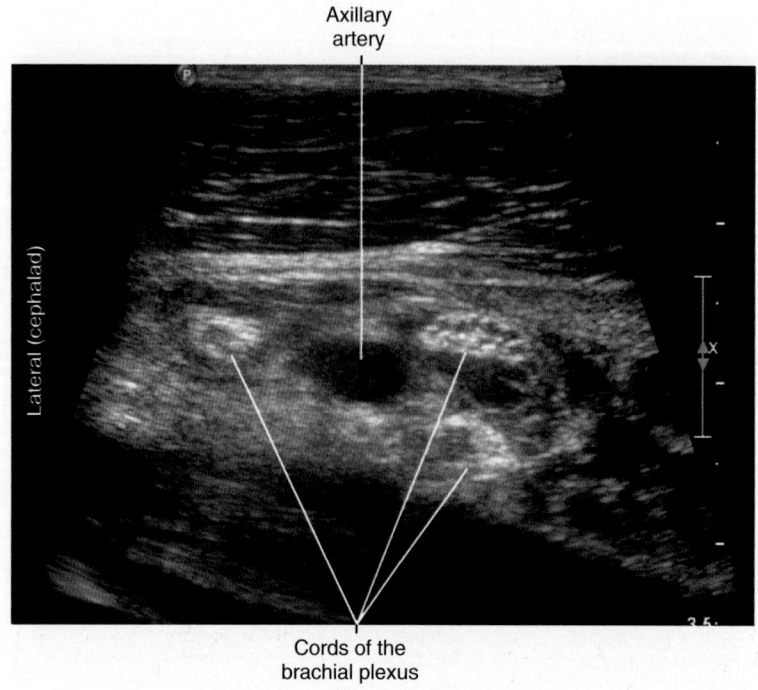

FIGURE 32.4 Sonographic assessment of the distribution after infraclavicular block. The local anesthetic surrounds the cords and separates them from the walls of the axillary artery.

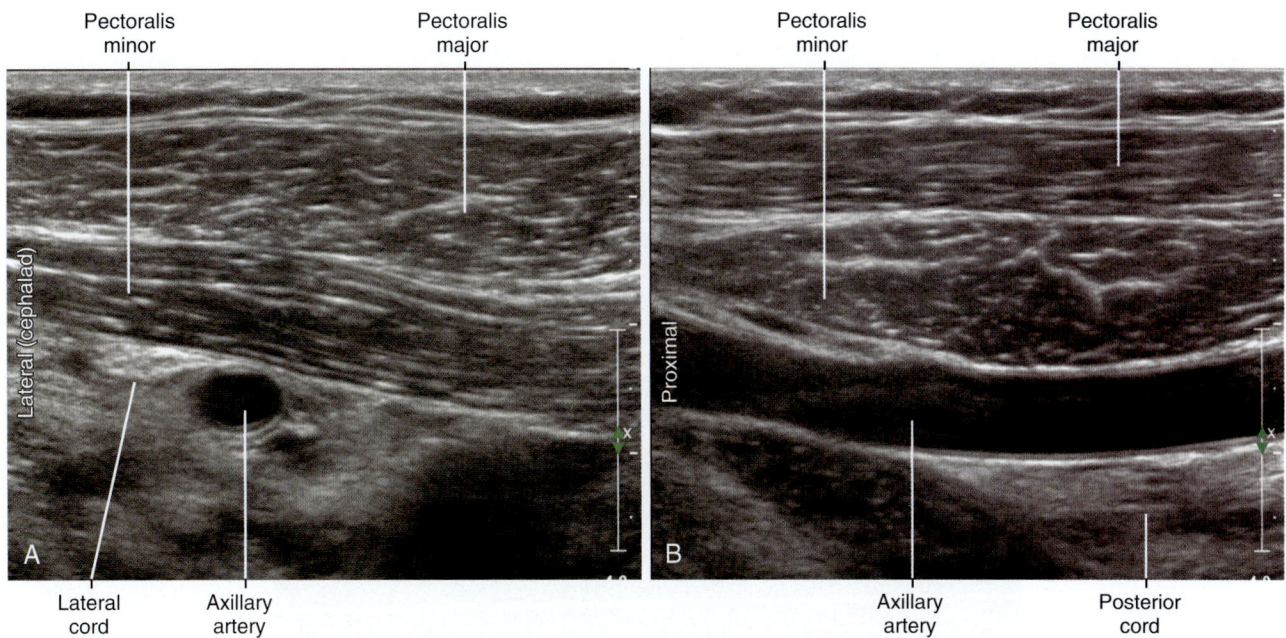

FIGURE 32.5 Short-axis (A) and long-axis (B) view of the axillary artery under the pectoralis minor muscle. The course of the posterior cord of the brachial plexus can be seen under the axillary artery.

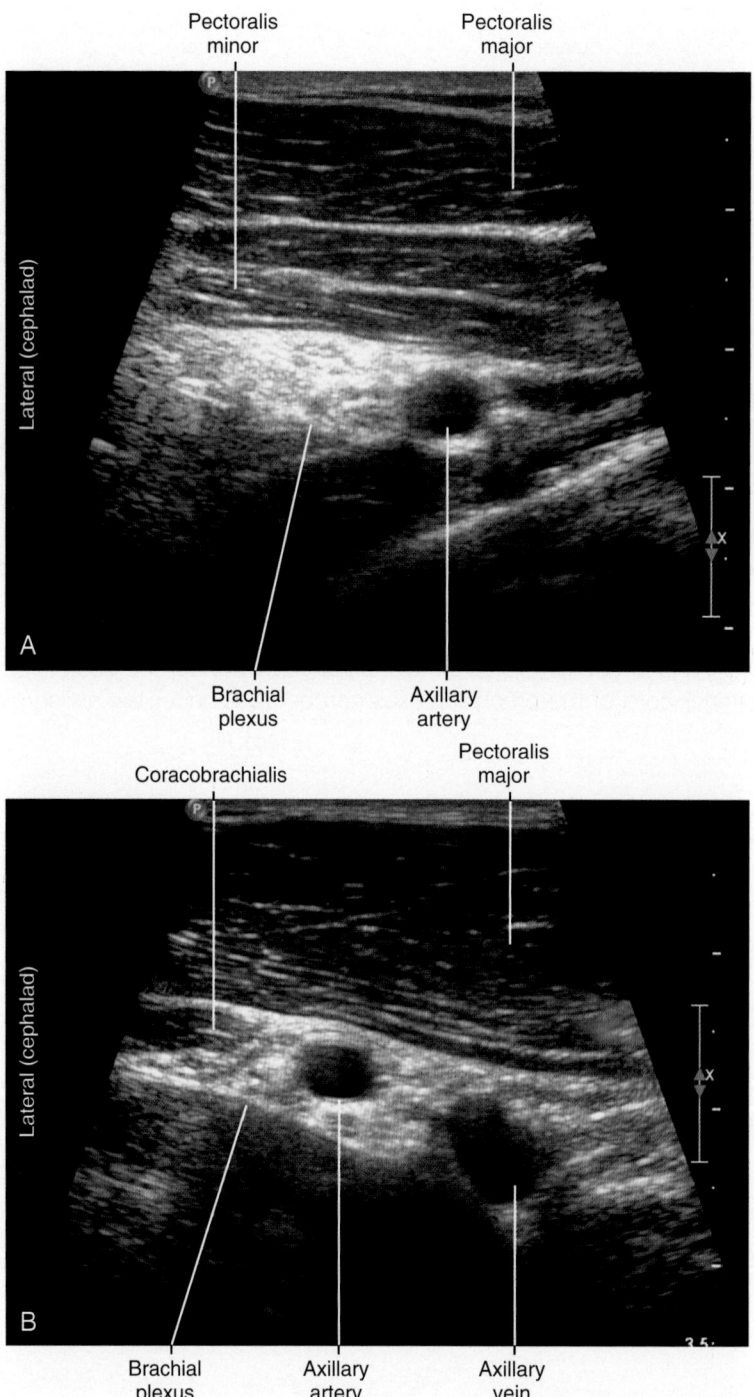

FIGURE 32.6 Sonograms illustrating aberrant transducer positions for infraclavicular block. (A) The transducer is placed too medial (proximal or central). In this sonogram, all cords of the brachial plexus lie on the lateral side of the axillary artery. (B) The transducer is placed too lateral (distal or peripheral). In this sonogram, the coracobrachialis muscle is seen on the lateral aspect of the axillary.

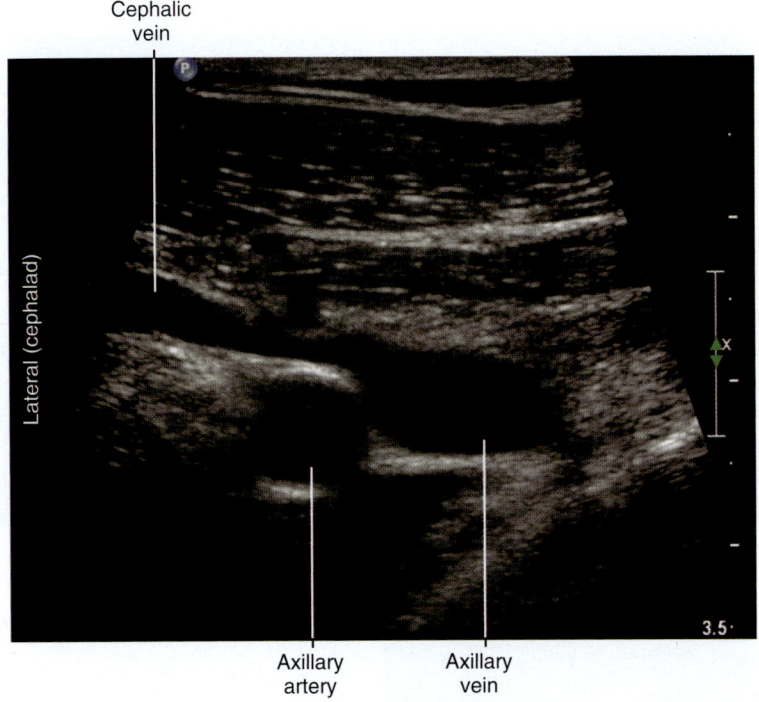

FIGURE 32.7 The "tadpole" sign of the cephalic vein entering the axillary vein. Because the cephalic vein enters the axillary vein at 90 degrees, it is seen in long axis, whereas the axillary vein is seen in short axis.

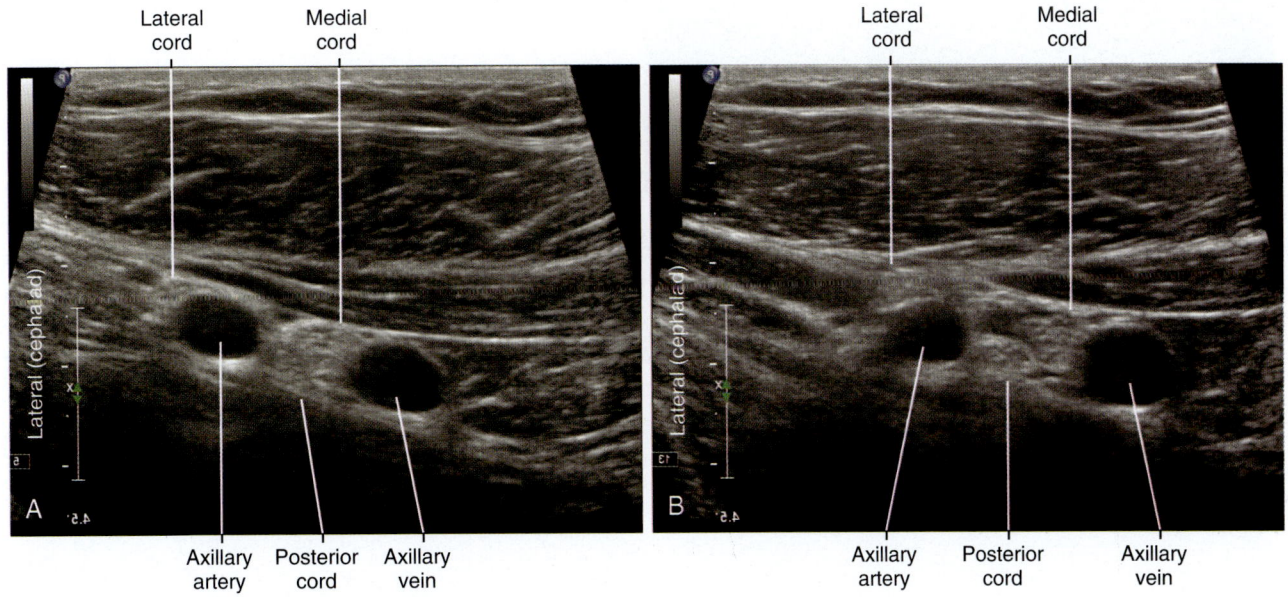

FIGURE 32.8 Separation of the axillary artery and vein by cords of the brachial plexus. When the walls of the axillary artery and vein are not touching in the infraclavicular region, the medial cord of the brachial plexus usually separates them. In this example, both the medial cord and posterior cord lie between the two vessels. Sonograms are shown before (A) and after (B) injection for infraclavicular block.

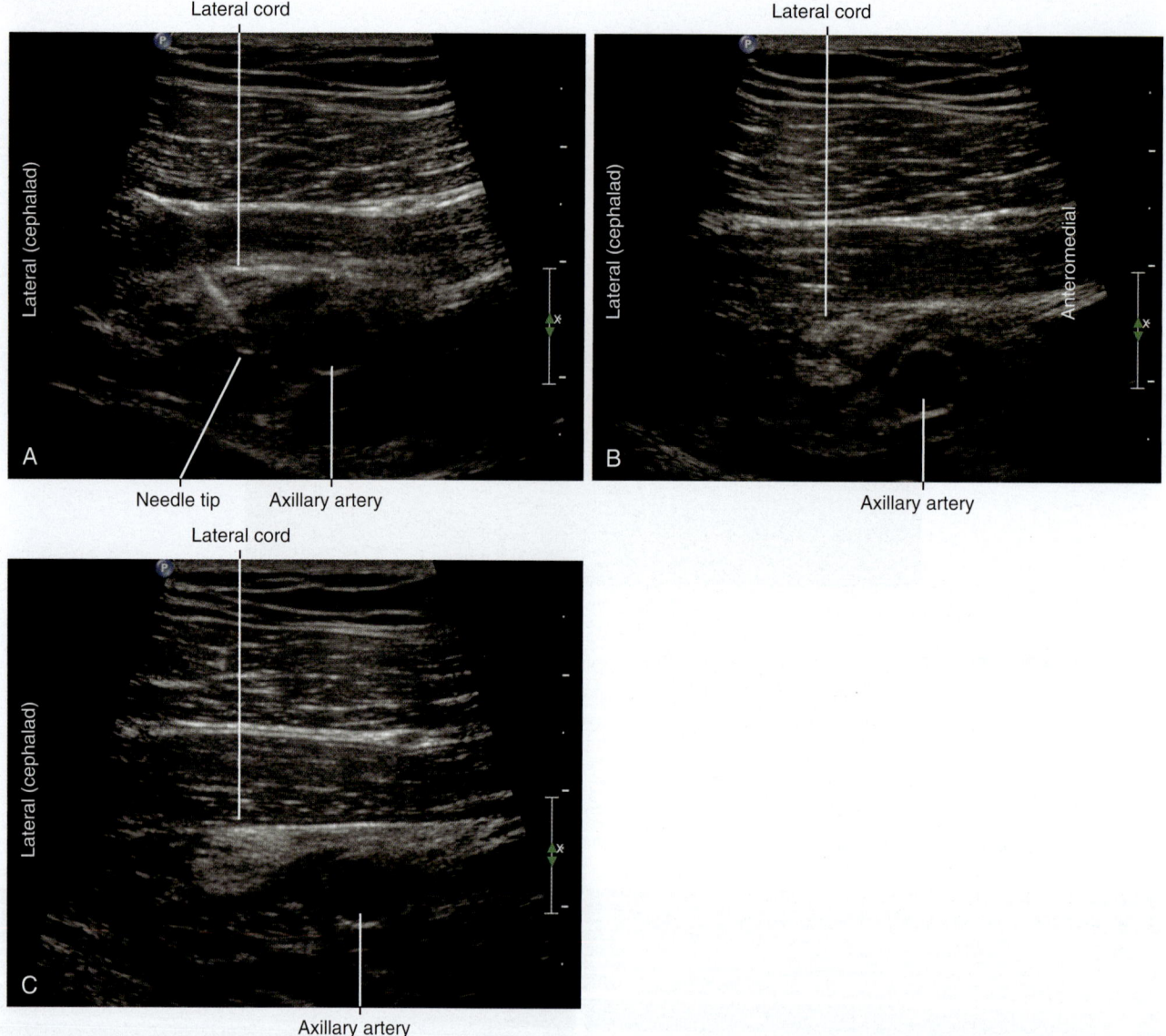

FIGURE 32.9 Sonograms illustrating intraneural injection during infraclavicular block. To access the posterior aspect of the axillary artery, the block needle was inadvertently placed through the lateral cord of the brachial plexus (A). Intraneural injection in a fracture pattern is noted after the block (B). Sliding the transducer away from the site verified nerve integrity was intact (C), and there were no neurologic sequelae.

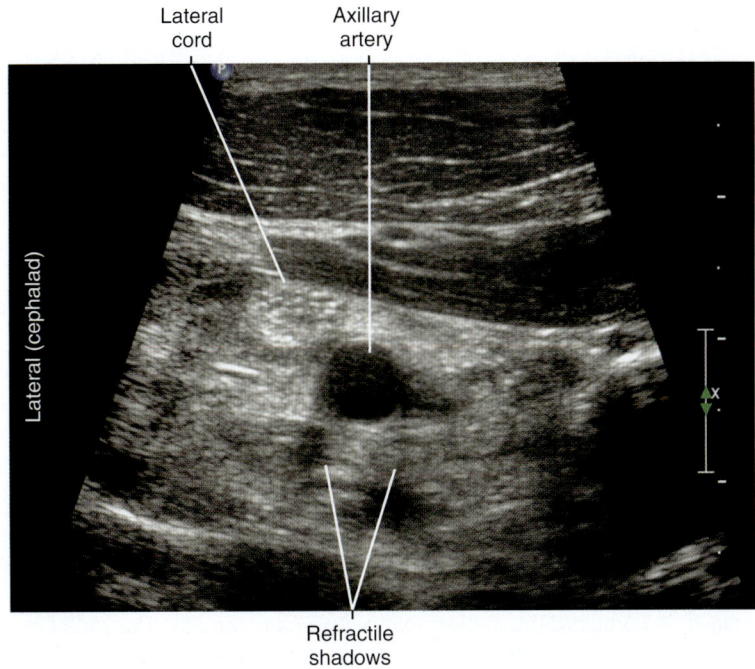

FIGURE 32.10 Sonogram illustrating artifacts during imaging for infraclavicular block. In this example, refractile shadowing from the sides of the axillary artery is seen. Refractile shadows are the linear hypoechoic artifacts that emanate down from the sides of vessels and are formed by refraction of ultrasound waves. Posterior acoustic enhancement (amplification of echoes deep to the artery) typically occurs when this is noted. This enhancement artifact can resemble nerves (although the cords themselves frequently occupy this position).

CHAPTER 33

Axillary Block

 See Video 33.1 on ExpertConsult.com.

Three terminal branches of the brachial plexus (the median, radial, and ulnar nerves) lie close to the axillary artery in the axilla (Table 33.1). This makes the axilla a convenient place to block the brachial plexus (Table 33.2). Axillary block is traditionally performed by transarterial injection of local anesthetic around the axillary artery or by the use of nerve stimulation to evoke motor responses. Transarterial block necessitates puncturing the axillary artery. Another weakness is failure to anesthetize the musculocutaneous nerve, which leaves the neurovascular bundle proximally underneath the pectoralis minor muscle at the level of the coracoid process.

Ultrasound imaging improves axillary block of the brachial plexus. Many institutions have reported advantages to using ultrasound to guide this procedure.[1,2] Ultrasound can be used to guide injections around the axillary artery. In addition, the musculocutaneous nerve can be directly imaged to complete the axillary block (see Chapter 34). The radial nerve is the most difficult terminal branch of the brachial plexus to image in the axilla.[3]

SUGGESTED TECHNIQUE

The transpectoral approach for proximal axillary block is performed with the needle tip just inside the chest before the nerves of the brachial plexus diverge. With this lateral to medial approach, the needle enters through the pectoralis major muscle.

Axillary block is performed with the patient in supine position. The arm should be slightly hyperabducted to allow the needle placement to be as proximal as possible, and slightly more than 90 degrees of abduction is optimal for probe positioning. Because the pectoralis major inserts

TABLE 33.1 Characteristics of Terminal Branches of the Brachial Plexus in the Axilla

Nerve	Characteristics
Axillary	Accompanies posterior circumflex humeral artery Takeoff is proximal to teres major and latissimus dorsi tendons
Musculocutaneous	Lateral course through coracobrachialis Flat shape when inside this muscle If not visible, rule out median-musculocutaneous nerve fusion
Radial	Accompanies profunda brachii artery Travels to spiral groove of humerus Takeoff is distal to teres major and latissimus dorsi tendons
Median	Can be displaced to side of axillary artery with compression Accompanies brachial artery
Ulnar	Lies between axillary artery and vein Acoustic window through axillary vein Most consistent position (at 2- to 3-o'clock position with respect to artery) Travels to cubital tunnel
Medial antebrachial cutaneous	Lies between median nerve and ulnar nerve
Intercostobrachial and medial brachial cutaneous	Lie within the subcutaneous tissue of the medial arm Medial to axillary artery

TABLE 33.2 Clinical Considerations for Axillary Block With Ultrasound	
Advantages	**Disadvantages**
Shallow nerves	Divergent plexus
Working room	Anatomic variation
Compressible site	Arm positioning
Remote from the lung	Multiple veins
No risk for phrenic nerve block	Catheters problematic

on the humerus, hyperabduction of the arm reduces the pectoral ridge by retracting the pectoralis major toward the midline. A Mayo stand can be used to support the arm in this position. The operator should stand at the head of the bed to view the ultrasound display across the patient's arm.

The pectoral ridge separates the needle entry point and the transducer for this proximal axillary block. This can allow for coverless imaging, because the needle entry site is remote from the transducer. The skin preparation is over the pectoralis major muscle. Tilting and rotating the angle of the transducer slightly into the chest torso allow for more proximal imaging. The axillary veins can be used as a manometer to measure the amount of probe compression, and the correct amount of pressure for this procedure just coapts the walls of the veins.

Structures potentially in the needle path when approaching the axillary neurovascular bundle are the cephalic vein, the tendon of the pectoralis major, and the musculocutaneous nerve. The cephalic vein lies in the deltopectoral groove; therefore, there is a low potential for venous puncture as the needle enters the skin.

The conjoint tendon of the latissimus dorsi and teres major inserts on the humerus and is a valuable landmark for this procedure. The radial nerve takeoff from the axillary artery is always distal to this tendon. The needle should enter the skin away from the transducer so that it approaches slightly deep to the artery and can easily be placed between the artery and conjoint tendon for injection. The latissimus dorsi is the more shallow and proximal layer of the conjoint tendon, whereas the teres major is the deeper and more distal overlapping layer.

Because the axillary artery and wall-hugging branches of the brachial plexus (median, radial, and ulnar nerves) are surrounded by common connective tissue, the ideal place for block needle tip placement is between these nerves and the artery. If this is done, the perivascular injections will separate the nerves from the artery. Injections at the outside corner of the nerves (away from the axillary artery) also can be successful, but careful assessment must show that the injection actually encircles the nerves.

Local anesthetic injections are made in front and in back of the axillary artery. The injection in back of the artery is typically done first. This brings the neurovascular bundle even closer to the skin surface. The musculocutaneous nerve is blocked separately (see Chapter 34).

It is especially important for the front-wall injection to be between the median nerve and the axillary artery. The median nerve crosses the front surface of the axillary artery. If local anesthetic tracks proximally along the median nerve to its medial and lateral cord contributions, two-thirds of the brachial plexus should be anesthetized. The median, ulnar, medial antebrachial cutaneous, and musculocutaneous nerves all derive from the medial and lateral cords. The medial antebrachial cutaneous nerves are small and lie between the median nerve and ulnar nerve in the axilla. These nerves can sometimes be imaged after axillary block because anechoic fluid surrounds them to provide acoustic contrast. Medial antebrachial cutaneous nerve distally travel with the basilic vein in the arm.

The intercostobrachial nerves (from T1 and T2) are not part of the brachial plexus, but they contribute to sensory innervation of the medial arm. Intercostobrachial nerve block can be achieved by subcutaneous infiltration of the medial arm at the axillary crease. Imaging guidance is usually not necessary for this procedure, but it is sometimes used in obese patients.

KEY POINTS

Axillary Block	The Essential Points
Anatomy	There are three wall-hugging nerves in the axilla (MN, RN, UN). All terminal branches lie superficial to the CT in the axilla (MN, RN, UN, MCN). The nerves are about 3 mm in diameter.
Image orientation	The CT has a medial (superficial) to lateral (deep) inclination.
Positioning	Supine, with arm abducted. A blue foam headrest provides working room.
Operator	Standing on the lateral (cephalad) side of armboard (for laptop system). At the side of the patient (for system with movable display)
Display	Across the armboard (for laptop system). Across the table (for system with movable display)
Transducer	High-frequency linear, 23- to 38-mm footprint. Initial depth setting: 25 mm
Needle	20–21 gauge, 70 mm in length
Anatomic location	Begin by scanning the axilla to identify the AA in SAX view. Slide transducer to obtain view of CT underneath AA
Approach	SAX view of AA, in-plane from lateral to medial. Place the needle tip between the nerves and AA.
Sonographic assessment	The injections should separate the nerves from artery. Anatomic variation MCN-median fusion (5%–10%). The MCN can be fused with the median nerve in the axilla. This is sometimes referred to as a low-lying lateral cord. Duplicate axillary artery can occasionally be observed.

AA, Axillary artery (third part); *CT*, conjoint tendon of teres major and latissimus dorsi muscles; *MCN*, musculocutaneous nerve; *MN*, median nerve; *RN*, radial nerve; *SAX*, short axis; *UN*, ulnar nerve.

Clinical Pearls

- With this proximal approach to axillary block, the needle is naturally channeled into the space between the axillary artery and conjoint tendon of the latissimus dorsi and teres major for the posterior injection. A slight upward trajectory is all that is needed to steer the needle along and above this tendon complex.
- With classic approaches to axillary block, the radial nerve and musculocutaneous nerves are often spared.[4]
- If there is any question as to whether the ulnar nerve has been surrounded by local anesthetic, it is easy to trace the ulnar nerve from the cubital tunnel to the axilla using a trail of gel along the known course of the nerve.

References

1. Soeding PE, Sha S, Royse CE, et al. A randomized trial of ultrasound-guided brachial plexus anaesthesia in upper limb surgery. *Anaesth Intensive Care*. 2005;33:719–725.
2. Lo N, Brull R, Perlas A, et al. Evolution of ultrasound guided axillary brachial plexus blockade: retrospective analysis of 662 blocks. *Can J Anaesth*. 2008;55:408–413.
3. Frkovic V, Ward C, Preckel B, et al. Influence of arm position on ultrasound visibility of the axillary brachial plexus. *Eur J Anaesthesiol*. 2015;32(11):771–780.
4. Lanz E, Theiss D, Jankovic D. The extent of blockade following various techniques of brachial plexus block. *Anesth Analg*. 1983;62:55–58.

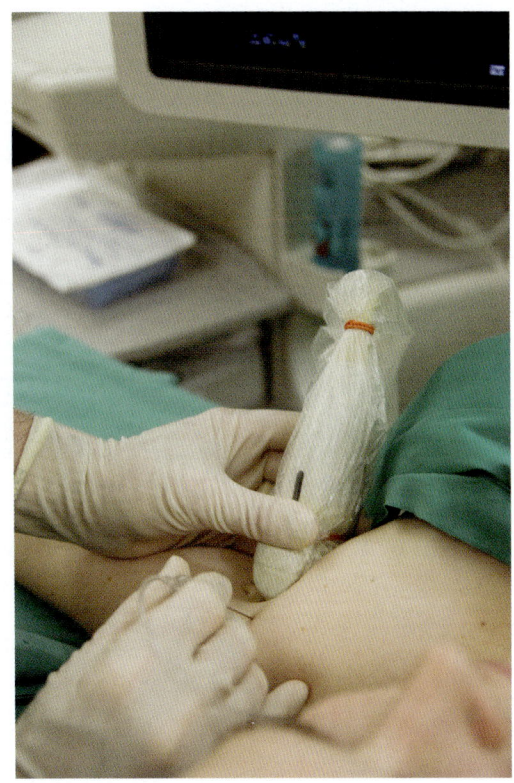

FIGURE 33.1 External photograph showing an in-plane approach to axillary block from the lateral aspect of the arm. In this example, the display is placed across the armboard and the operator stands at the head of the bed.

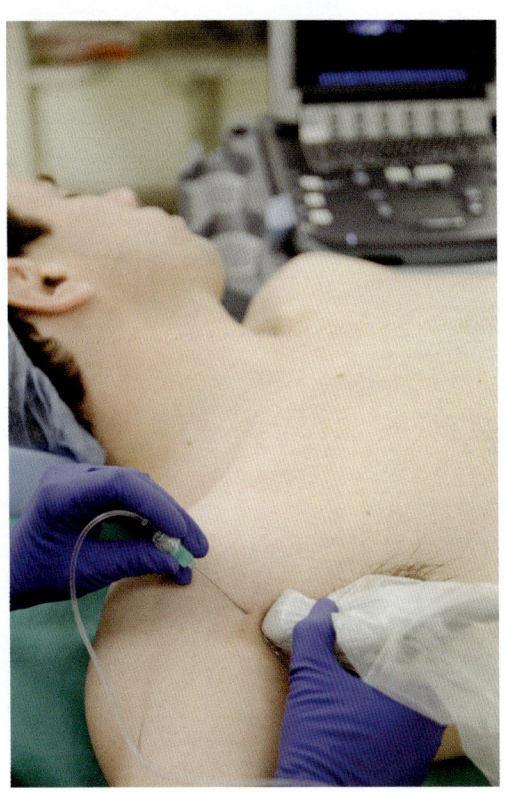

FIGURE 33.2 External photograph showing an in-plane approach to axillary block from the lateral aspect of the arm. In this example, the display is placed across the table, and the operator stands at the side of the bed.

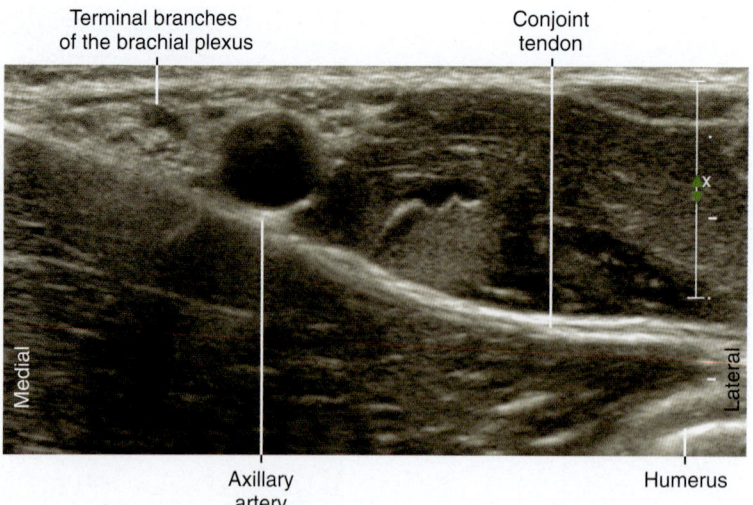

FIGURE 33.3 Short-axis view of the axillary artery and surrounding branches of the brachial plexus in the axilla. The conjoint tendon of the teres major and latissimus dorsi lies under the neurovascular bundle. Because the radial nerve takeoff is distal to the conjoint tendon, visualization of this structure ensures a compact brachial plexus suitable for complete block.

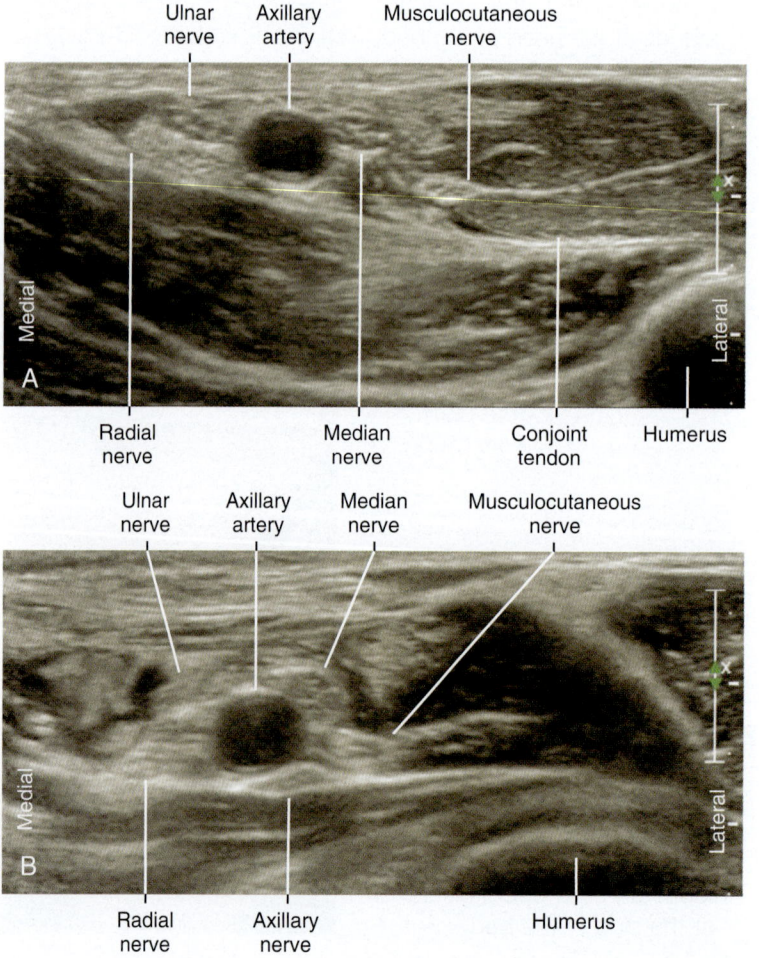

FIGURE 33.4 Short-axis views of the brachial plexus from probe manipulation in the axilla. With some subjects, the axillary nerve can be viewed posterior to the axillary artery by tilting the probe into the chest. Both distal (A) and proximal (B) views are shown.

AXILLARY BLOCK 109

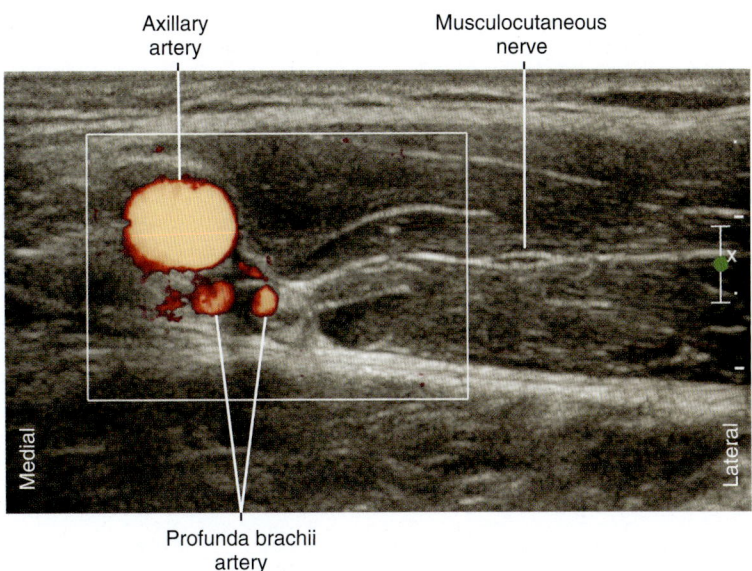

FIGURE 33.5 The profunda brachii artery shown in short-axis view with power Doppler imaging. The profunda brachii artery exits the back wall of the axillary artery to accompany the radial nerve into the spiral groove of the humerus.

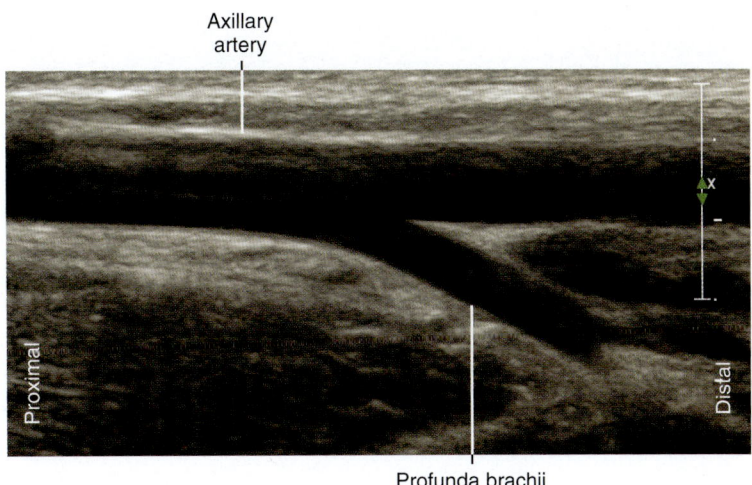

FIGURE 33.6 The profunda brachii artery shown in long-axis view with B-mode imaging.

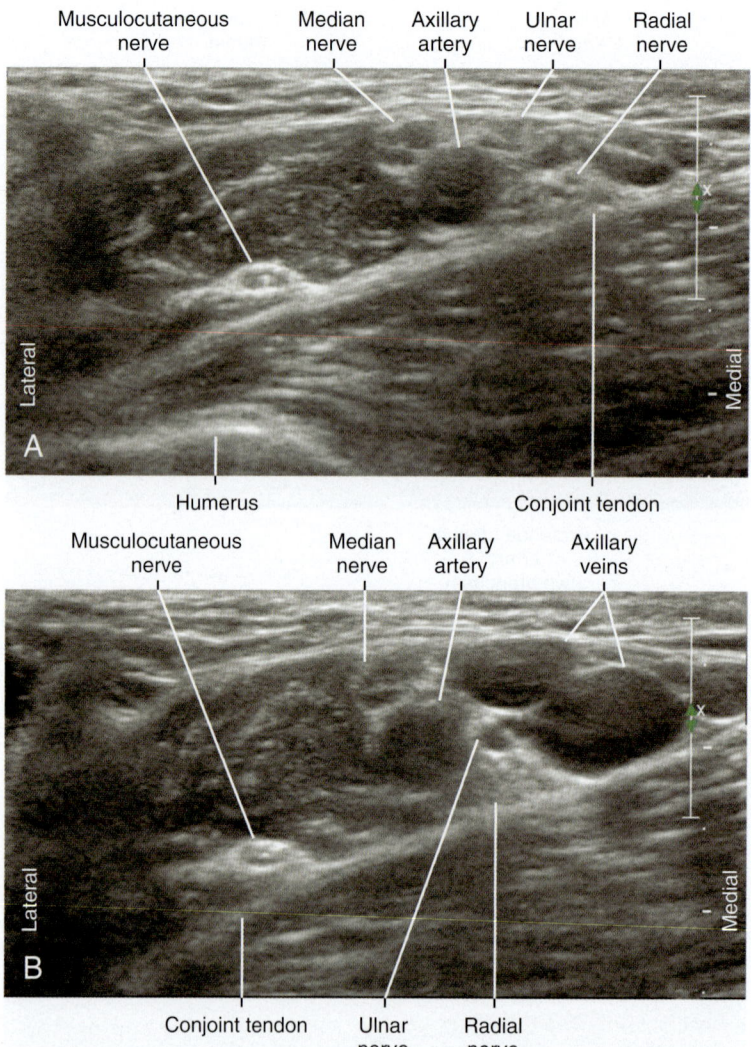

FIGURE 33.7 Axillary scout view imaging to look for veins before needle placement. Images are shown with (A) and without (B) probe compression. During needle placement, the vein walls are maintained coapted to reduce the chance of venous puncture.

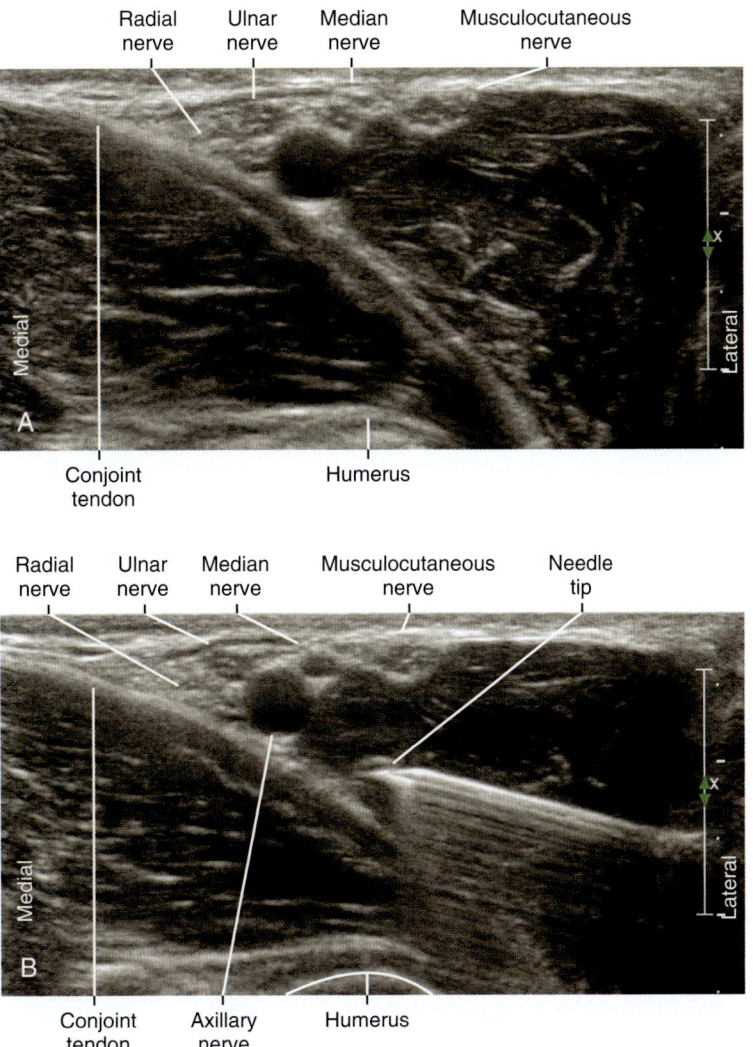

FIGURE 33.8 In-plane approach to axillary block. Sonograms are shown before (A) and after (B) needle placement. With this approach, the needle is naturally channeled into the space between the axillary artery and conjoint tendon of the latissimus dorsi and teres major for the posterior injection. A slight upward trajectory is all that is needed to steer the needle along and above the tendon complex.

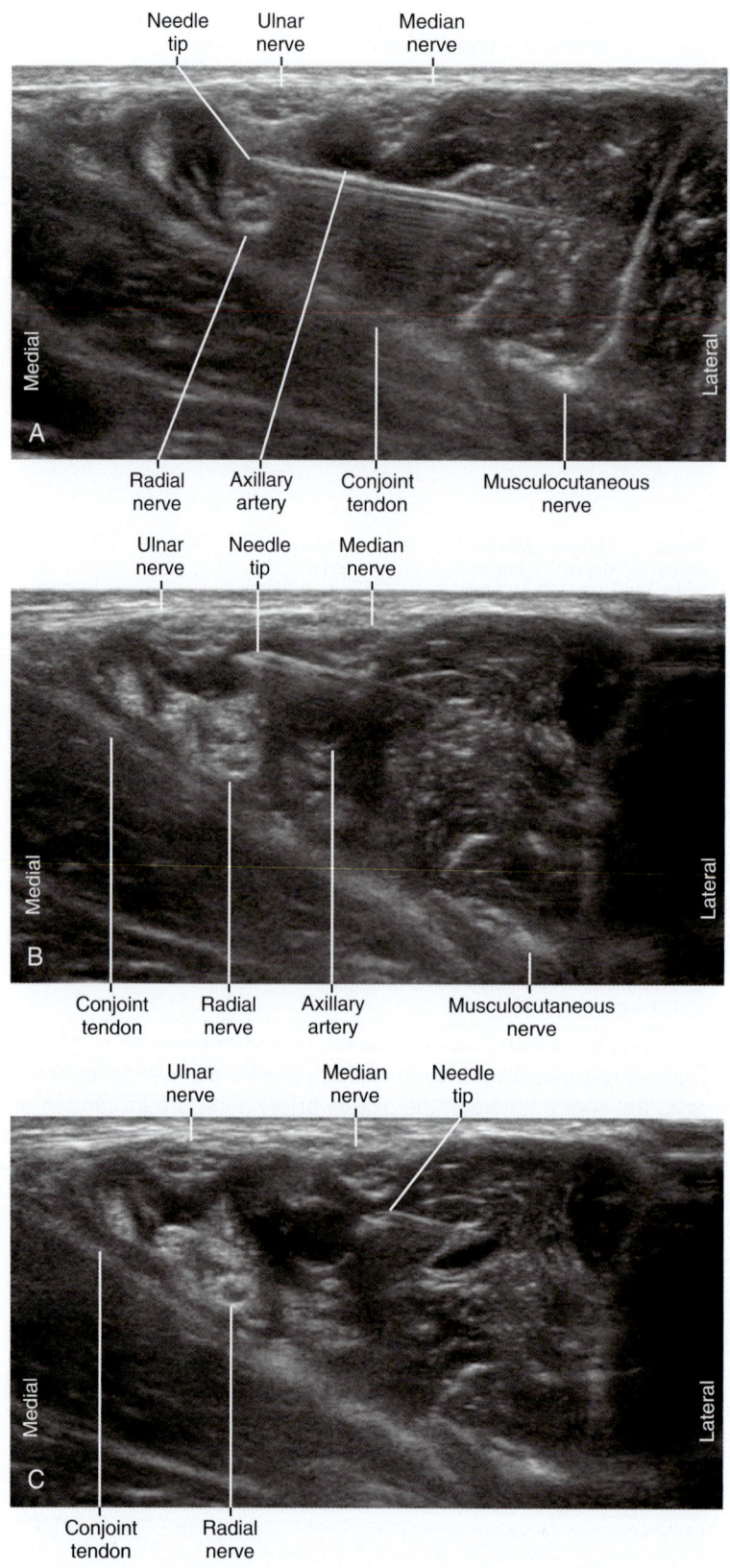

FIGURE 33.9 Axillary block image sequence showing back-wall injection (A), front-wall injection (B), and front-wall injection as the needle is removed (C).

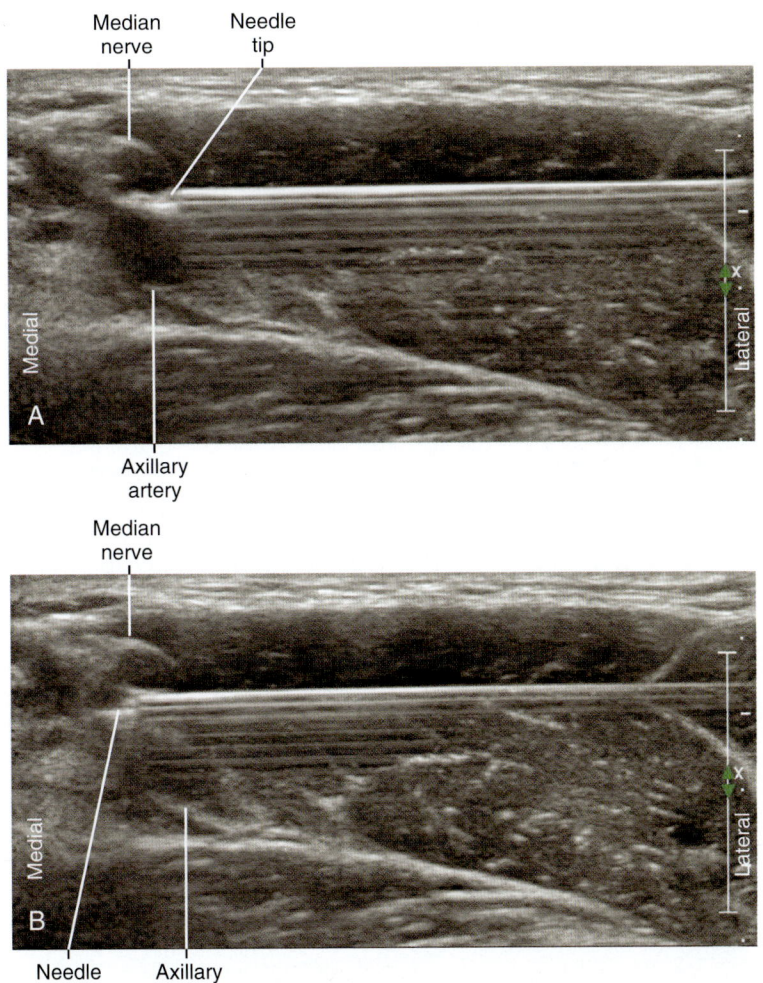

FIGURE 33.10 Axillary block image sequence. The block needle approaches the gap between the median nerve and axillary artery (A). As the needle is advanced and local anesthetic is slowly injected, the nerve and artery are separated (B). The beveled needle can be used as a shovel to scoop up the peripheral nerve and displace it away from adjacent structures (e.g., arteries or other peripheral nerves).

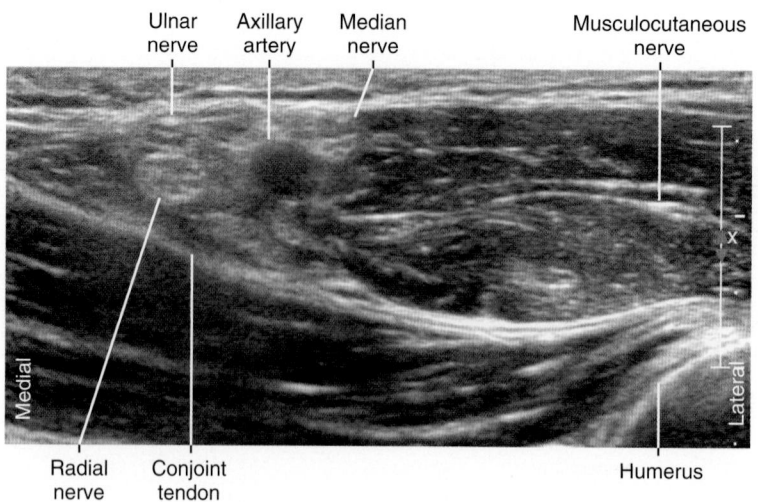

FIGURE 33.11 Short-axis view of the axillary artery after axillary block. After successful injection, the local anesthetic separates the nerves from the axillary artery.

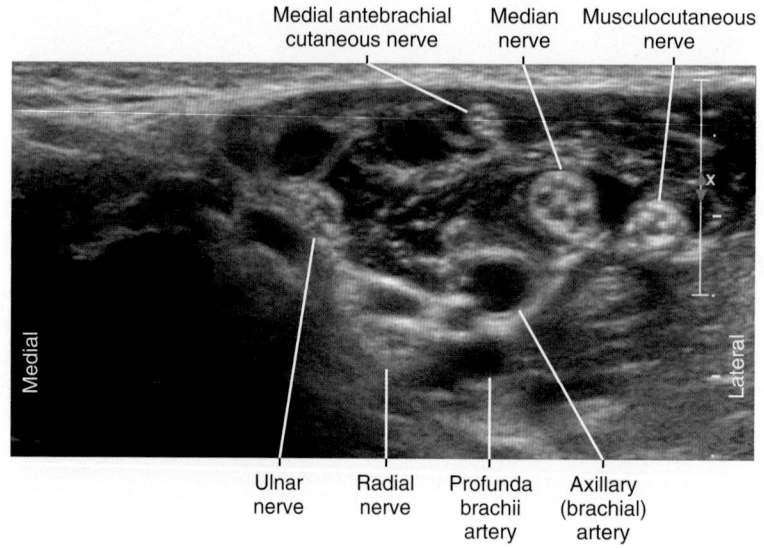

FIGURE 33.12 Short-axis view of the medial antebrachial cutaneous nerve after axillary block. After injection, this small nerve can often be identified between the median and ulnar nerves toward the skin surface. Visible separation of the wall-hugging nerves from the axillary artery ensures successful axillary block.

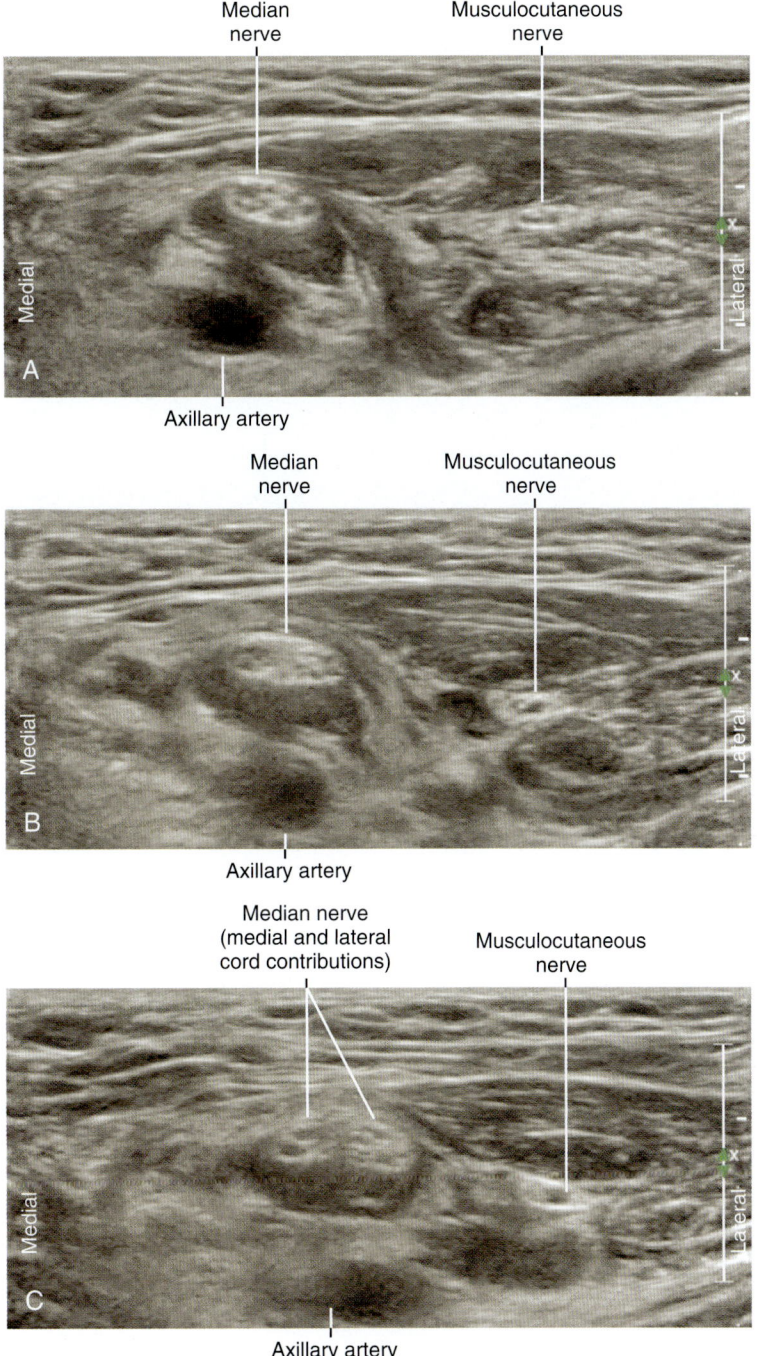

FIGURE 33.13 Median nerve after axillary block in short-axis view from distal (A) and proximal (B and C). The median nerve derives from both the medal and lateral cords, and these contributions can often be identified after successful axillary block because the local anesthetic tracks proximally to provide reverse acoustic contrast to outline the nerve borders.

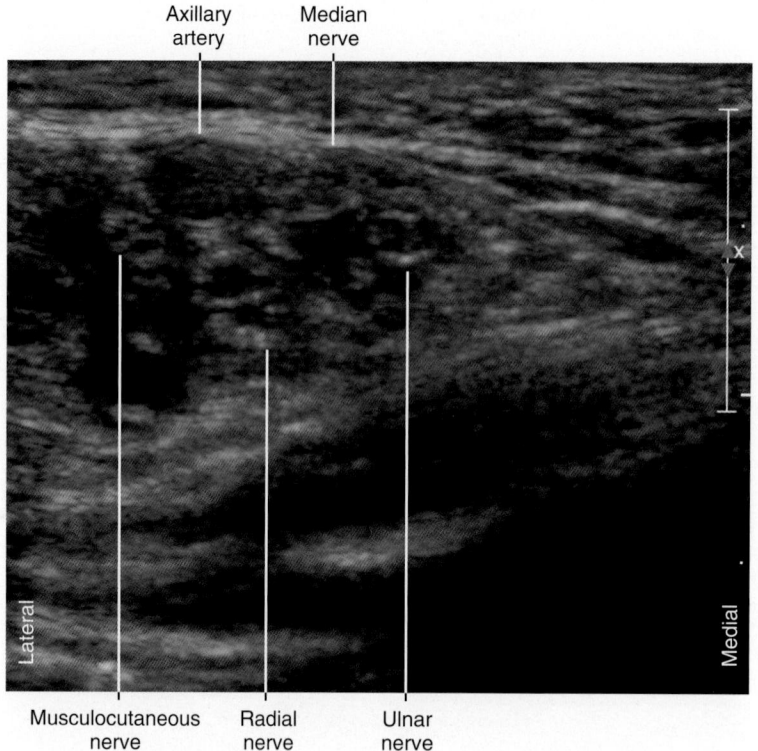

FIGURE 33.14 Short-axis view after axillary block in a young child. The axillary block is a versatile block applicable in many clinical circumstances.

Musculocutaneous Nerve Block

CHAPTER 34

The musculocutaneous nerve is a branch of the lateral cord of the brachial plexus. The nerve innervates all the flexors of the arm at the elbow (biceps brachii, brachialis, and coracobrachialis muscles). The nerve also gives rise to the lateral cutaneous nerve of the forearm.

The musculocutaneous nerve usually passes through the coracobrachialis muscle. The musculocutaneous nerve exits the coracobrachialis between its two parts and the short head of the biceps, forming a triangle with these three muscular components.[1] The musculocutaneous nerve lies between the biceps and the brachialis more distally.

SUGGESTED TECHNIQUE

Ultrasound imaging of the musculocutaneous nerve in the axilla can be used to facilitate regional block.[2] This directly addresses one of the primary weaknesses of traditional axillary block.

The lateral course of the nerve and its changes in shape as it passes through the coracobrachialis muscle are characteristic features that allow ultrasound identification of the nerve.[3] The nerve typically has a flat shape within the coracobrachialis muscle; therefore, this is a desirable location for regional block. The relatively high surface area–to–volume ratio may improve onset kinetics of the block.

The block is performed with the arm abducted, and the needle approaches from the lateral side of the arm. The choices of transducer and block needle are not critical. The needle tip is positioned at the lateral corner of the musculocutaneous nerve within the fascial plane of the coracobrachialis muscle that contains the nerve in the axilla.

The lateral cutaneous branch of the musculocutaneous nerve can be more selectively blocked distal to the nerve exit from the coracobrachialis muscle. The point of exit is usually easy to identify, because the nerve has a triangular shape in that location. Blockade of the more proximal motor fibers of the musculocutaneous nerve is unlikely with this approach. However, the nerve to the biceps brachii continues for about 4 cm after the exit from the coracobrachialis before branching off.[4]

The estimated incidence of pass-over musculocutaneous nerve (musculocutaneous nerve passes over the coracobrachialis muscle rather than through it) ranges from 8% to 30%.[5] This usually does not present a problem, because the nerve can be directly imaged.

Fusion of the median nerve and musculocutaneous nerve is another common anomaly (a low-lying lateral cord). In these fusion products, the median contribution is typically larger and more superficial than the musculocutaneous contribution.[6] Small muscular branches can sometimes be identified that course medial to lateral from the musculocutaneous contribution.

In some patients, the lateral cutaneous nerve of the forearm extends to the dorsal aspect of the thumb (musculocutaneous dominance of the dorsum of the hand). Local anesthetic infiltration through the anatomic snuffbox blocks both superficial radial and musculocutaneous contributions to the dorsum of the hand. Alternatively, the lateral cutaneous nerve of the forearm can be blocked lateral to the biceps tendon at the antecubital fossa.[7]

KEY POINTS

Musculocutaneous Nerve Block	The Essentials
Anatomy	The MCN usually has a lateral course through the CBr.
	The MCN has a flat shape within the CBr.
	The MCN becomes triangular in shape where it exits the CBr.
	The MCN is about 2.5 mm in diameter.
Image orientation	The MCN lies lateral to the axillary artery.
Positioning	Arm supinated and abducted
Operator	Standing on lateral (cephalad) side of armboard (for laptop system)
	At the side of the patient (for system with movable display)
Display	Across the armboard (for laptop system)
	Across the table (for system with movable display)
Transducer	High-frequency linear, 38- to 50-mm footprint
Initial depth setting	25 mm
Needle	21–22 gauge, 50–70 mm in length
Anatomic location	Begin by scanning in the proximal axilla.
	Slide distally to observe MCN moving away from AA.
Approach	SAX view of MCN, in-plane from lateral to medial.
	Place the needle tip at lateral corner of MCN within CBr.
Sonographic assessment	The injection should track along the MCN within CBr.
Anatomic variation	Pass-over MCN (8%–30%)
	The MCN can travel over the CBr rather than through it.
	MCN-median fusion (5%–10%)
	The MCN can be fused with the median nerve in the axilla.
	This is sometimes referred to as a low-lying lateral cord.

AA, Axillary artery; *CBr*, coracobrachialis muscle; *MCN*, musculocutaneous nerve; *SAX*, short axis.

References

1. Tagliafico AS, Michaud J, Marchetti A, et al. US imaging of the musculocutaneous nerve. *Skeletal Radiol*. 2011;40(5):609–616. [Epub 2010, Oct 8].
2. Spence BC, Sites BD, Beach ML. Ultrasound-guided musculocutaneous nerve block: a description of a novel technique. *Reg Anesth Pain Med*. 2005;30:198–201.
3. Schafhalter-Zoppoth I, Gray AT. The musculocutaneous nerve: ultrasound appearance for peripheral nerve block. *Reg Anesth Pain Med*. 2005;30:385–390.
4. Macchi V, Tiengo C, Porzionato A, et al. Musculocutaneous nerve: histotopographic study and clinical implications. *Clin Anat*. 2007;20:400–406.
5. Remerand F, Laulan J, Couvret C, et al. Is the musculocutaneous nerve really in the coracobrachialis muscle when performing an axillary block? An ultrasound study. *Anesth Analg*. 2010;110:1729–1734.
6. Orebaugh SL, Pennington S. Variant location of the musculocutaneous nerve during axillary nerve block. *J Clin Anesth*. 2006;18:541–544.
7. Hasenkam CS, Hoy GA, Soeding PF. Sensory distribution of the lateral cutaneous nerve of forearm after ultrasound-guided block: potential implications for thumb-base surgery. *Reg Anesth Pain Med*. 2017;42:478–482.

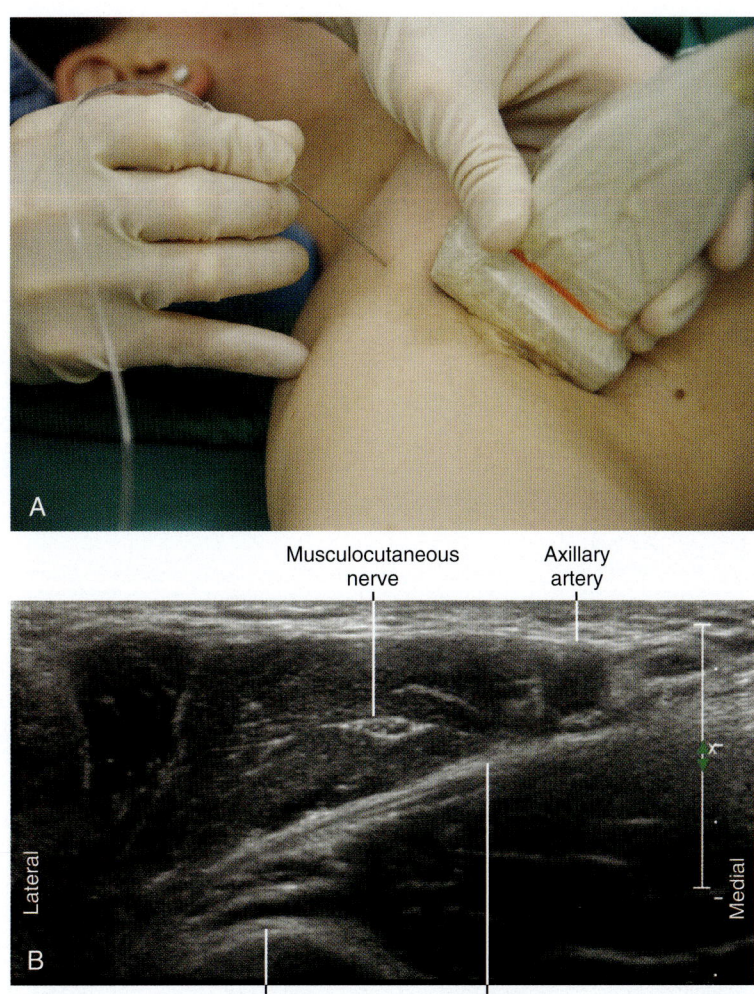

FIGURE 34.1 External photograph showing the approach to musculocutaneous nerve block in the axilla (A). An in-plane approach from the lateral aspect of the forearm is shown. The corresponding sonogram before needle placement is shown (B).

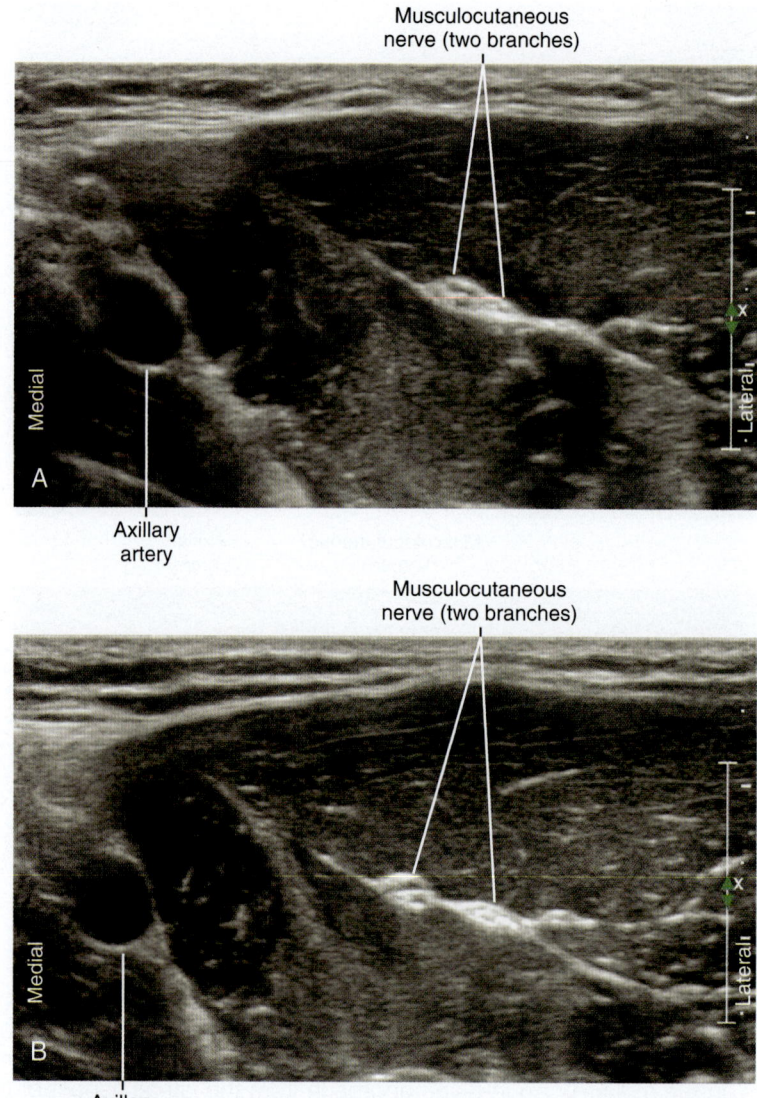

FIGURE 34.2 Division of the musculocutaneous nerve into anterior and posterior branches in the distal arm. Sonograms are shown proximal (A) and distal (B) to the division. Musculocutaneous nerve blocks are usually performed proximally for more complete anesthesia.

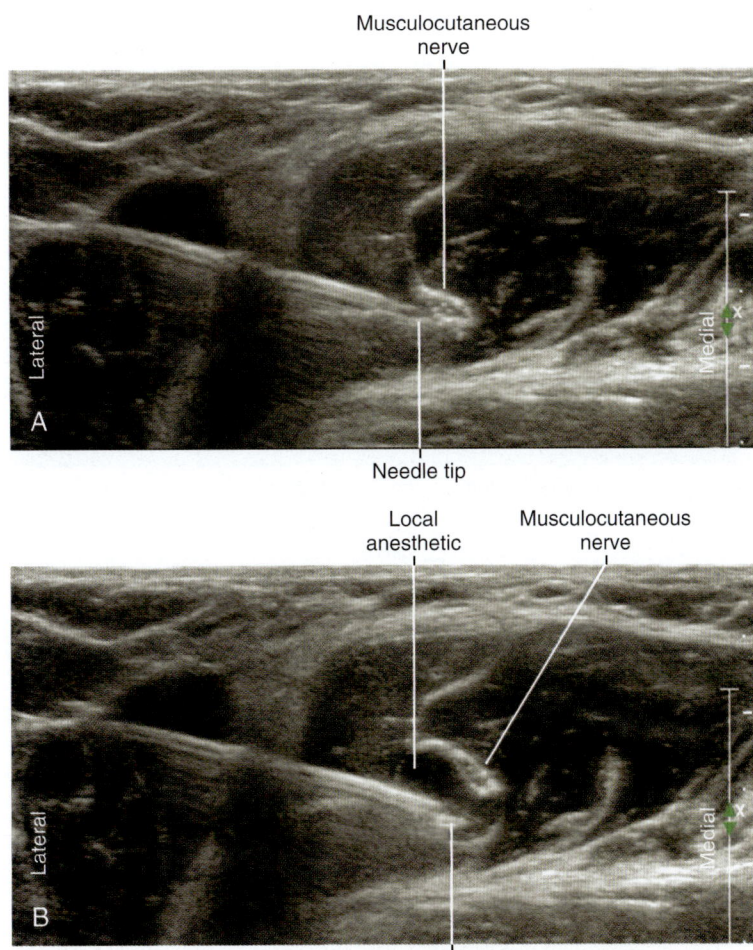

FIGURE 34.3 Image sequence showing musculocutaneous nerve block in the axilla. An in-plane approach is demonstrated where the needle tip is placed under the lateral aspect of the musculocutaneous nerve (A). After injection, local anesthetic is distributed around the musculocutaneous nerve (B).

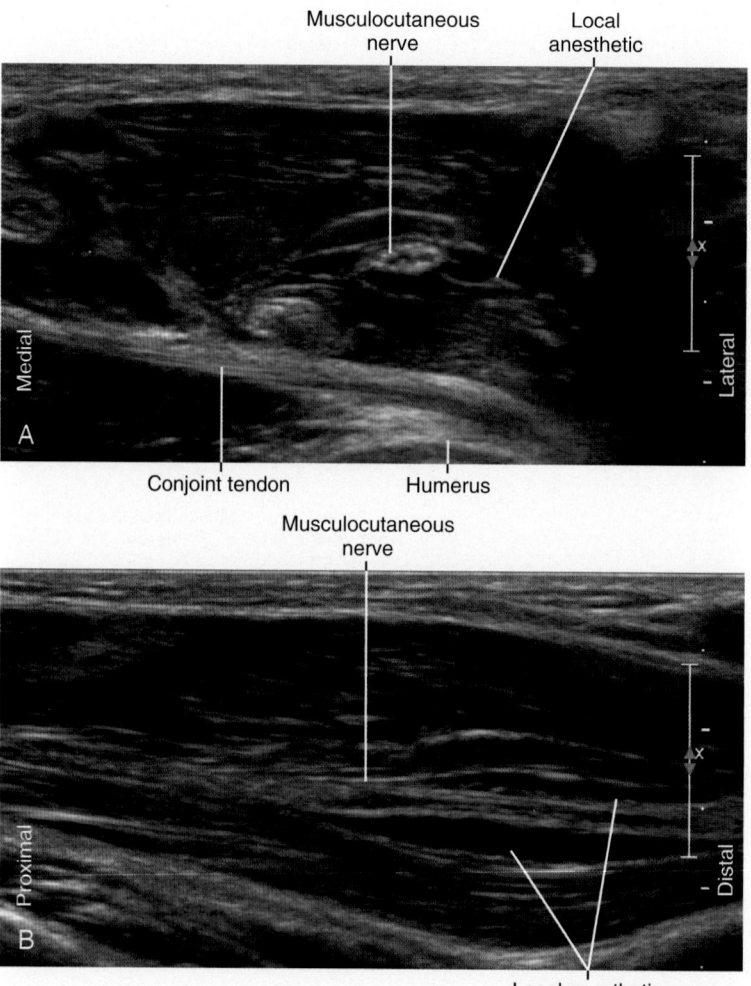

FIGURE 34.4 Distribution of local anesthetic after musculocutaneous nerve block in the axilla. After injection, local anesthetic is distributed around the musculocutaneous nerve as seen in short-axis view (A) and tracks along the nerve as seen in long-axis view (B).

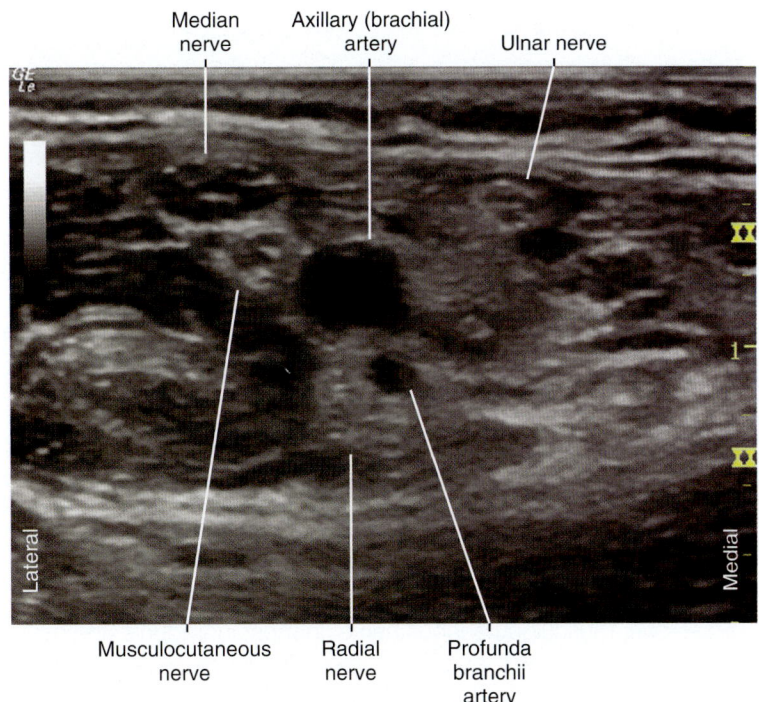

FIGURE 34.5 Musculocutaneous-median nerve fusion (low-lying lateral cord). In this variation, the two nerves are together in the axilla. Muscular and cutaneous branches may split off directly from the fusion product more distally in the arm.

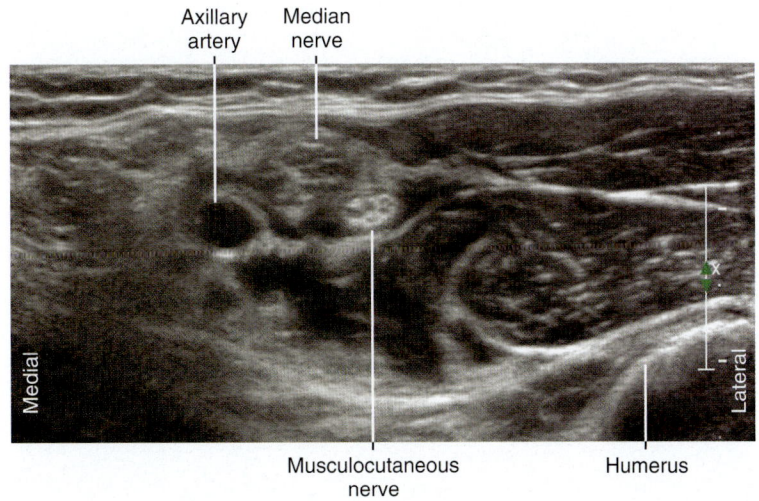

FIGURE 34.6 Musculocutaneous-median nerve fusion (low-lying lateral cord). After regional block, local anesthetic separates this fusion product.

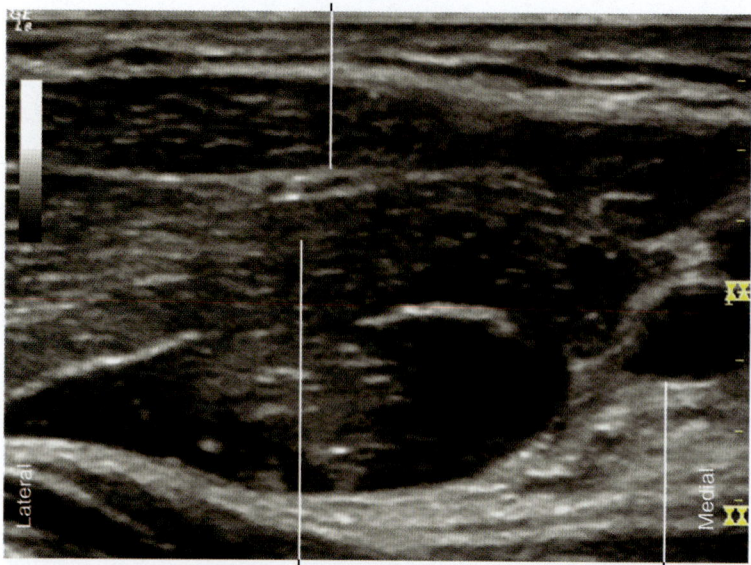

FIGURE 34.7 Pass-over musculocutaneous nerve. In most individuals, the musculocutaneous nerve passes through the coracobrachialis muscle. However, in some individuals, the musculocutaneous nerve passes over the muscle. Under most circumstances, the nerve can be directly imaged, thereby facilitating regional block.

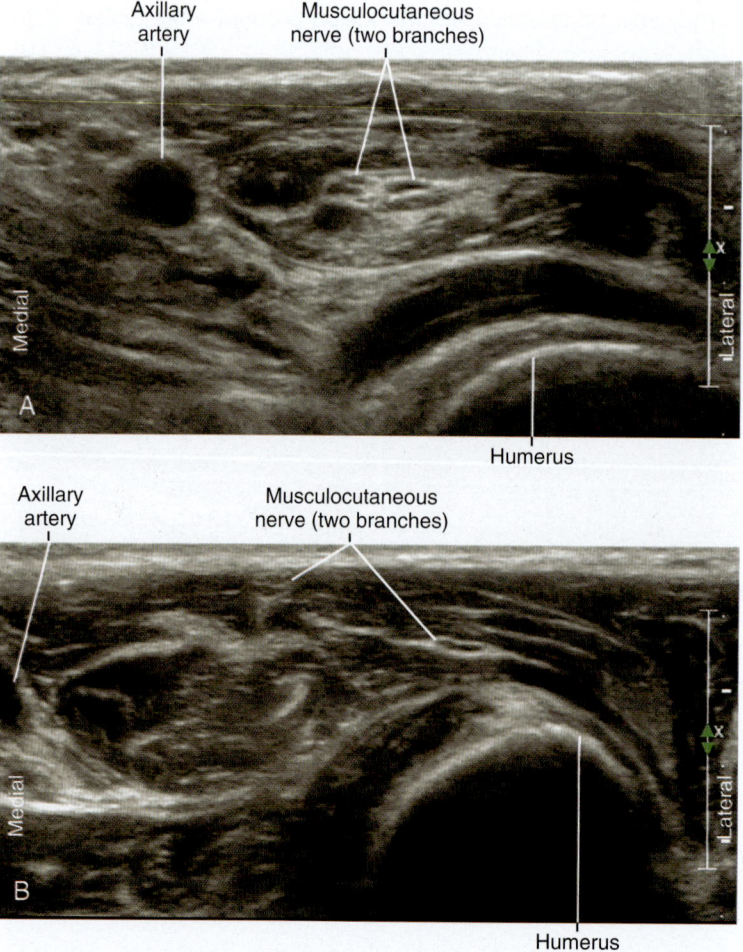

FIGURE 34.8 In some individuals, a large cutaneous branch of the musculocutaneous nerve can be identified that travels to the skin of the lateral arm (A and B). When present, this branch may be important for arm tourniquet tolerance.

Forearm Blocks

CHAPTER 35

See Video 35.1 on ExpertConsult.com.

Peripheral blocks of terminal branches of the brachial plexus (median, radial, and ulnar nerves) can offer benefits in terms of patient disposition.[1,2] These procedures can be used to prevent and treat postoperative pain. Ultrasound-guided nerve blocks of the radial, ulnar, and median nerves are also useful in the emergency department to provide anesthesia for hand procedures.[3]

Forearm blocks are a sonographic approach similar to traditional wrist block. These ultrasound-guided blocks are typically performed in the mid-forearm (between the bulk of the flexor muscles and the flexor tendons that form near the wrist). Because forearm blocks anesthetize the proximal palmar and dorsal cutaneous nerves of the hand, these blocks are usually more complete than wrist blocks are. Another advantage of using ultrasound guidance is that puncture of adjacent blood vessels and tendons should be less likely. A small-footprint linear transducer is used for these relatively shallow blocks.

Forearm blocks provide sensory anesthesia of the hand and block the intrinsic muscles of the hand. However, the extrinsic muscles (the more proximal branches to the flexors and extensors of the digits) are spared, and therefore some hand motion is possible. Forearm blocks are useful for trigger finger release when some active motion is desired and for other minor surgical procedures of the hand that do not require an arm tourniquet. Because the flexors and extensors of the arm at the elbow are spared, no arm sling is necessary following forearm blocks.

References

1. Gebhard RE, Al-Samsam T, Greger J, Khan A, Chelly JE. Distal nerve blocks at the wrist for outpatient carpal tunnel surgery offer intraoperative cardiovascular stability and reduce discharge time. *Anesth Analg.* 2002;95:351–355.
2. Gray AT, Schafhalter-Zoppoth I. Ultrasound guidance for ulnar nerve block in the forearm. *Reg Anesth Pain Med.* 2003;28:335–339.
3. Liebmann O, Price D, Mills C, et al. Feasibility of forearm ultrasonography guided nerve blocks of the radial, ulnar, and median nerves for hand procedures in the emergency department. *Ann Emerg Med.* 2006;48:558–562.

Radial Nerve Block

The radial nerve is a branch of the posterior cord of the brachial plexus. It provides motor innervation to the extensor-supinator group of muscles. Of the three nerves that surround the axillary artery in the axilla (median, radial, and ulnar), the radial nerve is the most difficult to visualize and access with the block needle.[1]

The radial nerve has branches all along its course, including the posterior cutaneous branch of the forearm (sensory), deep radial nerve (motor), and superficial radial nerve (sensory).

The posterior cutaneous branch of the forearm diverges from the radial nerve about 16 cm proximal to the lateral epicondyle of the humerus.[2] This branch provides sensation to both the elbow joint and posterior forearm.

The radial nerve divides into its superficial and deep branches in the antecubital fossa over the lateral epicondyle of the humerus. The radial nerve often has a "snake-eyes" appearance before this separation. The superficial radial nerve is slightly medial to the deep radial nerve within a fascial plane in this location. The deep radial nerve can be easily viewed crossing through the supinator muscle by sliding the transducer back and forth just distal to the lateral epicondyle with the arm pronated. This is a useful starting point to help find the common radial nerve and its superficial branch, which can be more difficult to visualize.

The superficial radial nerve joins the lateral side of the radial artery in the middle third of the forearm. The superficial radial nerve travels the lateral forearm just deep to the brachioradialis muscle. Most patients have radial dominance of sensation of the dorsal aspect of the hand, as primarily supplied by the superficial branch of the radial nerve.[3] The superficial radial nerve (cross-sectional area 2.7 mm^2)[4] is substantially smaller than the median and ulnar nerves.

SUGGESTED TECHNIQUE

The superficial radial nerve can be blocked in the proximal third of the forearm before it joins the lateral side of the radial artery and divides into smaller branches.[5,6] In this location the superficial radial nerve is covered by the brachioradialis as it travels over the supinator muscle. An in-plane approach from the lateral side of the forearm works well with the block needle tip placed under the nerve. The arm is pronated to facilitate placement of the needle. This approach to superficial radial nerve block can be used for single shot and catheter techniques.[7] Similarly, the radial nerve can be blocked slightly more proximally in the antecubital fossa before the nerve divides into superficial (sensory) and deep (motor) branches.

The radial nerve can also be blocked in the distal arm after the nerve emerges from the spiral groove of the humerus. The radial nerve lies within the fascia that divides the brachioradialis from the underlying brachialis muscle. The arm is pronated and elevated to facilitate imaging of the nerve in the posterolateral arm for the block procedure. The radial nerve is round or oval in this location. The injection targets the fascial plane between the brachialis (deep) and brachioradialis (superficial). The posterior cutaneous nerve of the forearm lies superficial and posterior to the radial nerve above the elbow, so injection on pullback of the needle is advised to ensure complete block.

The radial nerve emerges from the spiral groove where the lateral intermuscular septum inserts on the humerus. This insertion creates the lateral supracondylar ridge along the bone. Because the lateral intermuscular septum separates the brachioradialis from the triceps, the ridge will point behind to the radial nerve. The radial nerve travels anteriorly after emerging from the spiral groove of the humerus. The nerve travels within the fascia between the brachialis and brachioradialis muscles.

NEUROLOGIC ASSESSMENT

Sensory block of the radial nerve can be tested at the dorsal web between the index finger and thumb. Motor block of the deep radial nerve results in wrist drop.

KEY POINTS

Superficial Radial Nerve Block	The Essential Points
Anatomy	The brachioradialis muscle covers the SRN in the forearm
Image orientation	The SRN lies lateral to the RA
Positioning	Arm pronated
Operator	Standing on the lateral (cephalad) side of the arm board
Display	Across the arm board
Transducer	High-frequency linear, 23- to 38-mm footprint
Initial depth setting	25 mm
Needle	25 gauge, 38 mm in length
Anatomic location	Proximal third of the forearm
Approach	SAX view of SRN, in-plane from lateral to medial
	Place the needle tip through BR adjacent to the SRN
	Local anesthetic should layer under the BR and around the SRN
Sonographic assessment	The injection should track along the SRN
Anatomic variation	Proximal branching of SRN is possible

BR, Brachioradialis muscle; *RA*, radial artery; *SAX*, short axis; *SRN*, superficial radial nerve.

Clinical Pearls

- The superficial radial nerve supplies the majority of the dorsum of the hand in most individuals.
- The superficial radial nerve travels in the lateral forearm. The nerve lies deep to the brachioradialis muscle, lateral to the radial artery, and underneath the cephalic vein.
- On average, the superficial radial nerve first branches 5 cm proximal to the radial styloid, but with variability.
- The superficial radial nerve joins the radial artery in the proximal third of the forearm, travels with the radial artery in the mid-forearm, and leaves the radial artery in the distal third of the forearm (the rule of thirds).

References

1. Chan VW, Perlas A, McCartney CJ, Brull R, Xu D, Abbas S. Ultrasound guidance improves success rate of axillary brachial plexus block. *Can J Anaesth*. 2007;54:176–182.
2. MacAvoy MC, Rust SS, Green DP. Anatomy of the posterior antebrachial cutaneous nerve: practical information for the surgeon operating on the lateral aspect of the elbow. *J Hand Surg Am*. 2006;31:908–911.
3. Auerbach DM, Collins ED, Kunkle KL, Monsanto EH. The radial sensory nerve. An anatomic study. *Clin Orthop Relat Res*. 1994;308:241–249.
4. Meng S, Tinhofer I, Weninger WJ, Grisold W. Anatomical and ultrasound correlation of the superficial branch of the radial nerve. *Muscle Nerve*. 2014;50(6):939–942.
5. Ikiz ZA, Ucerler H. Anatomic characteristics and clinical importance of the superficial branch of the radial nerve. *Surg Radiol Anat*. 2004;26:453–458.
6. Visser LH. High-resolution sonography of the superficial radial nerve with two case reports. *Muscle Nerve*. 2009;39(3):392–395.
7. Henshaw DS, Kittner SL, Jaffe JD. Ultrasound-guided continuous superficial radial nerve block for complex regional pain syndrome. *J Pain Palliat Care Pharmacother*. 2016;30:118–123.

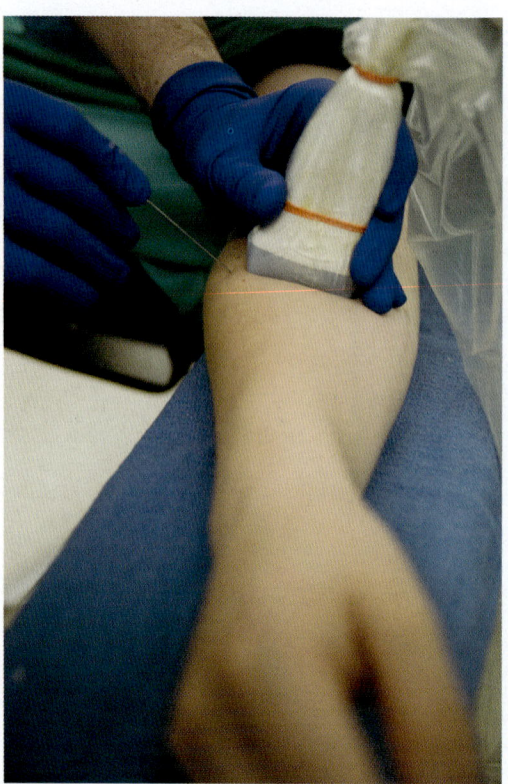

FIGURE 36.1 External photograph showing the approach to superficial radial nerve block in the proximal forearm. An in-plane approach from the lateral aspect of the forearm is shown.

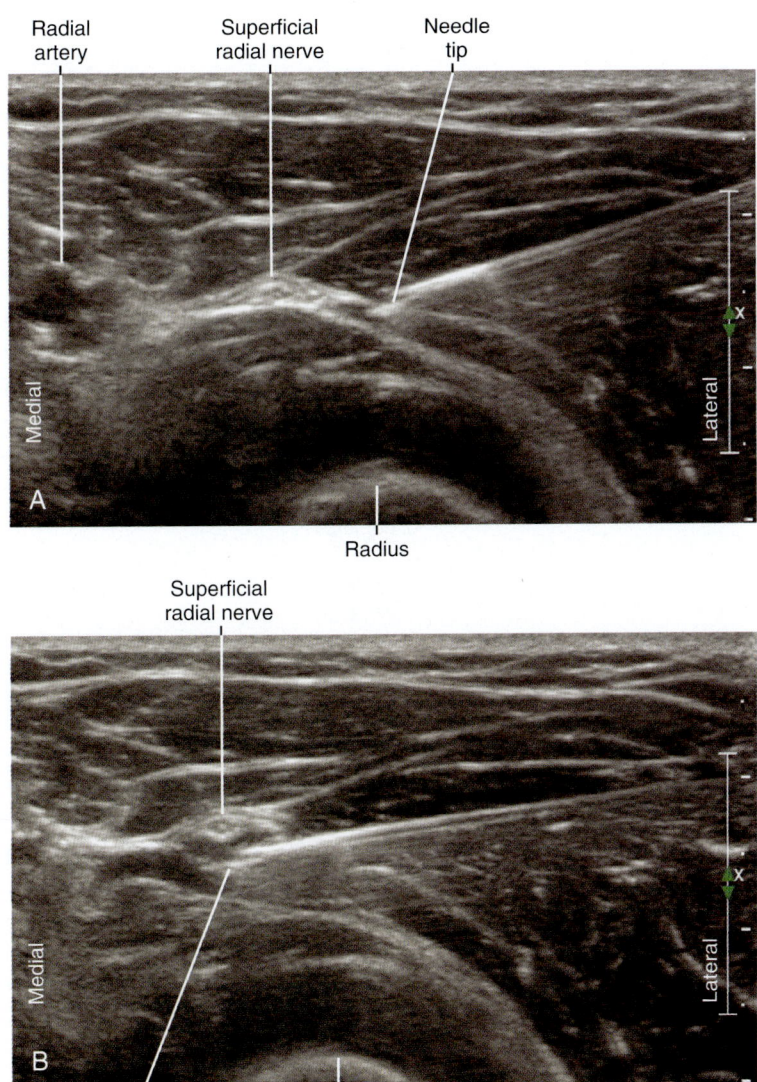

FIGURE 36.2 Image sequence showing a superficial radial nerve block in the forearm. An in-plane approach is demonstrated where the needle tip is placed under the superficial radial nerve (A). After injection, local anesthetic is distributed around the superficial radial nerve, resulting in sensory block of the dorsum of the hand (B).

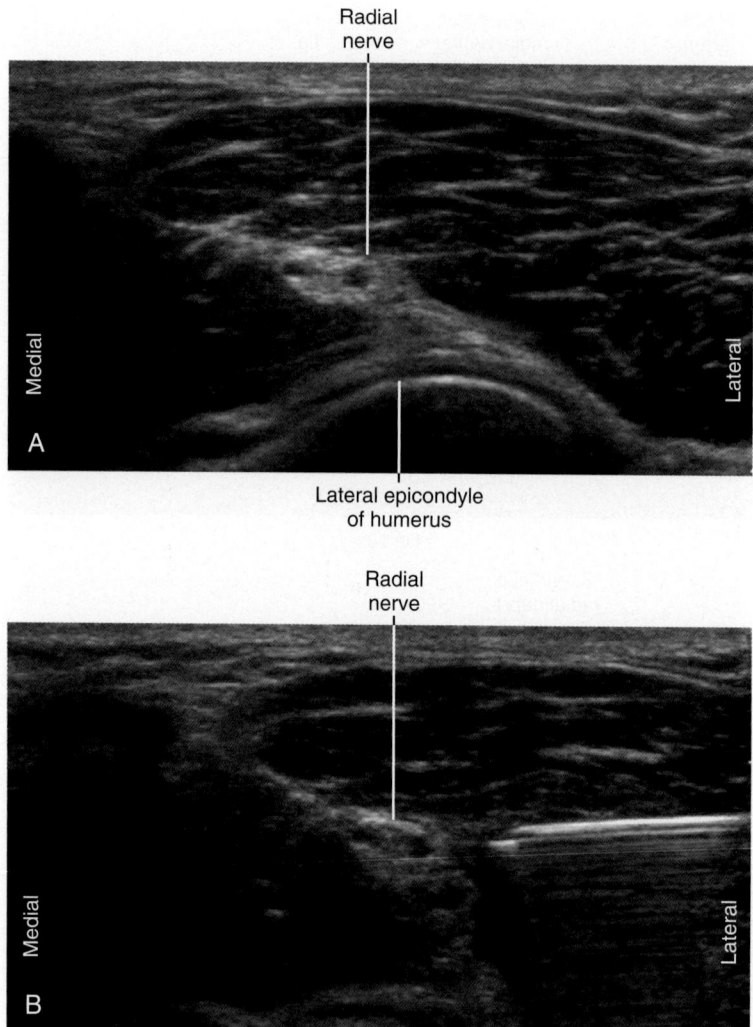

FIGURE 36.3 Snake-eyes appearance of the radial nerve in the antecubital fossa (A). The snake-eyes appearance consists of both the superficial (sensory) and deep (motor) branches before the deep branch dives through the supinator muscle. In-plane approach to radial nerve block from the lateral aspect of the arm (B). If the radial nerve is blocked in this location, the motor block will result in wrist drop.

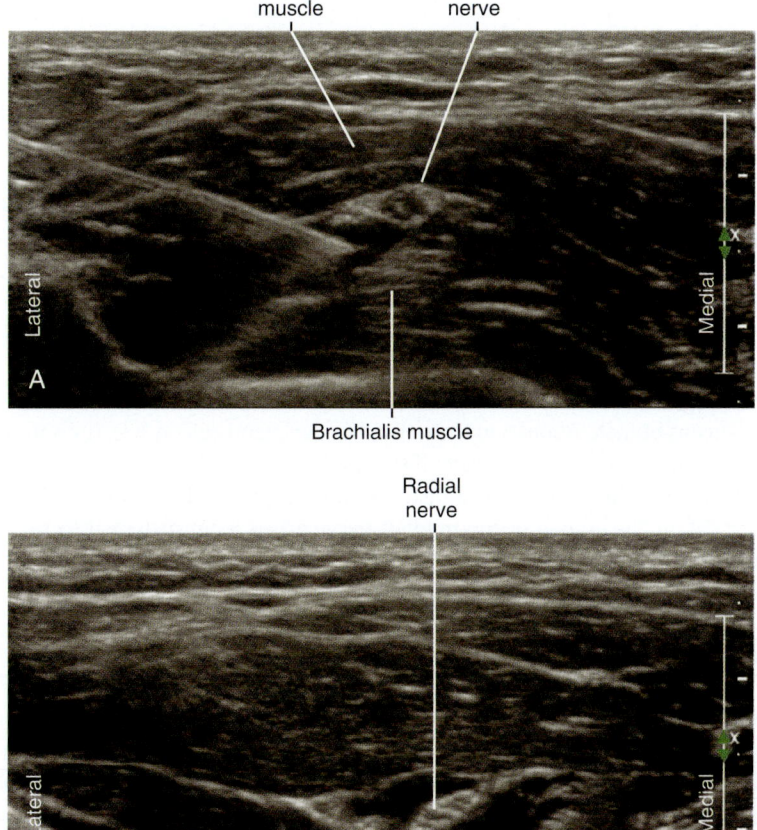

FIGURE 36.4 Short-axis view of the radial nerve in the distal arm between the spiral groove and the lateral epicondyle of the humerus showing the block needle in place (A). The brachialis muscle separates the radial nerve from the underlying bone. The brachioradialis muscle covers the radial nerve. After injection, local anesthetic is seen to surround the radial nerve (B). Radial nerve block in this location results in both sensory and motor block.

CHAPTER 37

Median Nerve Block

The median nerve is a branch of the medial and lateral cords of the brachial plexus. The median nerve provides most of the sensory innervation to the palm of the hand. It is part of the neurovascular bundle in the axilla and continues with the brachial artery on its medial side proximal to the elbow.

In the forearm, the median nerve lies between the flexor digitorum profundus and the flexor digitorum superficialis muscles. This is where the median nerve is usually brightest on ultrasound scans.

The two largest branches of the median nerve are the anterior interosseous nerve and the palmar cutaneous branch. About 5 to 8 cm distal to the lateral epicondyle, the anterior interosseous nerve (a purely motor nerve) branches off the median nerve. It travels deep to the median nerve between the flexor pollicis longus and flexor digitorum profundus (both of which it innervates). The palmar cutaneous branch of the median nerve arises 5 cm proximal to the wrist crease on the radial side of the nerve.[1,2]

SUGGESTED TECHNIQUE

With ultrasound, the median nerve is usually blocked in the mid-forearm because it is echobright without adjacent tendons. This location is also chosen because it is away from the carpal tunnel, proximal to the palmar cutaneous branch takeoff, but distal to the anterior interosseous motor branch takeoff. In the mid-forearm, the median nerve lies within the fascial plane between the flexor digitorum superficialis and profundus, which provides a means for targeting drug injections without nerve contact. The block is performed on the volar side of the forearm with the arm supinated. Both in-plane and out-of-plane approaches can be used for these blocks. A steep in-plane approach to the median nerve from the lateral aspect of the forearm avoids the radial artery and the superficial radial nerve.

The hand should be relaxed so that the median nerve is mobile and not under tension. Wrist hyperextension stretches the median nerve and can lead to impairment of nerve function if prolonged. Therefore, median nerve block should be performed with the wrist in a neutral position.

Near the elbow, the median nerve lies medial to the brachial artery. Median nerve block proximal to the elbow is often used in the recovery room following surgery because of the presence of surgical dressings covering the forearm. If this approach is used, care must be taken to avoid puncturing the brachial artery because this can result in median epineurial hematoma.[3,4]

Although the median artery normally evolutes during development, persistent median artery can be detected with high-resolution ultrasound in about 25% of asymptomatic individuals.[5] Persistent median artery is sometimes associated with high division or bifid median nerve, in which cases the artery is often in the middle of the divided nerve.[6] When the persistent median artery is eccentrically located with respect to the nerve, the block should target the nonarterial side of the nerve to avoid intraneural hematoma.

Ultrasound guidance can be useful for placement of indwelling median nerve catheters to provide prolonged pain relief following hand surgery.[7]

NEUROLOGIC ASSESSMENT

Sensory block of the median nerve can be tested at the palmar web near the base of the index finger. Motor block of the opponens pollicis can be tested by having the patient touch the base of the small finger with the thumb against resistance. Alternatively, the abductor pollicis brevis can be tested.

KEY POINTS

Median Nerve Block	The Essential Points
Anatomy	The MN lies between the FDS and FDP in the mid-forearm. The MN is about 3 mm in diameter.
Positioning	Arm supinated
Operator	Standing on the lateral (cephalad) side of the arm board
Display	Across the arm board Transducer, high-frequency linear, 23- to 38-mm footprint
Initial depth setting	25 mm
Needle	25 gauge, 38 mm in length
Anatomic location	Mid-forearm on the volar surface
Approach	SAX view of MN, in-plane from lateral to medial Place the needle tip between the FDS and FDP at the lateral corner of the MN.
Sonographic assessment	The injection should track distally along the MN to its palmar cutaneous branch.
Anatomic variation	PMA (25%) Bifid median nerve (5%) These two anomalies are associated with each other. A PMA can divide a bifid median nerve.

FDP, Flexor digitorum profundus muscle; *FDS*, flexor digitorum superficialis muscle; *MN*, median nerve; *PMA*, persistent median artery; *SAX*, short axis.

Clinical Pearls

- The median nerve provides most of the sensory innervation to the palm of the hand.
- The median nerve lies in the center of the forearm and lies within the fascia separating the flexor digitorum superficialis and flexor digitorum profundus muscles.
- Median nerve block is typically performed distal to the bulk of the flexor muscles in the forearm.
- Bifid median nerve is a common anatomic variation and may require two injections for complete block. Bifid median nerves are often divided by a persistent median artery.

References

1. Bezerra AJ, Carvalho VC, Nucci A. An anatomical study of the palmar cutaneous branch of the median nerve. *Surg Radiol Anat*. 1986;8:183–188.
2. Tagliafico A, Pugliese F, Bianchi S, et al. High-resolution sonography of the palmar cutaneous branch of the median nerve. *AJR Am J Roentgenol*. 2008;191:107–114.
3. Macon WL 4th, Futrell JW. Median-nerve neuropathy after percutaneous puncture of the brachial artery in patients receiving anticoagulants. *N Engl J Med*. 1973;288:1396.
4. Chuang YM, Luo CB, Chou YH, et al. Sonographic diagnosis and treatment of a median nerve epineural hematoma caused by brachial artery catheterization. *J Ultrasound Med*. 2002;21:705–708.
5. Gassner EM, Schocke M, Peer S, Schwabegger A, Jaschke W, Bodner G. Persistent median artery in the carpal tunnel: color Doppler ultrasonographic findings. *J Ultrasound Med*. 2002;21:455–461.
6. Klauser AS, Halpern EJ, Faschingbauer R, et al. Bifid median nerve in carpal tunnel syndrome: assessment with US cross-sectional area measurement. *Radiology*. 2011;259(3):808–815.
7. Maxwell BG, Hansen JA, Talley J, et al. Ultrasound-guided continuous median nerve block to facilitate intensive hand rehabilitation. *Clin J Pain*. 2013;29(1):86–88.

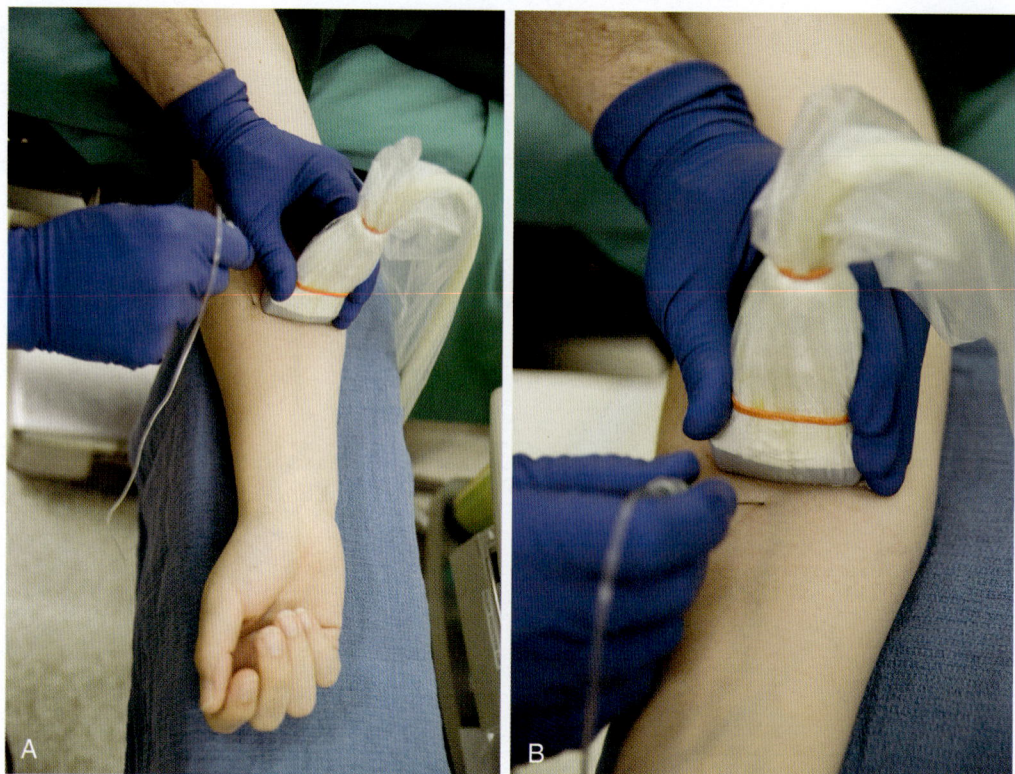

FIGURE 37.1 External photograph showing the in-plane (A) and out-of-plane (B) approaches to median nerve block in the forearm. For the in-plane technique, the needle approaches from the lateral aspect of the forearm. For the out-of-plane technique, the needle approaches from distal to proximal.

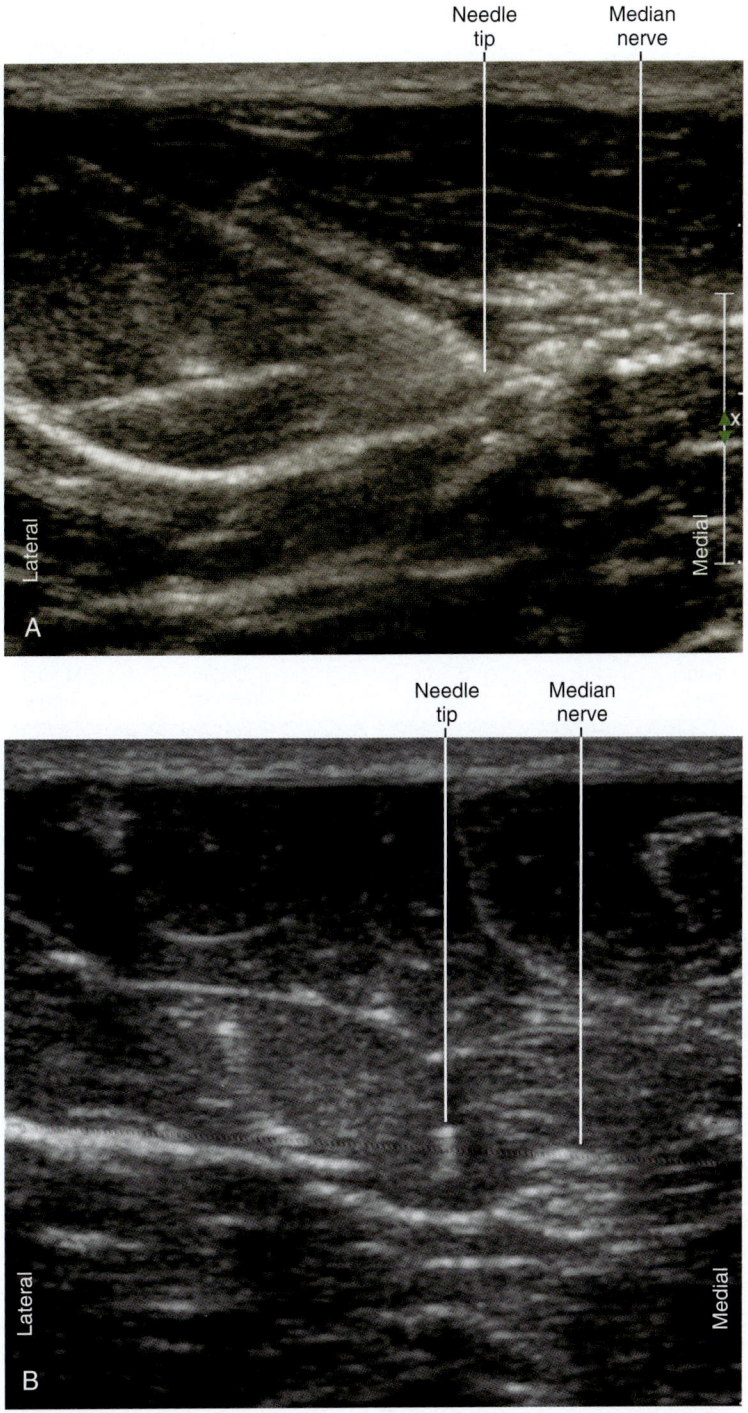

FIGURE 37.2 Sonograms illustrating the in-plane (A) and out-of-plane (B) approaches to median nerve block.

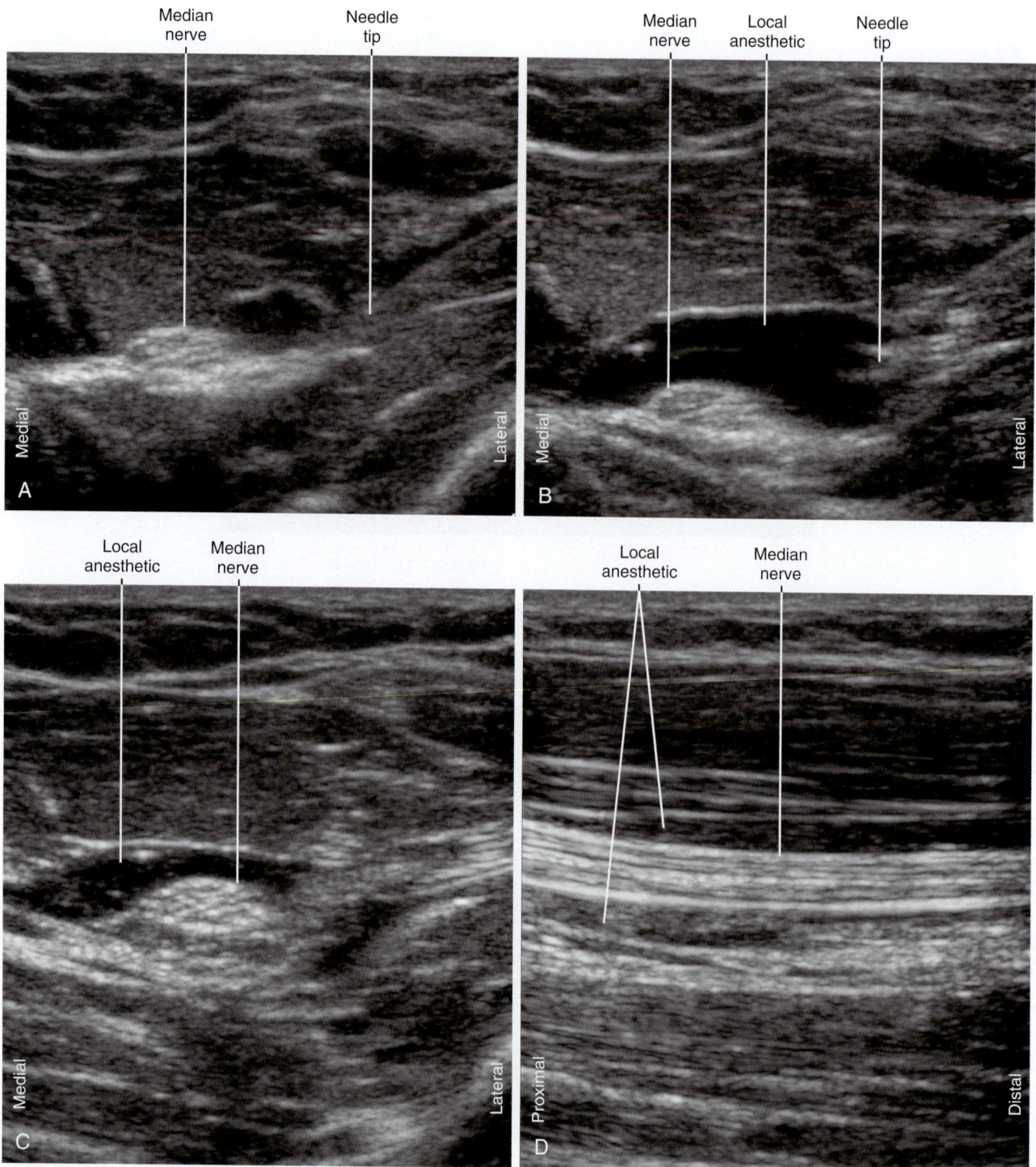

FIGURE 37.3 Image sequence showing median nerve block in the forearm. An in-plane approach is demonstrated whereby the needle tip is placed between the flexor digitorum superficialis and profundus at the lateral corner of the median nerve (A and B). Because the local anesthetic is primarily distributed over the surface of the nerve, additional local anesthetic is then deposited underneath the nerve. After completing the injection, local anesthetic is distributed around the median nerve (C) and tracks along the nerve (D).

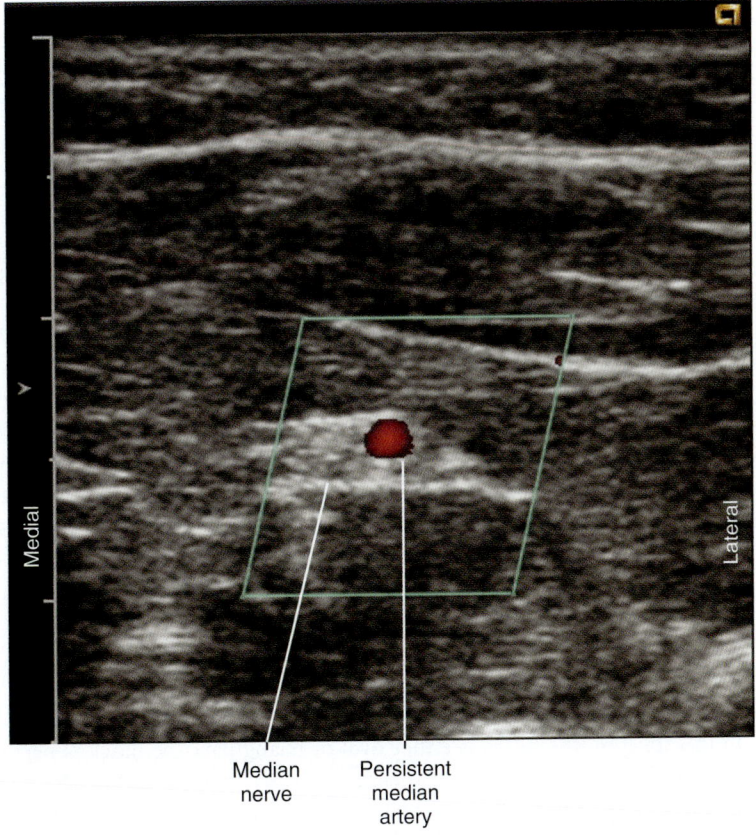

Median nerve   Persistent median artery

FIGURE 37.4 A relatively common anatomic variant is persistent median artery. In this variation the persistent median artery lies within the same connective tissue bundle as the median nerve and can divide it into two parts. When this condition is identified, the needle tip is placed on the side of the nerve away from the artery.

CHAPTER 38

Ulnar Nerve Block

The ulnar nerve is a branch of the medial cord of the brachial plexus. The ulnar nerve provides sensation of the dorsal and palmar sides of the ulnar aspect of the hand (including the fifth digit and the ulnar side of the fourth digit). It leaves the neurovascular bundle in the axilla to travel through the cubital tunnel. In the forearm it joins the ulnar artery on its medial side. The ulnar nerve usually lies between the ulnar artery and the flexor carpi ulnaris (FCU) tendon in the forearm. The palmar cutaneous branch of the ulnar nerve arises in the middle of the forearm. The dorsal cutaneous (DCUN) branch leaves the ulnar nerve in the forearm proximal to the wrist.[1,2] The DCUN takes off medially underneath the FCU about 55 mm proximal to the ulnar styloid process.[3] At the level of the hamate, the ulnar nerve divides into its superficial sensory branch and its deep motor branch. Identification of the ulnar nerve and its dorsal and palmar cutaneous branches is possible with ultrasound scanning in the forearm.[4]

SUGGESTED TECHNIQUE

The ulnar nerve is usually blocked just proximal to its juncture with the ulnar artery in the forearm.[5] In this location the nerve is either oval or triangular. The block is performed with the patient supine and the arm supinated. The needle tip is placed within the fascial plane that connects the ulnar nerve and ulnar artery using an in-plane approach from the lateral side of the forearm. To access this plane with the block needle it is best to puncture the fascia and slowly inject as the needle is pulled back.

A relatively common (3% to 10%) anatomic variant is the superficial ulnar artery, in which the ulnar artery lies superficial to the flexor muscles.[6]

NEUROLOGIC ASSESSMENT

Neurologic assessment of ulnar nerve block includes testing sensation of the ulnar side of the hand. Motor block assessment can be performed by testing the dorsal and palmar interossei functions. These muscles abduct and adduct the fingers, respectively.

KEY POINTS	
Ulnar Nerve Block	**The Essential Points**
Anatomy	The UN lies between the UA and FCU tendon.
	The UN is about 3 mm in diameter.
Image orientation	The UN lies on the ulnar (medial) side of the UA in the forearm.
Positioning	Arm supinated
Operator	Standing on the lateral (cephalad) side of the arm board
Display	Across the arm board
Transducer	High-frequency linear, 23- to 38-mm footprint
Initial depth setting	25 mm
Needle	25 gauge, 38 mm in length
Anatomic location	Mid-forearm, just proximal to where the UN and UA join
Approach	SAX view of UN, in-plane from lateral to medial
	Place the needle tip between the UN and UA at their juncture.

KEY POINTS—CONT'D	
Ulnar Nerve Block	**The Essential Points**
Sonographic assessment	The injection should track distally along the UN to the DCUN.
Anatomic variation	Superficial ulnar artery (3%–10%; when the UA lies superficial to the flexor muscles)
	Absent ulnar artery

DCUN, Dorsal cutaneous branch of the ulnar nerve; *FCU*, flexor carpi ulnaris; *SAX*, short axis; *UA*, ulnar artery; *UN*, ulnar nerve.

Clinical Pearls

- Ulnar nerve block is a more definitive alternative to digital block of the small finger.
- The ulnar nerve lies between the ulnar artery and the central tendon of the flexor carpi ulnaris in 90% of subjects. In the other 10%, the ulnar artery is either absent or lies superficial to the flexor muscles (superficial ulnar artery).
- The ideal needle path is between the ulnar artery and the ulnar nerve, so that the injection separates the two structures by splitting their common fascia.

References

1. Botte MJ, Cohen MS, Lavernia CJ, von Schroeder HP, Gellman H, Zinberg EM. The dorsal branch of the ulnar nerve: an anatomic study. *J Hand Surg Am*. 1990;15:603–607.
2. Grossman JA, Yen L, Rapaport D. The dorsal cutaneous branch of the ulnar nerve: an anatomic clarification with six case reports. *Chir Main*. 1998;17:154–158.
3. Le Corroller T, Bauones S, Acid S, Champsaur P. Anatomical study of the dorsal cutaneous branch of the ulnar nerve using ultrasound. *Eur Radiol*. 2013;23(8):2246–2251.
4. Kim KH, Lee SJ, Park BK, Kim DH. Sonoanatomy of sensory branches of the ulnar nerve below the elbow in healthy subjects. *Muscle Nerve*. 2017 [Epub ahead of print].
5. Gray AT, Schafhalter-Zoppoth I. Ultrasound guidance for ulnar nerve block in the forearm. *Reg Anesth Pain Med*. 2003;28:335–339.
6. Schafhalter-Zoppoth I, Gray AT. Ultrasound-guided ulnar nerve block in the presence of a superficial ulnar artery. *Reg Anesth Pain Med*. 2004;29:297–298.

UPPER EXTREMITY BLOCKS

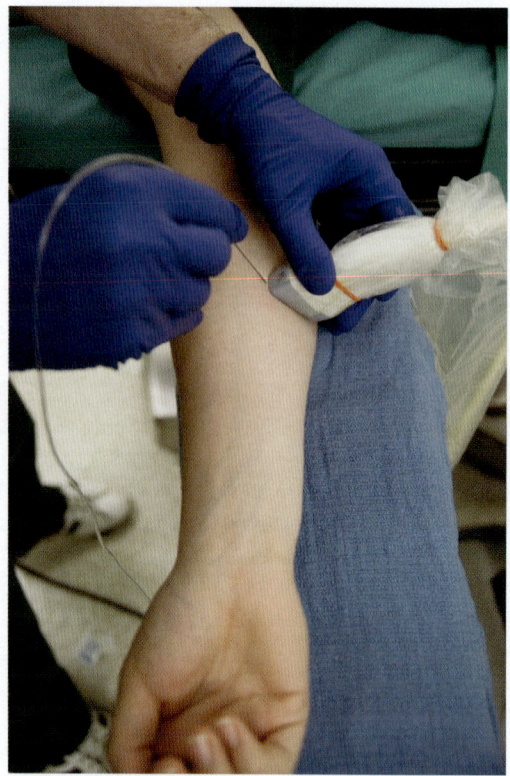

FIGURE 38.1 External photograph showing the approach to ulnar nerve block in the forearm. An in-plane approach from the lateral aspect of the forearm is shown.

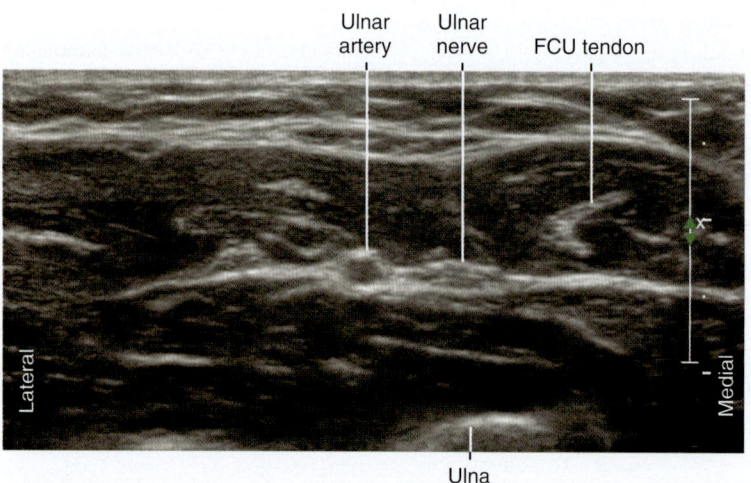

FIGURE 38.2 Short-axis view of the ulnar nerve in the forearm. The flexor carpi ulnaris *(FCU)* tendon and ulnar artery are shown.

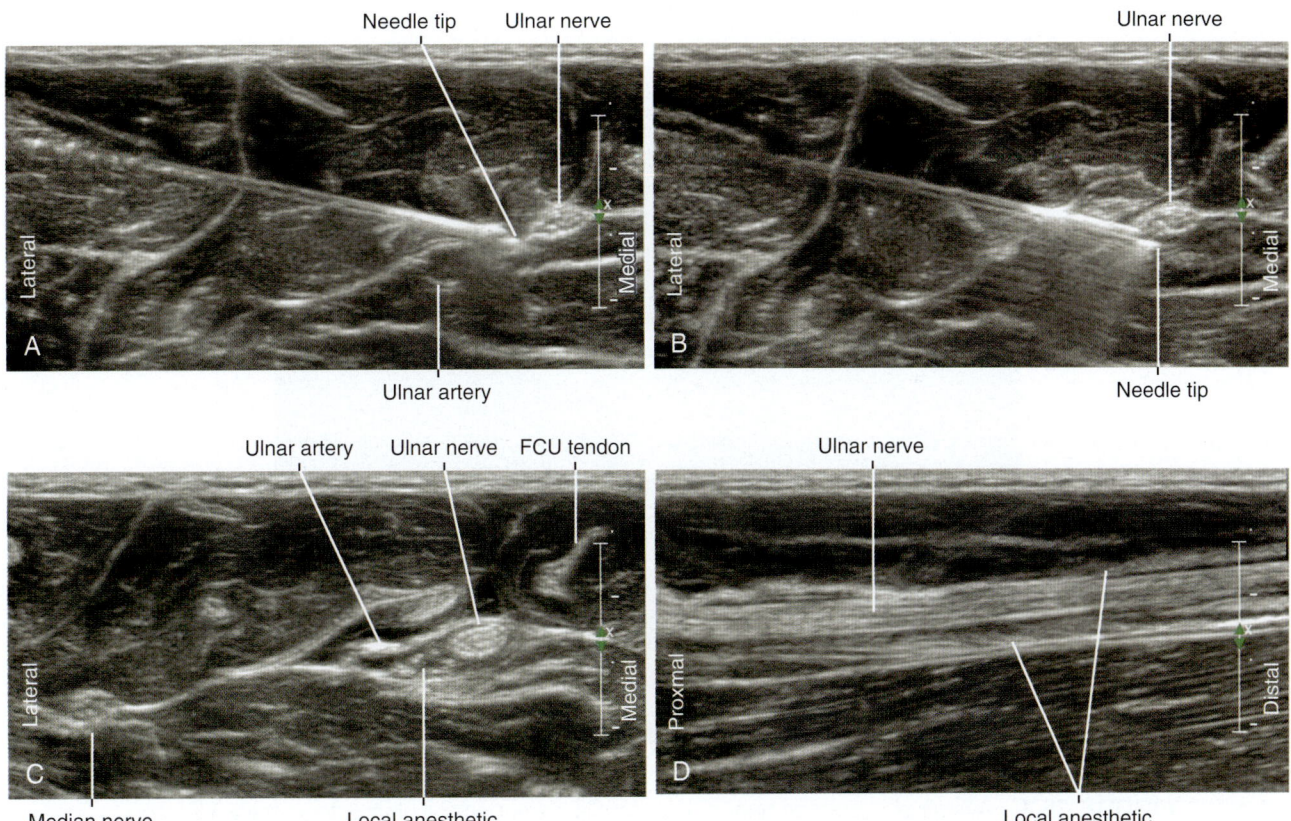

FIGURE 38.3 Image sequence showing ulnar nerve block in the forearm. An in-plane approach is demonstrated whereby the needle tip is placed between the ulnar artery and ulnar nerve (A and B). After injection, local anesthetic is distributed around the ulnar nerve (C) and tracks along the nerve (D). *FCU*, Flexor carpi ulnaris.

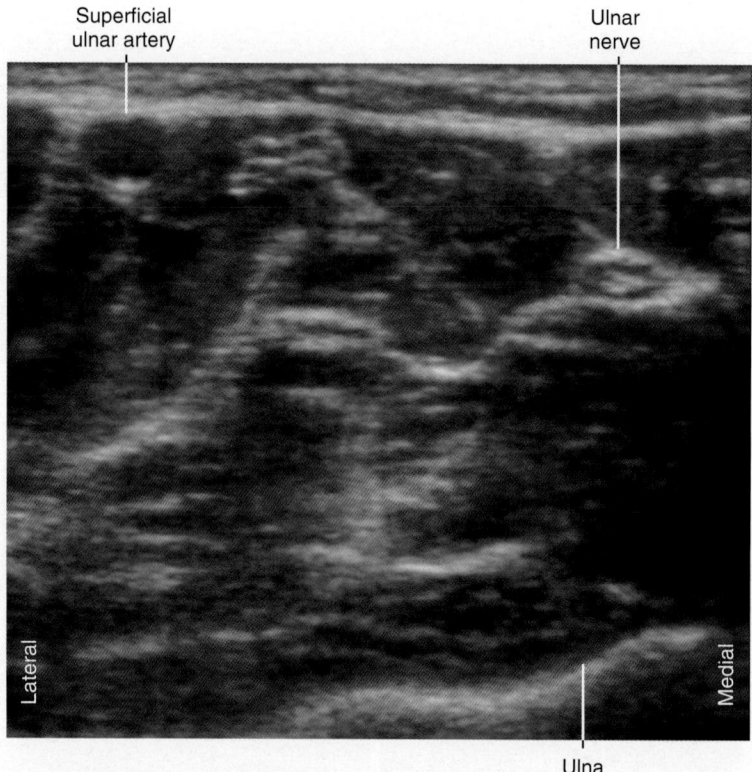

FIGURE 38.4 A relatively common anatomic variant is the superficial ulnar artery. In this variation, the ulnar artery lies superficial to the flexor muscles and is not adjacent to the ulnar nerve.

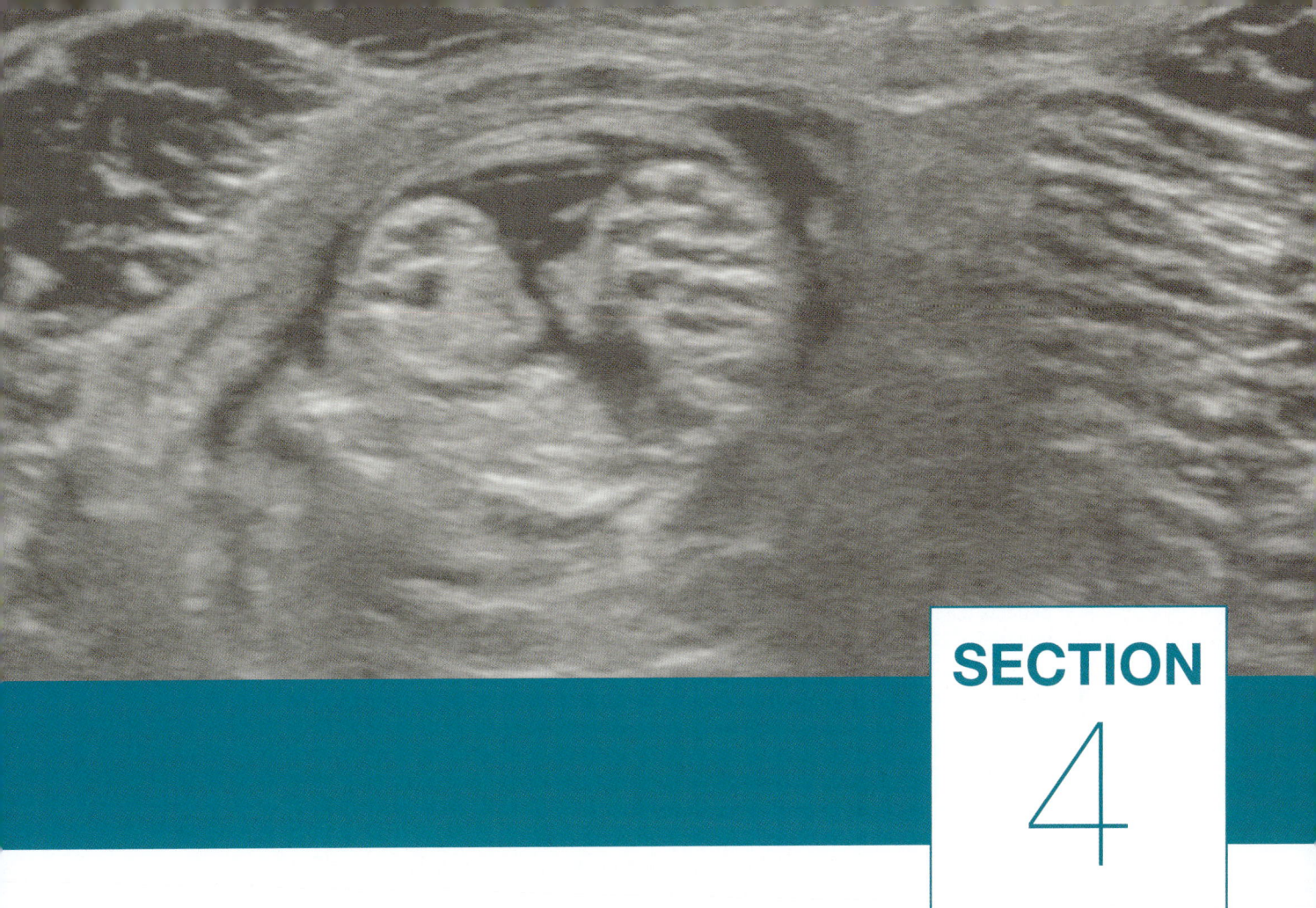

SECTION 4

Lower Extremity Blocks

CHAPTER 39
Lateral Femoral Cutaneous Nerve Block

The lateral femoral cutaneous nerve (LFCN) is a sensory nerve derived from the second and third lumbar nerve roots. The nerve is a branch of the lumbar plexus that provides cutaneous sensation from the lateral aspect of the thigh. The nerve emerges from the lumbar plexus to travel across the iliacus muscle and rise up toward the anterior-superior iliac spine (ASIS). The nerve usually enters the anterior thigh medial to the ASIS and then crosses over the sartorius muscle from medial to lateral.

Anatomic variation of the LFCN is common. The nerve may consist of as many as four branches where it exits the pelvis. The nerve passes medial to the ASIS by a variable distance and may cross the pelvic bone to reach the anterior thigh. Rather than passing over the sartorius, in some patients the LFCN can pass through the sartorius muscle. The estimated incidence of this ranges between 3% and 22%. Although the LFCN is referred to as a discrete nerve, this designation can indicate a collective set of nerves. Like other cutaneous nerves, the LFCN branches extensively when it enters the subcutaneous tissue. In rare cases (≈7%), the LFCN is absent, and its territory is covered by the ilioinguinal and femoral nerves. The sensory territory of the LFCN often extends distal to the knee.[1,2]

High-resolution ultrasound imaging can identify the LFCN superficial to the sartorius muscle in the proximal thigh.[3] The nerve has a characteristic medial-to-lateral course over this muscle. The nerve and muscle are best visualized just medial and distal to the ASIS. As with other small nerves, it is necessary to scan along the length of the nerve to confirm nerve identity. The best imaging technique is to slide the transducer along the known course of the nerve with the nerve viewed in short axis. LFCNs that pass through the sartorius are easier to image because the nerve is surrounded by hypoechoic muscle that provides better acoustic contrast than echo-bright subcutaneous tissue. Although ultrasound imaging of the LFCN has been reported, the nerve is normally small (1 to 2 mm in diameter, cross-sectional area of 0.8 mm^2),[4] and sonographic visualization can be difficult within the echo-bright subcutaneous tissue of the anterior thigh.

LFCN block can be used alone or in conjunction with other lower extremity blocks. It is useful for skin graft harvests and surgical procedures with lateral incisions of the thigh. It is one of the few lower extremity blocks for weight-bearing patients (this group also includes ankle block and saphenous block). LFCN block can improve thigh tourniquet tolerance when combined with other lower extremity blocks.[5]

If adequate volume is administered, a separate LFCN block is not normally necessary after ultrasound-guided femoral block. However, as volume reduction for femoral blocks becomes more feasible because of more targeted injections, sparing of the other nerves, such as the LFCN, will occur.

Ultrasound imaging may be useful for the diagnosis and treatment of meralgia paresthetica (from Greek meros for "thigh," and algos for "pain"). Meralgia can result from mechanical stretch or compression injury of the LFCN. Abnormal nerve morphology has been described in patients with meralgia paresthetica. Fusiform enlargement of the LFCN, loss of fascicular discrimination, and hyperemia can all occur in this condition.[6] With meralgia paresthetica, LFCN compression is usually at the level of the inguinal ligament.

SUGGESTED TECHNIQUE

LFCN blocks are performed in the supine position. The sartorius muscle is imaged in short-axis view near its insertion on the ASIS. By sliding the ultrasound transducer back and forth between proximal and distal locations, the LFCN is identified by its characteristic lateral course over the sartorius muscle. The in-plane approach can be used from the lateral aspect of the thigh. Acoustic standoff may be advantageous in thin patients to image the LFCN close to the ASIS, so that the conforming gel pad forms around the bone.

It may not be critical to directly visualize the LFCN for block success. When the nerve is not sonographically visible, our recommendation for performing LFCN block is to image the sartorius muscle in short-axis view near the ASIS. The sartorius muscle has a triangular shape near its origin on the ASIS. The fascial planes that lie over the anterolateral border of the sartorius muscle (in particular, the fascia lata) can be separated by infiltrating local anesthetic between these layers. The LFCN consistently runs within an oval-shaped, fat-filled fascial tunnel between the sartorius and tensor fascia lata muscles, which is identified with light touch of the transducer.[7,8] After injection, scan to verify local anesthetic tracking along the course of the LFCN within the tunnel.

KEY POINTS

Lateral Femoral Cutaneous Nerve Block

	The Essentials
Anatomy	The LFCN usually crosses over the Sa.
	The LFCN lies in the space between the Sa and TFL.
	The Sa is usually triangularly shaped near its ASIS insertion.
	The LFCN is about 1–2 mm in diameter.
Positioning	Supine
Operator	Standing on side of patient
Display	Across the table
Transducer	High-frequency linear, 23- to 38-mm footprint
Initial depth setting	20 mm
Needle	25 gauge, 38 mm in length
Anatomic location	Proximal lateral thigh, 1–2 cm distal to ASIS
	Begin by sliding the transducer back and forth (proximal and distal). Look for the LFCN crossing over the Sa.
Approach	SAX view of LFCN, in-plane from lateral to medial
	Place the needle tip between the LFCN and Sa.
	Alternatively, place the needle tip in the space between the Sa and the TFL.
Sonographic assessment	The injection should track distally along the LFCN.
Anatomic variation	The LFCN can travel through the Sa.
	The LFCN can divide proximally and be difficult to visualize.

ASIS, Anterior superior iliac spine; *LFCN*, lateral femoral cutaneous nerve; *Sa*, sartorius; *SAX*, short axis; *TFL*, tensor fascia lata.

Clinical Pearls

- The LFCN can be imaged between the fascia iliaca and the fascia lata. If light transducer pressure is applied, the nerve can be seen within the tissue between these two fascial layers for needle tip placement. The fat-filled fascial tunnel between the sartorius and tensor fascia lata muscles can be more difficult to identify in thin subjects.
- LFCN block is assessed by cutaneous anesthesia midway between the ASIS and the lateral knee joint line.
- In some patients, the crossing of the LFCN with the deep circumflex iliac artery can be identified on sagittal oblique sonograms.[9] This view is parallel to the course of the nerve and perpendicular to the course of the artery.

ASIS, Anterior superior iliac spine; *LFCN*, lateral femoral cutaneous nerve.

References

1. Bodner G, Bernathova M, Galiano K, Putz D, Martinoli C, Felfernig M. Ultrasound of the lateral femoral cutaneous nerve: normal findings in a cadaver and in volunteers. *Reg Anesth Pain Med*. 2009;34(3):265–268.
2. Corujo A, Franco CD, Williams JM. The sensory territory of the lateral cutaneous nerve of the thigh as determined by anatomic dissections and ultrasound-guided blocks. *Reg Anesth Pain Med*. 2012;37(5):561–564.
3. Thain LM, Downey DB. Sonography of peripheral nerves: technique, anatomy, and pathology. *Ultrasound Q*. 2002;18:225–245.
4. Tagliafico A, Cadoni A, Fisci E, Bignotti B, Padua L, Martinoli C. Reliability of side-to-side ultrasound cross-sectional area measurments of lower extremity nerves in healthy subjects. *Muscle Nerve*. 2012;46(5):717–722.
5. Morin AM, Pandurovic M, Eberhart LH, et al. Is a blockade of the lateral cutaneous nerve of the thigh an alternative to the classical femoral nerve blockade for knee joint arthroscopy? A randomised controlled study. *Anaesthesist*. 2005;54:991–999.
6. Klauser AS, Abd Ellah MM, Halpern EJ, et al. Meralgia paraesthetica: ultrasound-guided injection at multiple levels with 12-month follow-up. *Eur Radiol*. 2016;26(3):764–770.
7. Ng I, Vaghadia H, Choi PT, Helmy N. Ultrasound imaging accurately identifies the lateral femoral cutaneous nerve. *Anesth Analg*. 2008;107:1070–1074.
8. Zhu J, Zhao Y, Liu F, Huang Y, Shao J, Hu B. Ultrasound of the lateral femoral cutaneous nerve in asymptomatic adults. *BMC Musculoskelet Disord*. 2012;13:227.
9. Damarey B, Demondion X, Boutry N, Kim HJ, Wavreille G, Cotten A. Sonographic assessment of the lateral femoral cutaneous nerve. *J Clin Ultrasound*. 2009;37:89–95.

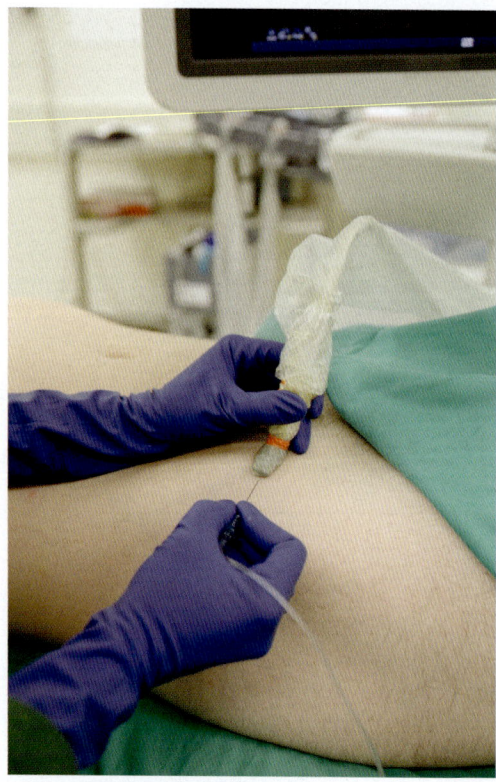

FIGURE 39.1 External photograph showing the in-plane approach to lateral femoral cutaneous nerve block from the lateral aspect of the thigh.

LATERAL FEMORAL CUTANEOUS NERVE BLOCK 147

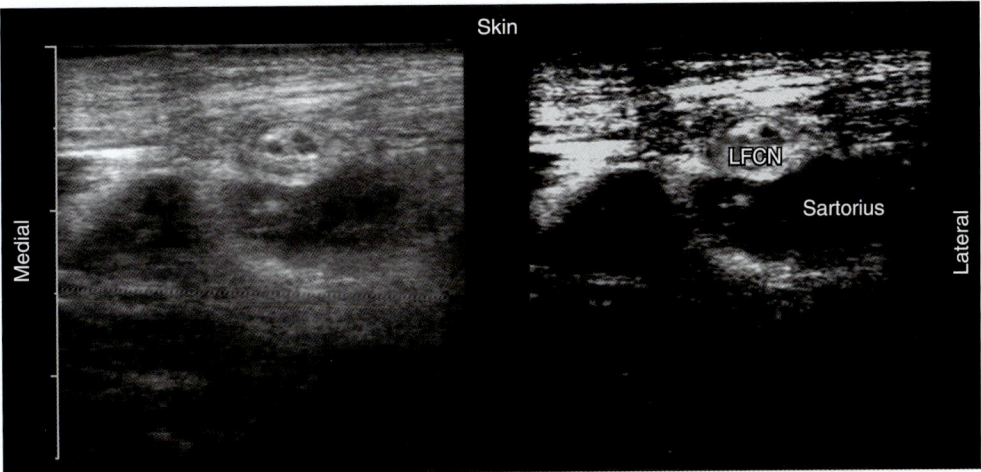

FIGURE 39.2 Short-axis view of the lateral femoral cutaneous nerve over the sartorius muscle near its proximal insertion on the anterior superior iliac spine. This large bifascicular nerve divides more distally in the thigh.

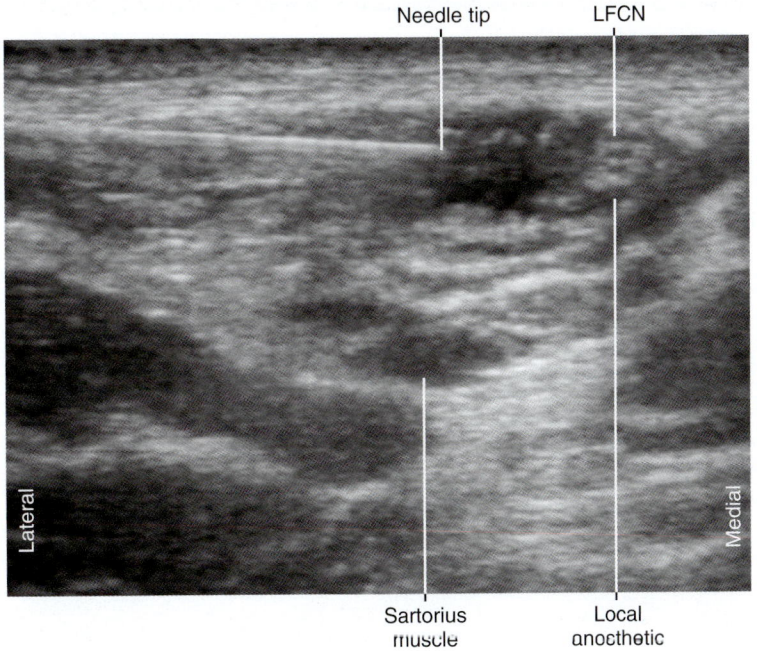

FIGURE 39.3 Needle tip in place for injection of local anesthetic for in-plane lateral femoral cutaneous nerve (LFCN) block. In this example the nerve is pushed against the sartorius muscle.

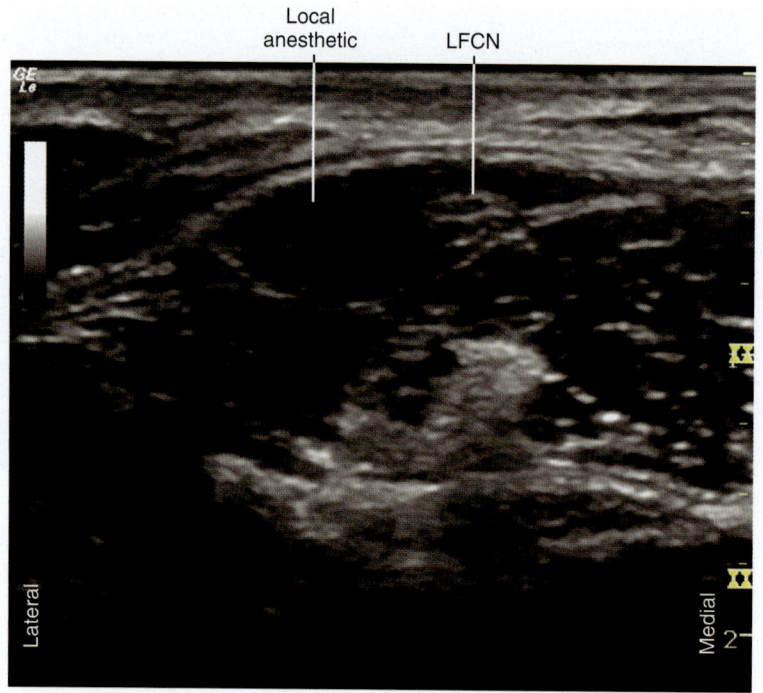

FIGURE 39.4 An in-plane approach demonstrates local anesthetic distributed around a fascicular lateral femoral cutaneous nerve (LFCN).

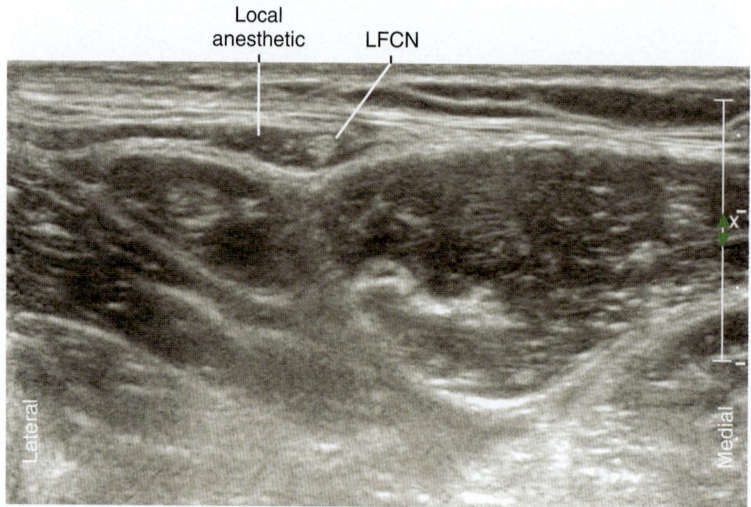

FIGURE 39.5 After injection, local anesthetic is seen to surround the lateral femoral cutaneous nerve (LFCN) in the fat-filled fascial tunnel between the sartorius and tensor fascia lata muscles of the thigh.

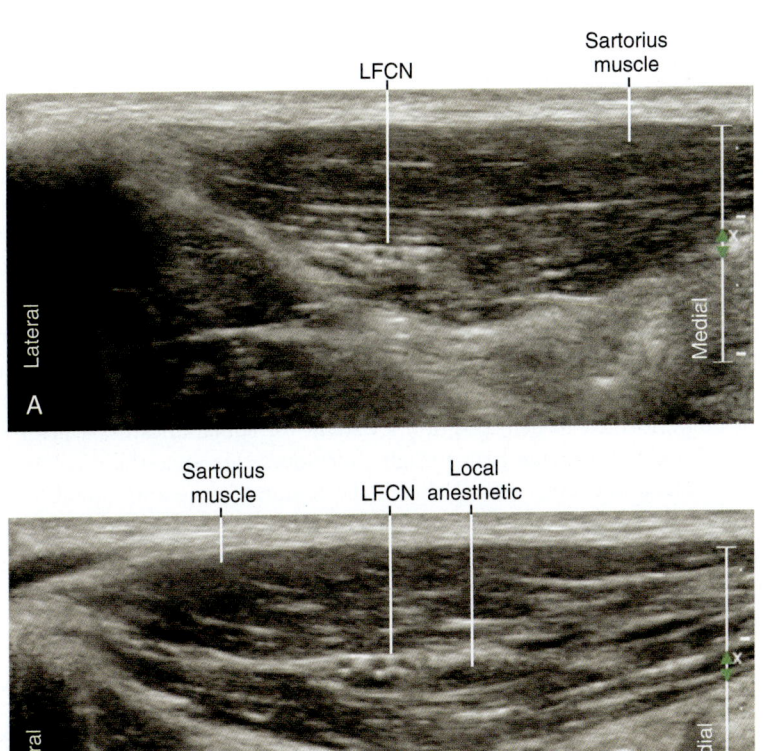

FIGURE 39.6 Pass-through lateral femoral cutaneous nerve (LFCN). In this anatomic variation, the LFCN passes through the sartorius muscle rather than over it. Although relatively uncommon, this variant is easily recognized. The nerve is shown before (A) and after (B) injection of local anesthetic.

CHAPTER 40

Fascia Iliaca Block

 See Video 40.1 on ExpertConsult.com.

The fascia iliaca block is an anterior approach to lumbar plexus block that can result in extensive anesthesia and analgesia of the lower extremity. This block can provide analgesia following hip surgeries involving a lateral incision. Fascia iliaca block can also provide pain relief following hip fracture or be performed to help position a patient for spinal anesthesia prior to surgery. The fascia iliaca block may provide better thigh tourniquet tolerance than isolated femoral nerve blocks. Fascia iliaca injections reliably block the femoral nerve and lateral femoral cutaneous nerve (LFCN). Block of some of the adjacent nerves is also possible (including the ilioinguinal, genitofemoral, obturator, and accessory obturator nerves). Classically, fascia iliaca block is guided by tactile sensation (feeling two pops as a dull block needle is advanced through the fascia lata and fascia iliaca of the thigh).

SUGGESTED TECHNIQUE

Fascia iliaca block is performed between the femoral nerve and LFCN. The patient is placed in supine position (flat with slight extension of the hip). Pannus retraction or reverse Trendelenburg position may be necessary in overweight patients. Place the transducer longitudinally to image the iliacus muscle lateral to the femoral nerve. Because of the inclination of the iliacus muscle, this region is slightly more superficial than the femoral nerve. The iliacus muscle forms a ridge because of the underlying bone of the superior pubic ramus. The deep circumflex artery lies superficial to the fascia iliaca 1 to 2 cm proximal to the inguinal ligament. This artery is 2 to 3 mm in diameter and lies on the central side of the iliacus ridge. Tilting the transducer laterally enhances imaging of the fascia iliaca due to its inclination.[1]

The in-plane approach from distal to proximal is used. For this block it is critical that the needle tip be positioned between the fascia iliaca and iliacus muscle,[2] just distal to the position of the deep circumflex iliac artery. The needle travels under the inguinal ligament, which lies over the ridge of the iliacus muscle. There is a handedness to this longitudinal approach (right handed for right-sided block, left handed for left-sided block).

Hold the needle with the hand over the hub to allow a shallow angle of approach for fascia iliaca block (similar to intravenous catheter placement). Enter the skin with the needle bevel facing up to promote needle tip visibility and puncture of the fascia iliaca. Pierce the fascia iliaca at the peak of the iliacus muscle. Once the needle tip is confirmed to be just deep to the fascia iliaca by injection, rotate the needle so that the bevel faces down. Now the needle can be advanced proximally and remain in the correct tissue plane, with less chance of the needle tip entering the substance of the iliacus muscle.

The initial injection under the fascia iliaca forms a lens shape. As volume is administered, the injected distribution should curve along the surface of the iliacus muscle, resembling a hill shape. A long block needle can be used to hydrodissect down into the injected fluid to promote proximal distribution. Most practitioners use high volumes of dilute local anesthetic (e.g., 25 to 30 mL for average-sized adult patients) to provide extensive distribution to the multiple nerves of the lumbar plexus. The deep circumflex iliac artery arises as a recurrent branch from the external iliac artery and can be a valuable landmark for proximal fascia iliaca block. The LFCN lies between the deep circumflex iliac artery and the iliacus muscle. Therefore, the fluid injected for the proximal fascia iliaca block should distribute under the deep circumflex iliac artery and around the lateral femoral cutaneous and femoral nerves.

The fascia iliaca block can also be approached with a transverse plane of imaging, and results similar to the longitudinal approach have been reported. If the transverse approach is used, perform the block proximally, near the inguinal ligament. The key to either approach is identification of the fascia iliaca by direct imaging or by observing a lens-shaped distribution of injected fluid just deep to this fascia.

Clinical Pearls

- Regional blocks are often used as part of hip fracture pathways. Both continuous femoral and fascia iliaca blocks provide effected analgesia for elderly patients undergoing hip replacement.[3]
- Suprainguinal injection under the fascia iliaca is an effective way to anesthetize the lateral femoral cutaneous nerve and femoral nerve. The correct injection has a lens (or spindle) shape.
- High volumes of dilute local anesthetic are recommended for fascia iliaca block (25–30 mL).
- The deep circumflex iliac artery is an important landmark for needle tip placement. It can be identified superficial to the fascia iliaca 1–2 cm proximal to the inguinal ligament.
- Recent studies suggest that fascia iliaca block does not consistently anesthetize the obturator nerve.[4]
- Fascia iliaca block can be performed before sciatic nerve block to reduce patient discomfort during needle insertion. In thin patients, local anesthetic can be seen to track over the retroperitoneal surface of the iliacus muscle.[5]

References

1. Hebbard P, Ivanusic J, Sha S. Ultrasound-guided supra-inguinal fascia iliaca block: a cadaveric evaluation of a novel approach. *Anaesthesia.* 2011;66(4):300–305.
2. Dalens B, Vanneuville G, Tanguy A. Comparison of the fascia iliaca compartment block with the 3-in-1 block in children. *Anesth Analg.* 1989;69(6):705–713. [Erratum in: *Anesth Analg.* 1990;70(4):474].
3. Yu B, He M, Cai GY, Zou TX, Zhang N. Ultrasound-guided continuous femoral nerve block vs continuous fascia iliaca compartment block for hip replacement in the elderly: a randomized controlled clinical trial (CONSORT). *Medicine (Baltimore).* 2016;95(42):e5056.
4. Swenson JD, Davis JJ, Stream JO, Crim JR, Burks RT, Greis PE. Local anesthetic injection deep to the fascia iliaca at the level of the inguinal ligament: the pattern of distribution and effects on the obturator nerve. *J Clin Anesth.* 2015;27(8):652–657.
5. Eastburn E, Hernandez MA, Boretsky K. Technical success of the ultrasound-guided supra-inguinal fascia iliaca compartment block in older children and adolescents for hip arthroscopy. *Paediatr Anaesth.* 2017;27:1120–1124.

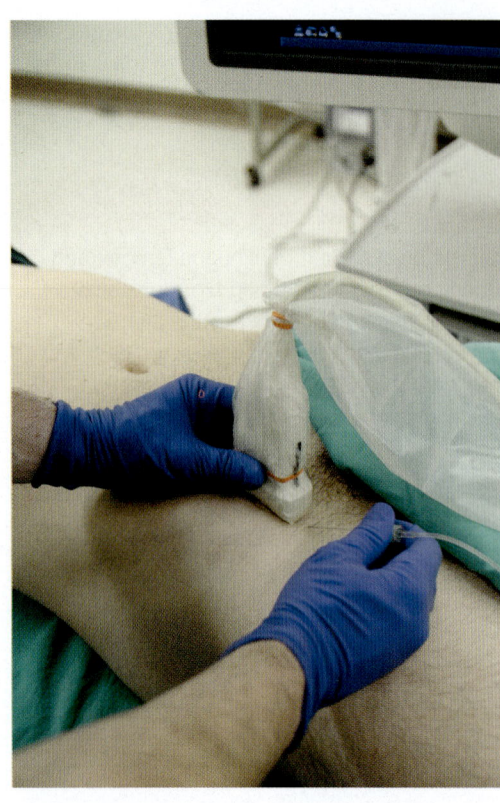

FIGURE 40.1 Positioning for ultrasound-guided proximal fascia iliaca block. In-plane approach with longitudinal imaging is shown.

FASCIA ILIACA BLOCK 153

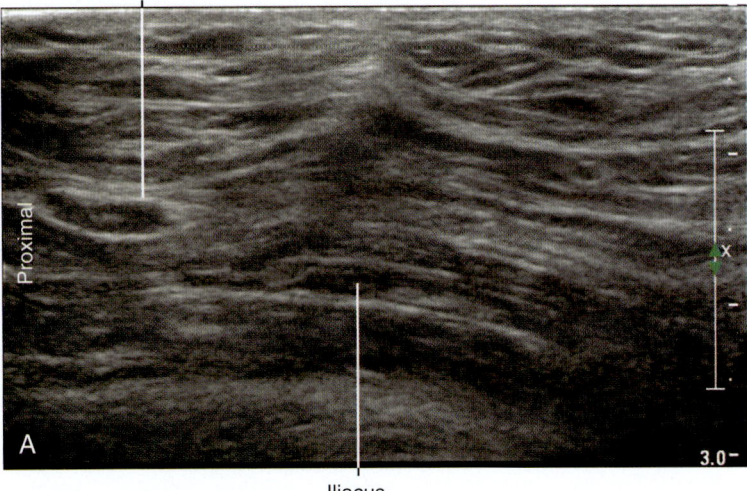

FIGURE 40.2 Longitudinal (coronal) imaging for ultrasound-guided fascia iliaca block. The deep circumflex iliac artery is shown in short-axis view (A). Verification that the deep circumflex arises from the external iliac artery is shown by rotating the transducer to obtain a long-axis view of the artery (B).

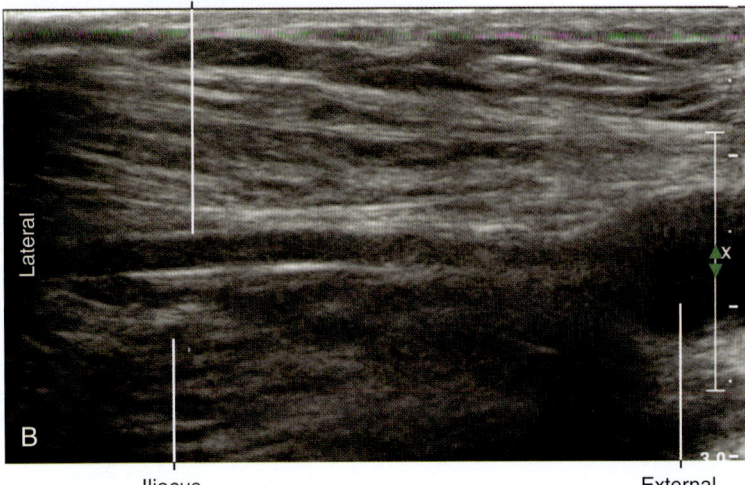

FIGURE 40.3 Longitudinal in-plane approach to ultrasound-guided fascia iliaca block. The needle tip pierces the fascia iliaca just distal to the peak of the iliacus muscle and the deep circumflex iliac artery. The injection tracks proximally and down toward nerves of the lumbar plexus.

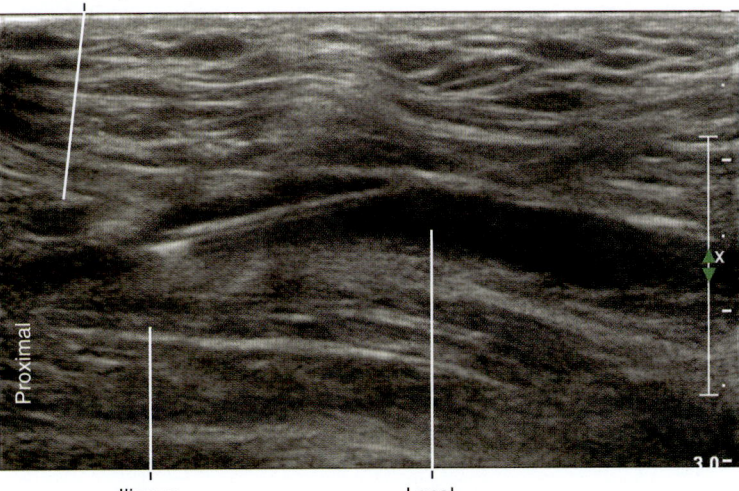

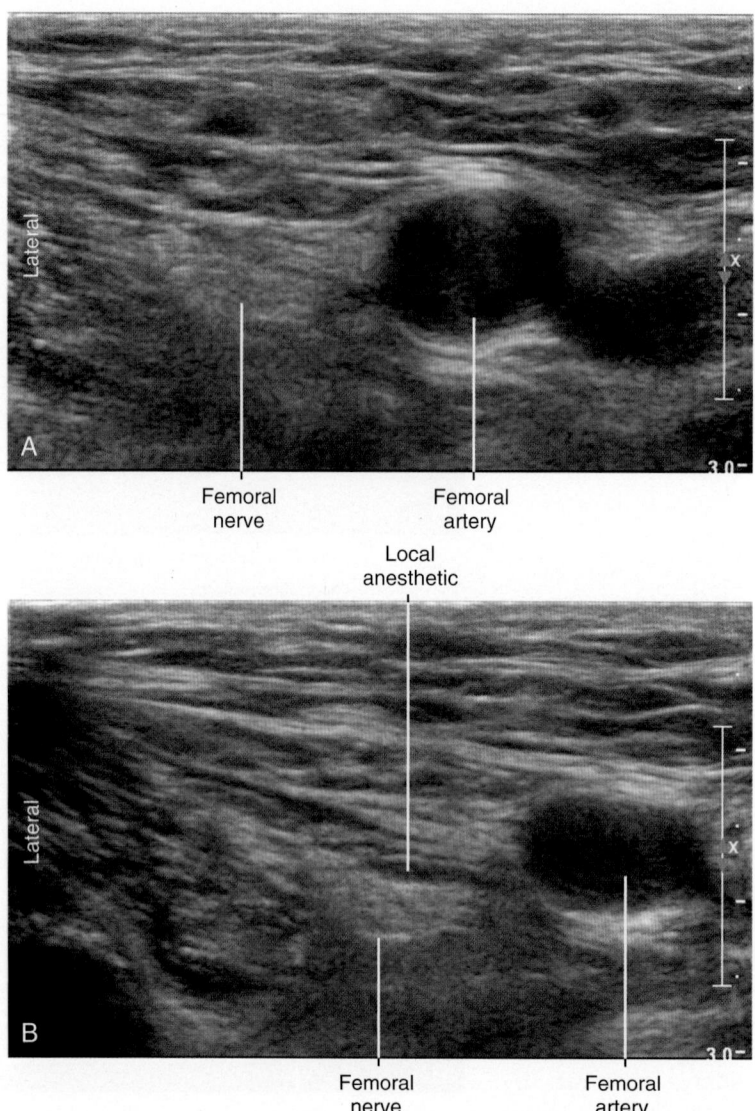

FIGURE 40.4 Verification of distribution of the injection to the femoral nerve as assessed in short-axis view. Sonograms are shown before (A) and after (B) injection. Local anesthetic has distributed over the anterior surface of the femoral nerve.

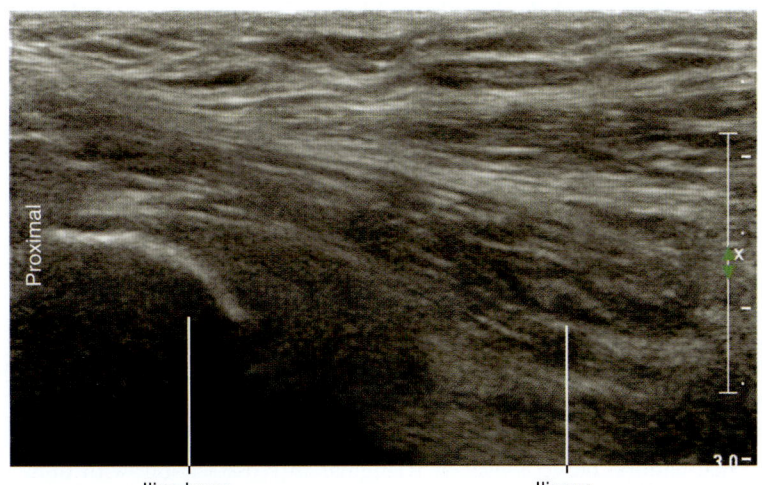

FIGURE 40.5 Longitudinal reference images for proximal fascia iliaca block. The anterior superior iliac spine is shown in coronal imaging, indicating the probe is too lateral for fascia iliaca block.

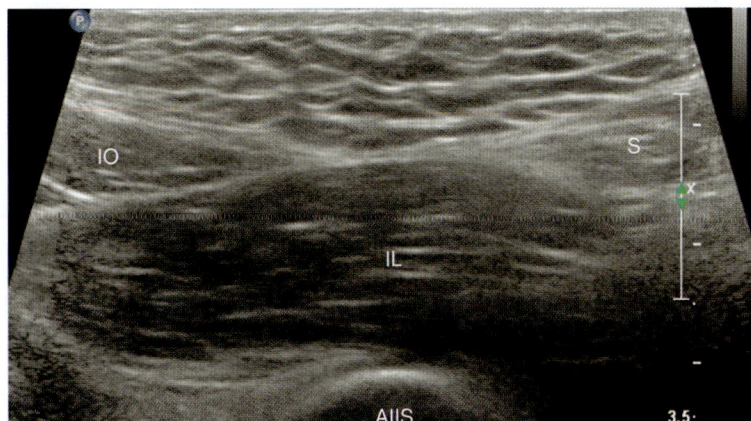

FIGURE 40.6 The "X" or "bowtie" appearance to the internal oblique *(IO)* and sartorius *(S)* muscles at the level of the anterior inferior iliac spine *(AIIS)* for fascia iliaca block via longitudinal approach (the fascia iliaca connects these two muscles and this is the approximate location for needle tip placement). The iliacus muscle *(IL)* lies over the shelf of bone.

CHAPTER 41

Femoral Nerve Block

 See Video 41.1 on ExpertConsult.com.

The femoral nerve is the largest branch of the lumbar plexus. It provides motor innervation to the quadriceps, sartorius, and pectineus muscles. The sensory branches include the anterior cutaneous nerve of the thigh, the infrapatellar nerve, and the saphenous nerve. These nerves innervate the anterior thigh, the patella, and the medial leg and foot, respectively.

The normal femoral nerve is oval or triangular in cross section, with dimensions of about 3 mm in anteroposterior diameter and 10 mm in mediolateral diameter in the inguinal region.[1] The femoral nerve usually lies lateral to the femoral artery but can contact or lie underneath the femoral artery in 15% of cases. In about one-third of individuals, the femoral nerve is triangular in the suprainguinal region on short-axis scans.

The femoral nerve is covered by echogenic subcutaneous tissue and fascia. The nerve lies on the hypoechoic iliopsoas muscle, which has a characteristic mediolateral inclination. This incline positions the lateral side of the nerve slightly closer to the skin surface. At this interface of bright fascia and dark muscle, the nerve can be difficult to visualize. The best nerve visibility is proximal to the inguinal crease before the femoral nerve and femoral artery divide into smaller branches distally. In this proximal location, the femoral nerve puts a small dent in the surface of the iliopsoas muscle. This occurs because the femoral nerve usually lies in the groove between the iliacus (lateral) and psoas (medial) components of the muscle. The tilt of the transducer strongly influences femoral nerve visibility owing to anisotropic effects.[2] With ultrasound guidance it may be possible to perform more proximal drug injections and therefore more complete resultant femoral nerve blocks.

SUGGESTED TECHNIQUE

Femoral nerve block is performed in the supine position with the nerve in short-axis view. The lateral corner of the nerve is targeted to avoid the femoral vessels and to make the injection closest to the skin surface. Both out-of-plane (from distal to proximal) and in-plane (from lateral to medial) approaches can be used. It is critical that the needle tip be positioned between the fascia iliaca and iliopsoas muscle.[3] It is not important to position the needle tip immediately adjacent to the nerve.

The needle tip should be placed in the layer under the femoral nerve so that the injection lifts the nerve toward the surface. This is especially important when catheters are placed. Successful injections not only surround the femoral nerve but also track along its small distal branches. If there is any question that the injection has not surrounded the femoral nerve, the distal tracking of local anesthetic can be verified by sliding the transducer along the nerve path. If local anesthetic appears to only layer over the femoral nerve, be concerned that the fascia iliaca is still intact.

Dull block needles can be used to detect tissue layers, both by visual inspection of the tent and recoil with needle advancement and by tactile sense. If sharp needles are used, the operator's hand motion and needle tip position will be more closely correlated. It may be necessary to combine ultrasound and nerve stimulation for femoral nerve blocks in morbidly obese patients. In these patients the femoral artery can be imaged to give an approximate location for nerve stimulation.

Posterior acoustic enhancement can occur deep to the femoral artery.[4] This artifact should not be confused with the femoral nerve. The femoral nerve and iliopsoas tendon can be distinguished because the iliopsoas tendon lies deep within the iliopsoas muscle.

The lateral-to-medial in-plane approach to femoral block has potential disadvantages because of the longer needle path, which can be near the lateral femoral cutaneous nerve. In addition, the needle has a tendency to skim along the fascia iliaca, deforming it rather than puncturing it. This can be particularly frustrating as the needle tip approaches the femoral artery.

Many institutions have found the out-of-plane approach to be very safe and effective. However, the operator must be cognizant of the unimaged needle path. Branches of the femoral artery may lie within the unimaged needle path short of the scan plane. Scanning before needle placement can be advantageous.

The incidence of vascular puncture rates with nerve stimulation–guided femoral nerve catheters is about 6%.[5] Ultrasound guidance likely reduces that incidence. Puncture of the inguinal vessels can result in blood tracking into the retroperitoneum, even if the puncture occurs distal to the inguinal ligament.[6]

KEY POINTS

Femoral Nerve Block

	The Essential Points
Anatomy	The FN lies lateral to the FA on the surface of the iliopsoas muscle. The FN lies in the groove between the iliacus and psoas muscles. The LCFA can lie over the FN. The FN is about 3 by 10 mm in diameter.
Image orientation	The iliopsoas muscle has an inclined surface from lateral to medial.
Positioning	Supine with leg slightly abducted. Some pannus retraction may be necessary
Operator	Standing on the side of the patient
Display	Across the table
Transducer	High-frequency linear, 38- to 50-mm footprint
Initial depth setting	25–30 mm
Needle	20–21 gauge, 70 mm in length
Anatomic location	Begin by scanning with the probe along the inguinal crease. Slide proximally until the common FA and FN are seen in SAX view. Best FN imaging is usually 1–2 cm proximal to the inguinal crease.
Approach	SAX view of the FN, in-plane from the lateral side. Place the needle tip through the fascia iliaca at lateral corner of the FN. Inject underneath the FN (between the FN and iliopsoas muscle).
Sonographic assessment	The injection should track along the FN branches (SAX slide).
Anatomic variation	Distance of the FN from the FA is variable. Different nerve morphologies (commonly oval or triangular shape). The FN can lie deep within the groove between iliacus and psoas muscles.

FA, Femoral artery; *FN*, femoral nerve; *LCFA*, lateral circumflex femoral artery; *SAX*, short axis.

Clinical Pearls

- The iliopsoas tendon lies under the femoral artery and should not be mistaken for the femoral nerve.[7]
- Transducer location is of paramount importance to femoral nerve visibility. If the transducer is too distal, the femoral nerve and artery will divide.[8] This compromises nerve visibility because it is difficult to image small femoral nerve branches, particularly those that branch to the surface, within the echo-bright subcutaneous tissue (only after injection of anechoic fluid can these branches be seen). If the transducer is too proximal, the nerve and artery will dive away from the transducer on the surface on the iliacus muscle.

Continued

Clinical Pearls—cont'd

- The transducer rotation can be varied to optimize visibility of the femoral nerve from along the inguinal crease and ligament to a straight transverse view.
- The fascia iliaca can often be seen merging with the lateral side of the femoral nerve after injection (the "string sign" or "tadpole sign").
- Femoral nerve blocks can be clinically assessed by testing quadriceps strength. Saphenous vein dilation is observed after femoral or saphenous nerve block.

References

1. Gruber H, Peer S, Kovacs P, Marth R, Bodner G. The ultrasonographic appearance of the femoral nerve and cases of iatrogenic impairment. *J Ultrasound Med.* 2003;22:163–172.
2. Soong J, Schafhalter-Zoppoth I, Gray AT. The importance of transducer angle to ultrasound visibility of the femoral nerve. *Reg Anesth Pain Med.* 2005;30:505.
3. Dalens B, Vanneuville G, Tanguy A. Comparison of the fascia iliaca compartment block with the 3-in-1 block in children. *Anesth Analg.* 1989;69:705–713.
4. Filly RA, Sommer FG, Minton MJ. Characterization of biological fluids by ultrasound and computed tomography. *Radiology.* 1980;134:167–171.
5. Wiegel M, Gottschaldt U, Hennebach R, Hirschberg T, Reske A. Complications and adverse effects associated with continuous peripheral nerve blocks in orthopedic patients. *Anesth Analg.* 2007;104:1578–1582.
6. Spies JB, Berlin L. Complications of femoral artery puncture. *AJR Am J Roentgenol.* 1998;170:9–11.
7. Mulroy RD. The iliopsoas muscle complex: iliacus muscle, psoas tendon release. *Clin Orthop.* 1965;38:81–85.
8. Lonchena TK, McFadden K, Orebaugh SL. Correlation of ultrasound appearance, gross anatomy, and histology of the femoral nerve at the femoral triangle. *Surg Radiol Anat.* 2016;38(1):115–122.

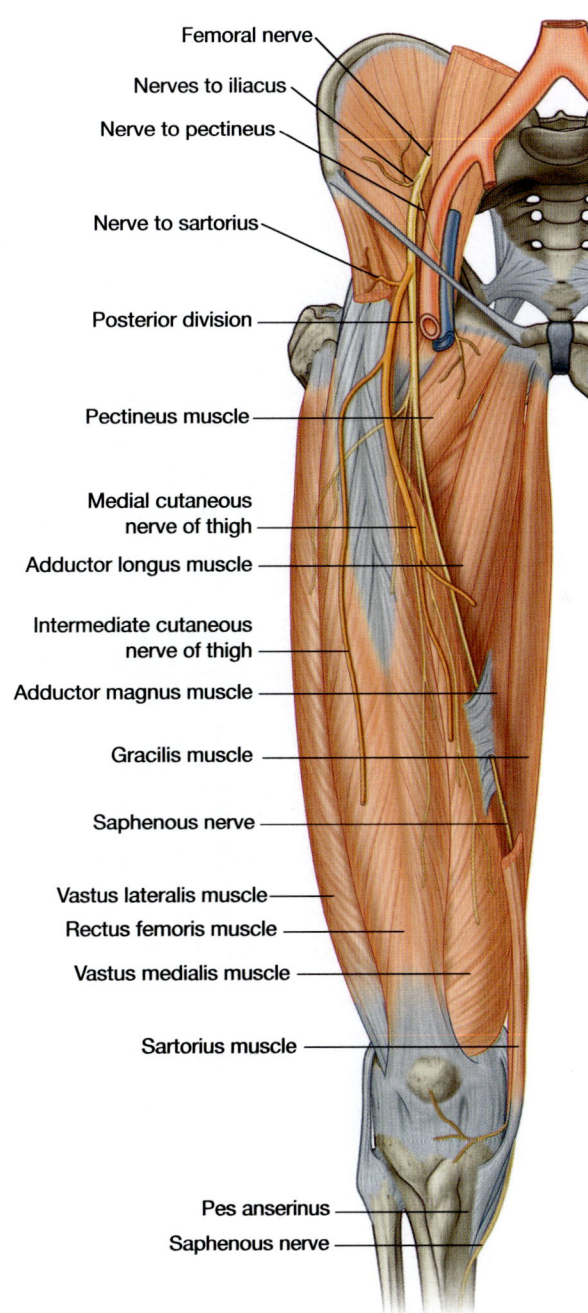

FIGURE 41.1 Course of the femoral nerve. (From Drake RL, Vogl W, Mitchell AWM. *Gray's anatomy for students*. Philadelphia: Churchill Livingstone; 2004.)

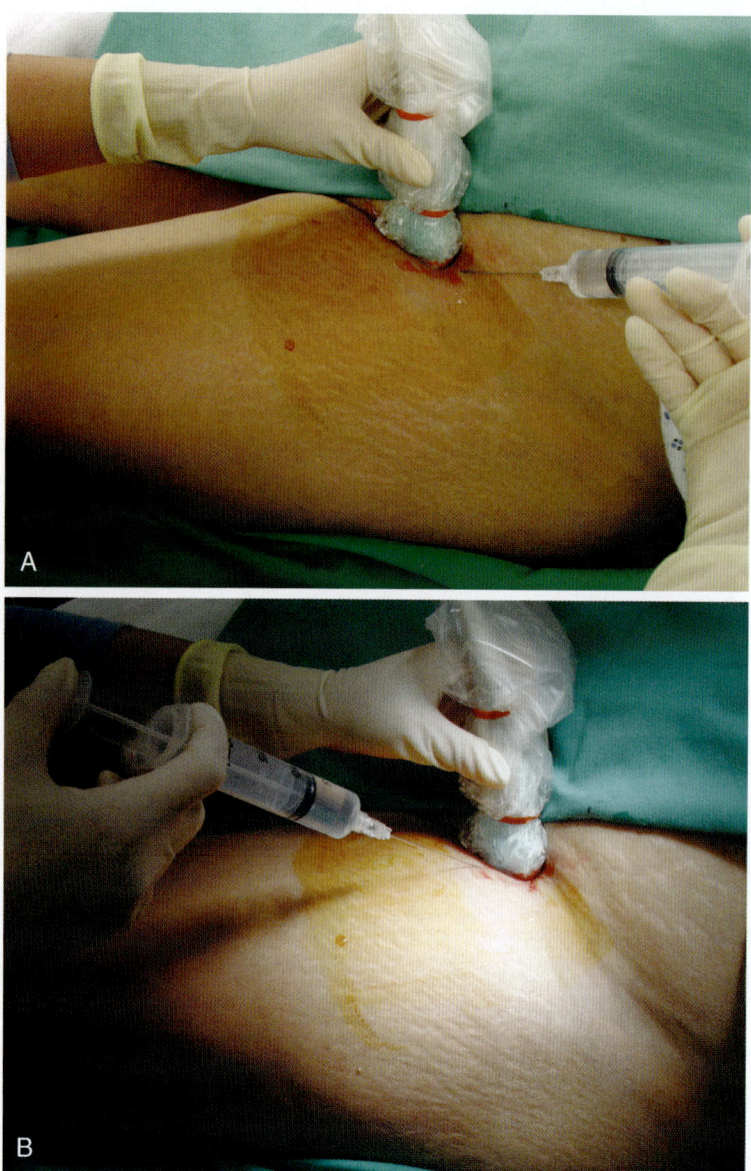

FIGURE 41.2 External photograph showing approaches to femoral nerve block in the inguinal region. An in-plane approach from the lateral aspect of the thigh is shown (A). An out-of-plane approach is also shown (B).

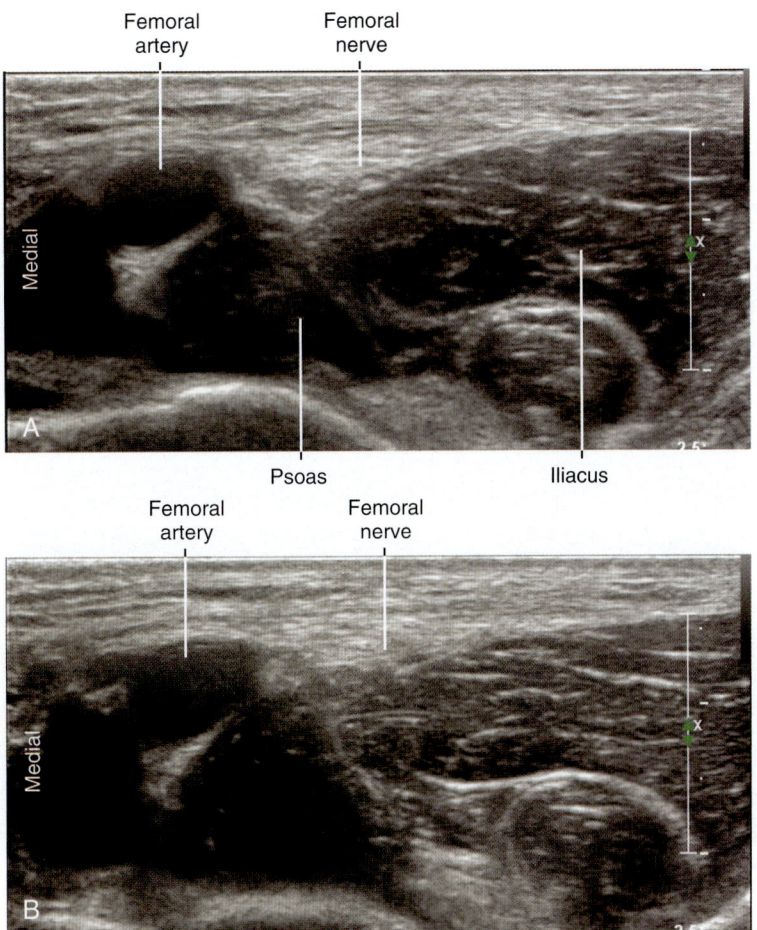

FIGURE 41.3 Short-axis views of the femoral nerve in the inguinal region. The inclination of the transducer is critical to visibility of the femoral nerve (A and B). In this example the echoes from a triangular femoral nerve disappear when the transducer is tilted (the property of anisotropy).

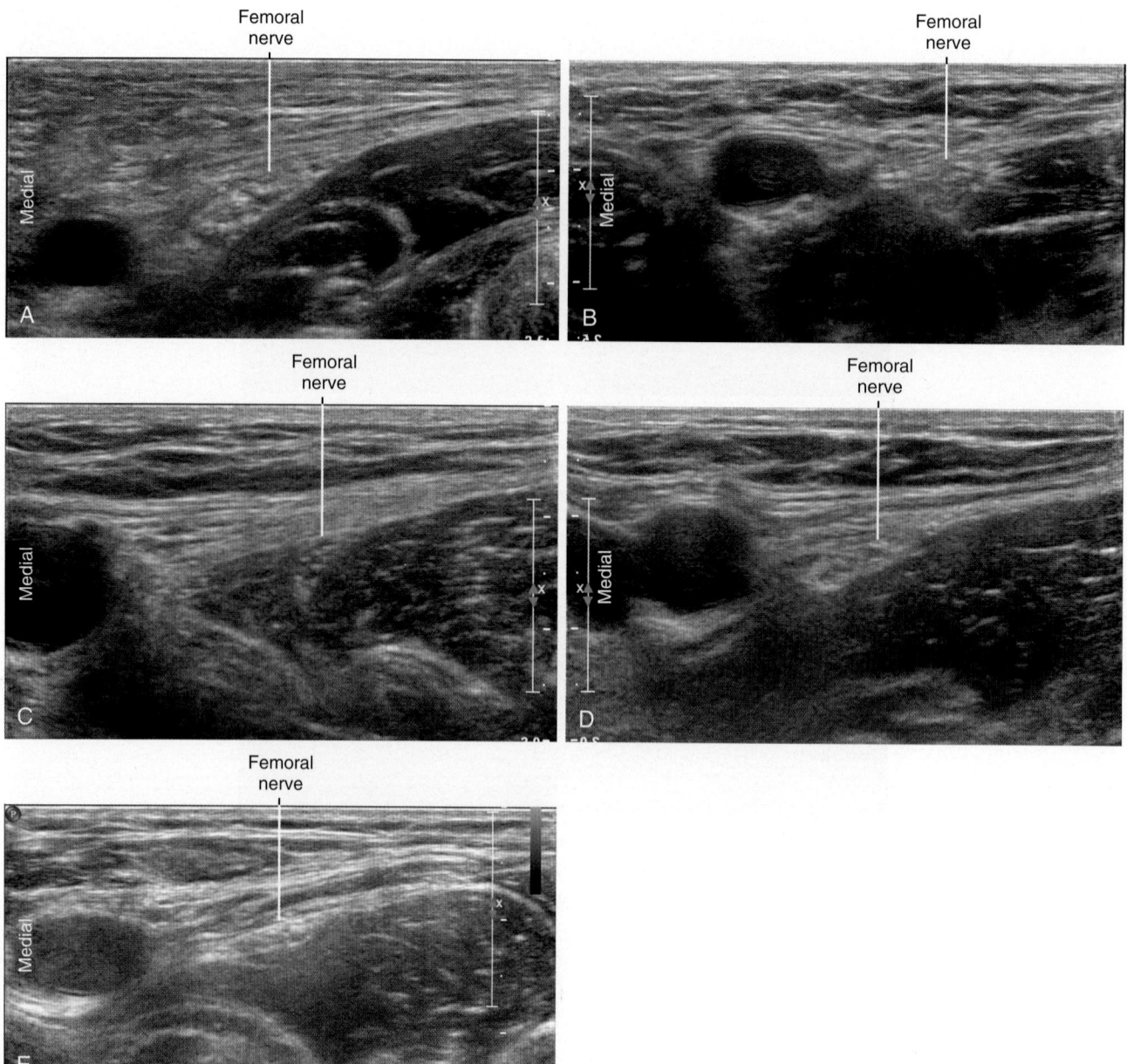

FIGURE 41.4 Morphologies of the femoral nerve in the inguinal region. Short-axis views are shown with foil (A), triangle (B), crescent (C), oval (D), and indented (E) shapes of the femoral nerve. Ultrasound visibility of the femoral nerve is complicated by the fact that the nerve lies at the interface of hyperechoic subcutaneous tissue and hypoechoic muscle. In many cases the femoral nerve is only visible as an indentation in the surface of the iliopsoas muscle.

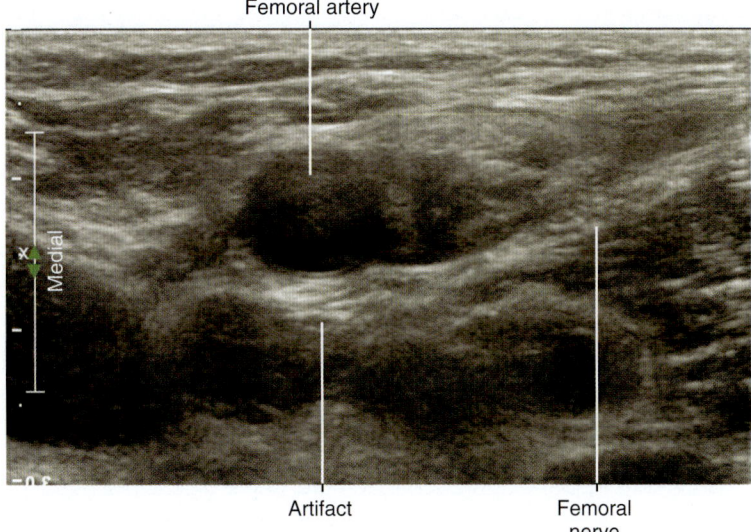

FIGURE 41.5 Posterior acoustic enhancement artifact occurs deep to the femoral artery and can resemble the femoral nerve.

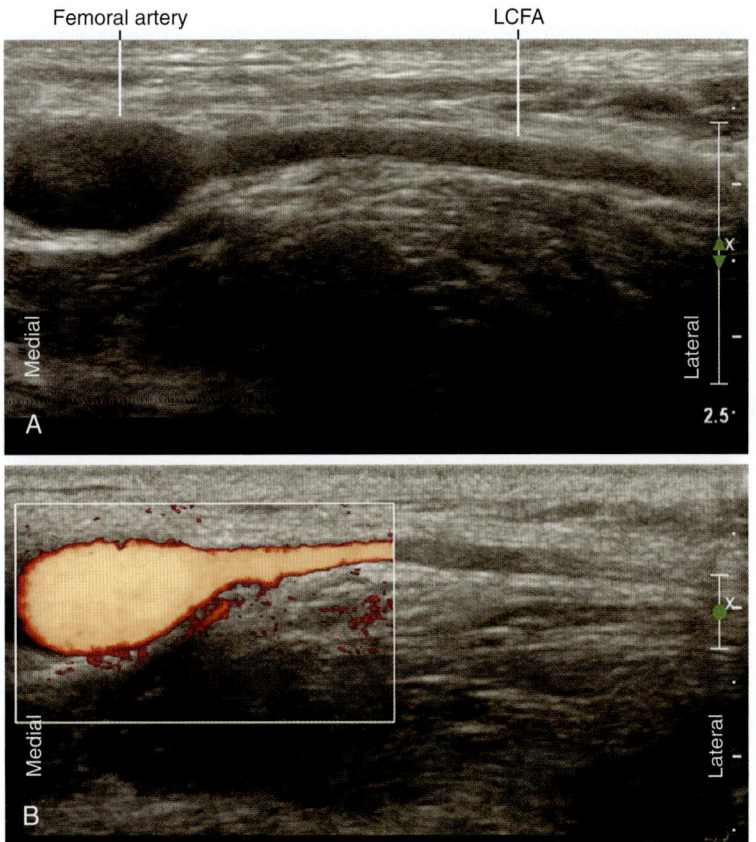

FIGURE 41.6 The femoral artery is seen in short-axis view with the lateral circumflex femoral artery in long-axis view (A). A duplex image is shown with power Doppler verifying color encoding of the vessels (B).

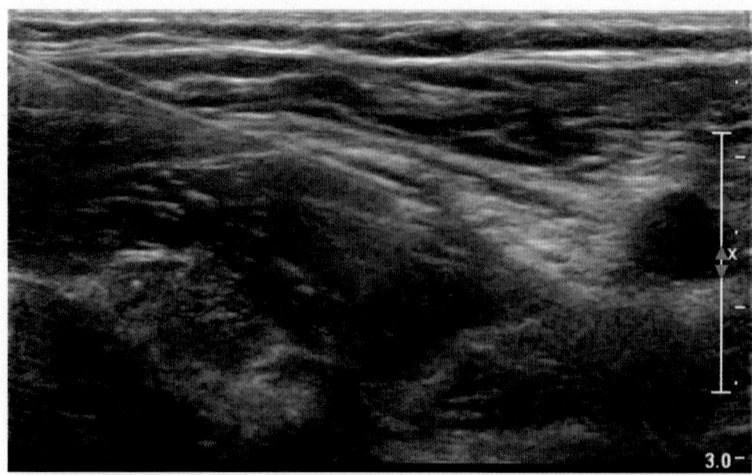

FIGURE 41.7 Short-axis in-plane approach to femoral nerve block. The needle tip approaches the femoral nerve from the lateral side to cross the fascia iliaca at the lateral border of the nerve.

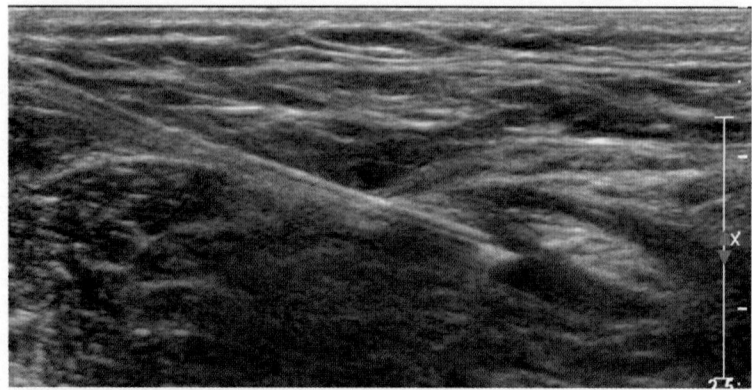

FIGURE 41.8 Femoral nerve visibility after injection of local anesthetic. The nerve visibility is improved by posterior acoustic enhancement and better definition of the nerve borders. Local anesthetic is seen to completely surround the nerve.

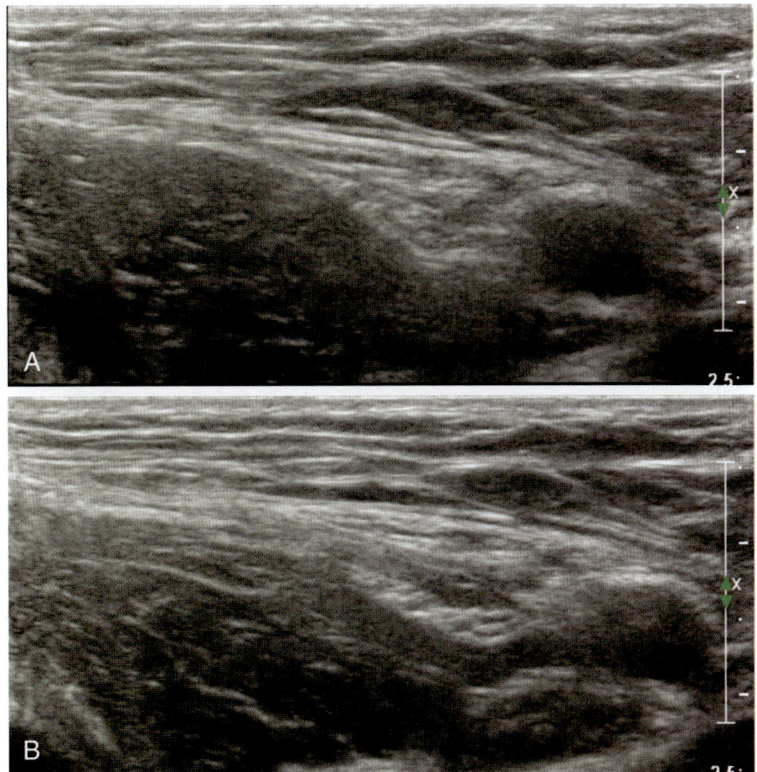

FIGURE 41.9 Femoral nerve in short-axis view before (A) and after (B) injection of local anesthetic. In this example a triangular femoral nerve is observed to lie in the groove between the iliacus and psoas muscles. After injection the nerve fascicles are more clearly seen.

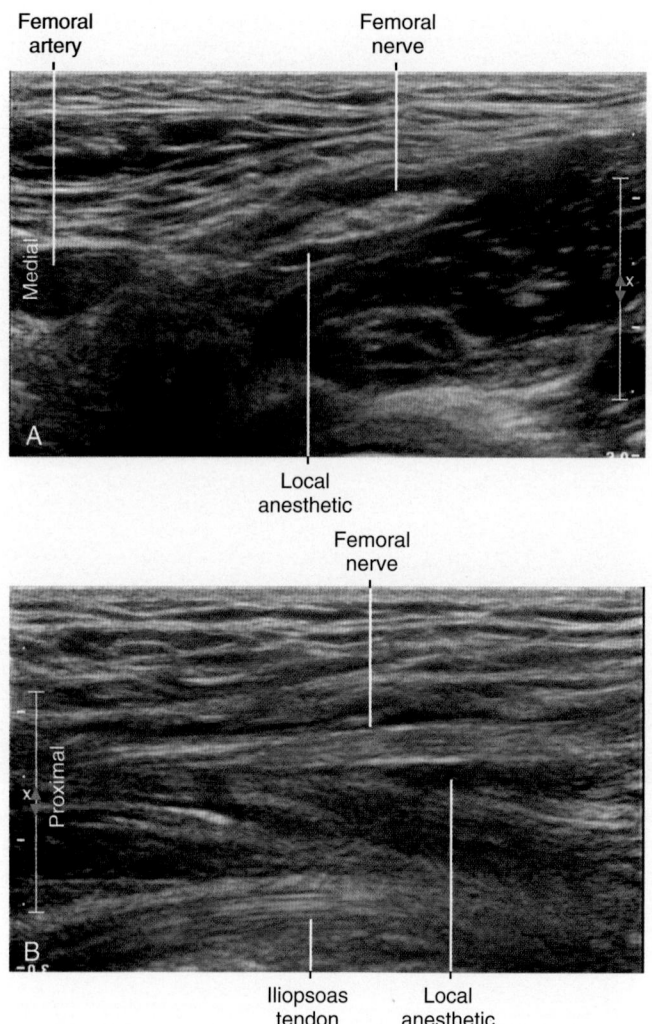

FIGURE 41.10 Femoral nerve in short-axis (A) and long-axis (B) views after injection of local anesthetic. This tracking pattern of local anesthetic verifies a successful block.

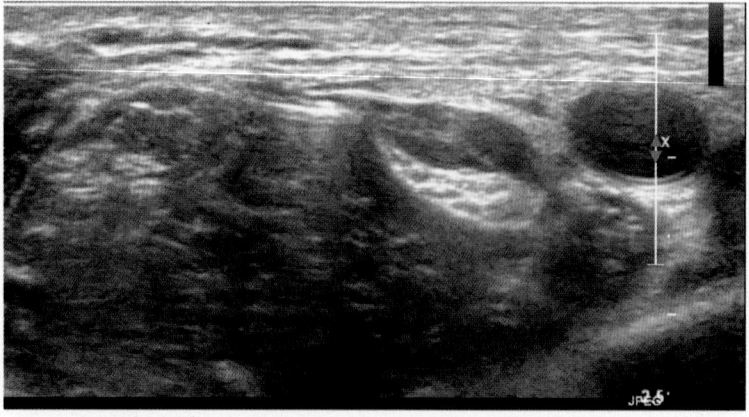

FIGURE 41.11 Femoral nerve in short-axis view after injection of local anesthetic. In this example, local anesthetic has separated the femoral nerve from the iliopectineal arch, resulting in a "paisley" shape of the femoral nerve.

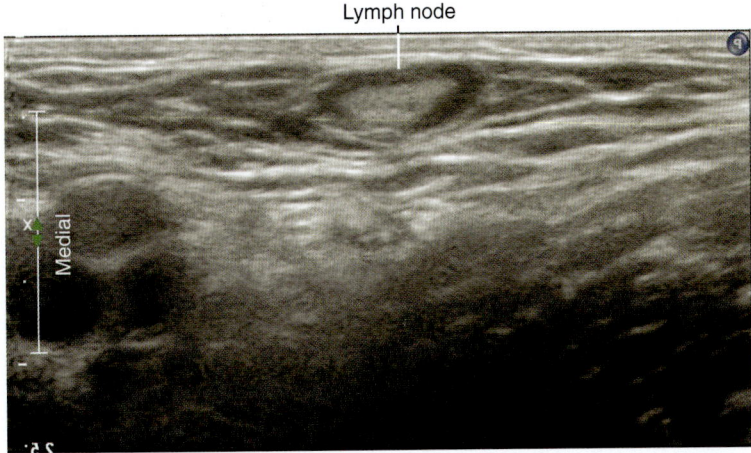

FIGURE 41.12 Inguinal lymph nodes are commonly observed during femoral nerve block. Lymph nodes can be recognized by their oval shape and echogenic hilum.

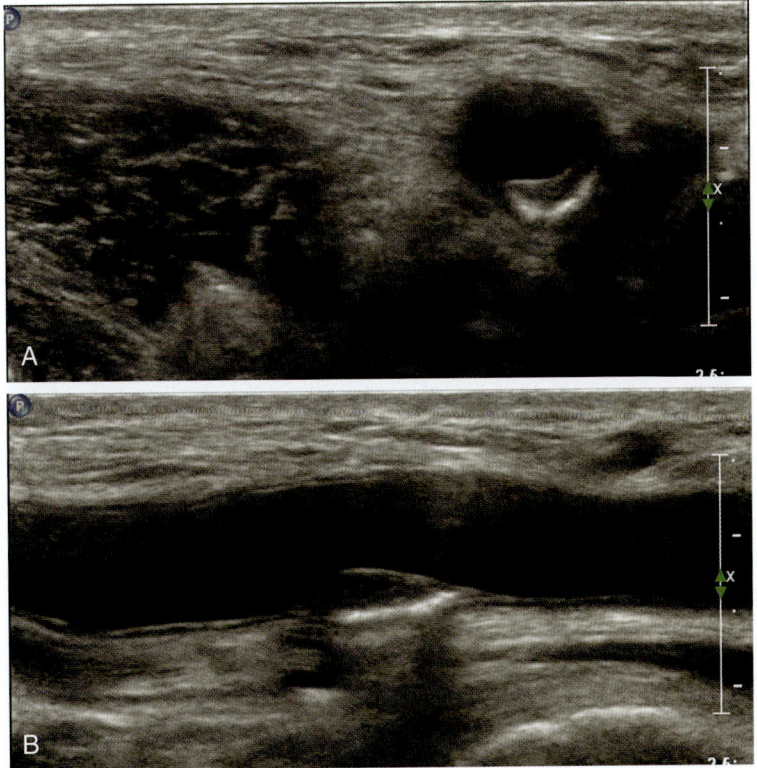

FIGURE 41.13 Femoral artery plaque observed in short-axis (A) and long-axis (B) views during femoral nerve block. This pathology is a common incidental finding that may warrant further medical workup.

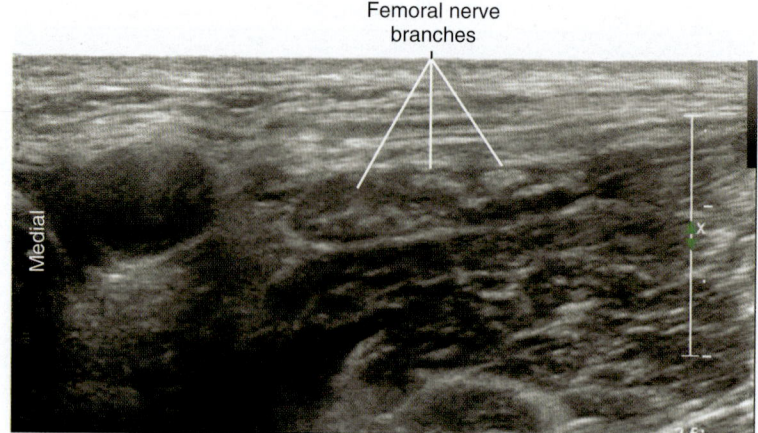

FIGURE 41.14 Femoral nerve branches observed after injection of local anesthetic. In this example the transducer slides distally with the nerve viewed in short axis. Local anesthetic is observed to track around and along the small nerve branches, confirming successful distribution for regional block.

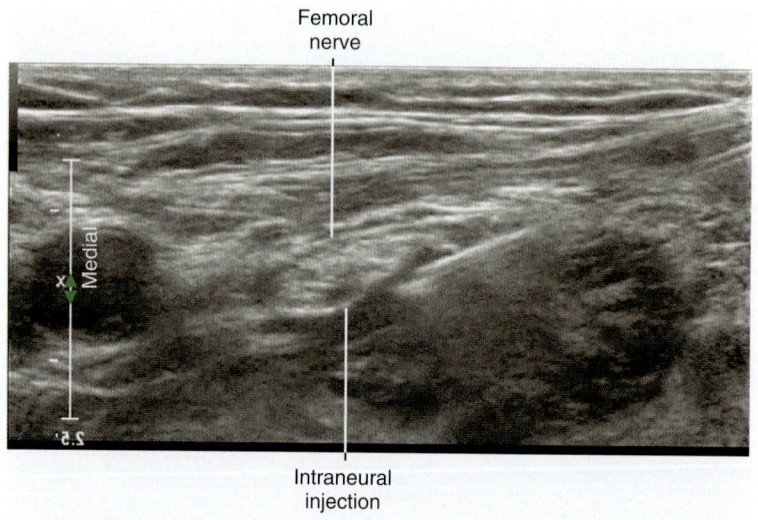

FIGURE 41.15 Intraneural injection observed during femoral nerve block. In this example, local anesthetic was inadvertently injected into the femoral nerve, resulting in small cystic collection of fluid inside the nerve. There were no neurologic sequelae.

Adductor Canal Block

Jeffrey Ghassemi

CHAPTER 42

See Video 42.1 on ExpertConsult.com.

The adductor canal (Hunter's canal, subsartorial canal) is a musculoaponeurotic space, triangular in cross section, that runs from the apex of the femoral triangle (defined by the crossing of the medial margin of the adductor longus muscle and the medial margin of the sartorius muscle) to an opening in the adductor magnus known as the adductor hiatus.[1,2] The adductor hiatus is the distal extent of the canal, identified as the sonographic point at which the femoral artery dives deep away from the sartorius and vastus medialis muscles in the distal thigh.[3] The canal is bounded anteriorly by the sartorius, anterolaterally by the vastus medialis, and posteromedially by the adductor longus/magnus (Fig. 42.1).

The distal part of the canal is covered by a strong, thickened fascia known as the vastoadductor membrane (VAM). This aponeurotic roof forms a subcompartment within the subsartorial canal, connecting the medial edge of the vastus medialis to the lateral edge of the adductor magnus muscle.[4]

The adductor canal consistently contains the femoral vessels, the saphenous nerve (SN), and the nerve to the vastus medialis (NVM). Other nerves found in the adductor canal include the medial femoral cutaneous nerve, articular branches from the obturator, infrapatellar branch of the SN, and anterior and medial genicular nerves (from branches of the SN and NVM)—the extent to which they travel in some form through the canal may vary.[5,6]

The SN is the largest and longest branch of the femoral nerve. From the proximal thigh, it courses lateral to the femoral artery under the roof of the adductor canal. As it descends in the canal, the SN crosses anteriorly over the femoral artery to lie medial to it in the distal thigh.[3] The SN, a purely sensory nerve, enters the adductor canal after the motor branches of the femoral nerve have divided, with the exception being the NVM. The NVM is a motor nerve that travels with the SN in the adductor canal under the sartorius muscle and anterolateral to the femoral artery.[3]

The SN may either divide within the canal or distally in the subsartorial fat. It gives off the infrapatellar branch and other cutaneous branches that may join with cutaneous branches from the obturator nerve and deep genicular nerves to form a subsartorial plexus.[7] Only a few of the nerves of the subsartorial plexus, namely the SN, infrapatellar nerve, and the NVM muscle, can be identified with ultrasound imaging.

Though the complete analgesic effect of an adductor canal block has been attributed to anesthetizing the SN, the degree of analgesia reported in clinical studies seems disproportionate to that expected from an isolated block of the SN.[6] Contributions to knee innervation—specifically the anteromedial joint capsule—of the SN, NVM, obturator, and deep genicular nerves (SN and NVM) suggest that an adductor canal block is more than just an SN block.[6] Moreover, volunteer and cadaveric studies have shown interfascial spread extending distally into the popliteal fossa following an adductor canal block, suggesting a potential sciatic contribution.[8,9]

Although injection of local anesthetic within the adductor canal is a means of blocking the SN for surgeries of the foot and ankle, the notion that this technique does more than block the SN has lent itself to applications in knee surgery, including total knee arthroplasty (TKA). The adductor canal block can provide effective postoperative analgesia and preserve quadriceps strength, compared to a femoral nerve block.[10] Several studies now show the superiority of adding the adductor canal block to local infiltration analgesia or pericapsular injection when compared to either technique alone.[11–13] In the era of enhanced early mobilization after surgery and expedited care pathways, the adductor canal block has become an attractive option to achieve meaningful analgesia without significantly compromising motor function.

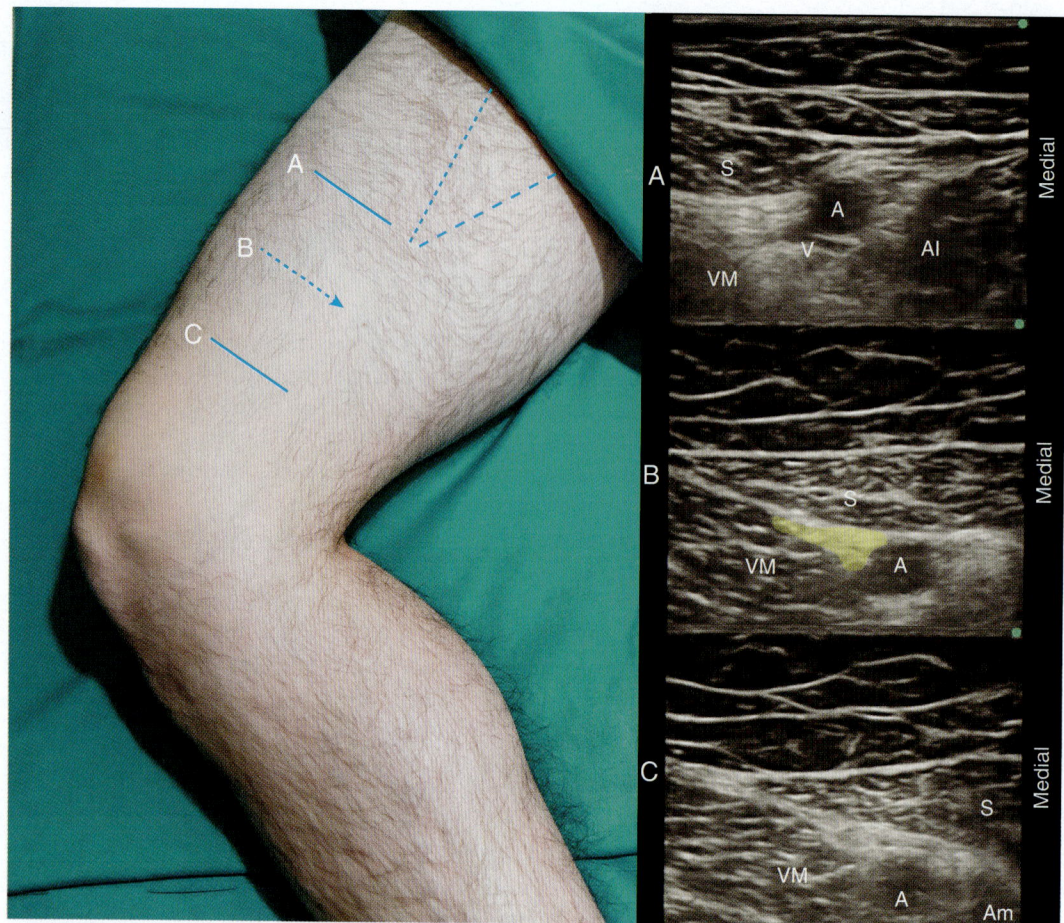

FIGURE 42.1 Surface anatomy of the right thigh with corresponding sonograms. The apex of the femoral triangle is denoted by the intersection of the medial borders of the sartorius *(dotted line)* and adductor longus *(broken line)* muscles. (A) shows the sonographic plane of the apex of the femoral triangle. (B) shows a sonographic plane that may be ideal for local anesthetic injection in the mid-AC canal. (C) shows a sonographic plane at the distal extent of the canal near the adductor hiatus. *A*, femoral artery; *AC*, adductor canal; *Al*, adductor longus; *Am*, adductor magnus; *S*, sartorius muscle; *V*, femoral vein; *VM*, vastus medialis muscle; the area shaded in *yellow* represents the likely location of the saphenous nerve and nerve to the vastus medialis, anterolateral to the femoral vessels.

SUGGESTED TECHNIQUE

Previous studies have suggested approaches to the adductor canal consistent with the subsartorial plexus block (mid-thigh) and VAM block (distal thigh).

The proximal and distal ends of the canal are anatomic sites that do not readily correlate with surface anatomic landmarks, but they can be easily identified with ultrasound imaging (Fig. 42.2). The proximal end of the canal is the site where the medial border of the sartorius muscle crosses over the medial border of the adductor longus muscle and can be located more distally in the thigh than is commonly appreciated. The distal end is the site where the femoral artery diverges from the sartorius muscle and becomes deep, passing through the adductor hiatus on its way to the popliteal fossa. Ideally, the proximal and distal ends of the canal should be identified before needle insertion to correctly ascertain that the injection site is within the adductor canal proper.[6]

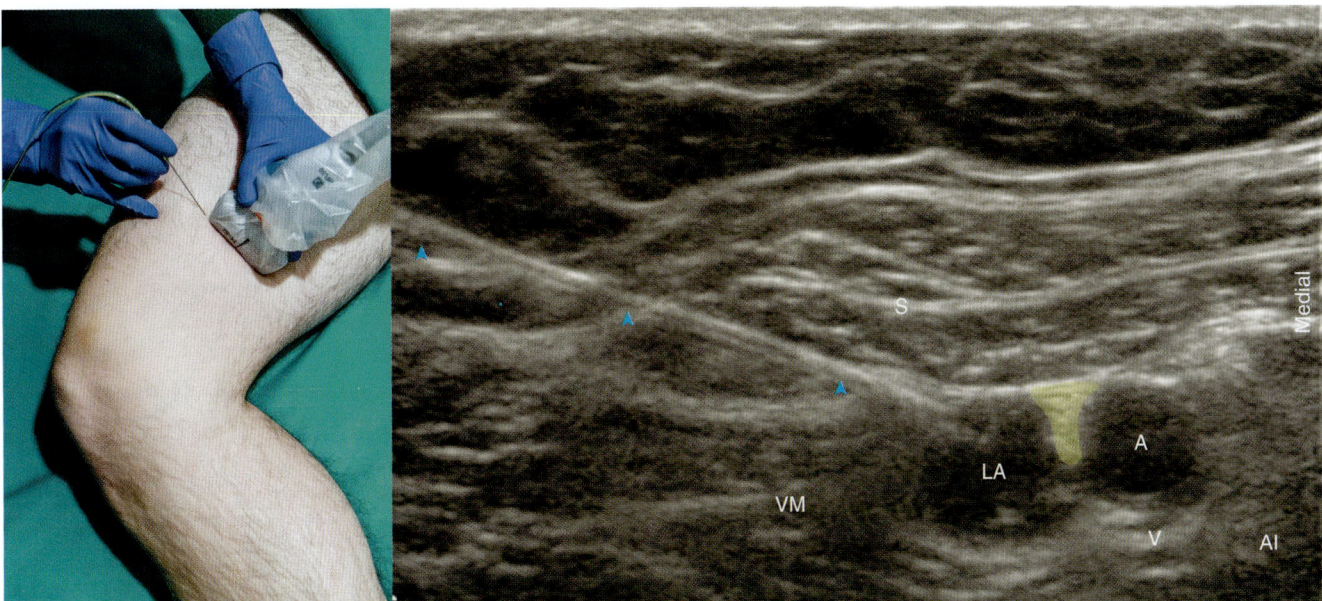

FIGURE 42.2 Suggested site and approach of block needle into the adductor canal with corresponding sonogram. *Arrows*, block needle in transsartorial approach; *A*, femoral artery; *Al*, adductor longus; *LA*, local anesthetic (hypoechoic); *S*, sartorius muscle; *V*, femoral vein; *VM*, vastus medialis muscle; the area shaded in *yellow* represents the likely location of the saphenous nerve.

Although differences in proximal-versus-distal injection in the adductor canal remain more theoretical, it has been suggested that the mid-portion of the adductor canal is an optimal site for local anesthetic administration because it is proximal enough to consistently block the SN and NVM and distal enough to avoid significant spread to the femoral triangle.[6,10,14–15]

This technique is most easily performed with the patient supine and the operative leg externally rotated and slightly flexed at the knee to facilitate coverage of the SN and superficial femoral artery by the sartorius muscle (see Fig. 42.1). Perform the block with the sartorius muscle viewed in short axis with in-plane advancement of the needle. The needle approach is from the anterior side at a level sonographically deemed within the adductor canal, i.e., with the superficial femoral artery deep to, and at the midpoint of, the sartorius muscle (see Fig. 42.2). The needle is advanced through the sartorius muscle to enter the plane deep to the muscle ("transsartorial approach").[16] Alternatively, the needle may be advanced in plane, with a short-axis view, through the superficial aspect of the vastus medialis muscle in a lateral-to-medial direction deep to the VAM and sartorius muscle. The local anesthetic injection should track within the plane deep to the sartorius muscle or VAM. Often, the local anesthetic may improve visibility of a previously indistinct SN following the injection.

QUADRICEPS WEAKNESS

The goal of an adductor canal block for surgeries about the knee is analgesia without impairment of ambulation. Given the location of the NVM (a motor branch of the femoral nerve) in the canal, an adductor canal block should produce only partial motor weakness of the quadriceps. Indeed, healthy subjects showed 92% retention of baseline quadriceps motor strength following an adductor canal block in the mid-thigh.[17] Motor function of the other three quadriceps components (rectus femoris, vastus lateralis, and vastus intermedius) should be spared because their motor nerves do not course in the adductor canal.[3]

The optimal dose or regimen of local anesthetic injection in the adductor canal has not yet been determined, though some have postulated that higher bolus dosing can lead to more proximal spread of local anesthetic to the motor fibers of the femoral nerve.[10] The minimal effective volume for an adductor canal block needed to fill the canal distally in at least 95% of patients, or ED_{95}, was determined in one study to be 20 mL.[18]

Although the adductor canal block is associated with greater preservation of quadriceps strength compared to the femoral nerve block, quadriceps dysfunction after knee surgery may ensue following an adductor canal block for other reasons, including prior weakness, surgical insult, age-related factors (even in the absence of a block), and even local anesthetic–induced myotoxicity.[10,19] As a result, patients undergoing this technique or surgery about the knee should be considered at risk for falling, and prevention measures should be implemented.

KEY POINTS

Adductor Canal Block	The Essentials
Anatomy	The SN lies lateral to the femoral artery in the proximal thigh, crossing anteriorly over the artery to lie medially to it in the distal thigh
Positioning	Supine, leg externally rotated and flexed at the knee
Operator	Standing to the side of the patient
Display	Across the table
Transducer	High-frequency linear, 28- to 50-mm footprint
Initial depth setting	35 mm
Needle	20–21 gauge, 50–100 mm in length (depending on the patient's body habitus)
Anatomic location	Mid-thigh, medial aspect
Approach	SAX view of the SN and Sa, in-plane from anterior to posterior Place the needle tip through the Sa on the anterior side of the SFA
Sonographic assessment	The injection should track distally along the SN under the Sa/VAM
Anatomic variation	Position of the SN and SFA can vary Inconsistent imaging of infrapatellar nerve and the NVM Variability of articular branch of obturator nerve within the adductor canal

NVM, Nerve to the vastus medialis; *Sa*, sartorius muscle; *SAX*, short axis; *SFA*, superficial femoral artery; *SN*, saphenous nerve; *VAM*, vastoadductor membrane.

Clinical Pearls

- The adductor canal is an anatomic canal bordered by muscle and fascia that contains the femoral vessels, saphenous nerve (SN), and nerve to the vastus medialis (NVM).
- The adductor canal block is more than just an SN block.
- Other nerves may travel through the adductor canal: the infrapatellar nerve (a branch of SN), the medial femoral cutaneous nerve, articular branches from the obturator nerve, and anterior and medial genicular nerves (from deep nerve plexus).
- SN is purely sensory; the NVM is the only motor nerve in the adductor canal.
- An adductor canal injection has the potential for spread into the popliteal fossa.
- The adductor canal block has gained popularity for effective analgesia around the knee while minimizing quadriceps motor blockade, compared to a femoral nerve block.
- For knee analgesia following total knee arthroplasty, an adductor canal block and local infiltration are better than either alone.
- Proximal and distal ends of the adductor canal do not correlate with external surface landmarks; therefore, ultrasound should be used to define its range.
- It has been suggested that an injection in the mid-portion of the adductor canal is optimal to consistently block the SN and NVM but avoid significant spread to the femoral triangle, although published reports suggest that anatomic location (proximal vs. distal) for this block may not matter.

> **Clinical Pearls—cont'd**
> - Externally rotate and flex the knee to facilitate sartorial coverage of the SN.
> - Confirm injection with ultrasound by tracking local anesthetic spread along the fascial plane deep to the sartorius/vastoadductor membrane.
> - Theoretically, significant motor blockade should be avoided with injections in the adductor canal, but potential for motor weakness still exists; providers should implement fall precautions.

References

1. Bendtsen TF, Moriggl B, Chan V, Pedersen EM, Børglum J. Redefining adductor canal block. *Reg Anesth Pain Med*. 2014;39(5):442–443.
2. Bendtsen TF, Moriggl B, Chan V, Pedersen EM, Børglum J. Defining adductor canal block. *Reg Anesth Pain Med*. 2014;39(3):253–254.
3. Manickam B, Perlas A, Duggan E, Brull R, Chan V, Ramlogan R. Feasibility and efficacy of ultrasound-guided block of the saphenous nerve in the adductor canal. *Reg Anesth Pain Med*. 2009;34(6):578–580.
4. Tubbs RS, Shoja MM, Oakes WJ. Anatomy and potential clinical significance of the vastoadductor membrane. *Surg Radiol Anat*. 2007;29:569–573.
5. Davis JJ, Bond TS, Swenson JD. Adductor canal block: more than just the saphenous nerve? *Reg Anesth Pain Med*. 2009;34(6):618–619.
6. Burckett-St. Laurant D, Peng P, et al. The nerves of the adductor canal and the innervation of the knee: an anatomic study. *Reg Anesth Pain Med*. 2016;41(3):321–327.
7. Horner G, Dellon A. Innervation of the human knee joint and implications for surgery. *Clin Orthop*. 1994;301:221–226.
8. Gautier PE, Hadzic A, Lecoq J, Brichant JF, Kuroda MM, Vandepitte C. Distribution of injectate and sensory-motor blockade after adductor canal block. *Anesth Analg*. 2016;122(1):279282.
9. Goffin P, Lecoq J, Ninane V, et al. Interfascial spread of injectate after adductor canal injection in fresh human cadavers. *Anesth Analg*. 2016;123(2):501503.
10. Mariano ER, Kim TE, Wagner MJ, et al. A randomized comparison of proximal and distal ultrasound-guided adductor canal catheter insertion sites for knee arthroplasty. *J Ultrasound Med*. 2014;33:1653–1662.
11. Andersen HL, Gyrn J, Møller L, Christensen B, Zaric D. Continuous saphenous nerve block as supplement to single-dose local infiltration analgesia for postoperative pain management after total knee arthroplasty. *Reg Anesth Pain Med*. 2013;38(2):106–111.
12. Sawhney M, Mehdian H, Kashin B, et al. Pain after unilateral total knee arthroplasty: a prospective randomized controlled trial examining the analgesic effectiveness of a combined adductor canal peripheral nerve block with periarticular infiltration versus adductor canal nerve block alone versus periarticular infiltration alone. *Anesth Analg*. 2016;122(6):2040–2046.
13. Nader A, Kendall MC, Manning DW, et al. Single-dose adductor canal block with local infiltrative analgesia compared with local infiltrate analgesia after total knee arthroplasty: a randomized, double-blind, placebo-controlled trial. *Reg Anesth Pain Med*. 2016;41(6):678–684.
14. Adoni A, Paraskeuopoulos T, Saranteas T, Sidiropoulou T, Mastrokalos D, Kostopanagiotou G. Prospective randomized comparison between ultrasound-guided saphenous nerve block within and distal to the adductor canal with low volume of local anesthetic. *J Anaesthesiol Clin Pharmacol*. 2014;30(3):378–382.
15. Head SJ, Leung RC, Hackman GP, Seib R, Rondi K, Schwarz SK. Ultrasound-guided saphenous nerve block—within versus distal to the adductor canal: a proof-of-principle randomized trial. *Can J Anaesth*. 2015;62(1):37–44.
16. Krombach J, Gray AT. Sonography for saphenous nerve block near the adductor canal. *Reg Anesth Pain Med*. 2007;32(6):536.
17. Jaeger P, Nielsen ZJ, Henningsen MH, Hilsted KL, Mathiesen O, Dahl JB. Adductor canal block versus femoral nerve block and quadriceps strength: a randomized, double-blind placebo-controlled, crossover study in healthy volunteers. *Anesthesiology*. 2013;118:409–415.
18. Jaeger P, Jenstrup MT, Lund J, et al. Optimal volume of local anaesthetic for adductor canal block: using the continual resassessment method to estimate the ED_{95}. *Br J Anaesth*. 2015;115(6):920–926.
19. Neal JM, Salinas FV, Choi DS. Local anesthetic-induced myotoxicity after continuous adductor canal block. *Reg Anesth Pain Med*. 2016;41(6):723–727.

CHAPTER 43

Obturator Nerve Block

 See Video 43.1 on ExpertConsult.com.

The obturator nerve arises from the lumbar plexus and innervates most of the adductors of the medial compartment of the thigh. The other adductors are the pectineus (innervated by the femoral nerve) and the adductor magnus (partially innervated by the sciatic nerve). The abundance of motor fibers makes the obturator nerve a frequent choice for electromyographic recording of compound motor action potentials (CMAPs).[1]

The cutaneous innervation by the obturator nerve is variable.[2] However, there are morphine-sparing effects of the obturator nerve block after major surgical procedures of the lower extremity. In blocks in which multiple lower extremity nerves are targeted (e.g., the posterior lumbar plexus block or the anterior 3-in-1 block), the obturator nerve has a relatively low block success rate. Therefore, the obturator nerve block is an important adjunct for lower extremity analgesia. Other indications for obturator nerve block include relief of hip pain, treatment of adductor spasticity, and prevention of obturator stimulation during transurethral resection of lateral bladder wall tumors. Change in adduction strength is the best method for assessing obturator nerve block. However, even with complete obturator nerve block, there is some residual adduction strength because the pectineus (femoral nerve innervation) and the hamstring component of the adductor magnus (sciatic nerve innervation) muscles remain intact.

SUGGESTED TECHNIQUE

The anterior and posterior divisions of the obturator nerve converge proximally along the rounded lateral border of the adductor brevis muscle. The obturator nerve divisions are thin and flat as the fascicles disperse to the muscle groups. The obturator nerve divisions have a "white bands" appearance on sonography.[3] It is important that the flat surfaces of the obturator nerve divisions are perpendicular to the sound beam to enhance their echo brightness. Note that although the anterior and posterior divisions converge along the lateral border of the adductor brevis, they do not actually meet there in most (75% to 80%) subjects because the divisions remain separated by the obturator externus muscle proximally.[4] Therefore, the obturator nerve block is usually performed as a multiple-injection technique targeting each of the two divisions separately.

The block is performed in supine position with the leg slightly abducted. The obturator divisions and adductor brevis are visualized in short-axis view in the medial thigh. This is best accomplished by sliding the transducer between proximal and distal locations to observe the convergence of the divisions along the lateral border of the adductor brevis. An out-of-plane approach is often used because of the proximity of the femoral vessels to the needle path for an in-plane approach. The block is usually performed where the anterior and posterior divisions are just separated by the adductor brevis, with the deeper posterior division targeted first. The local anesthetic distribution should be within the fascia that invests the adductor brevis and the obturator divisions. If the obturator nerve divisions cannot be visualized, a trans–adductor brevis injection can be performed. Care is taken to avoid puncture of the adjacent obturator arteries because puncture of these vessels can cause hemorrhage.[5]

KEY POINTS

Obturator Nerve Block	The Essentials
Anatomy	The ON divisions lie on the anterior and posterior sides of the adductor brevis muscle.
	The ON divisions are often accompanied by their respective arteries.
Image orientation	The ON divisions converge along the squared lateral edge of the adductor brevis muscle.
Positioning	Supine with leg slightly abducted
Operator:	Standing on the side of the patient
Display:	Across the table
Transducer:	Medium- to high-frequency linear, 38- to 50-mm footprint
Initial depth setting	40–50 mm (the posterior division of the obturator nerve lies at about twice the depth of the femoral nerve)
Needle:	20–21 gauge, 70 mm in length
Anatomic location:	Begin by scanning the thigh medial to the femoral vessels.
Approach:	SAX view of the ON divisions, in-plane from the lateral side
	Place the needle tip through the adductor brevis muscle and inject as the needle is slowly withdrawn.
	Local anesthetic should layer over posterior and anterior surfaces of the adductor brevis muscle.
Sonographic assessment:	The injection should track along the ON divisions (SAX slide).
Anatomic variation:	Relation of the ON divisions with obturator arteries is variable.
	ON divisions may be seen entering the adductor brevis muscle.

ON, Obturator nerve; *SAX*, short axis.

Clinical Pearls

- An accessory obturator nerve is present in about 8.7% of subjects.[6] When present, this nerve partially contributes to motor innervation of the pectineus.
- In some patients, branches entering the adductor brevis can be visualized, giving the appearance of three divisions of the obturator nerve. The position of the obturator arteries with respect to the obturator divisions is variable.

References

1. Atanassoff PG, Weiss BM, Brull SJ, et al. Compound motor action potential recording distinguishes differential onset of motor block of the obturator nerve in response to etidocaine or bupivacaine. *Anesth Analg*. 1996;82:317–320.
2. Bouaziz H, Vial F, Jochum D, et al. An evaluation of the cutaneous distribution after obturator nerve block. *Anesth Analg*. 2002;94:445–449.
3. Soong J, Schafhalter-Zoppoth I, Gray AT. Sonographic imaging of the obturator nerve for regional block. *Reg Anesth Pain Med*. 2007;32:146–151.
4. Choquet O, Capdevila X, Bennourine K, Feugeas JL, Bringuier-Branchereau S, Manelli JC. A new inguinal approach for the obturator nerve block: anatomical and randomized clinical studies. *Anesthesiology*. 2005;103:1238–1245.
5. Akata T, Murakami J, Yoshinaga A. Life-threatening haemorrhage following obturator artery injury during transurethral bladder surgery: a sequel of an unsuccessful obturator nerve block. *Acta Anaesthesiol Scand*. 1999;43:784–788.
6. Woodburne RT. The accessory obturator nerve and the innervation of the pectineus muscle. *Anat Rec*. 1960;136:367–369.

LOWER EXTREMITY BLOCKS

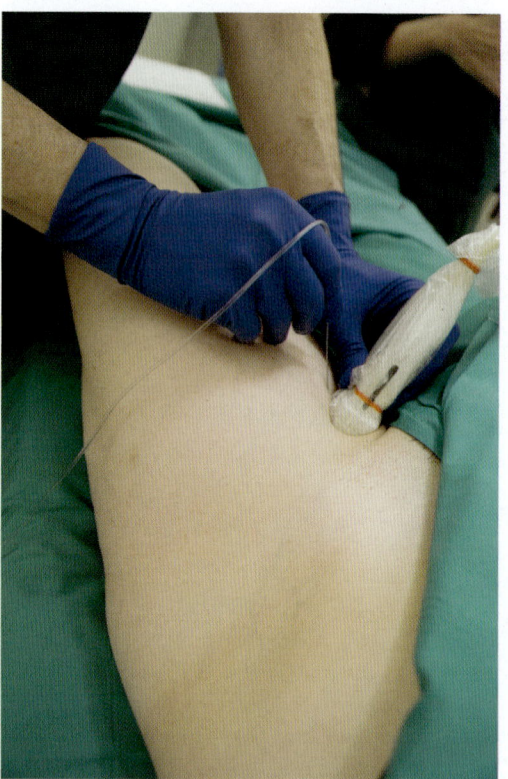

FIGURE 43.1 External photograph showing an out-of-plane approach to obturator nerve block in the medial thigh.

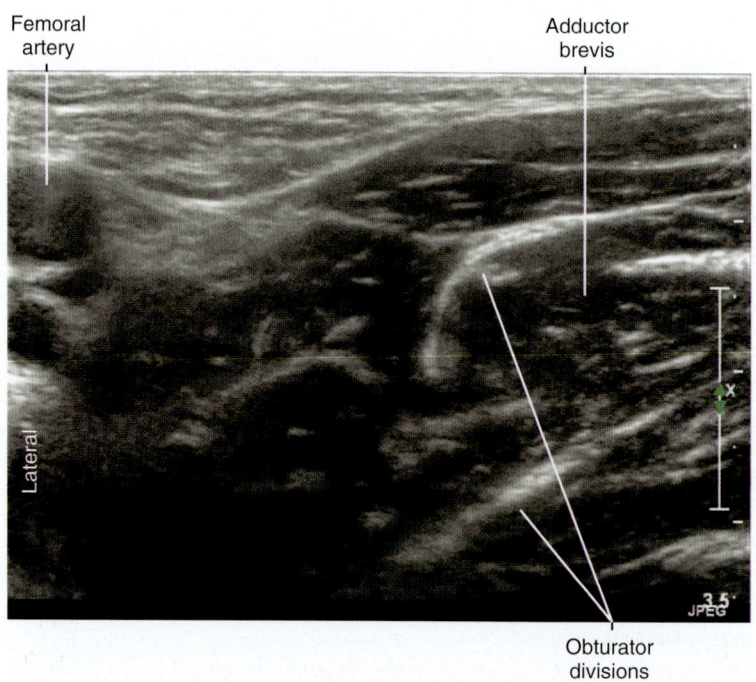

FIGURE 43.2 Sonogram of the medial thigh showing the divisions of the obturator nerve. The anterior and posterior divisions lie on the anterior and posterior sides of the adductor brevis muscle, medial to the femoral vessels.

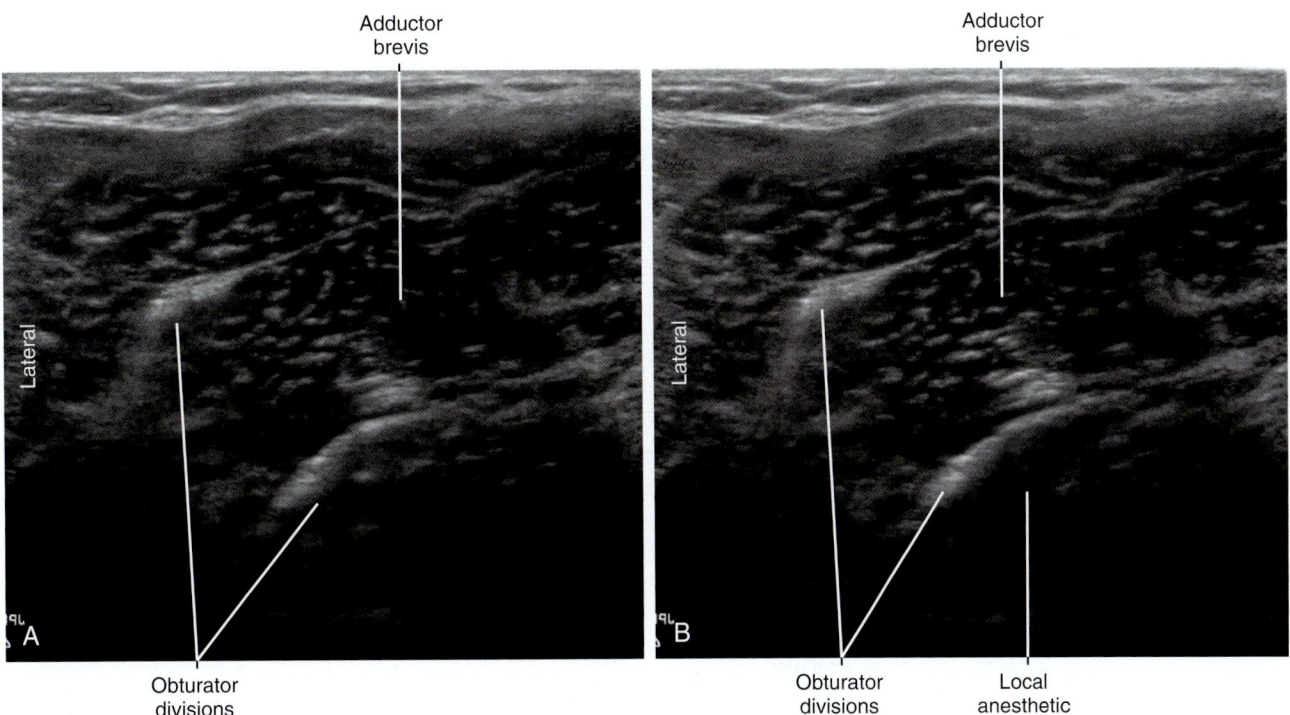

FIGURE 43.3 Image sequence showing an out-of-plane approach to obturator nerve block. The needle tip is placed through the adductor brevis muscle adjacent to the posterior division of the obturator nerve (A). After injection, local anesthetic is distributed around the posterior division (B).

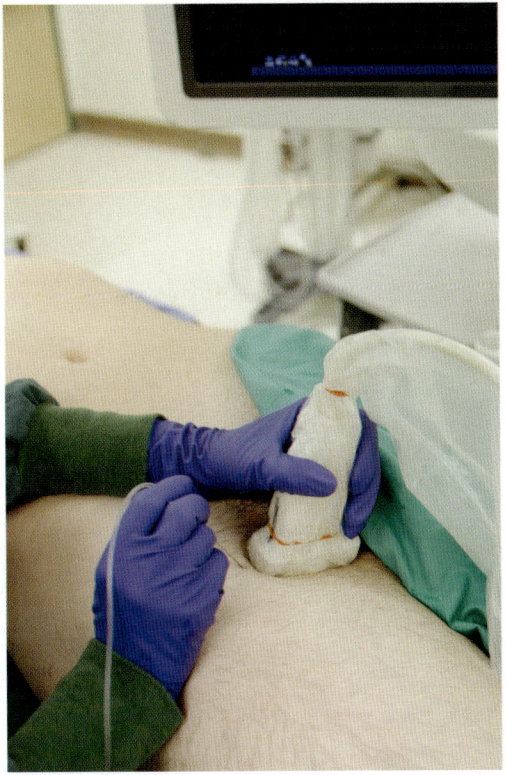

FIGURE 43.4 External photograph showing an in-plane approach to obturator nerve block in the medial thigh.

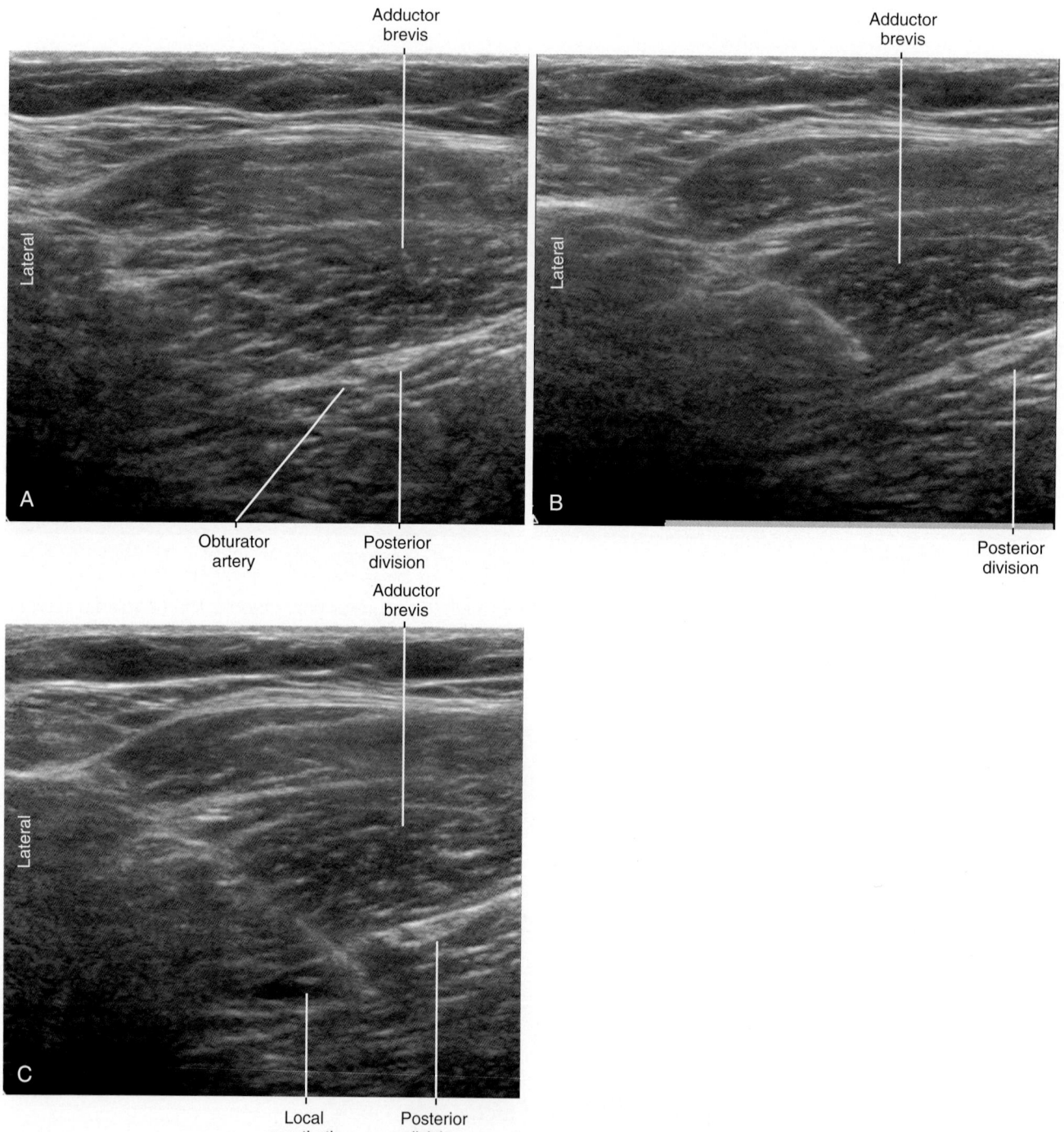

FIGURE 43.5 Image sequence showing an in-plane approach to obturator nerve block. The needle tip is placed through the adductor brevis muscle adjacent to the posterior division of the obturator nerve (A and B). After injection, local anesthetic is distributed around the posterior division (C). In this example, only the posterior division and its accompanying artery are well visualized.

Sciatic Nerve Block

CHAPTER 44

See Video 44.1 on ExpertConsult.com.

Proximal sciatic nerve block is a versatile regional anesthetic for lower extremity surgery. It is usually combined with femoral nerve block for more complete anesthesia of the leg. The sciatic nerve (L4 to S3) is the largest nerve in the body, with a transverse diameter of more than 17 mm on ultrasound scans.[1] However, despite its large size, the sciatic nerve can be difficult to visualize in the gluteal region and proximal thigh. Sonographic features of the regional anatomy are essential to identifying the nerve.

The subgluteal region has a "bright triangle" consisting of the hyperechoic sciatic nerve and adjacent tendons of the semitendinosus-biceps and semimembranosus. These proximal tendons can appear similar to the sciatic nerve on ultrasound scans. The sciatic nerve is always lateral to these ischiocrural tendons. The semimembranosus tendon is characterized by a large, flat proximal aponeurosis. The semitendinosus muscle forms a conjoint tendon with the biceps femoris that points to the medial aspect of the sciatic nerve. A short-axis view with sliding of the transducer is useful to confirm nerve identity and distinguish it from the adjacent tendons. The sciatic nerve can have a variety of shapes in the subgluteal region, including oval, triangle, and "banana boat or hammock" appearances.

Although we refer to the common sciatic nerve as a single entity, the common peroneal and tibial nerve fibers do not mix (there are no communicating branches or plexus formation between the ventral and dorsal divisions within the common sciatic nerve). The clinical implication is that even at the level of proximal sciatic block, there are actually two separate nerves present within the nerve bundle.

SUGGESTED TECHNIQUE

Prone position allows the most stable access for proximal sciatic nerve block. An in-plane technique from the lateral side of the leg is a relatively easy approach to proximal sciatic block. If prone positioning is difficult, a lateral approach can be used for this block. The leg should be relatively straight (and muscle not contracted) for proximal sciatic nerve block. A broad linear probe (5-cm footprint or larger) is best to provide a large field of view for this block because working room is not limited in this region.

Thick epineurial connective tissue invests the proximal sciatic nerve (the common investing extraneural layer).[2] Injections just deep to this layer or multiple injections may be necessary to promote block characteristics.[3] The lateral corner of the sciatic nerve lies on the thick intermuscular septum, and it can be difficult to split this fascia around the nerve. The posteromedial corner of the sciatic nerve lies in the space of the conjoint tendon of the biceps femoris and semitendinosus muscles. Both corners are natural targets for a multiple injection technique.

There are several sonographic signs of proximal sciatic nerve block success:
1. Distribution along the course of the nerve in the long-axis view (the "tram track" sign, with local anesthetic forming peeling edges on both sides of the nerve). This view is often useful because the sciatic nerve is relatively large with a straight course.
2. Echogenic fascia lifting away from the nerve with injection (the "orange peel" sign).
3. Clarity of the common peroneal and tibial nerve contributions to the sciatic nerve after injection (the "heart sign"), indicating injection deep to the investing fascia of the common sciatic nerve.

Anatomic variation of the sciatic nerve in the subgluteal region can consist of identification of separate contributions from the common peroneal and tibial nerves.[4,5] This indicates proximal division of the sciatic nerve by the piriformis muscle. If the anomaly is correctly identified, a multiple-injection technique guided by ultrasound can provide complete sciatic block. Persistent sciatic artery and different nerve morphologies are other possible variations.

More proximally the sciatic nerve lies between the greater trochanter (lateral) and the ischial tuberosity (medial). These bony reference points are useful landmarks for sciatic block in the gluteal region.[6] In some patients the inferior gluteal artery can be identified on the medial side of the proximal sciatic nerve.

KEY POINTS

Sciatic Nerve Block (Subgluteal) | **The Essentials**

Anatomy	The SN is about 6 by 18 mm in diameter.
	The conjoint ST-Bc tendon points to the medial side of the SN.
	The SM tendon lies medial to the SN.
	The PAs run over the anterior side of the SN (the AM side).
Image orientation:	The SN lies lateral to the ischiocrural tendons.
Positioning	Lateral or prone
Operator	Standing on the side of the patient
Display	Across the table
Transducer	Medium-frequency linear, 50-mm footprint
Initial depth setting	40–60 mm
Needle	20–21 gauge, 70–90 mm in length
Anatomic location	Begin by scanning the subgluteal region near the posterior midline.
	If imaging is difficult, trace the SN proximally from the popliteal fossa.
Approach	SAX view of the SN, in-plane from the lateral side.
	Place the needle tip between the SN and PA.
Sonographic assessment	The injection should track along the SN (LAX view).
Anatomic variation	Different nerve morphologies (commonly oval or triangular shape)
	Persistent sciatic artery
	Proximal division of the SN by the piriformis muscle (5%–10%)
	This may require separate injections.

AM, Adductor magnus; *Bc*, biceps femoris; *LAX*, long axis; *PA*, perforating artery; *SAX*, short axis; *SM*, semimembranosus; *SN*, sciatic nerve; *ST*, semitendinosus.

Clinical Pearls

- A number of patient positions can be used to approach the proximal sciatic nerve block. The prone position is favored because of the stable imaging for the in-plane technique from the lateral aspect of the thigh. Another relatively easy alternative is the lateral position with a hip bump to provide stability.
- One of the key landmarks for identification of the sciatic nerve in the proximal thigh is the intermuscular septum that separates the adductor magnus muscle from the hamstring muscles of the posterior thigh.
- The proximal semimembranosus tendon has a characteristic "teardrop" shape that tapers medially.
- The fascia surrounding the sciatic nerve in the subgluteal region is relatively thick. This emphasizes the importance of correct needle tip positioning and local anesthetic distribution.
- The sciatic nerve lies lateral to the tendon of the semimembranosus muscle. The conjoint tendon of the biceps femoris and semitendinosus points to the medial aspect of the sciatic nerve because the nerve lies in the crease between these two muscles.[7]

> **Clinical Pearls—cont'd**
>
> - Perforating arteries can usually be seen crossing the anterior side of the sciatic nerve through the intermuscular septum that separates the sciatic nerve from the adductor magnus muscle. The perforator arteries run oblique to the sciatic nerve (the perforator arteries will be seen in apparent short-axis view when the sciatic nerve is viewed in either short or long axis).
> - Sometimes the sciatic nerve must be traced proximally from its bifurcation in the popliteal fossa for identification.
> - Both proximal and distal sciatic nerve blocks reduce posterior and anterior knee pain following knee replacement surgery.[8]
> - In some subjects, the blood supply of the proximal sciatic nerve (arteria comitans) can be imaged with color Doppler and used to help establish nerve location.[9]

References

1. Heinemeyer O, Reimers CD. Ultrasound of radial, ulnar, median, and sciatic nerves in healthy subjects and patients with hereditary motor and sensory neuropathies. *Ultrasound Med Biol.* 1999;25:481–485.
2. Nader A, Kendall MC, De Oliveira GS Jr, et al. A dose-ranging study of 0.5% bupivacaine or ropivacaine on the success and duration of the ultrasound-guided, nerve-stimulator-assisted sciatic nerve block: a double-blind, randomized clinical trial. *Reg Anesth Pain Med.* 2013;38(6):492–502.
3. Yamamoto H, Sakura S, Wada M, Shido A. A prospective, randomized comparison between single- and multiple-injection techniques for ultrasound-guided subgluteal sciatic nerve block. *Anesth Analg.* 2014;119(6):1442–1448.
4. Benzon HT, Katz JA, Benzon HA, Iqbal MS. Piriformis syndrome: anatomic considerations, a new injection technique, and a review of the literature. *Anesthesiology.* 2003;98:1442–1448.
5. Pokorny D, Jahoda D, Veigl D, Pinskerová V, Sosna A. Topographic variations of the relationship of the sciatic nerve and the piriformis muscle and its relevance to palsy after total hip arthroplasty. *Surg Radiol Anat.* 2006;28:88–91.
6. Chan VW, Nova H, Abbas S, McCartney CJ, Perlas A, Xu DQ. Ultrasound examination and localization of the sciatic nerve: a volunteer study. *Anesthesiology.* 2006;104:309–314.
7. Bruhn J, Moayeri N, Groen GJ, et al. Soft tissue landmark for ultrasound identification of the sciatic nerve in the infragluteal region: the tendon of the long head of the biceps femoris muscle. *Acta Anaesthesiol Scand.* 2009;53(7):921–925.
8. Abdallah FW, Chan VW, Gandhi R, Koshkin A, Abbas S, Brull R. The analgesic effects of proximal, distal, or no sciatic nerve block on posterior knee pain after total knee arthroplasty: a double-blind placebo-controlled randomized trial. *Anesthesiology.* 2014;121(6):1302–1310.
9. Elsharkawy H, Kashy BK, Babazade R, Gray AT. Ultrasound detection of arteria comitans: a novel technique to locate the sciatic merve. *Reg Anesth Pain Med.* 2017. PMID: 29035937.

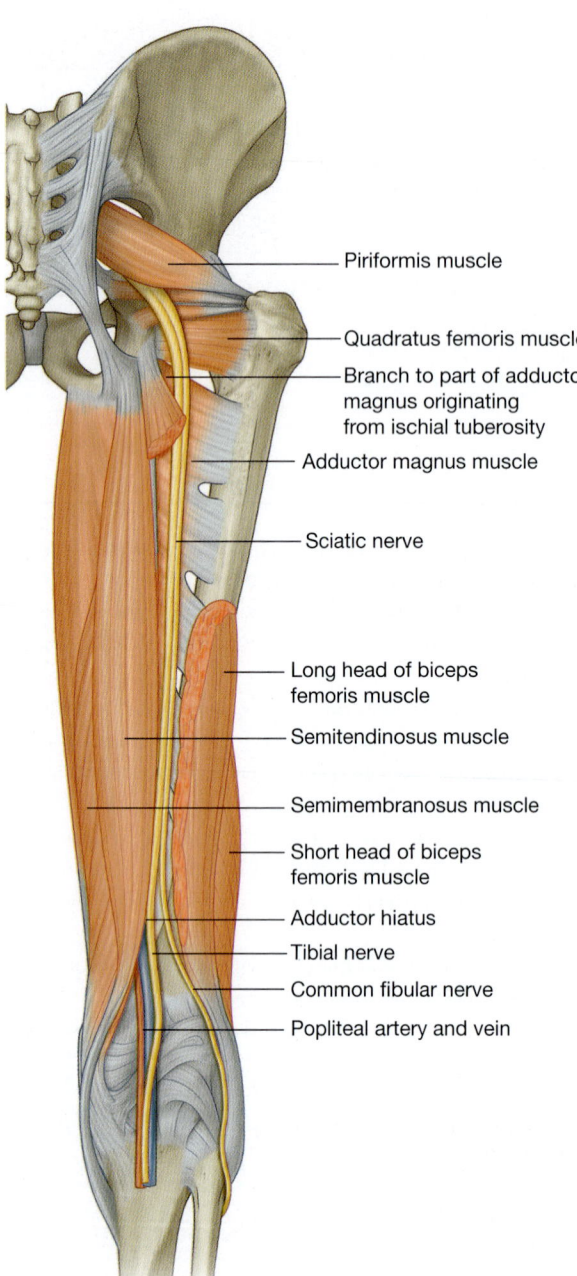

FIGURE 44.1 Course of the sciatic nerve. (From Drake RL, Vogl W, Mitchell AWM. *Gray's anatomy for students*. Philadelphia: Churchill Livingstone; 2004.)

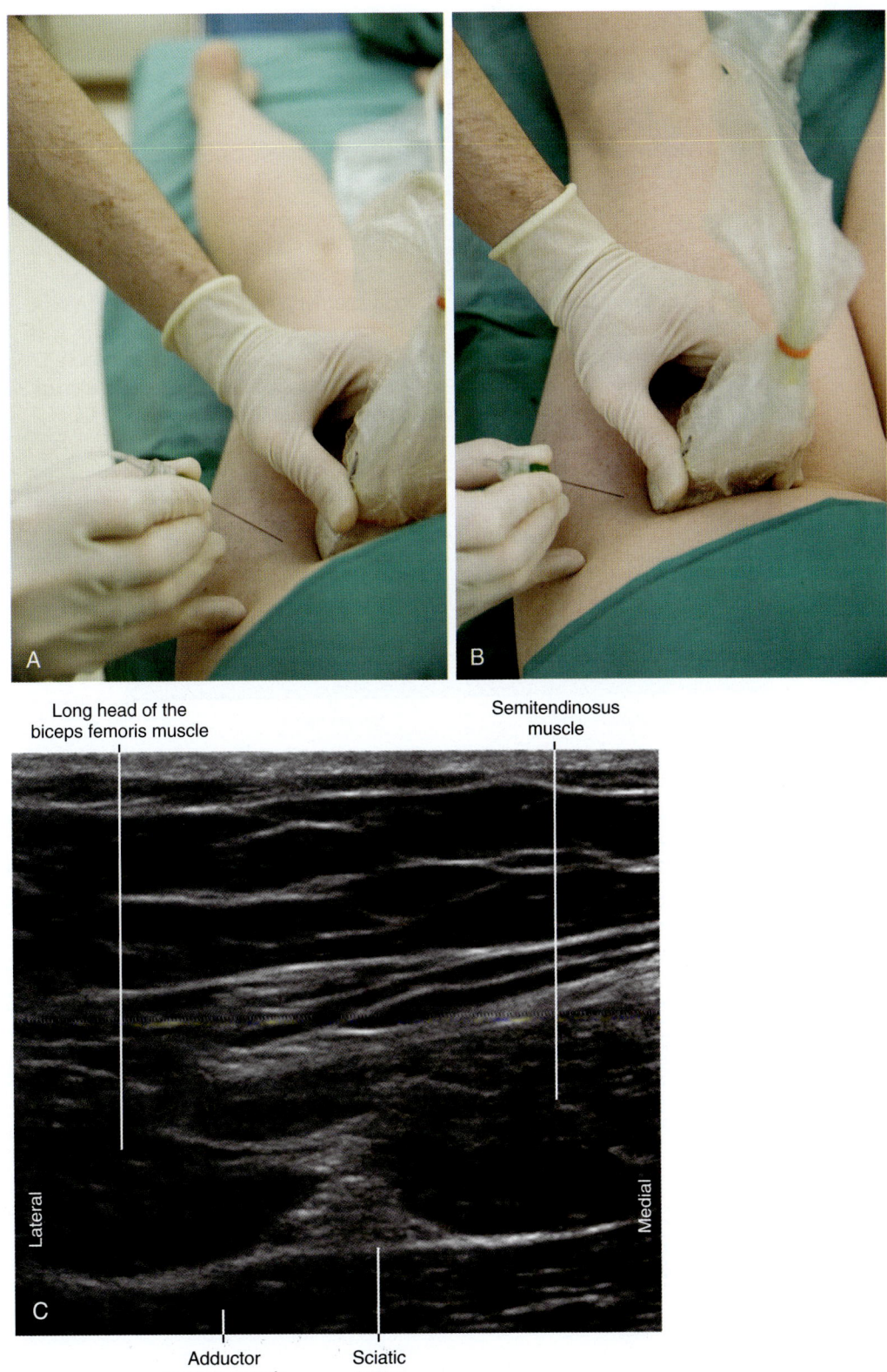

FIGURE 44.2 External photograph showing the approach to sciatic nerve block in the subgluteal region. An in-plane approach from the lateral aspect of the thigh is shown (A and B). The corresponding sonogram with the sciatic nerve in transverse view is shown (C). The subgluteal sciatic nerve often has a triangular shape defined by the following three borders: the long head of the biceps femoris (posterolateral), the semitendinosus (posteromedial), and the adductor magnus (anterior). Sciatic nerve block usually targets the lateral corner of the nerve.

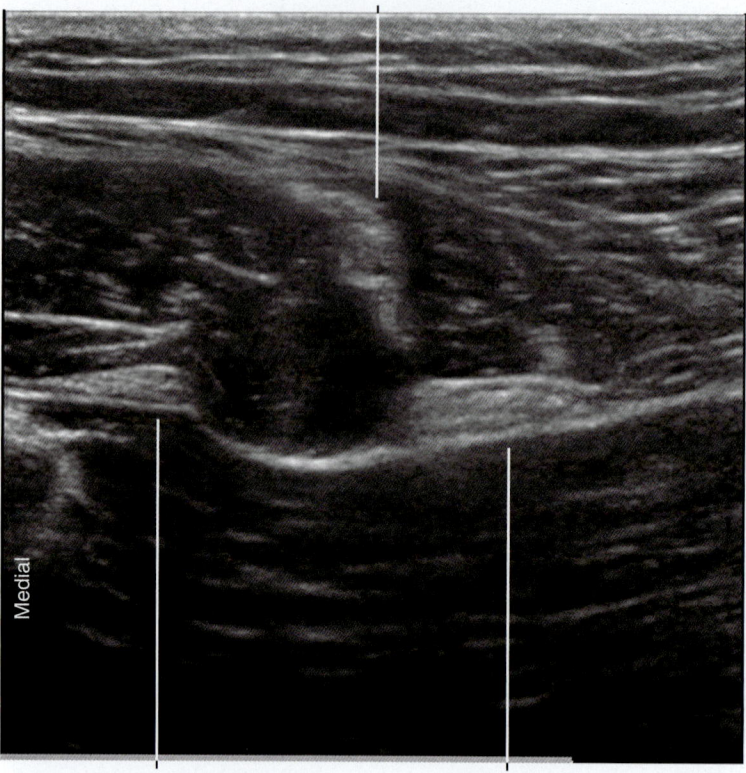

FIGURE 44.3 Short-axis view of the proximal sciatic nerve demonstrating its internal echotexture. The "comma" or "S"-shaped conjoint tendon of the biceps femoris and semitendinosus points to the medial side of the sciatic nerve. The semimembranosus tendon has a "teardrop" shape and is flattened medially. These ischiocrural tendons are valuable sonographic landmarks for proximal sciatic nerve block.

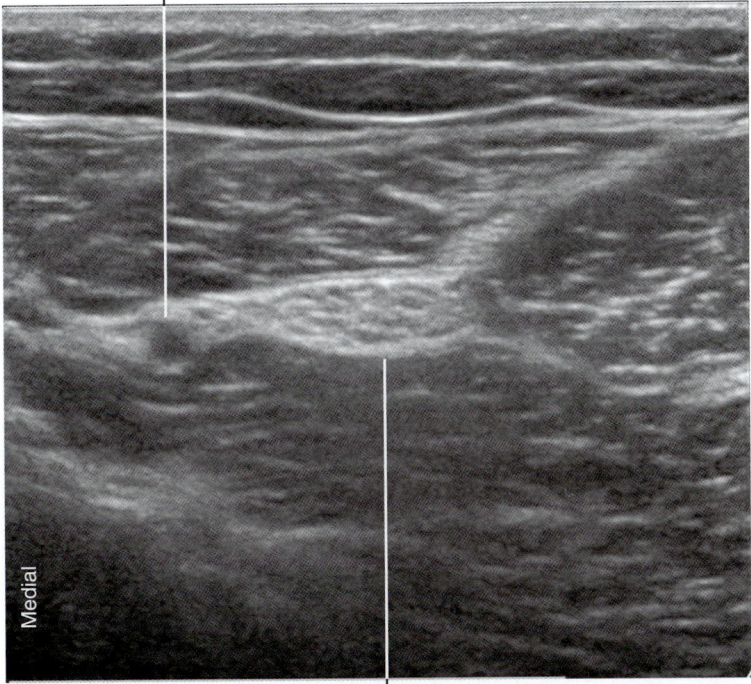

FIGURE 44.4 The perforating arteries have a characteristic oblique course over the anterior surface of the sciatic nerve in the proximal thigh. Because the perforator arteries have a 45-degree oblique course with respect to the sciatic nerve, the arteries appear in short-axis view regardless of whether the nerve is viewed in short axis or long axis. The perforating arteries travel through the intermuscular septum over the adductor magnus muscle.

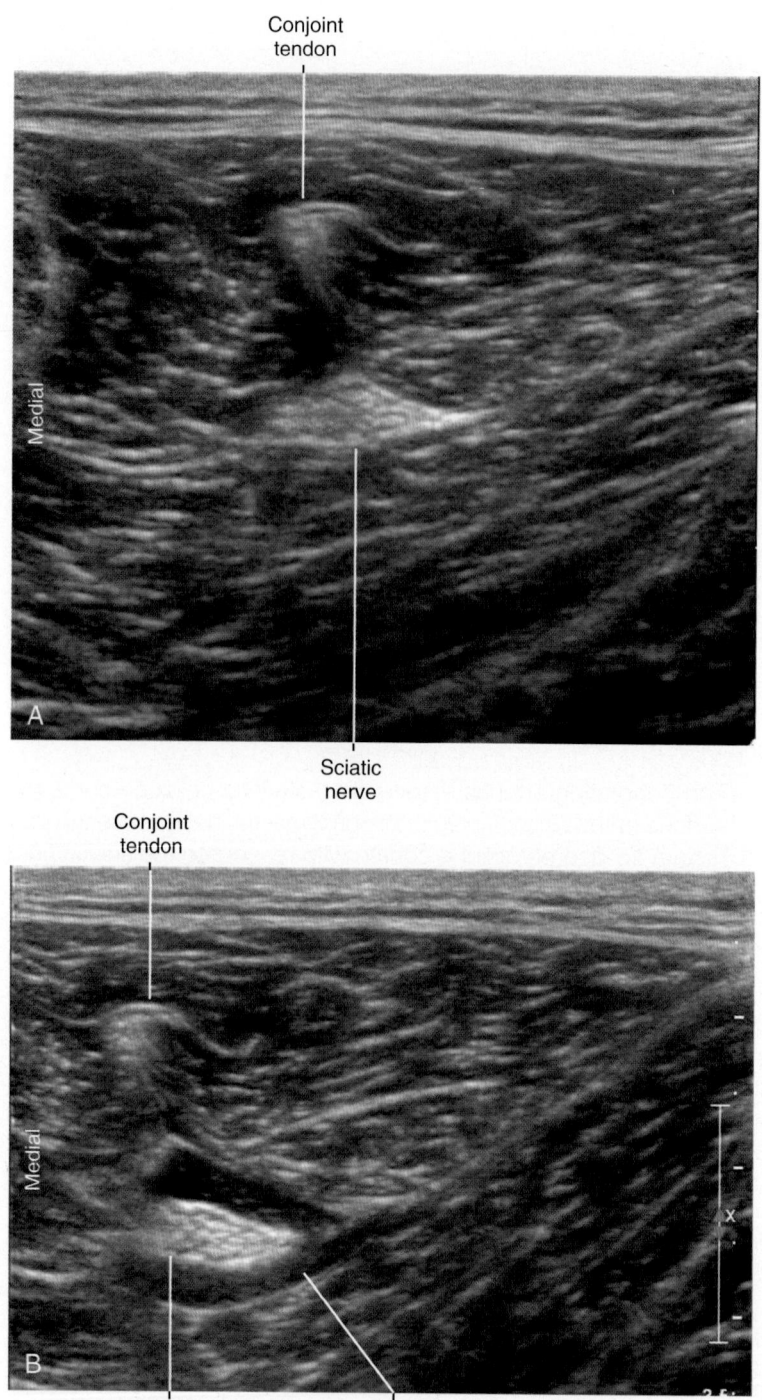

FIGURE 44.5 The sciatic nerve can have variable morphologies. The injection distribution around the sciatic nerve in the subgluteal region can have a triangular appearance, pointing toward the conjoint tendon of the semitendinosus and the biceps femoris. The term "subgluteal" is used to refer to the region distal to the gluteal crease. Sonograms are shown before (A) and after (B) injection.

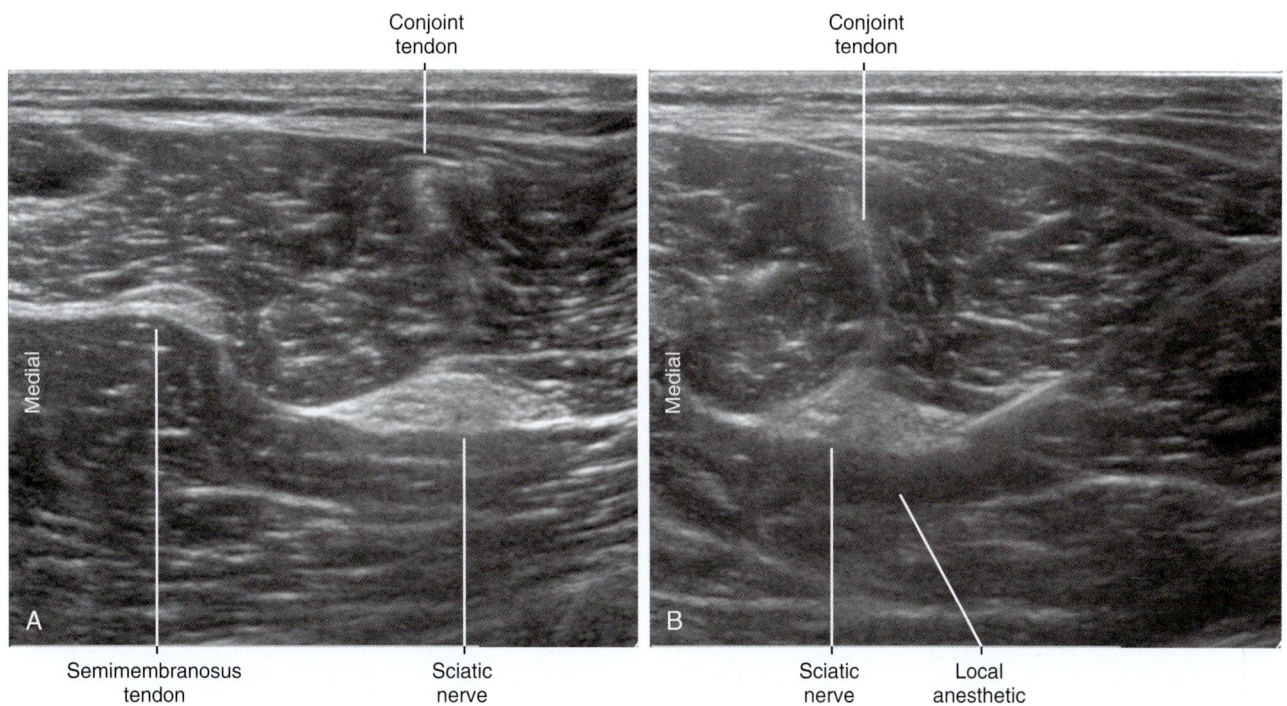

FIGURE 44.6 Short-axis in-plane approach to sciatic nerve block in the proximal thigh. The lateral corner of the nerve is targeted for local anesthetic injection. Sonograms are shown before (A) and after (B) injection.

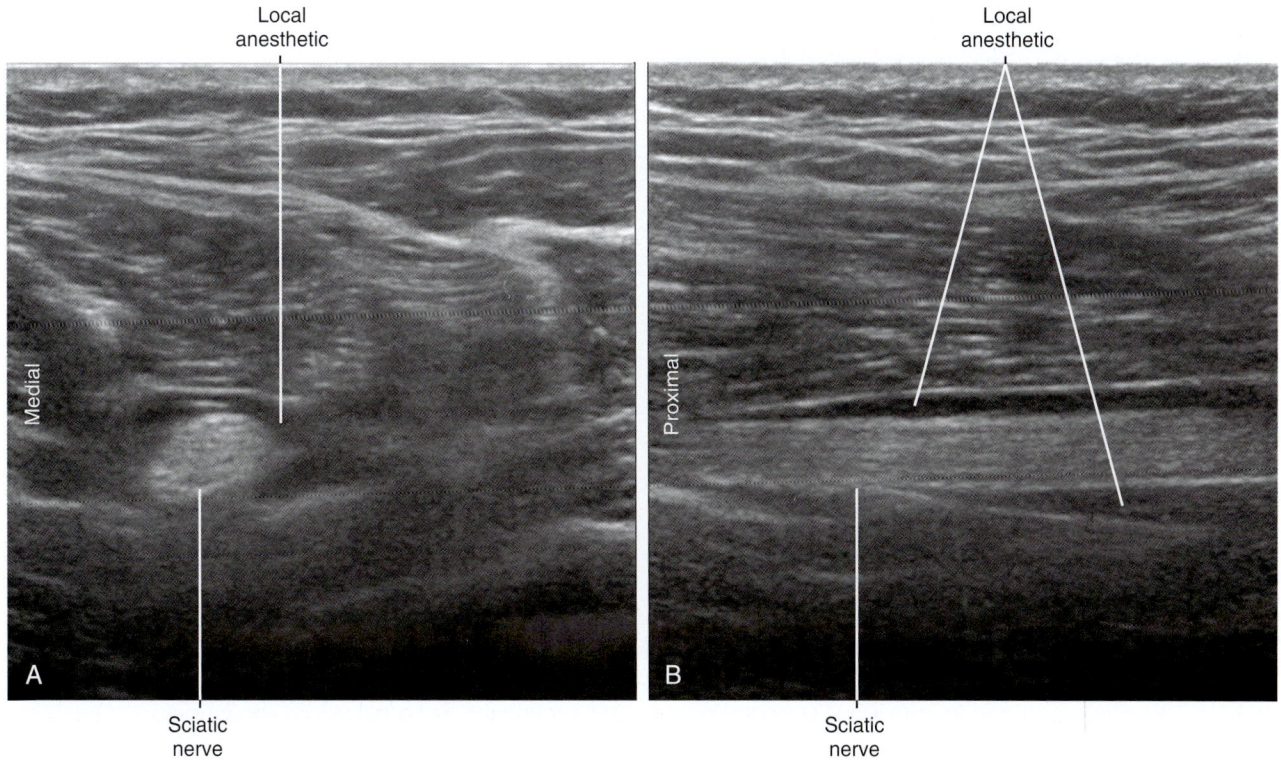

FIGURE 44.7 Because the sciatic nerve is large and straight, long-axis views can be useful for assessing the distribution along the course of the sciatic nerve. Local anesthetic should layer on both anterior and posterior sides of the nerve with the peeling edges of the distribution identified. Corresponding short-axis (A) and long-axis (B) views are shown.

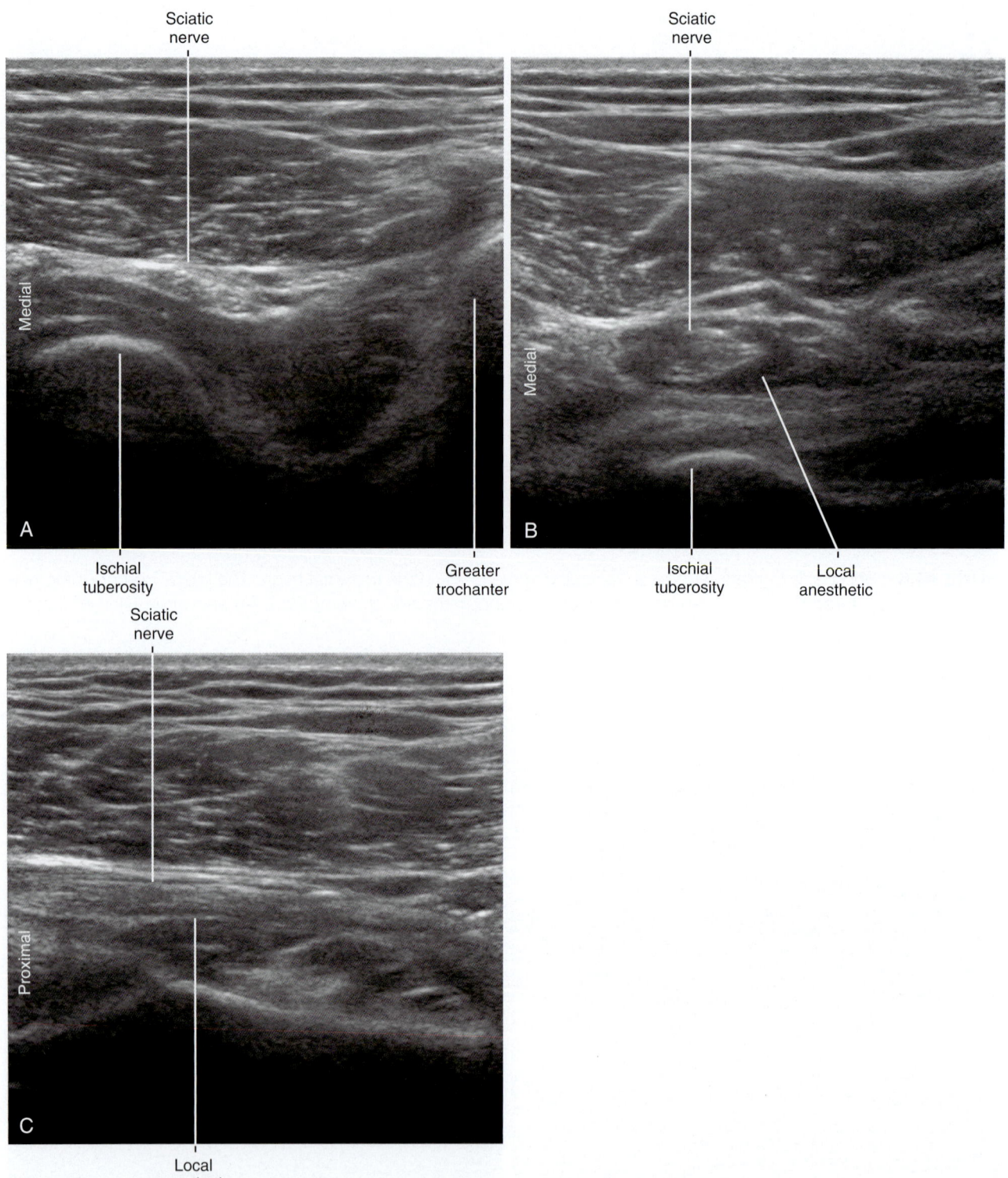

FIGURE 44.8 Sciatic nerve block can be performed in the gluteal region. In this location the ischial tuberosity (medial) and greater trochanter (lateral) serve as sonographic landmarks. The sciatic nerve lies between these two bony landmarks, usually closer to the ischial tuberosity. Sonograms are shown before (A) and after (B) injection in short-axis view, with the corresponding postinjection long-axis view shown (C).

Anterior Sciatic Nerve Block

CHAPTER 45

The anterior approach to the proximal sciatic nerve block can be used in patients who are difficult to situate in a lateral or prone position. This supine approach is deeper than other approaches because the sciatic nerve lies far from the anterior surface of the thigh and is therefore primarily used in thin patients.

SUGGESTED TECHNIQUE

First, obtain a long-axis view of the femur with the transducer placed on the anterior aspect of the thigh. The femur is easily identified by its bright cortical surface and acoustic shadowing. Next, slide the transducer medially to obtain a long-axis view of the sciatic nerve at approximately twice the depth of the femur. The sciatic nerve is wide and straight and therefore appears as an echogenic linear structure lying deep to the adductor magnus muscle. If the femoral artery is visible, then the transducer has slid too far medially.

The block needle approaches in-plane with the sciatic nerve in this long-axis view. The approach can be from proximal to distal or distal to proximal depending on the side of the block and the handedness of the operator. The sciatic nerve will bow like a string as the block needle approaches. When the local anesthetic is within the correct tissue plane, the injection will track along the proximal-distal course of the nerve and ideally on both the anterior and posterior sides of the nerve. Some practitioners elect to combine ultrasound imaging with nerve stimulation to confirm nerve identity for this block. Even though the sciatic nerve has a large diameter and a relatively straight course, it can still be difficult to simultaneously maintain a long-axis view of the nerve with the needle in-plane.

In many patients the sciatic nerve is easy to identify because it appears as a hyperechoic, linear (cable-like) structure deep to the clearly delineated border of the adductor magnus muscle that is formed by the intermuscular septum.[1] Because this block is performed distal to the lesser trochanter of the femur, external rotation of the leg promotes access to the sciatic nerve.[2]

The long-axis in-plane approach constrains the needle to a trajectory that can potentially puncture the nerve. Nerve stimulation may be used to help rule out intraneural needle tip placement by verifying that evoked motor responses are eliminated at low stimulation currents (e.g., ≤0.2 m Amp via cathodal stimulation).

Clinical Pearls

- The sciatic nerve is approximately 6–10 cm from the anterior surface of the thigh. Although the nerve is deep, its visibility is enhanced in long-axis view deep to the distinct border of the adductor magnus muscle.
- The anterior approach to sciatic nerve block is usually performed 2–5 cm distal to the lesser trochanter of the femur. The lesser trochanter is the bony prominence on the anteromedial aspect of the femur to which the iliopsoas tendon attaches.

References

1. Tsui BC, Ozelsel TJ. Ultrasound-guided anterior sciatic nerve block using a longitudinal approach: "expanding the view." *Reg Anesth Pain Med.* 2008;33(3):275–276.
2. Vloka JD, Hadžić A, April E, Thys DM. Anterior approach to the sciatic nerve block: the effects of leg rotation. *Anesth Analg.* 2001;92(2):460–462.

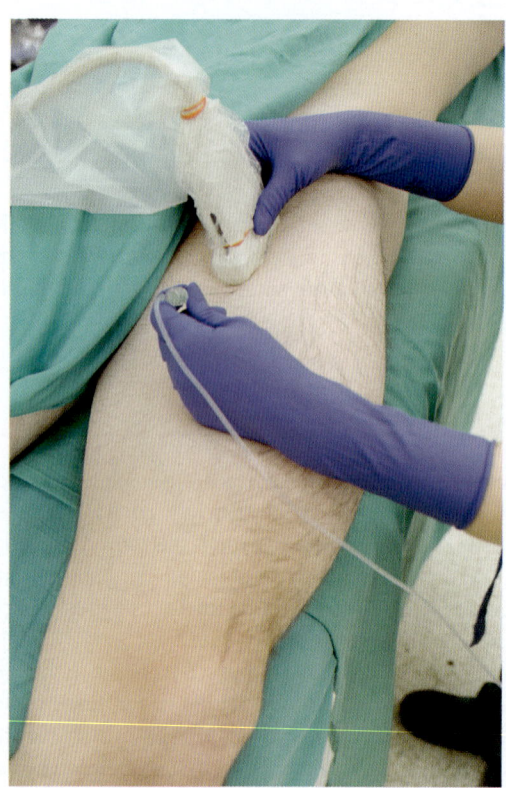

FIGURE 45.1 Positioning for ultrasound-guided anterior sciatic nerve block. An in-plane approach with longitudinal imaging is shown.

ANTERIOR SCIATIC NERVE BLOCK 191

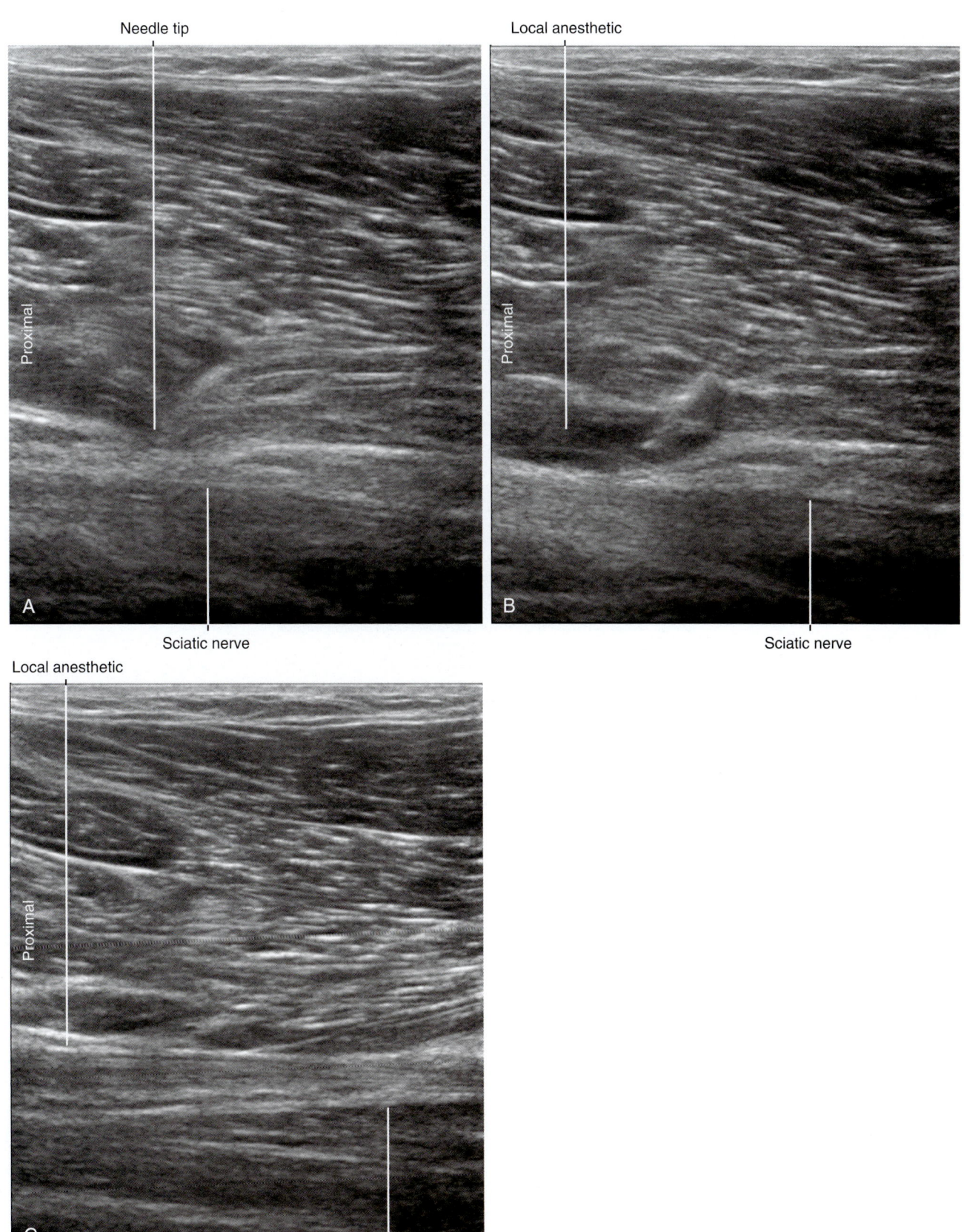

FIGURE 45.2 Long-axis view of the sciatic nerve with an in-plane approach of the block needle. From this anterior view the sciatic nerve can be seen deep to the adductor magnus muscle. Sonograms acquired before injection (A) and after injection (B), and longitudinal assessment of the distribution (C).

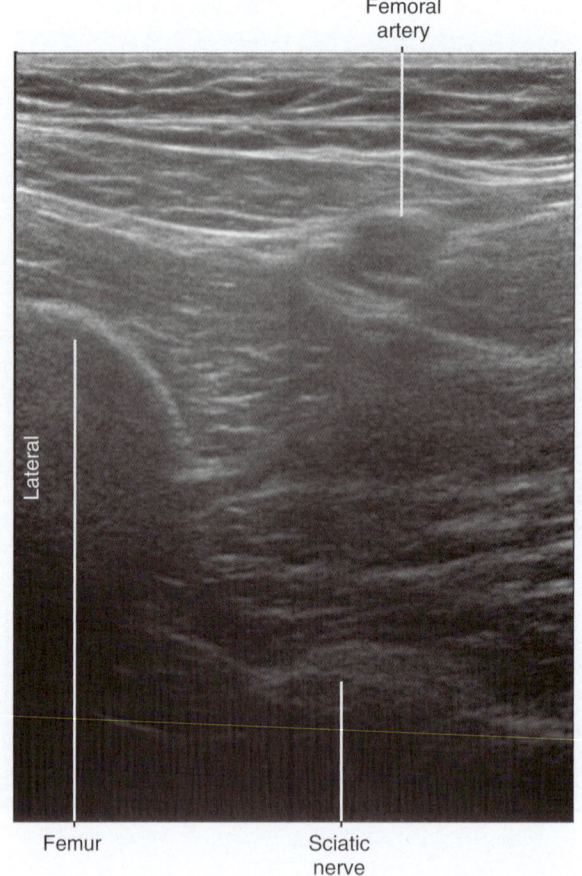

FIGURE 45.3 Transverse view from the anterior thigh showing the sciatic nerve lying between the femur and femoral vessels.

Popliteal Block

CHAPTER 46

See Video 46.1 on ExpertConsult.com.

Popliteal sciatic nerve blocks are versatile regional anesthetics that provide surgical anesthesia of the foot and ankle. These blocks are often combined with saphenous or femoral nerve blocks for complete anesthesia of the distal leg. The idea behind popliteal blocks is to perform the procedure just distal to where the sciatic nerve divides into its tibial and common peroneal nerve components. The only anatomic structure that bifurcates in the popliteal fossa is the sciatic nerve.

The tibial nerve visibility is best near the knee crease because of the relatively small extremity size. In that location, the typical anatomy comprises the popliteal artery, popliteal vein, and tibial nerve (listed from deep to superficial within a parasagittal plane). The tibial nerve is about twice the size of the common peroneal nerve in terms of cross-sectional area.[1] In addition, the tibial nerve has a straight course near the middle of the lower extremity, whereas the common peroneal nerve has a more oblique (lateral) course (Table 46.1).

The common peroneal nerve travels distally along the posterior or medial aspect of the conjoint tendon of the biceps femoris near the knee crease. With the foot in neutral position, the common peroneal nerve usually lies slightly closer to the posterior surface of the leg than the tibial nerve.[2] Because it is smaller and has fewer fascicles, the common peroneal nerve is more difficult to identify than the tibial nerve.[3]

SUGGESTED TECHNIQUE

Elevation of the leg and some internal rotation allow imaging of the popliteal fossa from the posterior surface.[4] A broad linear transducer (35- to 50-mm footprint, 10 MHz center frequency) is used for most adult patients. The choice of block needle (7- to 9-cm length, 20 to 22 gauge) is not critical.

Popliteal block is usually performed just distal to the sciatic nerve bifurcation in the popliteal fossa for several reasons. First, the nerves are close to the posterior skin surface. This makes nerve imaging and positioning the needle tip easier. Second, the needle can be aimed at the connective tissue space between the tibial and common peroneal nerves (rather than directly at the sciatic nerve).[5] The block is performed where the tibial and common peroneal nerves are about one

TABLE 46.1 Characteristics of the Bifurcation of the Sciatic Nerve in the Popliteal Fossa

Nerve	Common Peroneal Nerve	Tibial Nerve
Position	Lateral Posterior (superficial)	Medial Anterior (deep)
Diameter (mm)	4.0	6.5
Course	Oblique	Straight
Associated structures	Joins conjoint tendon of biceps femoris distally	Joins popliteal artery and vein distally
Echotexture	Less hyperechoic Fewer fascicles Larger fascicles	More hyperechoic More fascicles Smaller fascicles
Response to foot dorsiflexion	Moves anteriorly	Moves posteriorly

needle-width apart (about 1 mm). Third, there is a large amount of nerve surface area available for diffusion of local anesthetic to promote clinical block characteristics. The point of sonographic unity is closer to the knee crease than anatomic dissections would suggest because the tibial and common peroneal nerves run next to each other for some distance before visibly separating. The only potential disadvantage to this more distal popliteal block is that the popliteal vessels are closer to the nerves.

The needle bevel should face the transducer for optimal needle tip visibility (bevel down). Because the common peroneal nerve is slightly closer to the posterior surface than the tibial nerve is, it is best to approach the gap between the two nerves from the femur side (i.e., a slight posterior inclination of the block needle with the lateral approach).

Studies have suggested a limited ability of ultrasound to correctly assess circumferential distribution of local anesthetic around peripheral nerves. The reported predictive value of the "doughnut" sign is only about 90% for sciatic nerve blocks.[6] One major advantage to sciatic nerve block in the popliteal fossa is that it allows sliding assessment of the longitudinal distribution along the nerve branches (i.e., local anesthetic should not only surround the nerve but also track along the nerves).

The onset of blockade of the common peroneal nerve is usually faster than for the tibial nerve, which may reflect the smaller size of the common peroneal nerve.[7]

KEY POINTS

Popliteal Block	The Essentials
Anatomy	The TN is twice the size of the CPN.
	The TN is approximately 7 mm in diameter.
	The CPN is approximately 3.5 mm in diameter.
	The CPN is posterior and lateral to the TN.
	The TN lies posterior to the popliteal artery and vein at the knee crease (AVN).
	The CPN lies medial to the biceps femoris tendon at the knee crease.
Positioning	Supine with leg elevated
	This allows scanning from the posterior surface of thigh.
Operator	Standing at the side of the patient
Display	Across the table
Transducer	High-frequency linear, 38- to 50-mm footprint
Initial depth setting	35–45 mm
Needle	20–21 gauge, 70 mm in length
Anatomic location	Begin by scanning with the probe along the knee crease.
	Slide the transducer proximally from the knee crease.
	Identify the confluence of the TN and CPN to form the common SN.
Approach	SAX view, in-plane from lateral to medial
	Place the needle tip between the TN and CPN at point of bifurcation.
Sonographic assessment	The injection should track distally along the TN and CPN.
Anatomic variation	The nerves change position with foot motion.[2]

CPN, Common peroneal nerve; *SAX*, short axis; *SN*, sciatic nerve; *TN*, tibial nerve.

Clinical Pearls

- Leg elevation and internal rotation help ultrasound-guided popliteal blocks in the supine position.
- A hip bump helps rotate the leg into favorable position for popliteal block.
- Slight reverse Trendelenburg position levels the posterior surface of the leg for imaging.

> **Clinical Pearls—cont'd**
>
> - The only major branches of the sciatic nerve in the thigh are the tibial and common peroneal nerves. The connective tissue between these two branches is the target for the block needle tip, injection, and catheter placement. This paraneural sheath is the investing fascia of the common sciatic nerve and continues distally with these major branches.[8,9]
> - Movement of the foot induces characteristic nerve motion in the popliteal fossa that can improve nerve conspicuity (the "seesaw" sign).[2]
> - Ultrasound guidance is particularly useful for locating the bifurcation of the sciatic nerve into the tibial and common peroneal nerves. Most studies have confirmed that popliteal block performed just distal to the bifurcation improves clinical block characteristics.[10]

References

1. Heinemeyer O, Reimers CD. Ultrasound of radial, ulnar, median, and sciatic nerves in healthy subjects and patients with hereditary motor and sensory neuropathies. *Ultrasound Med Biol*. 1999;25:481–485.
2. Schafhalter-Zoppoth I, Younger SJ, Collins AB, et al. The " seesaw " sign: improved sonographic identification of the sciatic nerve. *Anesthesiology*. 2004;101:808–809.
3. Peeters EY, Nieboer KH, Osteaux MM. Sonography of the normal ulnar nerve at Guyon's canal and of the common peroneal nerve dorsal to the fibular head. *J Clin Ultrasound*. 2004;32:375–380.
4. Gray AT, Huczko EL, Schafhalter-Zoppoth I. Lateral popliteal nerve block with ultrasound guidance. *Reg Anesth Pain Med*. 2004;29:507–509.
5. Vloka JD, Hadžić A, Lesser JB, et al. A common epineural sheath for the nerves in the popliteal fossa and its possible implications for sciatic nerve block. *Anesth Analg*. 1997;84:387–390.
6. Perlas A, Brull R, Chan VW, et al. Ultrasound guidance improves the success of sciatic nerve block at the popliteal fossa. *Reg Anesth Pain Med*. 2008;33:259–265.
7. Paqueron X, Bouaziz H, Macalou D, et al. The lateral approach to the sciatic nerve at the popliteal fossa: one or two injections? *Anesth Analg*. 1999;89:1221–1225.
8. Karmakar MK, Shariat AN, Pangthipampai P, Chen J. High-definition ultrasound imaging defines the paraneural sheath and the fascial compartments surrounding the sciatic nerve at the popliteal fossa. *Reg Anesth Pain Med*. 2013;38(5):447–451.
9. Wolf FA, Gray AT. Sonography of the paraneural sheath of the sciatic nerve in the popliteal fossa: more than a bifurcation. *Reg Anesth Pain Med*. 2014;39(3):260–261.
10. Germain G, Lévesque S, Dion N, et al. Brief reports: a comparison of an injection cephalad or caudad to the division of the sciatic nerve for ultrasound-guided popliteal block: a prospective randomized study. *Anesth Analg*. 2012;114(1):233–235.

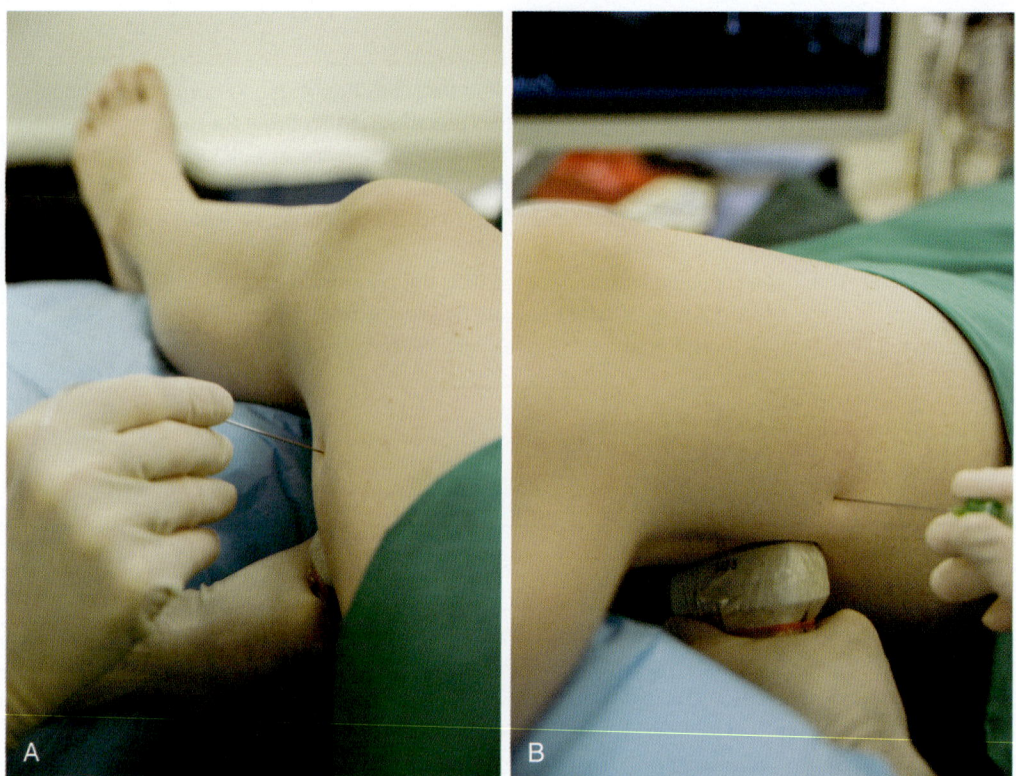

FIGURE 46.1 External photograph showing the approach to sciatic nerve block in the popliteal fossa (A and B). An in-plane approach from the lateral aspect of the thigh is shown. The patient is supine with the leg elevated to allow access for the transducer from the posterior aspect of the leg. Internal rotation of the leg also helps ultrasound-guided blocks in supine position.

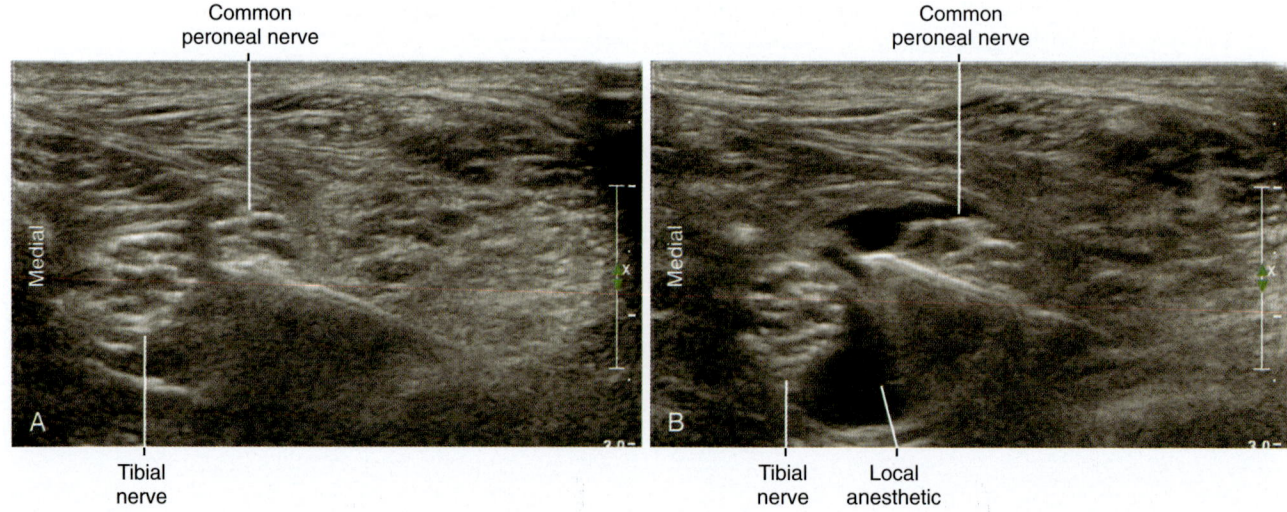

FIGURE 46.2 Image sequence showing popliteal block. An in-plane approach is demonstrated whereby the needle tip is placed between the common peroneal and tibial nerves (A). The block needle is then advanced until tent and recoil of the adjoining connective tissue are observed. After injection, local anesthetic is distributed around both nerves (B).

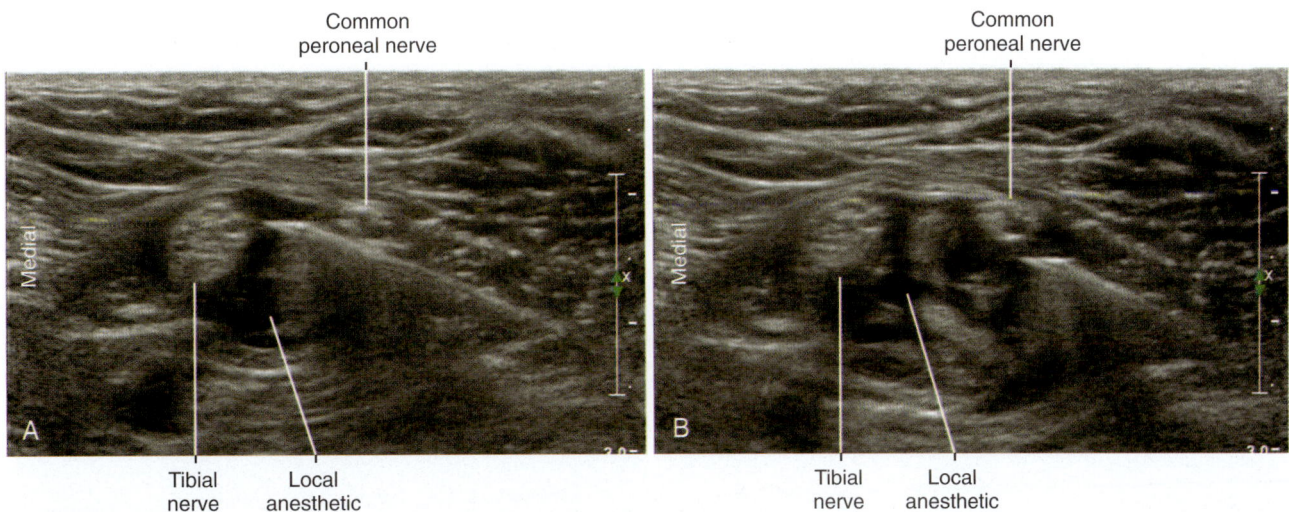

FIGURE 46.3 Image sequence showing popliteal block. An in-plane approach is demonstrated in which the needle tip is placed between the common peroneal and tibial nerves (A). Local anesthetic is distributed around both nerves by injecting as the needle is withdrawn (B).

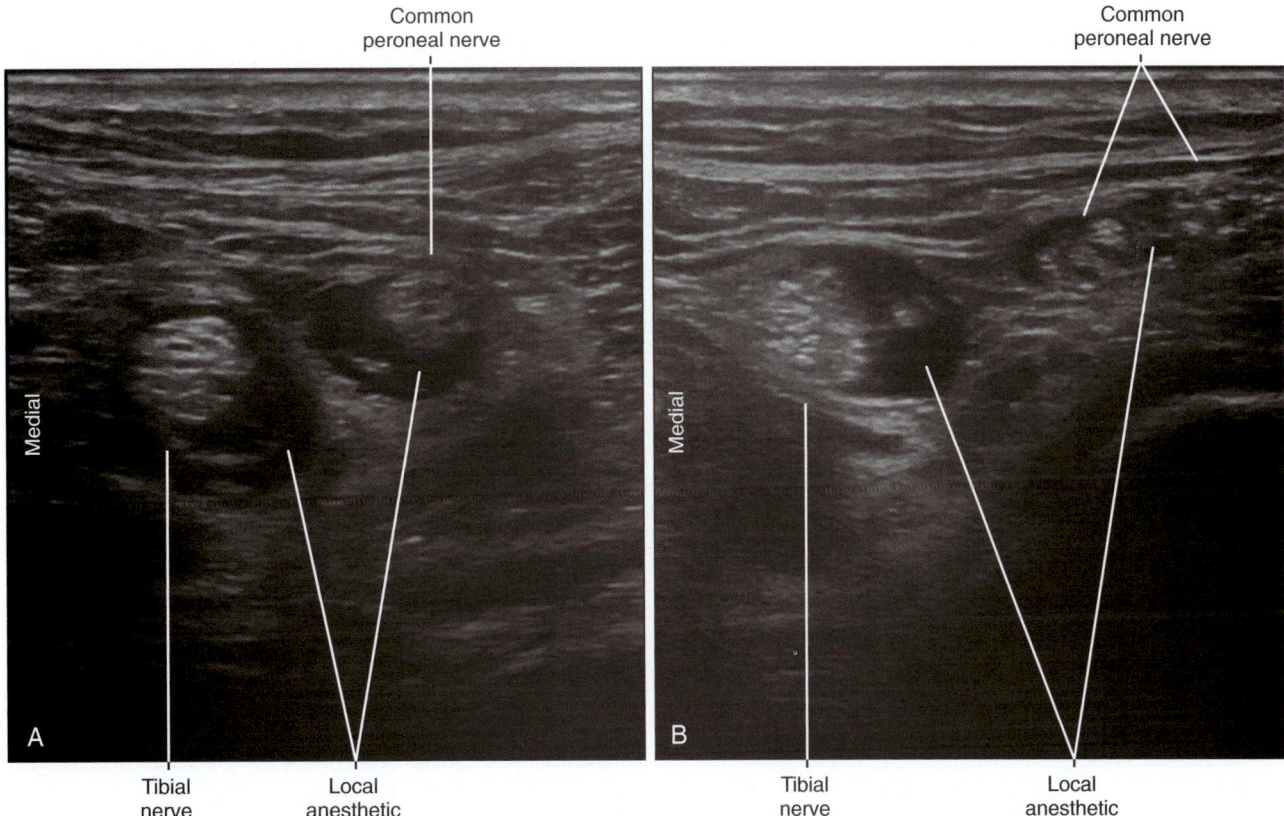

FIGURE 46.4 Sonographic assessment of popliteal block. Sliding the transducer distally along the course of the nerves demonstrates the local anesthetic distribution to both the tibial and common peroneal nerves (A). By sliding the transducer even more distally, the common peroneal nerve can be seen to give off a contributing branch to the sural nerve and lateral cutaneous nerve of the leg (B). The borders of this small nerve are clarified by the surrounding local anesthetic. When multiple rings of local anesthetic are identified that track along nerve branches, the resultant block is unequivocally established.

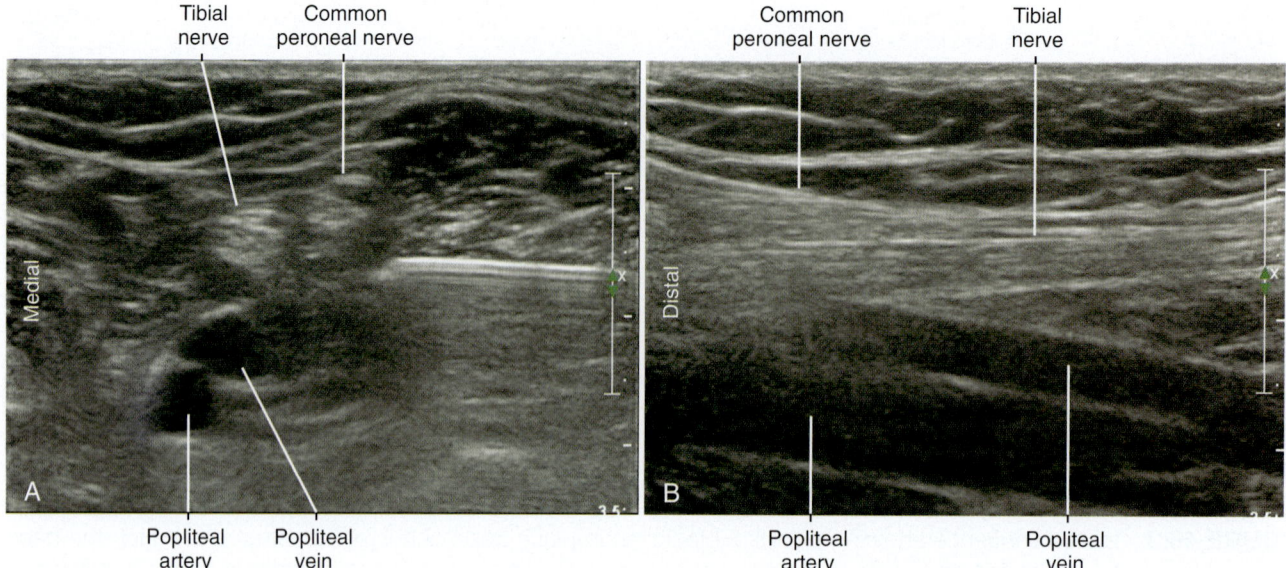

FIGURE 46.5 Sonographic anatomy of the popliteal fossa in short-axis (A) and long-axis (B) views. The nerves of the popliteal fossa lie closer to the posterior surface than the popliteal vessels (A). In the long-axis view (B), the usual courses of the common peroneal nerve, tibial nerve, popliteal vein, and popliteal artery are illustrated in one parasagittal plane of imaging (listed from posterior to anterior). In most cases, the common peroneal nerve lies closer to the posterior surface of the thigh than does the tibial nerve. However, the location of these nerves depends on foot position, and in some cases, the tibial nerve lies closer to the posterior surface.

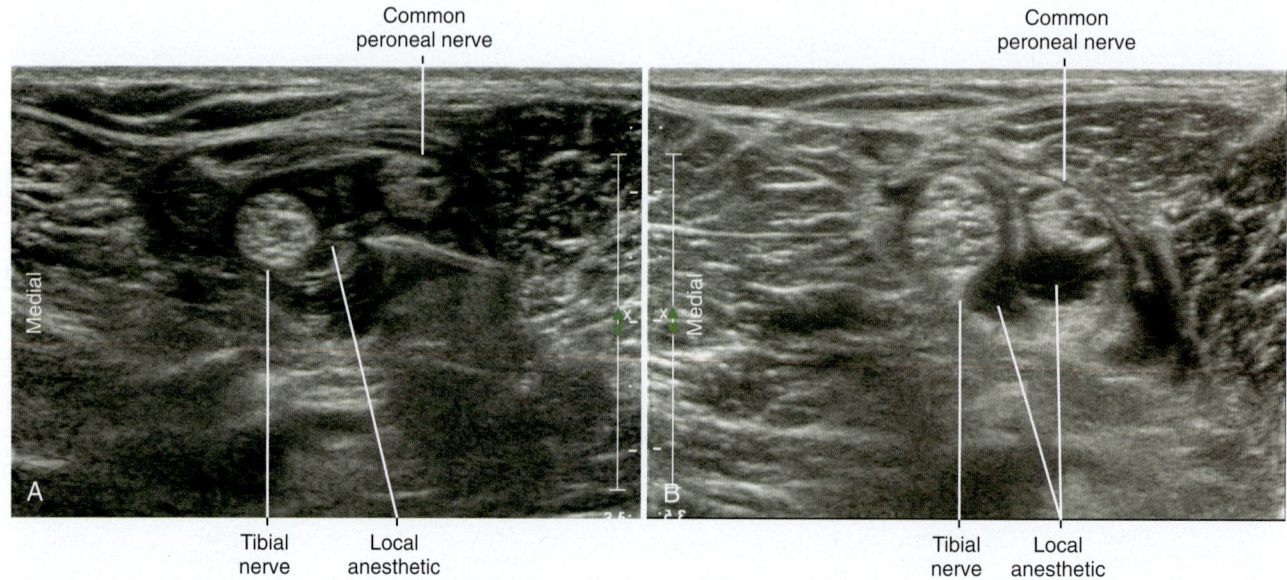

FIGURE 46.6 Echotexture of the common peroneal and tibial nerves. The tibial nerve is larger and has a straighter course than the common peroneal nerve. In addition, the tibial nerve has more fascicles and therefore usually appears brighter on ultrasound scans. In contrast, the common peroneal nerve can appear oligofascicular or even monofascicular with fewer, larger fascicles than the tibial nerve. Two separate examples are shown (A and B).

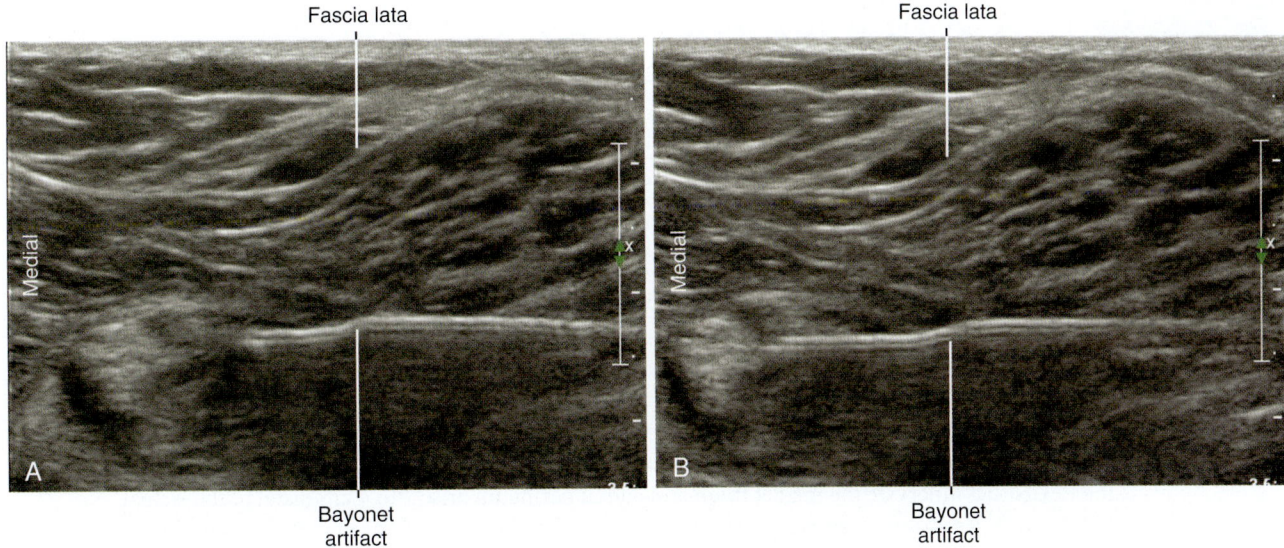

FIGURE 46.7 Bayonet artifact during popliteal block. Because the angle of approach is near-parallel to the active face of the transducer, bayonet artifacts can be observed during popliteal blocks. This speed-of-sound artifact causes apparent bending of the needle (although no actual mechanical bending of the needle exists). Bayonet artifacts observed during popliteal blocks are caused by the presence of adipose tissue near the midline of the popliteal fossa. The artifacts occur at this transition, because the speed of sound in adipose tissue is slower than the adjacent muscle. The end of the needle therefore appears to bend away from the transducer (A). As the needle is advanced, the bend of the bayonet remains in the same location (B).

Posterior Femoral Cutaneous Nerve Block

Bradley Lee

The posterior femoral cutaneous nerve (PFCN), also referred to as the posterior cutaneous nerve of the thigh, is a sensory nerve that derives from the sacral plexus (S1, S2, and S3). The main descending branch of the PFCN is approximately 2 mm diameter in the proximal thigh and has a relatively straight course, which is nearly parallel to the sciatic nerve.[1] The PFCN and the sciatic nerve are separated by the long head of the biceps femoris muscle (the PFCN runs over the posterior surface, whereas the sciatic nerve runs underneath the muscle). Perineal branches of the PFCN that innervate the medial thigh and lateral perineum arise 2 to 4 cm distal to the ischial tuberosity.[2,3] Recurrent branches of the PFCN form the inferior cluneal nerves that supply the gluteal region. End branches of the PFCN travel with the small saphenous vein in the proximal posterior leg.

Potential indications for PFCN block include surgical procedures of the posterior thigh (above the knee), skin graft harvests from the posterior thigh, diagnostic and therapeutic blocks,[4] and perhaps thigh tourniquet tolerance.

PFCN and lateral femoral cutaneous nerve (LFCN) blocks may be a way of improving thigh tourniquet tolerance without concomitant motor block (in combination with other blocks of the lower extremity). PFCN block has limited utility in clinical anesthesia, because few surgeries have an incision on the posterior thigh (above the knee amputation is one exception).

SUGGESTED TECHNIQUE

PFCN block can be approached in the subgluteal region or at the apex of the popliteal fossa.

PROXIMAL BLOCK OF THE POSTERIOR FEMORAL CUTANEOUS NERVE (SUBGLUTEAL REGION)

The PFCN lies on the posterior surface of the long head of the biceps femoris muscle. In the subgluteal region, the PFCN lies underneath the gluteus maximus muscle and over the biceps femoris muscle. On average, the nerve lies about 42% of the width of the thigh at the gluteal fold and almost exactly in the middle of the posterior thigh, slightly medial to the middle of the posterior thigh.[5] The PFCN lies medial to the femur near the center of the posterior thigh in the subgluteal region.

The PFCN can be blocked by placing the needle tip through the distal edge of the gluteus maximus over the long head of the biceps femoris (near the intersection of the gluteus maximus and conjoint tendon of the biceps femoris and semitendinosus, which points to the medial aspect of the sciatic nerve). The injection is slowly performed under low pressure as the needle is withdrawn through the distal edge of the muscle. The distal edge of the gluteus maximus is the thinnest part of this muscle, and it is close to the midline as defined by the interface of the biceps femoris and semitendinosus muscles.

NEUROLOGIC ASSESSMENT

There are recurrent branches of the PFCN (the perineal and inferior cluneal nerves derive from its S3 contributions). Cutaneous block can be tested both proximal and distal to the site of injection.

DISTAL BLOCK OF THE POSTERIOR FEMORAL CUTANEOUS NERVE (POPLITEAL REGION)

The PFCN travels in a flat fascial tunnel of the posterior thigh near the apex of the popliteal fossa. The PFCN runs medial to the sciatic nerve and then lies superficial to it. The PFCN lies in the groove between the biceps femoris and the semimembranosus/semitendinosus muscle complex.

The PFCN must be distinguished from the tendon of the semitendinosus in the popliteal fossa. The distal tendon of the semitendinosus is long and thin and lies posterior (superficial) to the semimembranosus muscle in the popliteal fossa. The distal tendon of the semitendinosus lies medially (it has a fibrillar echotexture with changes in size and shape along its course).

KEY POINTS

- Unlike the LFCN, PFCN distribution usually continues below the knee.
- Needle injection injury to the PFCN in the gluteal region is rare but has been reported.[6–8] In contrast, the sciatic nerve comprises over 80% of the reported cases of needle injection injury. There are no reports of PFCN injury from injections in the thigh.

Clinical Pearls

- The main descending branch of the PFCN lies between the biceps femoris and gluteus maximus muscles (usually just medial to the sciatic nerve). The PFCN emerges beneath the distal edge of gluteus maximus to follow the furrow/groove formed by the long head of the biceps and the semitendinosus muscles.[9]
- The PFCN remains subfascial in the subgluteal region: the nerve pierces the fascia lata after the distal edge of the gluteus maximus. There often appears a double layer of fascia lata within which the PFCN lies in the subgluteal region of the posterior thigh. Needle tip entry into this fascial space is accompanied by tactile response.[10]
- Do not mistake the PFCN for the conjoint tendon of the semitendinosus and biceps femoris muscles (the PFCN does not lie between these two muscles). Furthermore, do not mistake the PFCN for the proximal tendon of the semimembranosus muscle.
- The PFCN is usually blocked with parasacral approaches to the sciatic nerve but may be spared with more distal approaches to this block.[11]
- Cadaveric studies have demonstrated the potential for injectate isolated to PFCN without involving the sciatic nerve, which may spare motor weakness associated with sciatic nerve blockade.[12]

References

1. Meng S, Lieba-Samal D, Reissig LF, et al. High-resolution ultrasound of the posterior femoral cutaneous nerve: visualization and initial experience with patients. *Skeletal Radiol.* 2015;44(10):1421–1426. PMID: 26105014.
2. Tubbs RS, Miller J, Loukas M, et al. Surgical and anatomical landmarks for the perineal branch of the posterior femoral cutaneous nerve: implications in perineal pain syndromes. Laboratory investigation. *J Neurosurg.* 2009;111(2):332–335. PMID: 19361263.
3. Fritz J, Bizzell C, Kathuria S, et al. High-resolution magnetic resonance-guided posterior femoral cutaneous nerve blocks. *Skeletal Radiol.* 2013;42(4):579–586. PMID: 23263413.
4. Kasper JM, Wadhwa V, Scott KM, et al. CT-guided therapeutic posterior femoral cutaneous nerve block. *Clin Imaging.* 2014;38(4):540–542. PMID: 24667042.
5. Hawing K et al. Posterior cutaneous nerve of the thigh relating to the restoration of the gluteal fold. *Ann Plast Surg.* 2008;60(4):357–361. PMID 18362559.
6. Iyer VG, Shields CB. Isolated injection injury to the posterior femoral cutaneous nerve. *Neurosurgery.* 1989;25(5):835–838. PMID: 2586740.
7. Tong HC, Haig A. Posterior femoral cutaneous nerve mononeuropathy: a case report. *Arch Phys Med Rehabil.* 2000;81(8):1117–1118. PMID: 10943764.

8. Kim JE, Kang JH, Choi JC, et al. Isolated posterior femoral cutaneous neuropathy following intragluteal injection. *Muscle Nerve*. 2009;40(5):864–866. PMID: 19623639.
9. Arnoldussen WJ, Korten JJ. Pressure neuropathy of the posterior femoral cutaneous nerve. *Clin Neurol Neurosurg*. 1980;82(1):57–60. PMID: 6257441.
10. Hughes PJ, Brown TC. An approach to posterior femoral cutaneous nerve block. *Anaesth Intensive Care*. 1986;14(4):350–351. PMID: 3565724.
11. Fuzier R, Hoffreumont P, Bringuier-Branchereau S, et al. Does the sciatic nerve approach influence thigh tourniquet tolerance during below-knee surgery? *Anesth Analg*. 2005;100(5):1511–1514. PMID: 15845716.
12. Johnson C, Johnson R, Niesen A, et al. Ultrasound-guided posterior femoral cutaneous nerve block. *J Ultrasound Med*. 2017.

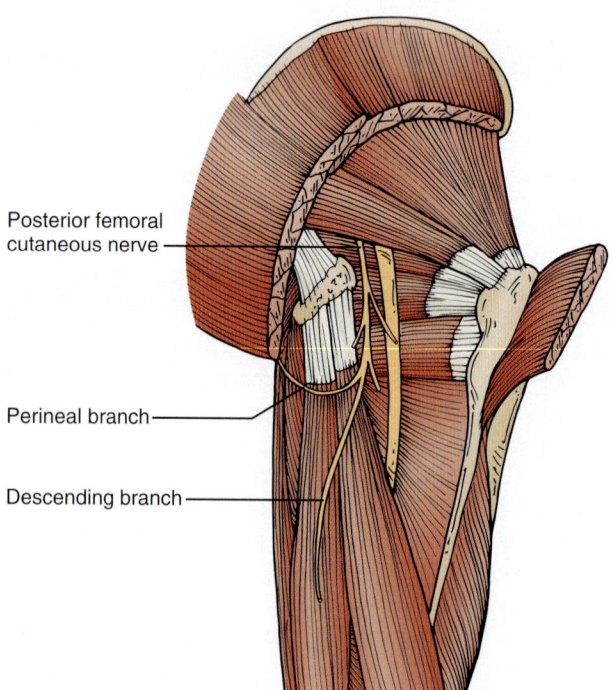

FIGURE 47.1 Course of the posterior femoral cutaneous nerve. (Redrawn from Fritz J, Bizzell C, Kathuria S, et al. High-resolution magnetic resonance-guided posterior femoral cutaneous nerve blocks. *Skeletal Radiol*. 2013;42(4):579–586.)

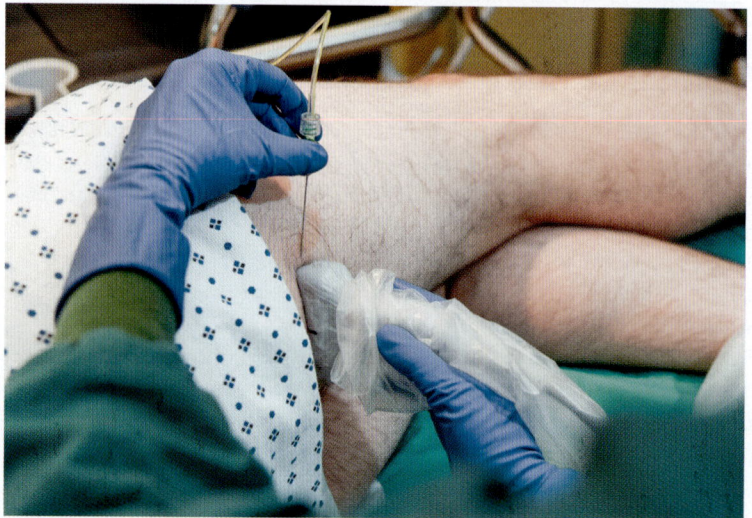

FIGURE 47.2 External photograph showing lateral to medial in-plane approach to posterior femoral cutaneous nerve block in the subgluteal region.

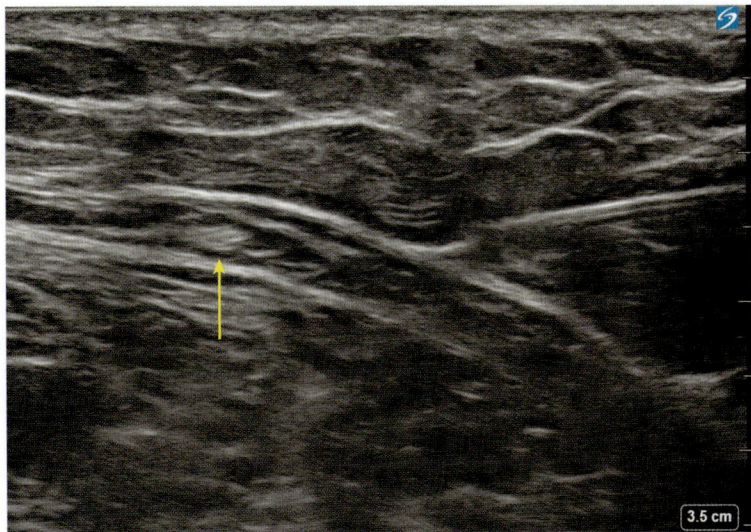

FIGURE 47.3 Short-axis view of the posterior femoral cutaneous nerve (PFCN, *yellow arrow*) in the subgluteal region of the thigh (before injection, showing the needle tip approaching the fascia that invests the PFCN).

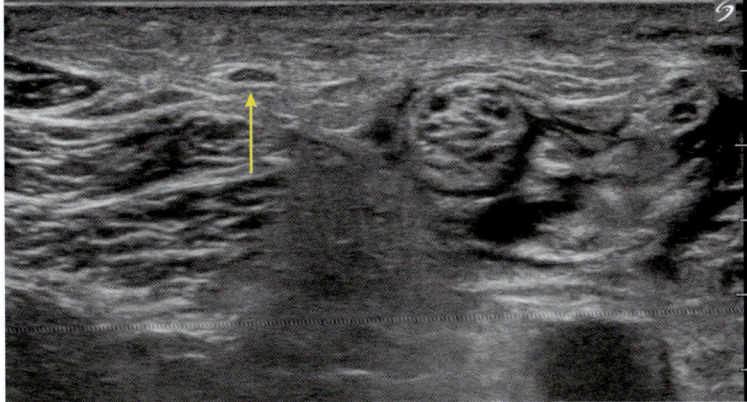

FIGURE 47.4 Short-axis view of the posterior femoral cutaneous nerve (PFCN) at the apex of the popliteal fossa. The PFCN *(yellow arrow)* lies medial to the tibial nerve.

CHAPTER 48

Ankle Blocks

 See Video 48.1 on ExpertConsult.com.

Ankle blocks are a useful regional anesthetic technique for foot surgery, especially in the ambulatory setting.[1,2] Additionally, ankle blocks provide excellent postoperative analgesia, which is important because foot surgeries often involve osteotomies that cause moderate to severe postoperative pain, which is difficult to manage with standard oral analgesic regimens.

The foot is innervated by five nerves: four are terminal branches of the sciatic nerve (deep peroneal, superficial peroneal, sural, and tibial), and one is the terminal branch of the femoral nerve (the saphenous nerve). All five nerves of the foot can be directly imaged with ultrasound. This approach is more targeted than traditional ankle blocks. Furthermore, although traditional ankle blocks are performed at the level of the malleoli, ultrasound-guided approaches are more proximal (usually in the mid-leg region). This can produce more complete blocks (a stocking distribution) and may improve calf or ankle tourniquet tolerance. More generally, ultrasound-guided ankle blocks can serve as a model of small nerve imaging for a variety of other regional blocks.

Some practitioners reserve the use of ultrasound for the deeper blocks of the ankle (deep peroneal, tibial) and elect to use subcutaneous infiltration for the more shallow blocks (saphenous, superficial peroneal, sural). Others use ultrasound for all five nerve blocks. The fascia that defines leg compartments is particularly thick and strong. For some blocks described here (e.g., superficial peroneal, tibial), it is critical that the injection is made within the correct compartment. When ankle blocks are performed with ultrasound, it is optimal for the operator and machine to remain in one location for block efficiency. The leg can be elevated with plastic basins to facilitate access for ankle blocks. One potential limitation of ultrasound imaging for ankle block is that optimal positioning for transducer placement requires some mobility of the lower extremity (especially for tibial and sural nerve blocks).

Using ultrasound guidance, it may be possible to improve patient comfort during the procedure and reduce the risk of puncture of adjacent anatomic structures. In addition, more proximal blocks may be indicated when edema or infection is present. In contrast to blocks of the sciatic nerve in the popliteal fossa, ankle blocks do not produce foot drop, and therefore patient disposition is potentially facilitated.

References

1. Monkowski DP, Egidi HR. Ankle block. *Tech Reg Anesth Pain Manag*. 2006;10:183–188.
2. Chin KJ, Wong NW, Macfarlane AJ, Chan VW. Ultrasound-guided versus anatomic landmark-guided ankle blocks: a 6-year retrospective review. *Reg Anesth Pain Med*. 2011;36(6):611–618.

Saphenous Nerve Block in the Leg

CHAPTER 49

See Video 49.1 on ExpertConsult.com.

The saphenous nerve is a terminal branch of the femoral nerve that provides sensation to the medial leg, malleolus, and foot. In some cases the sensory distribution extends to the great toe.[1] The saphenous nerve pierces the fascia lata between the tendons of the sartorius and gracilis of the pes anserinus. The saphenous nerve and vein then travel together within a common fascial compartment within the subcutaneous tissue of the leg (a common fascial tunnel or tent).[2] The saphenous nerve adheres to the saphenous vein in the lower 13 cm of the leg and branches approximately 6 cm proximal to the medial malleolus.[3] The saphenous nerve and vein consistently travel anterior to the medial malleolus.

Saphenous nerve block is important for surgical anesthesia of the foot and ankle. Importantly, recent anatomic studies have demonstrated articular branches of the saphenous nerve that supply the ankle joint from the subcutaneous tissue.[4,5]

SUGGESTED TECHNIQUE

The saphenous nerve can be blocked adjacent to the saphenous vein in the middle third of the leg (near the distal edge of the bulk of the calf muscles). Although the saphenous nerve is difficult to directly visualize with ultrasound imaging in the leg, in this location the block can be performed by injecting into the fascial compartment that contains both the saphenous nerve and vein. Injection within this fascial compartment will track along and compress the adjacent saphenous vein. This tubular conduit for longitudinal distribution is the anatomic basis for similar tumescent anesthetic techniques. In thin patients these fascial layers are more closely opposed.

Visible saphenous vein distention occurs following saphenous nerve block due to interruption of vascular tone (and any compression of the saphenous vein at the injection site).

An alternative technique is to infiltrate local anesthetic around the saphenous vein within the subcutaneous tissue at the level of the tibial tuberosity.[6] For this procedure, local anesthetic is infiltrated within the subcutaneous tissue near the saphenous vein using an in-plane or out-of-plane approach. If the saphenous vein is difficult to visualize, a proximal tourniquet can be applied with reverse Trendelenburg position.

KEY POINTS	
Saphenous Nerve Block	**The Essentials**
Anatomy	The SaN lies adjacent to the SV in a common fascial compartment. This fascial compartment is within the subcutaneous tissue of the medial leg.
Positioning	Supine
Operator	Standing on the side of the patient
Display	Across the table
Transducer	High-frequency linear, 23- to 38-mm footprint

Continued

KEY POINTS—CONT'D

Saphenous Nerve Block | **The Essentials**

Initial depth setting	20 mm
Needle	25 gauge, 38 mm in length
Anatomic location	Mid-leg, medial aspect
Approach	SAX view of SaN and SV, in-plane from either side of the transducer. Place the needle tip underneath the SV (but superficial to the fascia lata).
Sonographic assessment	The injection should track along and compress the SV.
Anatomic variation	Position of the SaN and SV can vary, but both lie deep within the subcutaneous tissue of the leg.

Sa, Sartorius muscle; *SaN*, saphenous nerve; *SAX*, short axis; *SV*, saphenous vein.

Clinical Pearls

- The saphenous nerve is a branch of the posterior division of the femoral nerve.
- Distal block of the saphenous nerve is potentially more selective and may carry less risk for vascular puncture. However, direct nerve imaging can be difficult with these distal approaches.
- The saphenous vein runs anterior to the medial malleolus. Follow the saphenous vein 5–10 cm proximally to identify the fascial tunnel in which the saphenous vein and saphenous nerve branches lie. This fascial tunnel sometimes has an "Egyptian eye" appearance on ultrasound scans.
- The saphenous vein sometimes has a "frosted donut" appearance from the adjacent branches of the saphenous nerve that lie on the side walls of the vein.
- Inject between the saphenous vein and fascia lata (underneath the vein in the medial aspect of the mid-leg). The fascia lata is slightly thicker than the overlying fascia (and therefore easier to identify on ultrasound scans).

References

1. Benzon HT, Sharma S, Calimaran A. Comparison of the different approaches to saphenous nerve block. *Anesthesiology*. 2005;102:633–638.
2. Caggiati A. Fascial relationships of the long saphenous vein. *Circulation*. 1999;100(25):2547–2549.
3. Dayan V, Cura L, Cubas S, Carriquiry G. Surgical anatomy of the saphenous nerve. *Ann Thorac Surg*. 2008;85(3):896–900.
4. Clendenen SR, Whalen JL. Saphenous nerve innervation of the medial ankle. *Local Reg Anesth*. 2013;6:13–16.
5. Eglitis N, Horn JL, Benninger B, Nelsen S. The importance of the saphenous nerve in ankle surgery. *Anesth Analg*. 2016;122:1704–1706.
6. Gray AT, Collins AB. Ultrasound-guided saphenous nerve block. *Reg Anesth Pain Med*. 2003;28:148.

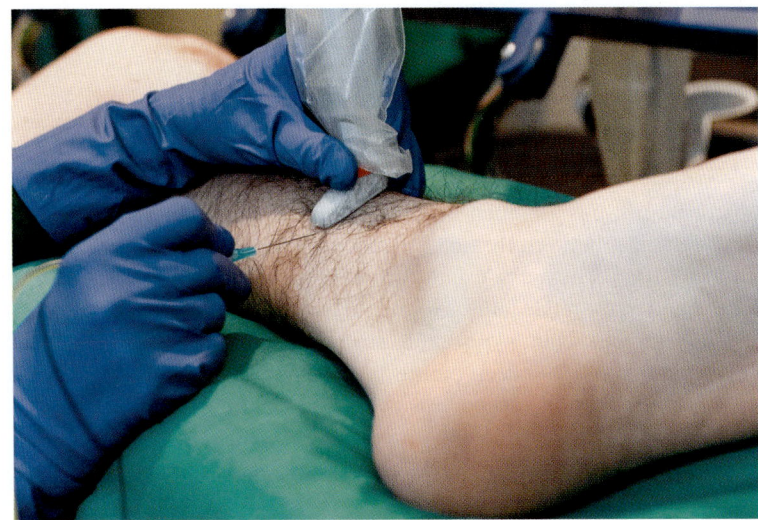

FIGURE 49.1 External photograph showing the approach to saphenous nerve block in the mid-leg. An in-plane approach from the posterior aspect of the leg is shown.

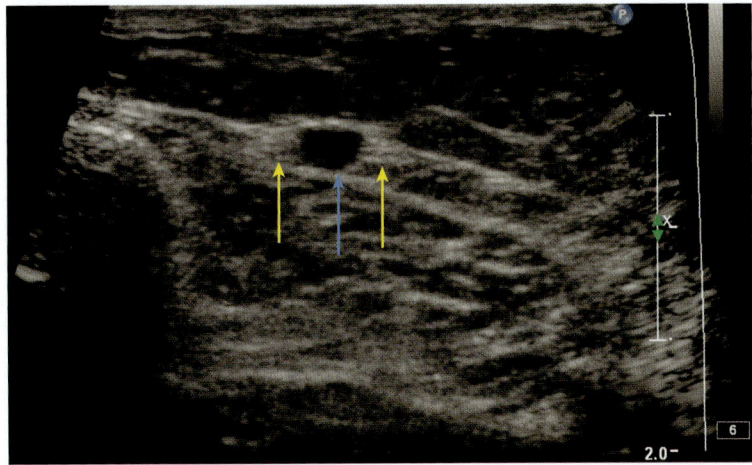

FIGURE 49.2 Sonogram illustrating the saphenous vein *(blue arrow)* with branches of the saphenous nerve *(yellow arrows)* on its walls (the "frosted donut" appearance). In the mid-leg the saphenous vein and nerve lie in a common fascial tunnel.

CHAPTER 50

Deep Peroneal Nerve Block

The deep peroneal nerve is a branch of the common peroneal nerve. The deep peroneal nerve innervates the web space between the first and second toes. In rare cases, it also provides innervation to the third toe (<10%). The nerve usually crosses over the anterior tibial artery from medial to lateral just proximal to the ankle joint near the surface of the distal tibia. The deep peroneal nerve can appear as a homogeneous hypoechoic structure surrounded by hyperechoic fat without polyfascicular echotexture. The deep peroneal nerve is more difficult to image in the proximal leg. This probably relates to the deep course of the nerve and its division into a large number of motor branches.

Ultrasound guidance may provide some advantages over landmark-based approaches to deep peroneal nerve block. One study reported that the use of ultrasound improved the onset of deep peroneal nerve block at the ankle, although the overall quality of this block was no different than the landmark-based technique.[1] Another study has reported high success rates with deep peroneal nerve blocks that combine ultrasound with nerve stimulation.[2]

SUGGESTED TECHNIQUE

The deep peroneal nerve and anterior tibial artery can be located by following the anterior surface of the tibia distally in transverse view. These anatomic structures will be visible about 3 cm proximal to the malleoli.[3] The deep peroneal nerve is about 1 mm in diameter. Medial and lateral branches of the deep peroneal nerve can sometimes be identified flanking the sides of the anterior tibial artery.

The deep peroneal nerve and anterior tibial artery lie between the surface of the tibia and the extensor hallucis longus muscle. Because of its superficial location and proximity to bone, the anterior tibial artery is easily compressed by the transducer over the dorsum of the foot and ankle. Light touch with the transducer is necessary to image the anterior tibial artery and its adjacent flanking veins. By sliding the transducer back and forth from proximal to distal, the crossing of the deep peroneal nerve over the anterior tibial artery can be identified. Both in-plane and out-of-plane approaches are useful for this block. An in-plane approach from lateral to medial can help avoid the large tibialis anterior and extensor hallucis longus tendons. Furthermore, the deep peroneal nerve is most likely to lie on the lateral side of the anterior tibial artery. The injection can either separate the nerve from the artery or layer underneath the artery for successful deep peroneal nerve block.

Of the five nerves for the ankle block, the deep peroneal nerve block is the most distal. A superficial peroneal nerve block is often performed first to anesthetize the skin over the site for deep peroneal nerve block.

KEY POINTS

Deep Peroneal Nerve Block	The Essentials
Anatomy	The DPN often crosses over the AT. This crossing point is near where the AT lies on the surface of the tibia.
Positioning	Supine
Operator	Standing on the side of the patient
Display	Across the table
Transducer	High-frequency linear, 23- to 38-mm footprint
Initial depth setting	20 mm
Needle	25 gauge, 38 mm in length
Anatomic location	Begin by scanning between the malleoli over the dorsum of the foot. Slide the probe proximal and distal to identify the DPN and AT. Light touch is needed to avoid compressing the AT.
Approach	SAX view of DPN, in-plane from either side of the transducer. Place the needle tip between the DPN and AT. Alternatively, place the needle tip underneath the AT.
Sonographic assessment	The injection should separate the DPN and AT. Layering underneath the AT also indicates successful block.
Anatomic variation	The DPN can divide into medial and lateral branches proximally. The AT can be absent (about 5% of normal subjects, plus cases of vascular insufficiency).

AT, Anterior tibial artery; *DPN*, deep peroneal nerve; *SAX*, short axis.

Clinical Pearls

- Because the deep peroneal nerve is small, it is often difficult to visualize where it branches off from the common peroneal nerve in the proximal leg.
- The point at which the deep peroneal nerve crosses over the anterior tibial artery is typically proximal to the ankle joint where the artery lies on the surface of the tibia.
- The deep peroneal nerve divides into medial and lateral branches. These branches lie on their respective sides of the anterior tibial artery.
- The deep peroneal nerve can be blocked by peeling off the nerve from the anterior tibial artery where it lies in the 12-o'clock position with respect to the artery (at the crossing point). The injection should separate the deep peroneal nerve from the surface of the anterior tibial artery. Alternatively, inject in the layer just deep to the anterior tibial artery over the surface of the tibia.

References

1. Antonakakis JG, Scalzo DC, Jorgenson AS, et al. Ultrasound does not improve the success rate of a deep peroneal nerve block at the ankle. *Reg Anesth Pain Med*. 2010;35(2):217–221.
2. Benzon HT, Sekhadia M, Benzon HA, Yaghmour ET, Chekka K, Nader A. Ultrasound-assisted and evoked motor response stimulation of the deep peroneal nerve. *Anesth Analg*. 2009;109(6):2022–2024.
3. Üçeyler N, Schäfer KA, Mackenrodt D, Sommer C, Müllges W. High-resolution ultrasonography of the superficial peroneal motor and sural sensory nerves may be a non-invasive approach to the diagnosis of vasculitic neuropathy. *Front Neurol*. 2016;7:48.

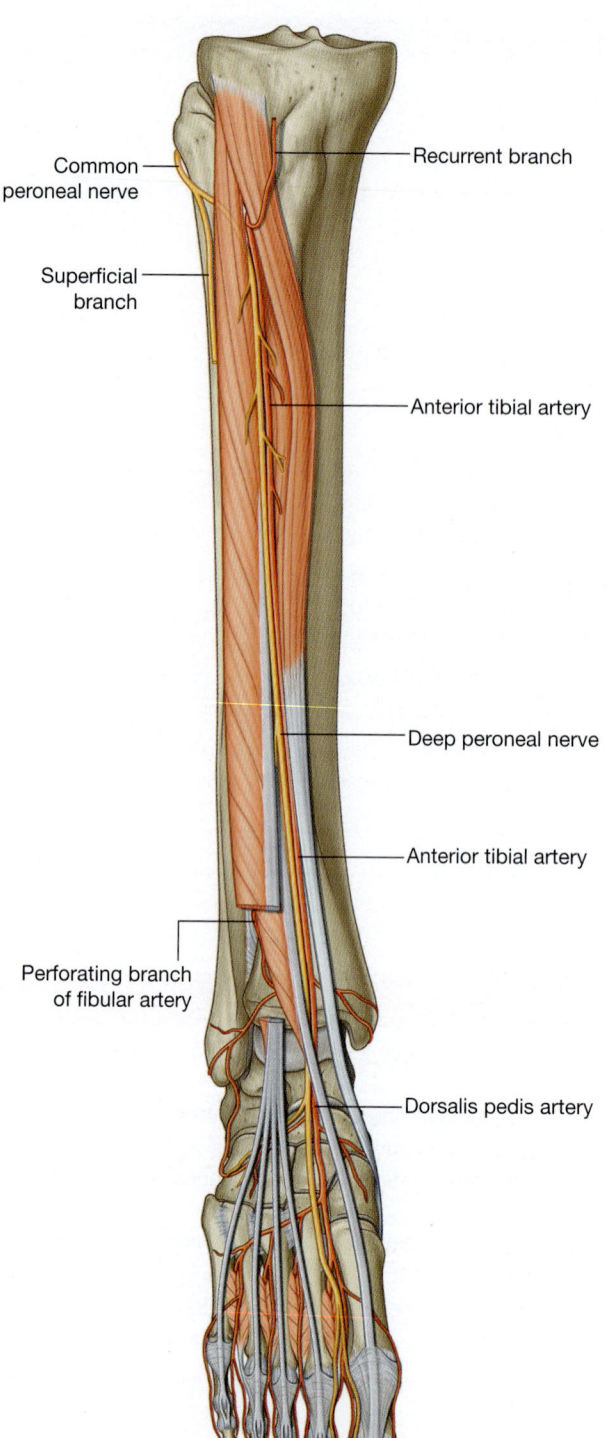

FIGURE 50.1 Course of the deep peroneal nerve. (Modified from Drake RL, Vogl W, Mitchell AWM. *Gray's anatomy for students*. Philadelphia: Churchill Livingstone; 2004.)

DEEP PERONEAL NERVE BLOCK

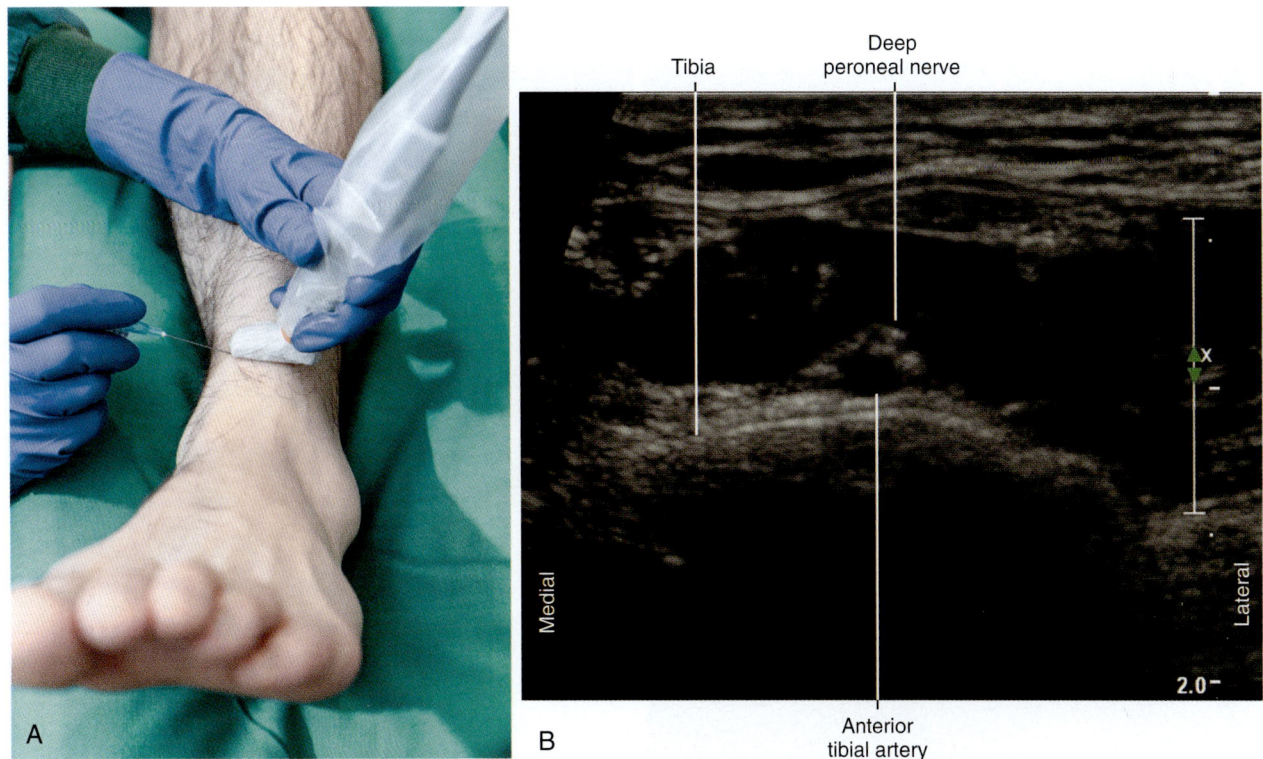

FIGURE 50.2 External photograph showing the approach to deep peroneal block in the distal leg. An in-plane approach from the medial aspect of the leg is shown (A). The corresponding sonogram is shown before needle placement (B). The deep peroneal nerve crosses over the surface of the anterior tibial artery proximal to the ankle joint.

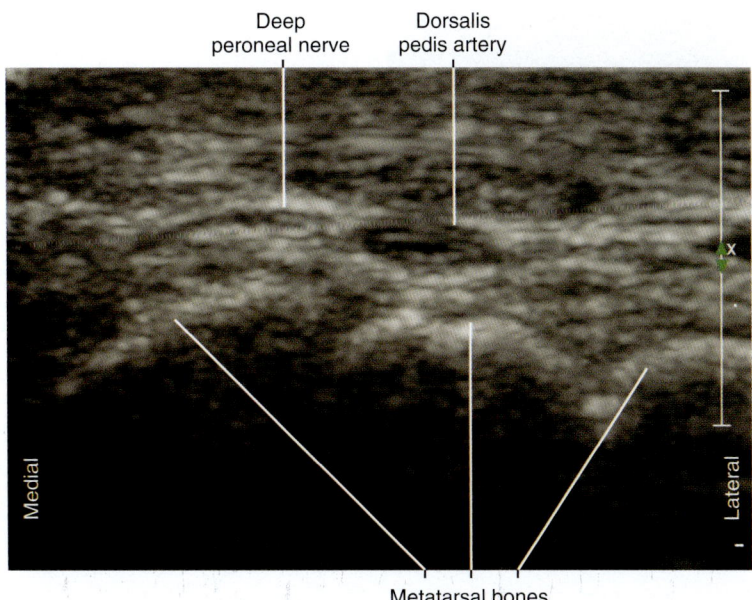

FIGURE 50.3 Short-axis view of the deep peroneal nerve over the dorsum of the foot. In this more distal location, the metatarsal bones lie under the nerve. This location is too distal for a complete block.

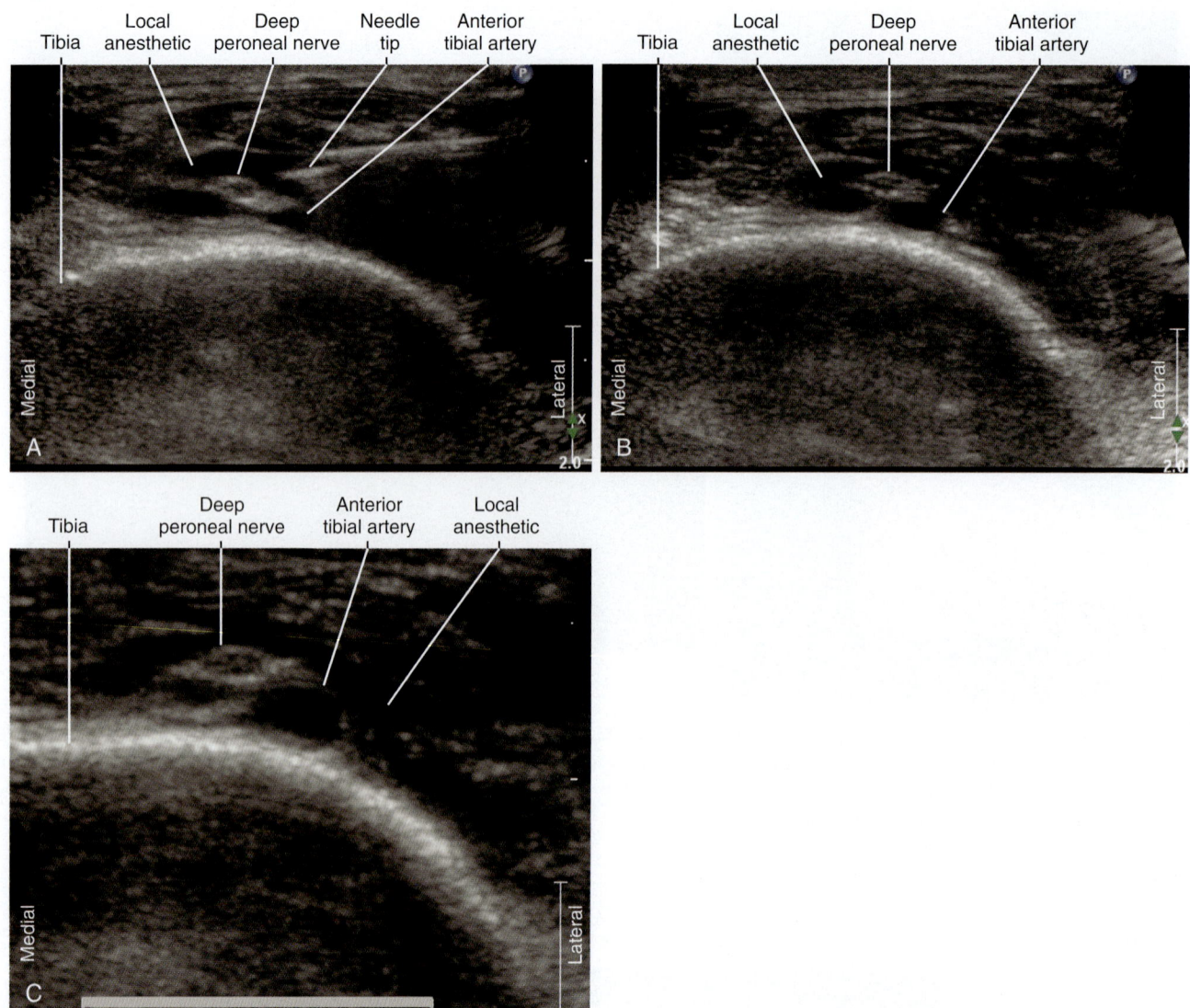

FIGURE 50.4 Image sequence showing deep peroneal nerve block in the distal leg. At this location the deep peroneal nerve lies over the anterior tibial artery. An in-plane approach is demonstrated in which the needle tip is placed adjacent to the anterior tibial artery and the deep peroneal nerve with the nerve in the 12-o'clock position (A). After injection, local anesthetic is distributed around the deep peroneal nerve and begins to separate the nerve from the artery (B), also shown at higher magnification (C).

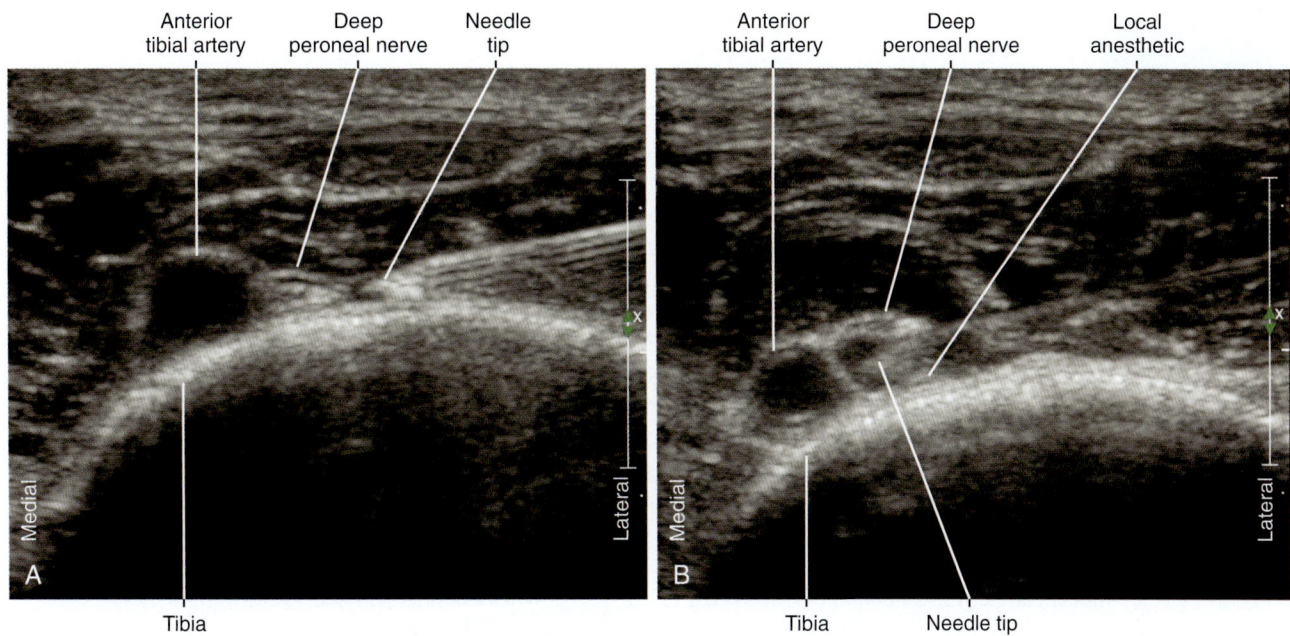

FIGURE 50.5 Image sequence showing deep peroneal nerve block in the distal leg. At this location the deep peroneal nerve lies on the side of the anterior tibial artery. An in-plane approach is demonstrated in which the needle tip is placed under the deep peroneal nerve (A). After injection the local anesthetic lifts the nerve from the surface of the bone (B).

CHAPTER 51
Superficial Peroneal Nerve Block

The superficial peroneal nerve is a branch of the common peroneal nerve that emerges at the neck of the fibula between the extensor digitorum longus and peroneal muscles to enter the subcutaneous tissue of the lateral leg. When emerging from the fibular neck, the superficial peroneal nerve most commonly lies in the lateral compartment of the leg (about 70% of subjects). In other cases, the superficial peroneal nerve lies partly or completely within the anterior compartment. The superficial peroneal nerve ascends along the anterior intermuscular septum to pierce the fascia lata at the juncture of the middle and lower thirds of the leg. The nerve usually flattens and divides into its medial and intermediate dorsal branches in the subcutaneous tissue.[1-3] The superficial peroneal (fibular) nerve is closely associated with the fibula in the distal leg, so scanning proximally from the lateral malleolus can be a useful technique to identify the nerve.

Some surgeons elect to infiltrate local anesthetic over the dorsum of the foot for superficial peroneal nerve block and reserve ultrasound for the deeper nerves of the ankle block.[4] However, superficial peroneal nerve block in the leg can be useful when edema or infection contraindicates more distal ankle block. Proximal ultrasound-guided superficial peroneal nerve block (along with sural block) can provide surgical anesthesia for hardware removal from the lateral ankle in weight-bearing patients. In addition, ultrasound-guided superficial peroneal nerve block in the leg is more complete and less painful than subcutaneous infiltration across the dorsum of the foot and does not pierce the extensor tendons of the foot. The superficial peroneal nerve is an important nerve for foot surgery, because most surgical incisions are made on the dorsum.

SUGGESTED TECHNIQUE

The superficial peroneal nerve can be difficult to image within the subcutaneous tissue of the distal lateral leg. By sliding the transducer along the known course of the nerve, the nerve can be identified where it emerges from the muscular compartment against the fascia lata. An in-plane approach from either side of the leg can then be used for needle tip placement adjacent to the nerve.

With the patient in supine position, the leg is elevated and internally rotated. Then it is scanned from distal to proximal, beginning just proximal and anterior to the lateral malleolus. The superficial peroneal nerve tracks superficial to the fibula along the fascia between the anterior and lateral compartments of the leg, and the anterior border (ridge) of the fibula is formed by the insertion of the anterior intermuscular septum. Because the nerve tracks along the anterior intermuscular septum, the anterior border of the fibula points toward the superficial peroneal nerve (the "mountain" sign). The intermuscular septum can be difficult to directly image with ultrasound because it is viewed nearly en face.

Because the superficial peroneal nerve most often lies in the lateral compartment side of the intermuscular septum, it is important for the block needle tip to puncture this septum when approaching from the anterior side. The block needle tip crosses the anterior intermuscular septum underneath the nerve, with injection of local anesthetic as the needle is pulled back. Injection of a small amount of local anesthetic as the needle is withdrawn will cover any branches that may lie in the anterior compartment.

The key to completely surrounding the superficial peroneal nerve with local anesthetic is passing the needle over the nerve (between the superficial peroneal nerve and fascia lata). This can usually be achieved by rotating the needle bevel to face away from the transducer and advancing with light transducer pressure. Alternatively, perform the block proximally where there is small amount of space between the fascia lata and the nerve. When the nerve is blocked close to the surface of the fascia lata, its deeper motor branches to the peroneus longus and peroneus brevis will be spared.

KEY POINTS

Superficial Peroneal Nerve Block	The Essentials
Anatomy	The SPN emerges between the EDL and PL along the intermuscular septum.
	The fibular ridge and intermuscular septum point to the SPN (the "mountain" sign).
	The cortical surface of the fibula appears bright on its posterior side ("snow on the mountainside").
	The fibular artery and vein often lie adjacent to the SPN (zoom or power Doppler, "pulsating dot" sign).
Positioning	Supine with leg elevated and internally rotated.
Operator	Standing on the side of the patient
Display	Across the table
Transducer	High-frequency linear, 23- to 38-mm footprint
Initial depth setting	25 mm
Needle	25 gauge, 38 mm in length
Anatomic location	Begin imaging the leg just proximal and anterior to the lateral malleolus.
	Scan proximally to identify the point just proximal to where the SPN pierces the FL.
Approach	SAX view of SPN, in-plane from either side of the transducer.
	Place the needle tip between the FL and SPN.
Sonographic assessment	The injection should track proximally to descend along the course of the SPN.
Anatomic variation	The SPN can divide proximally in the leg.

EDL, Extensor digitorum longus; *FL*, fascia lata; *PL*, peroneus longus; *SAX*, short axis; *SPN*, superficial peroneal nerve.

Clinical Pearls

- Begin by scanning anterior and proximal to the lateral malleolus with the probe, sliding proximally with the transducer perpendicular to the known course of the superficial peroneal nerve.
- The superficial peroneal nerve emerges in the groove between the extensor digitorum longus and peroneal muscles. The nerve is most visible where it emerges to lie against the fascia lata (about 10 cm proximal to the lateral malleolus).
- When the superficial peroneal nerve is divided by the intermuscular septum, it continues distally as the medial and intermediate dorsal cutaneous nerves of the foot.
- The diameters of the superficial peroneal nerve and its branches are approximately 3 mm and 2 mm, respectively. The superficial peroneal nerve is often accompanied by a small fibular artery and vein.
- The flat tendon of the peroneus longus muscle can appear similar to the superficial peroneal nerve on ultrasound scans in the leg (although the tendon will continue posterior to the fibula).
- Conditions that contraindicate ankle block (e.g., edema and infection) are not common in outpatients. Popliteal blocks are much more commonly used than more distal blocks in these settings because patient disposition is not an issue.

References

1. Canella C, Demondion X, Guillin R, et al. Anatomic study of the superficial peroneal nerve using sonography. *AJR Am J Roentgenol.* 2009;193(1):174–179.
2. Solomon LB, Ferris L, Tedman R, et al. Surgical anatomy of the sural and superficial fibular nerves with an emphasis on the approach to the lateral malleolus. *J Anat.* 2001;199:717–723.
3. Üçeyler N, Schäfer KA, Mackenrodt D, et al. High-resolution ultrasonography of the superficial peroneal motor and sural sensory nerves may be a non-invasive approach to the diagnosis of vasculitic neuropathy. *Front Neurol.* 2016;30(7):48.
4. Chin KJ, Wong NW, Macfarlane AJ, et al. Ultrasound-guided versus anatomic landmark-guided ankle blocks: a 6-year retrospective review. *Reg Anesth Pain Med.* 2011;36(6):611–618.

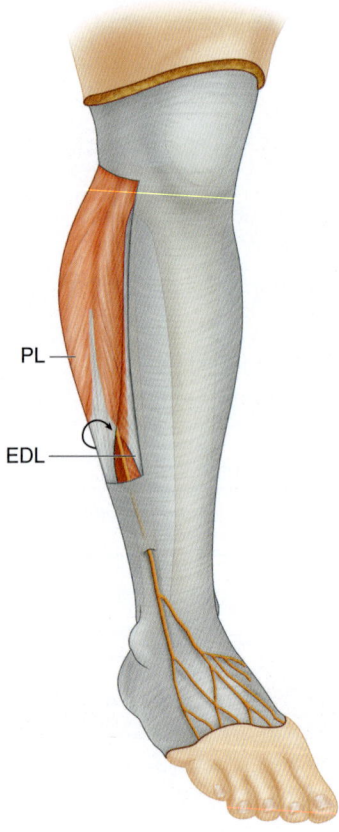

FIGURE 51.1 Anatomic course of the superficial peroneal nerve in the leg. *EDL*, Extensor digitorum longus; *PL*, peroneus longus. (Modified from Canella C, Demondion X, Guillin R, et al. Anatomic study of the superficial peroneal nerve using sonography. *AJR Am J Roentgenol.* 2009;193(1):174–179.)

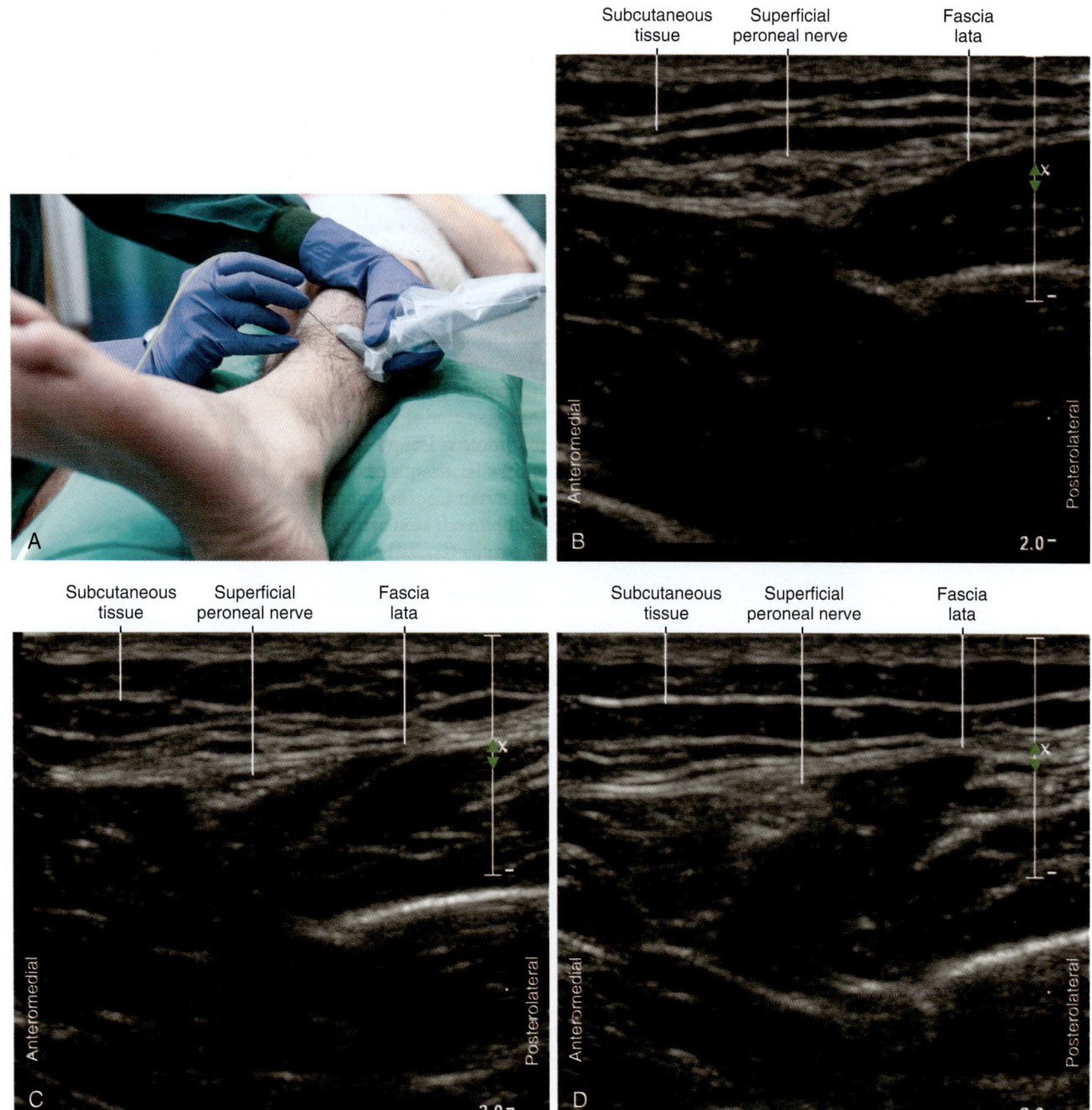

FIGURE 51.2 External photograph showing the approach to superficial peroneal nerve block in the distal leg. An in-plane approach from the anterolateral aspect of the leg is shown (A). The corresponding sonogram shows the nerve within the subcutaneous tissue of the lateral leg (B). More proximal sonograms show the nerve emerging from the muscular compartment (C and D).

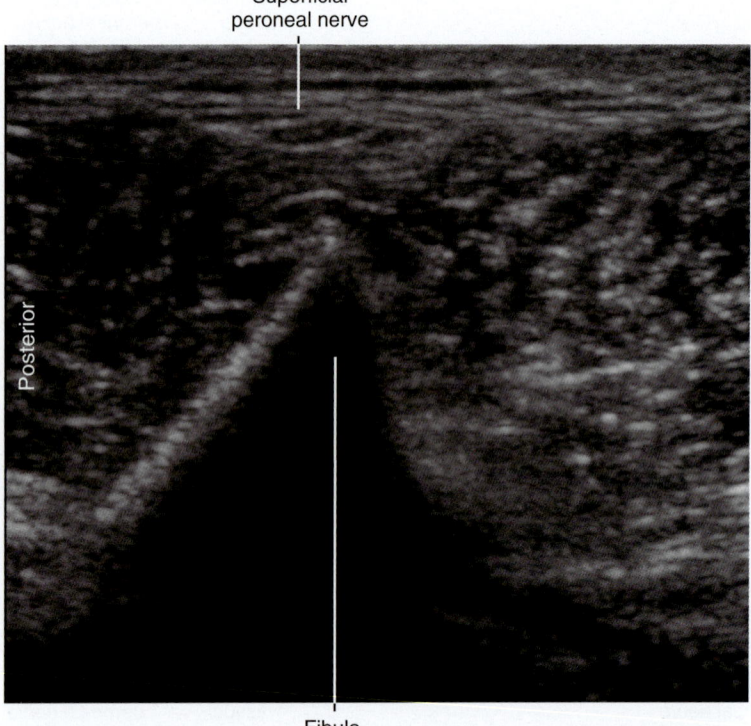

FIGURE 51.3 The superficial peroneal nerve arises from the common peroneal nerve near the neck of the fibula in the proximal leg. The edge of the bone is sharp and points to the superficial peroneal nerve because the nerve emerges within or adjacent to the intermuscular septum.

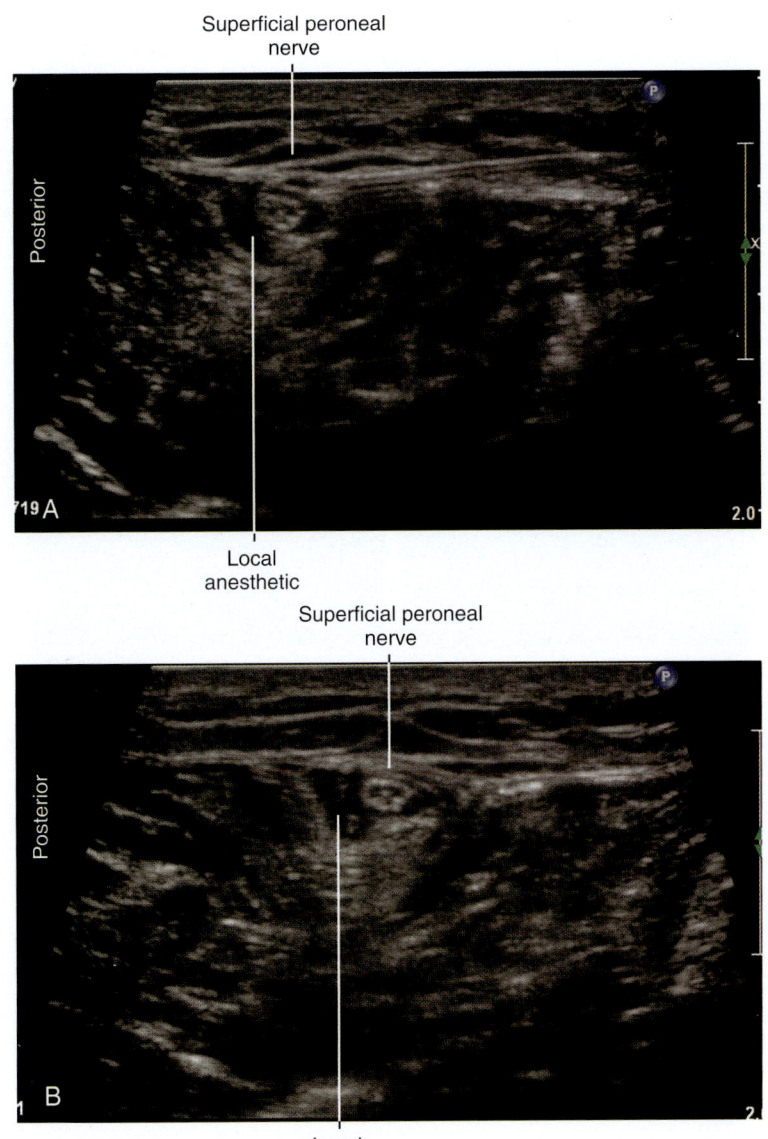

FIGURE 51.4 Image sequence showing superficial peroneal nerve block in the distal leg. An in-plane approach is demonstrated where the needle tip is placed adjacent to the nerve (A). After injection, local anesthetic is distributed around the superficial peroneal nerve (B).

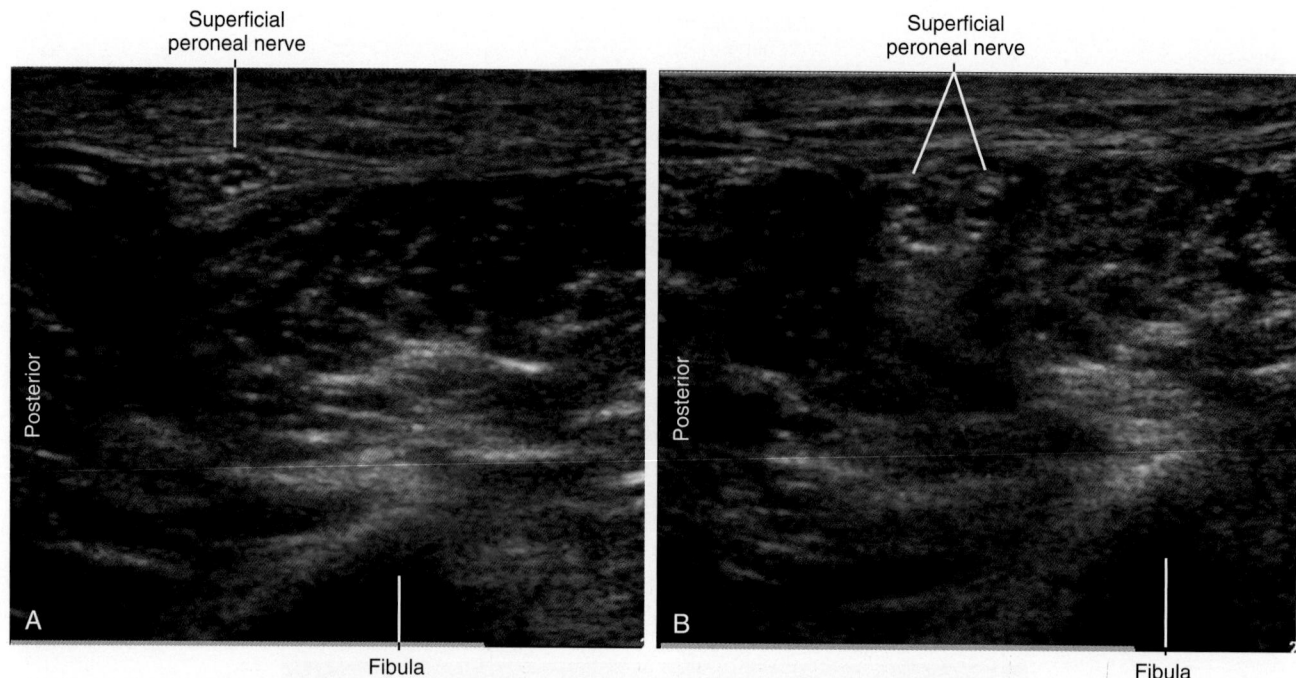

FIGURE 51.5 Image sequence showing superficial peroneal nerve dividing in the distal leg. The superficial peroneal nerve is shown proximally (A) and distally (B). After injection, local anesthetic is distributed along the branches of the superficial peroneal nerve.

Sural Nerve Block

CHAPTER 52

The sural nerve (from *sura*, Latin for calf) is a sensory nerve that typically derives from both peroneal (lateral) and tibial (medial) contributions (fibers of S1 origin, from the sciatic nerve). Although the sural usually receives both contributions, anatomic variation in its composition is common.[1] The sural nerve innervates the lateral aspect of the foot and the fifth toe,[2] and the sural nerve also gives rise to a small lateral calcaneal branch. The cross-sectional area of the sural nerve approximately is 3 mm^2 (approximately 2 mm diameter).[3]

The sural nerve emerges between the medial and lateral heads of the gastrocnemius muscle to join the small saphenous vein within a common fascial compartment of the subcutaneous tissue of the lateral leg (a common fascial tunnel or tent).[4] Because it is a sensory nerve, the sural nerve is sometimes used for biopsy or harvest. Although subcutaneous infiltration is an effective means of blocking the distal sural nerve, more proximal block may be indicated in patients with infection or edema of the foot.[5]

SUGGESTED TECHNIQUE

Because of its small size, the sural nerve can be difficult to image. The sural nerve can be blocked proximal to the lateral malleolus by applying a calf tourniquet to help identify the small saphenous vein. In this location, the sural nerve lies adjacent to the vein within the subcutaneous tissue of the leg, and an in-plane approach can be used to distribute local anesthetic around the sural nerve.

A sural contribution from the tibial nerve can often be imaged between the medial and lateral heads of the gastrocnemius muscle. This contribution emerges between these muscles to pierce the fascia lata and join the lesser saphenous vein and the common peroneal nerve contribution within the subcutaneous tissue of the lateral aspect of the lower leg. The sural nerve can be blocked with an in-plane approach from the lateral aspect of the leg with the patient in supine position and the leg elevated. Although prone position is optimal for sural nerve imaging, the former approach is more practical and useful in most patients.

KEY POINTS

Sural Nerve Block	The Essentials
Anatomy	The SuN emerges between the medial and lateral heads of the GC.
	The SuN lies adjacent to the SSV within SQ tissue of the lateral leg.
	The SuN is about 2 mm in diameter.
Positioning	Supine with leg elevated
Operator	Standing at side of patient
Display	Across the table
Transducer	High-frequency linear, 23- to 38-mm footprint
Initial depth setting	25 mm
Needle	25 gauge, 38 mm in length
Anatomic location	Apply a calf tourniquet to help identify the SSV.
	Begin by scanning the lateral leg proximal to the lateral malleolus.
Approach	Perform the block proximal to the lateral malleolus.
	SAX view of SuN, in-plane from anterior to posterior

Continued

KEY POINTS—CONT'D	
Sural Nerve Block	**The Essentials**
Sonographic assessment	The injection should track along the SuN and SSV.
Anatomic variation	The SuN may divide proximally.

GC, Gastrocnemius muscle; *SAX*, short axis; *SSV*, small saphenous vein; *SQ*, subcutaneous; *SuN*, sural nerve.

Clinical Pearls

- The sural nerve emerges between the medial and lateral heads of the gastrocnemius to enter the subcutaneous tissue of the lower calf.
- In this location, the sural nerve lies adjacent to the small saphenous vein. When the sural nerve consists of separate branches, they typically flank either side of the small saphenous vein.
- Because common fascia covers both the small saphenous vein and sural nerve in the leg, inject just below the small saphenous vein for sural nerve block. Injections within the fascial compartment will compress the adjacent small saphenous vein.
- The sural nerve and small saphenous vein pass posterior to the lateral malleolus. Because the sural nerve lies in subcutaneous tissue in the lower calf, it is not mistaken for a nearby tendon.
- Surgeries of the fifth (small) toe also require superficial peroneal and tibial blocks because these nerves often contribute innervation.

References

1. Zhu J, Li D, Shao J, et al. An ultrasound study of anatomic variants of the sural nerve. *Muscle Nerve*. 2011;43(4):560–562.
2. Solomon LB, Ferris L, Tedman R, et al. Surgical anatomy of the sural and superficial fibular nerves with an emphasis on the approach to the lateral malleolus. *J Anat*. 2001;199:717–723.
3. Üçeyler N, Schäfer KA, Mackenrodt D, et al. High-resolution ultrasonography of the superficial peroneal motor and sural sensory nerves may be a non-invasive approach to the diagnosis of vasculitic neuropathy. *Front Neurol*. 2016;7:48.
4. Caggiati A. Fascial relationships of the short saphenous vein. *J Vasc Surg*. 2001;34(2):241–246.
5. Redborg KE, Sites BD, Chinn CD, et al. Ultrasound improves the success rate of a sural nerve block at the ankle. *Reg Anesth Pain Med*. 2009;34(1):24–28.

SURAL NERVE BLOCK 223

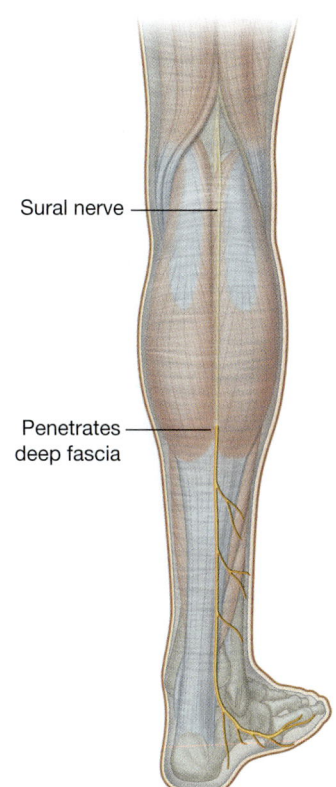

FIGURE 52.1 Course of the sural nerve. (From Drake RL, Vogl W, Mitchell AWM. *Gray's anatomy for students*. Philadelphia: Churchill Livingstone; 2004.)

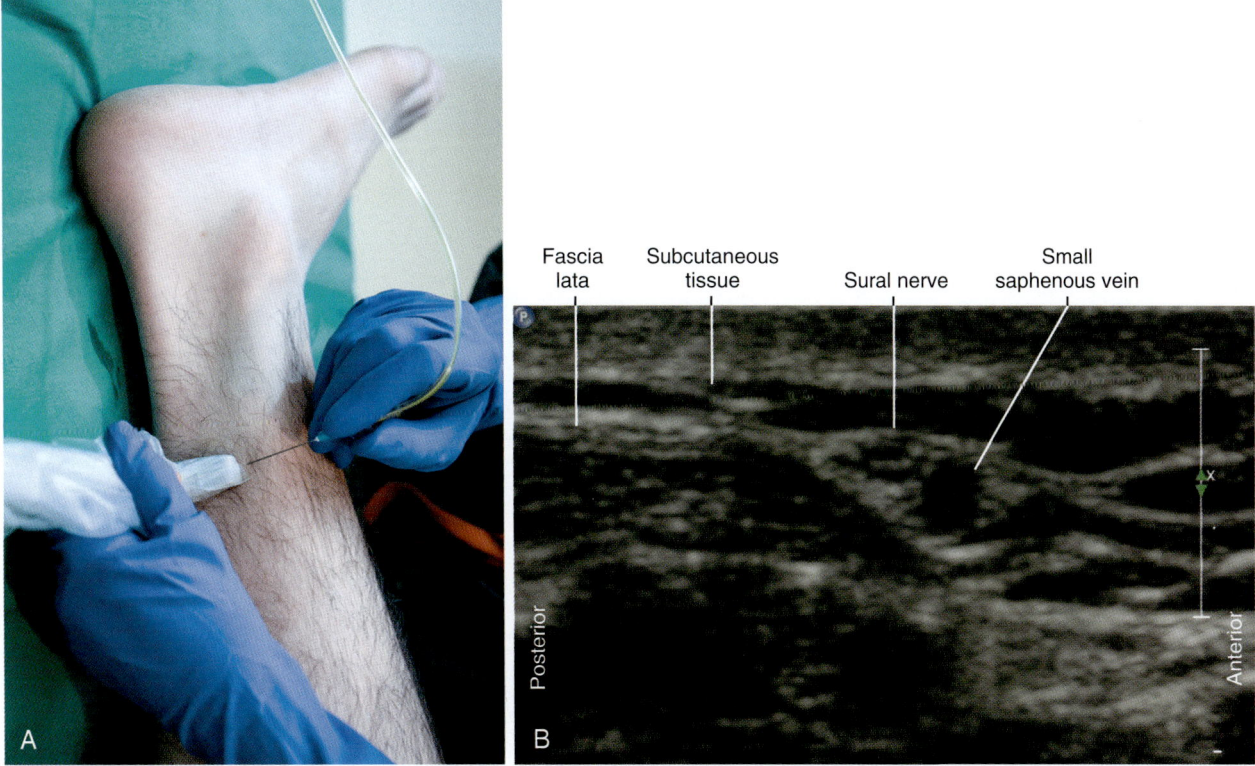

FIGURE 52.2 External photograph showing the approach to sural nerve block in the distal leg (A). The corresponding sonogram is shown (B). The sural nerve is adjacent to the small saphenous vein within a common fascial tunnel of the subcutaneous tissue of the posterolateral leg. The nerve and vein are viewed in short axis.

LOWER EXTREMITY BLOCKS

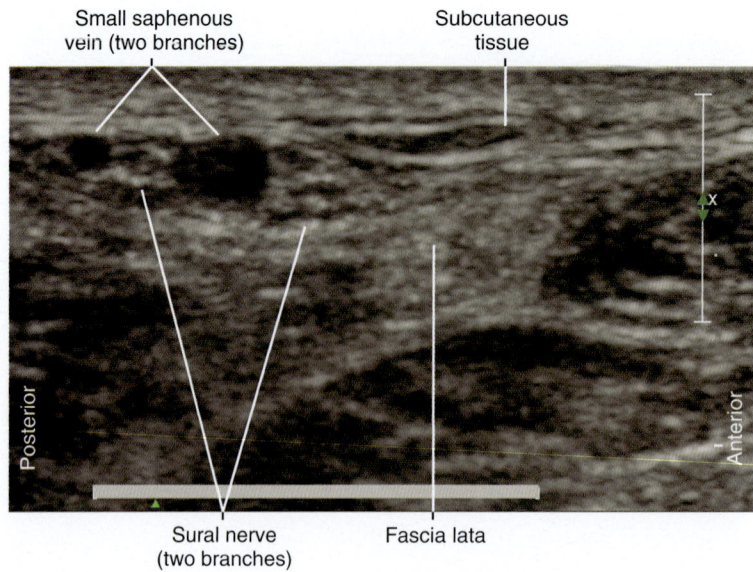

FIGURE 52.3 Short-axis view of the sural nerve in the distal leg. In some patients, the sural nerve and adjacent small saphenous vein are divided.

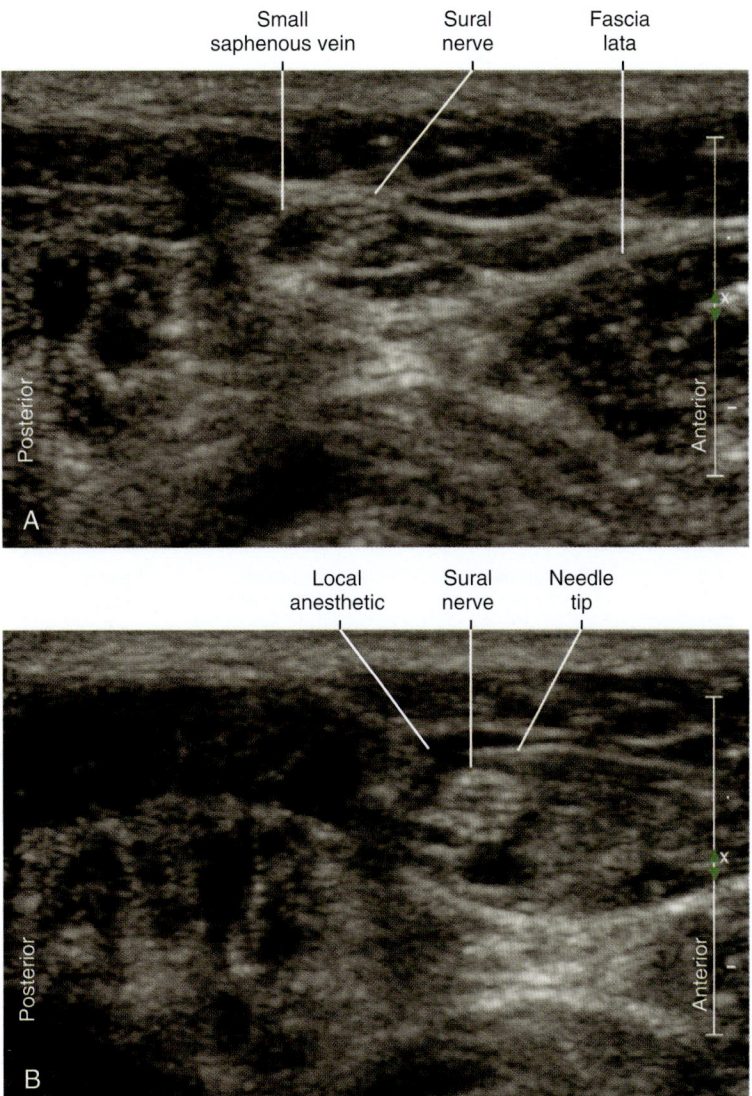

FIGURE 52.4 Image sequence showing sural nerve block in the distal leg. Before injection, the sural nerve is identified adjacent to the small saphenous vein (A). An in-plane approach is demonstrated where the needle tip is placed adjacent to the sural nerve within the subcutaneous tissue of the leg (B). Local anesthetic surrounds the sural nerve and compresses the small saphenous vein.

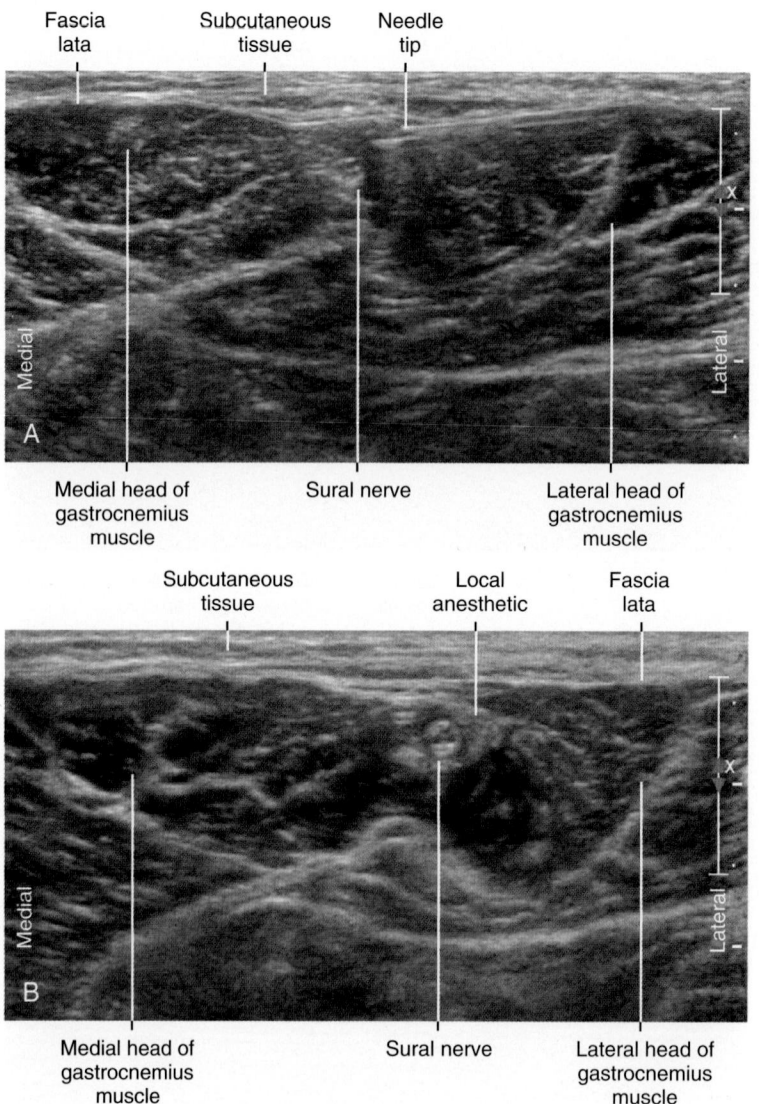

FIGURE 52.5 Proximal sural nerve block. The sural nerve also can be blocked in the posterior calf where it emerges between the medial and lateral heads of the gastrocnemius muscle into the subcutaneous tissue of the leg (A and B).

Tibial Nerve Block

CHAPTER 53

The tibial nerve is the largest branch of the sciatic nerve and the largest nerve for the ankle block (cross-sectional area of about 14 mm^2 in the leg). It provides sensory innervation to the heel region and sole of the foot. The tibial nerve innervates all five toes, including all five nail beds (similar to digital nerves, the distal fibers of the tibial nerve curve dorsally). The tibial nerve has a relatively straight course in the leg and divides into the medial calcaneal, medial plantar, and lateral plantar branches near the ankle. In some subjects, the takeoff of the medial calcaneal branch from the tibial nerve can be imaged above the ankle joint. The medial calcaneal branch travels directly inferior and medial to supply the heel region.

The order of anatomic structures from anterior to posterior at the medial malleolus is as follows: Tom, Dick, AVN, Harry (Tibialis posterior tendon, flexor Digitorum longus tendon, posterior tibial Artery and Veins, tibial Nerve, flexor Hallucis longus tendon). Therefore, the tibial nerve lies on the heel side of the posterior tibial artery. The posterior tibial artery is often accompanied by two or three flanking veins. This neurovascular bundle, typically consisting of one artery and two veins, can have a "Mickey Mouse" ears appearance if light touch with the transducer is applied (similar to the appearance of the brachial artery and veins near the elbow). The adjacent tendons can be similar in ultrasound appearance to the tibial nerve near the ankle but will be less prominent proximally in the leg. The tibial nerve moves considerably with foot motion, and this translational motion along the nerve path can be used to help identify the nerve.[1]

Edema or infection often makes routine ankle block ineffective or contraindicated.[2] However, tibial nerve imaging can be difficult in some surgical patients with peripheral vascular disease because vascular landmarks for the nerve are not present. Tibial nerve block in the leg avoids the foot-drop that occurs with more proximal popliteal block of the sciatic nerve,[3,4] and this can be an advantage for ambulatory surgery patients.

SUGGESTED TECHNIQUE

The tibial nerve can be approached in-plane from the posterior (Achilles) or anterior (tibial) side in supine position with the leg externally rotated using a short-axis view of the neurovascular bundle. The best point of tibial nerve imaging in the leg is usually halfway between the medial malleolus and the bulk of the gastrocnemius-soleus muscle complex in the calf. Place the block needle tip between the posterior tibial artery and the tibial nerve so as to enter the neurovascular compartment. For effective tibial nerve block, the needle tip must cross through the intermuscular septum to enter the deep compartment of the leg. With the posterior approach, the Achilles and plantaris tendons can lie close to the point of needle entry. With the anterior approach, the saphenous vein can be close to the needle path near the skin surface.

KEY POINTS	
Tibial Nerve Block	**The Essentials**
Anatomy	Two veins usually flank either side of the PTA.
	The TN is about 4 mm in diameter.
Image orientation	The TN lies on the heel side of the PTA in the leg.
Positioning	Externally rotate and support the leg.
	The heel points toward the operator.

Continued

KEY POINTS—CON'T

Tibial Nerve Block

	The Essentials
Operator	Standing on the contralateral side of the table
Display:	Across the table, on the ipsilateral side
Transducer:	High-frequency linear, 23- to 25-mm footprint
Initial depth setting	30 mm
Needle	21–25 gauge, 38–50 mm in length
Anatomic location	Begin by scanning the medial aspect of mid-leg.
	Optimal imaging of TN usually halfway between the gastrocnemius and malleoli.
Approach	SAX view of TN, in-plane from the Achilles side
	Place the needle tip between the TN and PTA.
Sonographic assessment	Injection should track distally along the TN to MCB (SAX slide).
Anatomic variation	Some anatomic variation of the TN position with respect to the PTA.
	Absent PTA (about 5% of normal subjects, plus cases of vascular insufficiency).
	Accessory soleus muscle.

MCB, Medial calcaneal branch of the tibial nerve; *PTA*, posterior tibial artery; *SAX*, short axis; *TN*, tibial nerve.

Clinical Pearls

- The ideal needle path is between the posterior tibial artery and the tibial nerve so that the injection separates the two structures.
- Tibial nerve block with ultrasound can be used for outpatient heel surgery to avoid foot-drop that occurs with more proximal popliteal block of the sciatic nerve.
- The medial calcaneal branch of the tibial nerve can sometimes be imaged, particularly after tibial nerve block in the leg. This nerve often has multiple branches.
- Be careful with long-axis assessments of local anesthetic distribution along peripheral nerves that lie close to arteries (e.g., the tibial nerve). Partial lineups containing the adjacent posterior tibial artery or vein can appear similar to the distributed fluid.
- The central aponeurosis of the tibialis posterior muscle lies deep to the tibial nerve in the leg. These two structures can have similar ultrasound appearance.
- When tibial nerve block is approached from the Achilles tendon side, position the patient with the leg elevated and slightly flexed.

References

1. Boyd BS, Dilley A. Altered tibial nerve biomechanics in patients with diabetes mellitus. *Muscle Nerve*. 2014;50(2):216–223.
2. Redborg KE, Antonakakis JG, Beach ML, Chinn CD, Sites BD. Ultrasound improves the success rate of a tibial nerve block at the ankle. *Reg Anesth Pain Med*. 2009;34(3):256–260.
3. Sobey JH, Franklin A. Ultrasound-guided tibial nerve block for definitive treatment of tarsal tunnel syndrome in a pediatric patient. *Reg Anesth Pain Med*. 2016;41(3):415–416.
4. Clattenburg E, Herring A, Hahn C, Johnson B, Nagdev A. ED ultrasound-guided posterior tibial nerve blocks for calcaneal fracture analgesia. *Am J Emerg Med*. 2016;34(6):1183.e1–1183.e3.

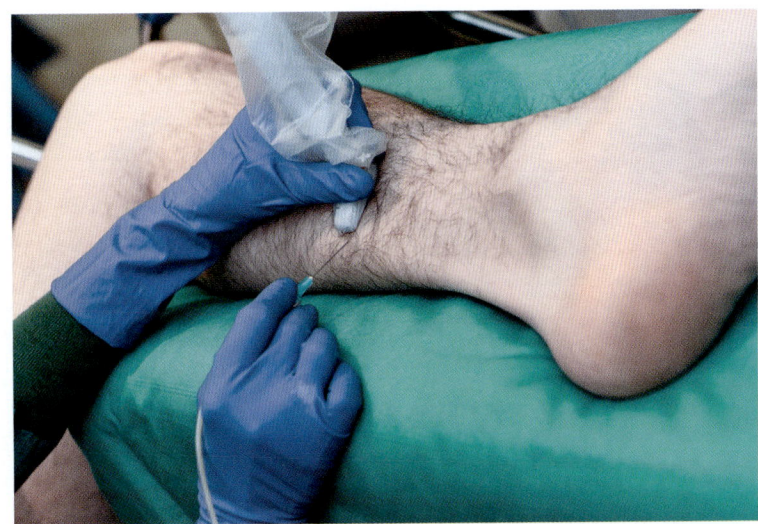

FIGURE 53.1 External photograph showing posterior-to-anterior in-plane approach to tibial nerve block in the distal leg. This location is proximal to where the tibial nerve divides into its medial plantar, lateral plantar, and medial calcaneal branches.

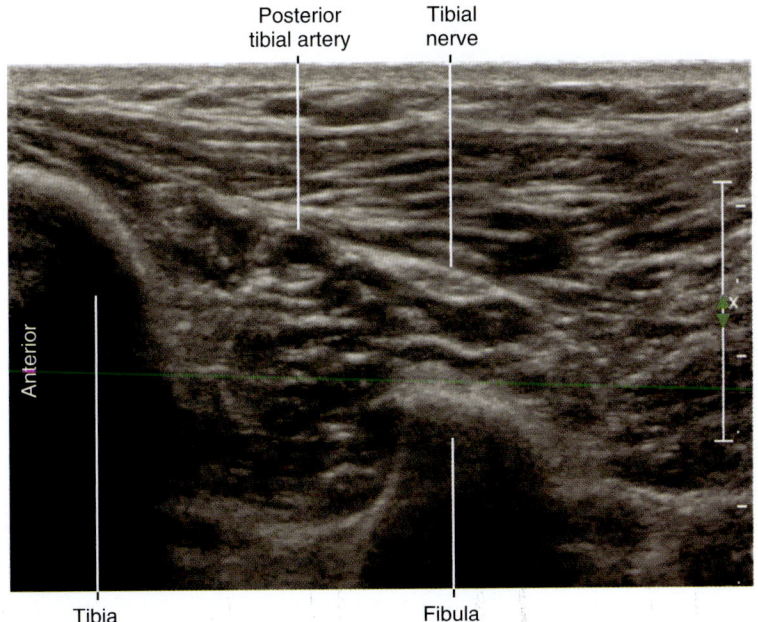

FIGURE 53.2 Short-axis view of the tibial nerve in the distal leg. With a broad footprint transducer, both the tibia and fibula can be imaged deep to the nerve.

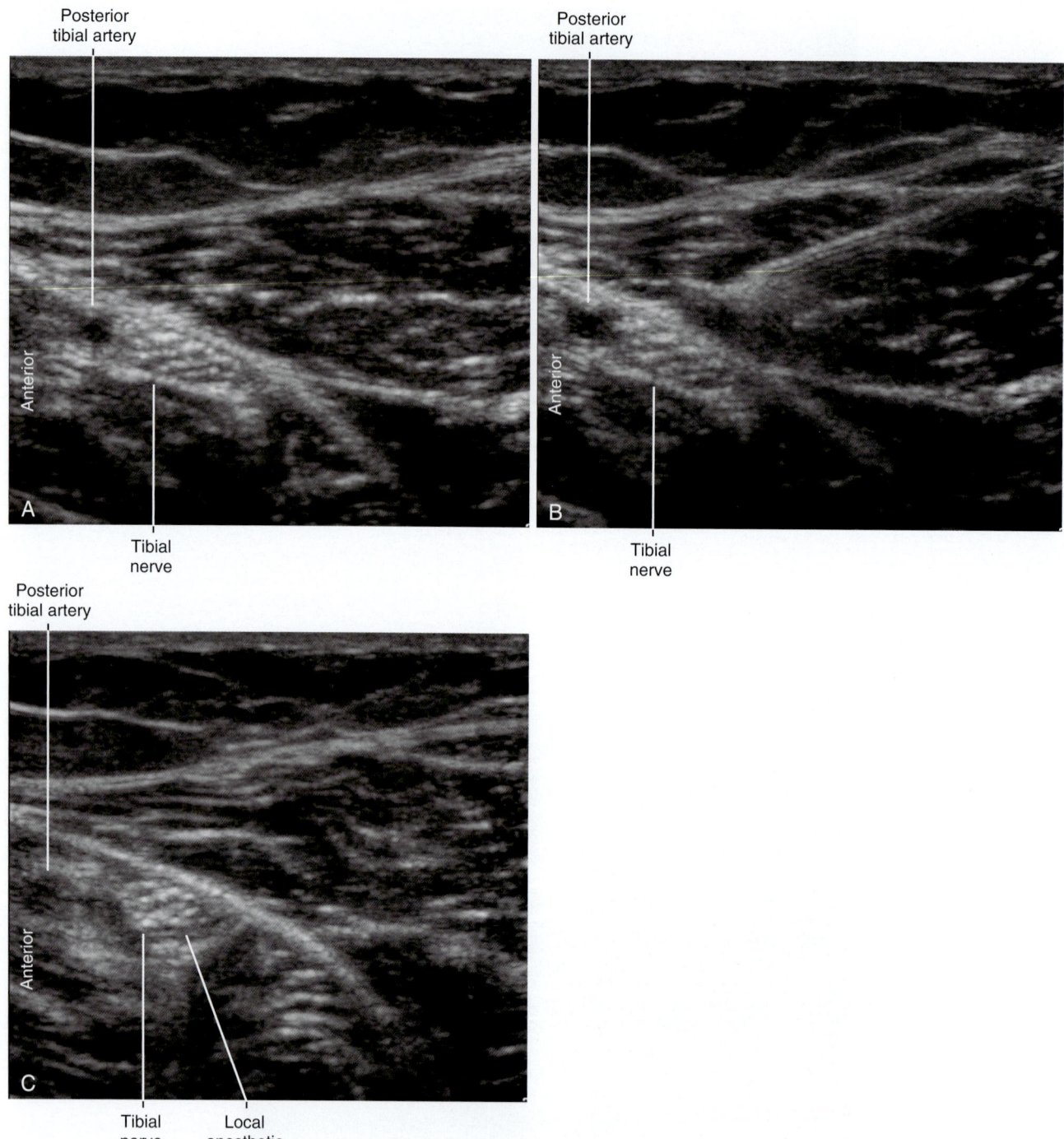

FIGURE 53.3 Tibial nerve block in the distal leg showing the in-plane approach from posterior to anterior. Image sequence is shown before (A), during (B), and after (C) injection. Local anesthetic surrounds the tibial nerve and separates it from the posterior tibial artery.

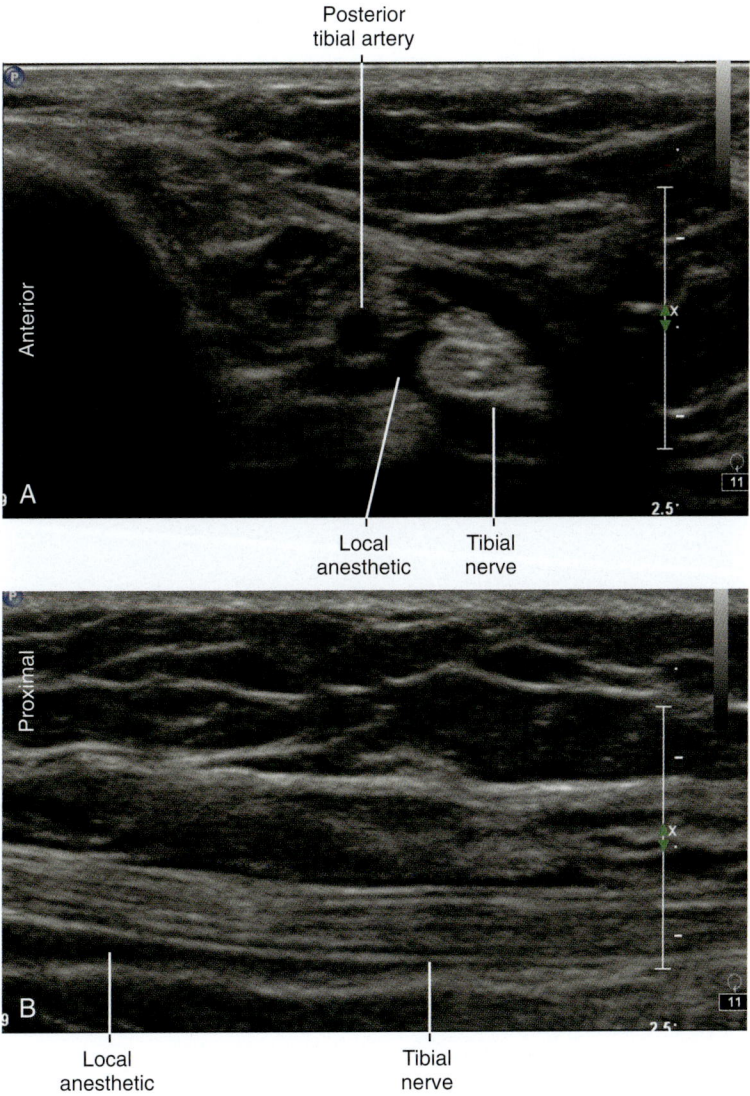

FIGURE 53.4 After injection, local anesthetic is distributed around the tibial nerve (A) and tracks along the nerve (B).

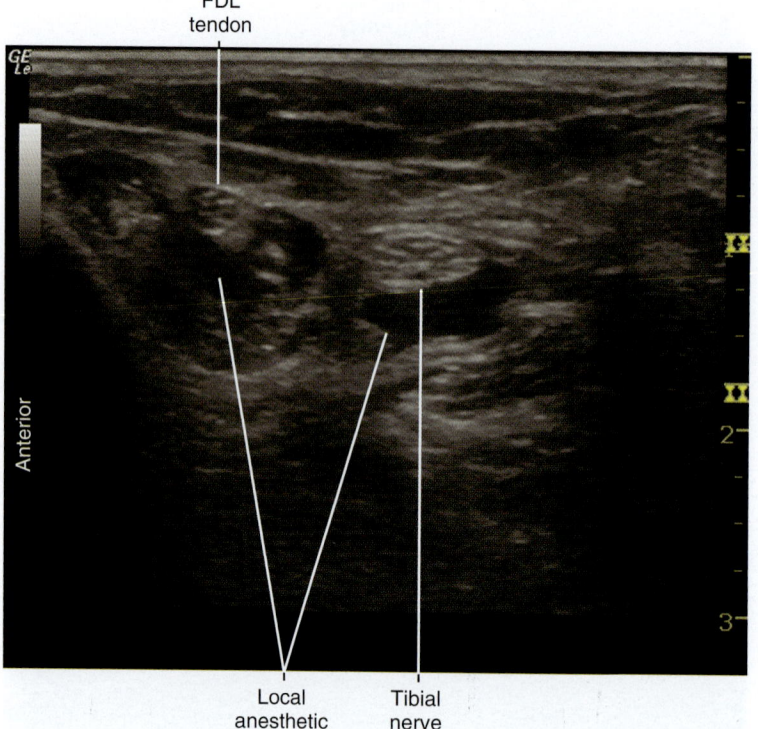

FIGURE 53.5 The flexor digitorum longus (FDL) tendon and tibial nerve can have similar ultrasound appearances. The FDL tendon is smaller than the tibial nerve and lies closer to the tibia. This sonogram was obtained after an ankle block was performed using surface landmarks (without ultrasound guidance). Local anesthetic is seen to surround both the tibial nerve and the FDL tendon.

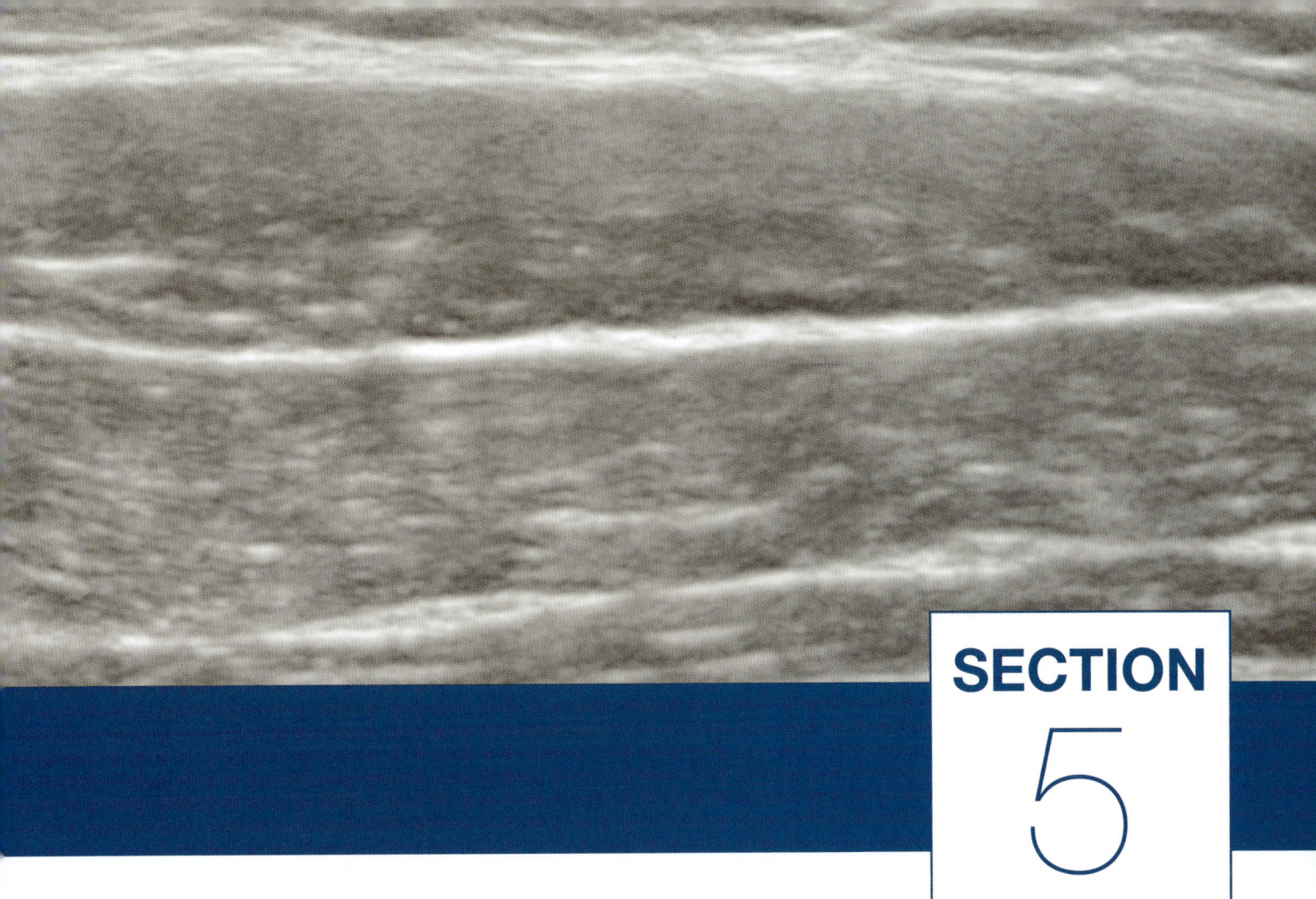

SECTION 5

Trunk Blocks

CHAPTER 54

Intercostal Nerve Block

Twelve pairs of intercostal nerves lie within or near the inferior groove of each corresponding rib. These nerves supply the skin and chest wall skeletal muscles. An intercostal artery and vein accompany each nerve and lie superior to it. Intercostal nerves are difficult to image with ultrasound because they are small and often covered by the caudal edge of the corresponding rib. Proximal intercostal nerves are found in the classic subcostal position in 17%, in the midzone in 73%, and in the inferior supracostal position in 10% of anatomic specimens. The intercostal nerves migrate away from their respective ribs near the midaxillary line. Although intercostal nerves are difficult to directly image with ultrasound, ultrasound guidance has advantages over landmark-based techniques.[1]

Doppler ultrasound has been used to locate intercostal arteries for intercostal block.[2] Intercostal arteries are 3 to 4 mm in diameter and can be detected in an acoustic window 4 cm lateral from the midline.[3] Doppler measurements of the intercostal arteries are possible from T4 and lower. Ultrasound-guided intercostal nerve blocks have been used for acute and chronic pain management.[4] Intercostal nerve blocks can be used for breast surgery and are best placed at T3, T4, and T5 for these surgical procedures. Another common application is for thoracic trauma, chest tube placement, open cholecystectomy, and open nephrolithotomy.[5-7]

The subcostal nerve (the anterior ramus of the spinal nerve T12) is a unique intercostal nerve. This nerve supplies the lower abdominal wall and is not closely associated with the 12th rib. The subcostal nerve is about 3 mm in diameter and passes over the iliac crest.

SUGGESTED TECHNIQUE

Intercostal nerve blocks are a viable alternative to paravertebral blocks for unilateral trunk anesthesia and analgesia, although more clinical investigations are needed.[8] There are 12 pairs of intercostal nerves that travel parallel to their respective ribs. Intercostal nerves and arteries are protected by the costal groove as they travel toward to the skin surface.

Intercostal nerve imaging can be performed in the sitting, lateral, or prone position, and the arms are positioned forward or hanging down to retract the scapulae laterally. This is particularly important when imaging the intercostal nerves above the fifth rib because of the overlying scapula. When intercostal blocks are performed in sitting position, the right-handed operator stands and turns to the patient's right to view the imaging display regardless of the side of the block.

It can be difficult to distinguish the intercostal muscle layers on ultrasound scans (external, internal, and innermost).[9] The fascia between the intercostal muscles is best seen in transverse view (an intercostal view between ribs, to image the external, internal and innermost intercostal muscles). If a thin dark layer is detected, this likely represents the innermost muscle layer (similar to the transversus abdominis muscle for transversus abdominis plane [TAP] block).

Intercostal blood vessels can be identified with B-mode and power Doppler imaging. Intercostal nerves lie caudal to the intercostal arteries, and division of an intercostal artery into main and collateral branches can be observed (injection central to the division of artery and nerve results in more complete block).[10] Intercostal nerves can sometimes be seen between adjacent ribs with small accompanying intercostal arteries (intercostal nerves are small flat nerves, echogenic with a few fascicles).

Perform intercostal nerve blocks near the angle of the ribs. In this location, the neurovascular bundle lies under the costal groove. The lateral cutaneous branches of the intercostal nerves emerge at the anterior edge of the latissimus dorsi and serratus anterior muscles (at about the mid-axillary line). Intercostal blocks performed central to this point are therefore more complete.

Long-axis view can be used to identify the angle of the rib. Block 2 cm medial to this point where the intercostal nerves divide and join the costal groove with their respective intercostal arteries.

Both hands of the operator rest on the back for optimal control of the needle and transducer during intercostal nerve block. In-plane intercostal approach can be used with the needle aimed centrally. The same intercostal approach can be used for both paravertebral block and intercostal nerve block (lateral to medial in-plane approach between adjacent ribs, with the intercostal nerve block performed at the angle of the ribs).

Injection distributions are usually confined to a single intercostal space. However, injections can travel medially to reach adjacent intercostal spaces by central spread. The intercostal nerves and vessels can serve as a tubular conduit to promote central distribution of the injection. Displacement of the pleura occurs with injection for intercostal block (the "pleural dent").

Injections at multiple levels are often used (many people use multiple injections for paravertebral blocks). At least three intercostal injections to achieve anesthesia at one level due to overlap in innervation from adjacent interspaces. Peak plasma levels after intercostal injections are high and occur rapidly, so carefully limit the total local anesthetic volume.

One of the potential benefits of ultrasound guidance is reduction of the risk for pneumothorax. The chance of developing a pneumothorax depends on the amount of aerated lung tissue traversed by the needle. The lung is particularly fragile in patients with chronic obstructive lung disease and emphysema. Demonstration of postinterventional lung sliding and comet-tail artifact from the pleura rule out pneumothorax. This examination is best performed over the nondependent portion of the lung (the anterior chest in supine position).

Another potential benefit of ultrasound guidance for intercostal block is the avoidance of arterial puncture, and this complication can result in hemothorax. This is particularly noteworthy because the tracking between the lower border of the ribs and the neurovascular bundle is not always precise. There is variability of the relationship between the caudal edge of the ribs and the neurovascular bundle, especially at the lower rib levels and farther lateral from the paravertebral region.

Clinical Pearls

- The easiest patient position to perform the block is prone, but lateral or sitting is also possible.
- Intercostal blocks are best performed near the posterior angulation of the ribs. In this location, the nerves are shallow and relatively centrally located before branching occurs.
- Both transverse and longitudinal in-plane approaches to intercostal injection result in similar distributions toward the paravertebral space.[11]
- With intercostal nerve blocks, rapid and high peak plasma levels of local anesthetic are expected. Therefore, careful attention to drug dosing is essential.
- Even with needle puncture of the pleura, the chance of pneumothorax is about 50%. This chance depends on the amount of aerated lung tissue traversed by the needle. The lung is particularly fragile in patients with chronic obstructive lung disease and emphysema.
- The tracking between the lower border of the ribs and the neurovascular bundle is not always matched. Discrepancies are sometimes observed along the course of the rib.
- One of the potential benefits of ultrasound guidance for intercostal block is the avoidance of arterial puncture, because this complication can result in hemothorax.

References

1. Bhatia A, Gofeld M, Ganapathy S, Hanlon J, Johnson M. Comparison of anatomic landmarks and ultrasound guidance for intercostal nerve injections in cadavers. *Reg Anesth Pain Med*. 2013;38(6):503–507.
2. Vaghadia H, Jenkins LC. Use of a doppler ultrasound stethoscope for intercostal nerve block. *Can J Anaesth*. 1988;35:86–89.
3. Koyanagi T, Kawaharada N, Kurimoto Y, et al. Examination of intercostal arteries with transthoracic doppler sonography. *Echocardiography*. 2010;27(1):17–20.
4. Eichenberger U, Greher M, Curatolo M. Ultrasound in interventional pain management. *Tech Reg Anesth Pain Manag*. 2004;8:171–178.

5. Stone MB, Carnell J, Fischer JW, et al. Ultrasound-guided intercostal nerve block for traumatic pneumothorax requiring tube thoracostomy. *Am J Emerg Med*. 2011;29(6):697.e1–679.e2.
6. Vandepitte C, Gautier P, Bellen P, Murata H, Salviz EA, Hadzic A. Use of ultrasound-guided intercostal nerve block as a sole anaesthetic technique in a high-risk patient with Duchenne muscular dystrophy. *Acta Anaesthesiol Belg*. 2013;64(2):91–94.
7. Ozkan D, Akkaya T, Karakoyunlu N, et al. Effect of ultrasound-guided intercostal nerve block on postoperative pain after percutaneous nephrolithotomy: prospective randomized controlled study. *Anaesthesist*. 2013;62(12):988–994.
8. Abrahams M, Derby R, Horn JL. Update on ultrasound for truncal blocks: a review of the evidence. *Reg Anesth Pain Med*. 2016;41(2):275–288.
9. Sakai F, Sone S, Kiyono K, et al. High-resolution ultrasound of the chest wall. *Rofo*. 1990;153:390–394.
10. Kuhlman DR, Khuder SA, Lane RD. Factors influencing the diameter of human anterior and posterior intercostal arteries. *Clin Anat*. 2015;28(2):219–226.
11. Paraskeuopoulos T, Saranteas T, Kouladouros K, et al. Thoracic paravertebral spread using two different ultrasound-guided intercostal injection techniques in human cadavers. *Clin Anat*. 2010;23(7):840–847.

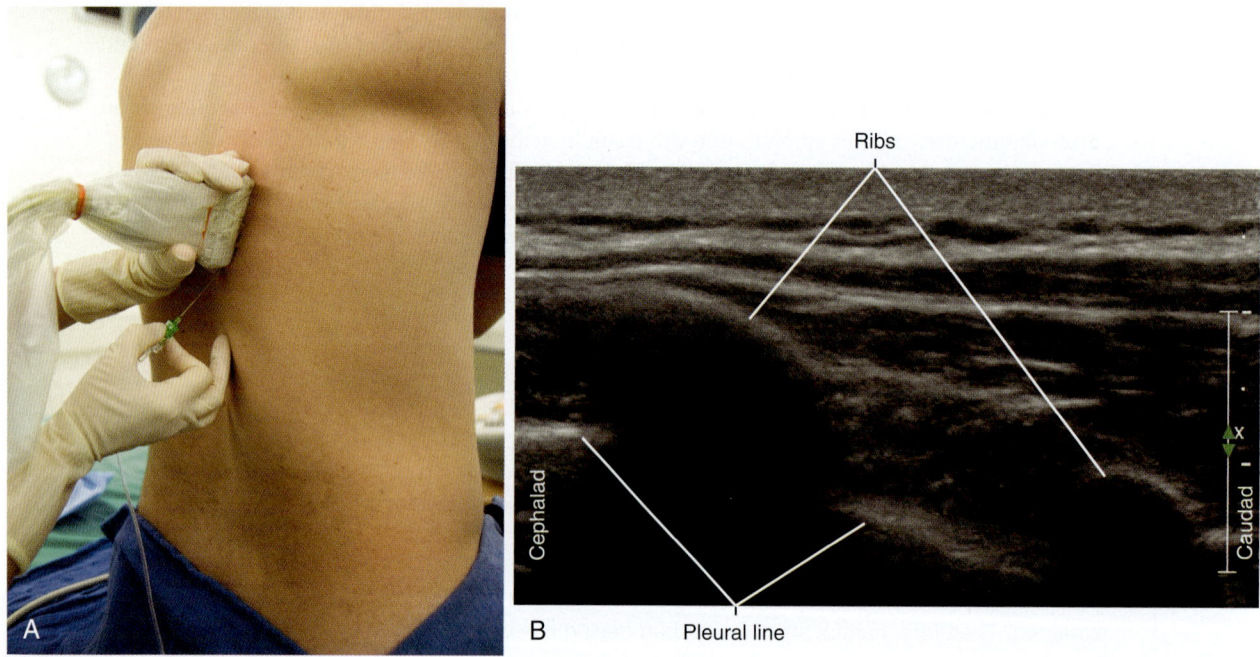

FIGURE 54.1 External photograph showing the approach to intercostal nerve block in sitting position (A). The corresponding sonogram of the intercostal interspace before needle placement is shown (B).

INTERCOSTAL NERVE BLOCK 237

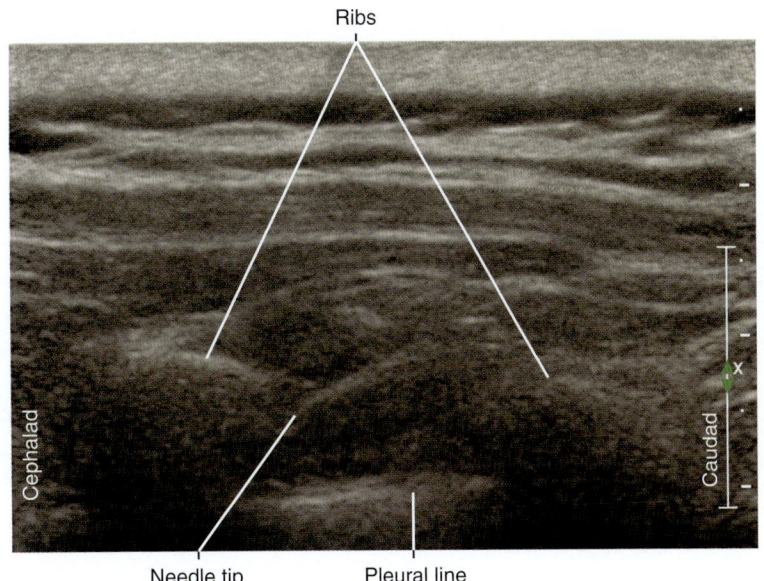

FIGURE 54.2 In-plane approach to intercostal nerve block. The needle tip advances between the ribs to place local anesthetic underneath the caudal edge of the superior rib.

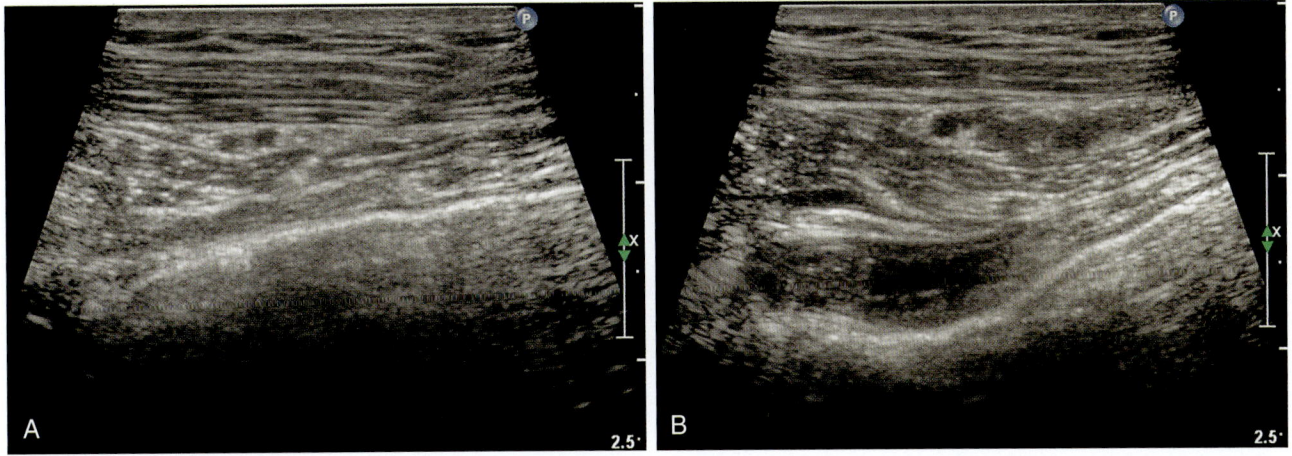

FIGURE 54.3 "Dent" in the pleural line after intercostal nerve block injection. Sonograms are shown before (A) and after (B) injection (approach between adjacent ribs).

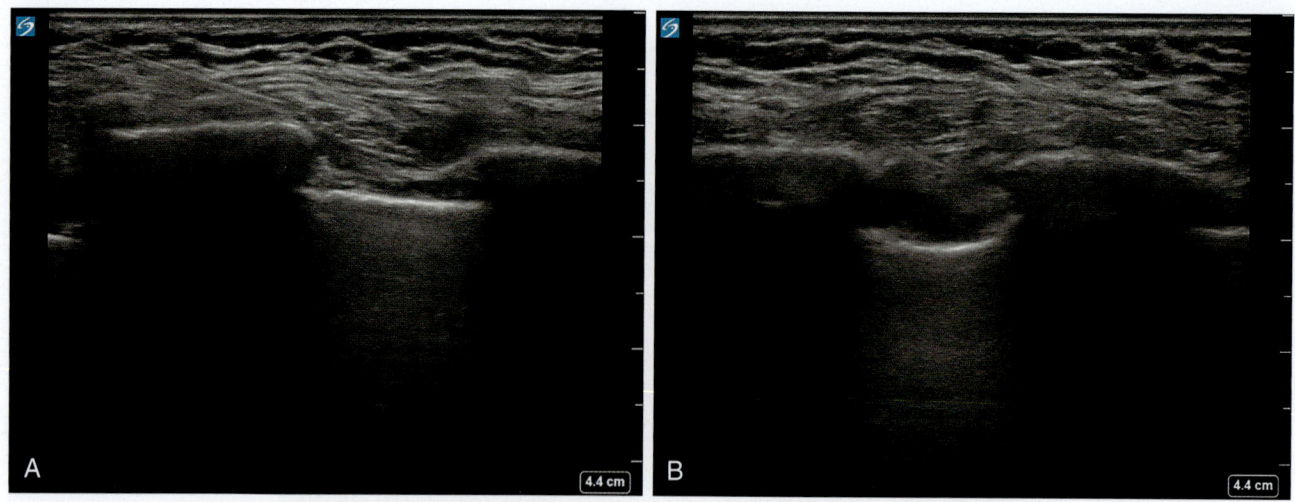

FIGURE 51.4 "Dent" in the pleural line after intercostal nerve block injection. Sonograms are shown before (A) and after (B) injection (approach over rib).

Pectoral Nerve Block (the Pecs Block)

CHAPTER 55

The pectoral nerves are branches of the brachial plexus that innervate the pectoral muscles. The lateral pectoral nerve (C5, C6, C7) is often a branch of the lateral cord and innervates the pectoralis major muscle. The medial pectoral nerve (C8, T1) is often a branch of the medial cord and innervates both the pectoralis major and minor muscles. The lateral and medial pectoral nerves communicate via the ansa pectoralis that crosses the second part of the axillary artery, just distal to the thoracoacromial takeoff.[1] The pectoral nerves have no cutaneous branches.

Several variations of pectoral nerve block have been described.[2,3] These blocks are often used to provide postoperative analgesia for surgeries of the chest wall and sub-pectoral breast implants.[4]

SUGGESTED TECHNIQUE

The approach for pectoral nerve block is similar to infraclavicular block of the brachial plexus. The lateral pectoral nerve travels with the pectoral branch of the thoracoacromial artery. The pectoral nerves can be blocked in the fascial plane between the pectoralis major and minor muscles adjacent to this artery. About 10 mL of local anesthetic in this plane is sufficient for block. Larger volumes of local anesthetic may cause brachial plexus block.

NEUROLOGIC ASSESSMENT OF BLOCK

Pectoral nerve block can be assessed by instructing the patient to push the arm forward against resistance (starting with the arm in the same position as for axillary block). The motor block from pectoralis nerve block is impressive (there often is profound relaxation of the pectoral muscles).

RELATION WITH OTHER BLOCKS

Interscalene, supraclavicular, and infraclavicular blocks are expected to cover the pectoral nerves because these nerves arise from the divisions or cords of the brachial plexus. The pectoral nerves are not blocked with axillary, thoracic paravertebral, or intercostal blocks. Pectoral nerve blocks are often combined with injections that layer over the surface of the serratus anterior muscle (serratus plane blocks) for more complete analgesia of the chest wall.

KEY POINTS

Pectoral Nerve Block	The Essentials
Anatomy	The pectoral nerves lie between the pectoralis major and minor muscles
	The LPN is often visible adjacent to the pectoral branch of the thoracoacromial artery (PTA)
	The diameter of the pectoral nerves is about 2 mm
Image orientation	Arbitrary
Positioning	Supine
Operator	Standing on either side of the table
Display	Across the table, on the ipsilateral side

Continued

KEY POINTS—CONT'D

Pectoral Nerve Block	The Essentials
Transducer	High-frequency linear, 38- to 50-mm footprint
Initial depth setting	30 mm
Needle	21 gauge, 50–70 mm in length
Anatomic location	Similar to infraclavicular block of the brachial plexus.
Approach	SAX view of artery, in-plane from either side.
	Place the needle tip in the fascial plane between the pectoralis major and minor muscles.
Sonographic assessment	Injection should split the fascial plane between the pectoral muscles.
	Sometimes the injection compresses the PTA.
Anatomic variation	Pectoral nerves can arise from brachial plexus divisions.
	The MPN can wrap around the lateral edge of the pectoralis minor muscle.

LPN, Lateral pectoral nerve; *MPN*, Medial pectoral nerve; *PTA*, pectoral branch of the thoracoacromial artery; *SAX*, short axis.

Clinical Pearls

- Pectoral nerve blocks can be performed with the arm in any position. However, the block is easiest if the arm is abducted (similar position as for axillary block).
- Pectoral nerve blocks are plane blocks that can be performed after induction of general anesthesia.
- The medial pectoral nerve often courses through the pectoralis minor muscle. This proximal portion of the nerve may be difficult to block.
- The cephalic vein lies over the pectoralis minor muscle, thoracoacromial artery, and lateral pectoral nerve, so this vessel is potentially in the needle path.
- For bilateral blocks, the operator and display remain in one location (the further side is typically blocked first).
- Complications from PECS blocks are rare, with only a few hematomas reported in a large clinical series.[5]

References

1. Porzionato A, Macchi V, Stecco C, Loukas M, Tubbs RS, De Caro R. Surgical anatomy of the pectoral nerves and the pectoral musculature. *Clin Anat.* 2012;25(5):559–575.
2. Blanco R. The "pecs block": a novel technique for providing analgesia after breast surgery. *Anaesthesia.* 2011;66(9):847–848.
3. Blanco R, Fajardo M, Parras Maldonado T. Ultrasound description of Pecs II (modified Pecs I): a novel approach to breast surgery. *Rev Esp Anestesiol Reanim.* 2012;59(9):470–475.
4. Bashandy GM, Abbas DN. Pectoral nerves I and II blocks in multimodal analgesia for breast cancer surgery: a randomized clinical trial. *Reg Anesth Pain Med.* 2015;40(1):68–74.
5. Ueshima H, Otake H. Ultrasound-guided pectoral nerves (PECS) block: Complications observed in 498 consecutive cases. *J Clin Anesth.* 2017;42:46.

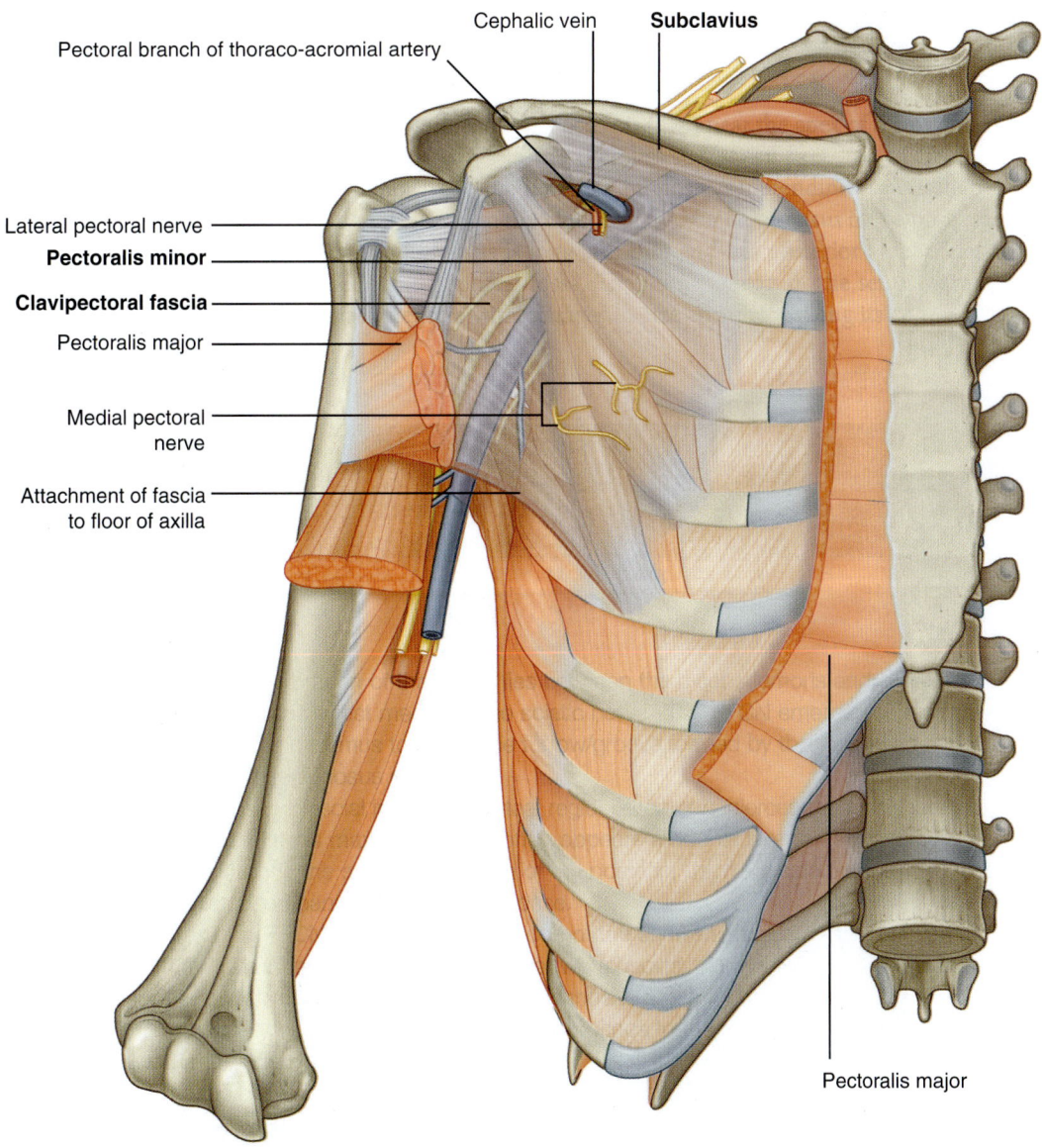

FIGURE 55.1 Course of the pectoral nerves. (From Drake RL, Vogl W, Mitchell AWM. *Gray's anatomy for students*. Philadelphia: Churchill Livingstone; 2004.)

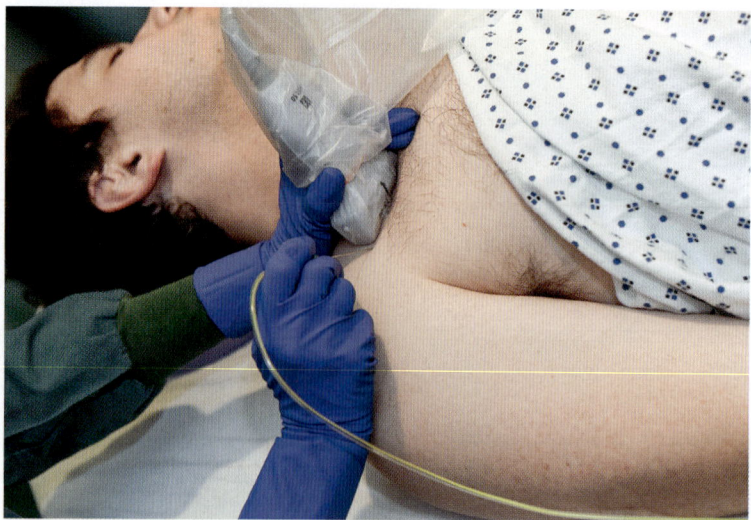

FIGURE 55.2 Transducer placement showing in-plane approach to pectoral nerve block.

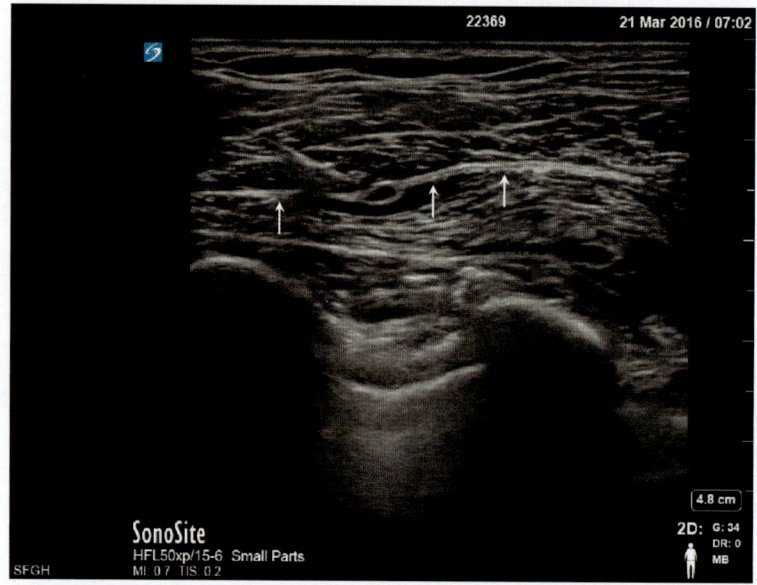

FIGURE 55.3 The lateral pectoral nerve identified between the pectoralis major and pectoralis minor muscles adjacent to the pectoral branch of the thoracoacromial artery. Local anesthetic is injected as the needle is withdrawn, attempting to split the double layer of fascia *(arrows)* that invests the lateral pectoral nerve and pectoral artery.

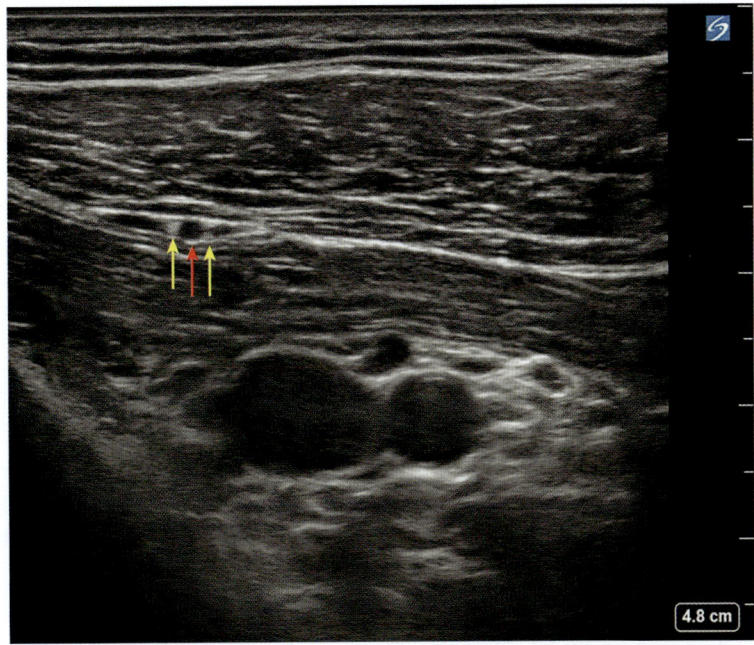

FIGURE 55.4 Short-axis view of the pectoral branch of the thoracoacromial artery *(red arrow)* and lateral pectoral nerve branches *(yellow arrows)* over the infraclavicular neurovascular bundle.

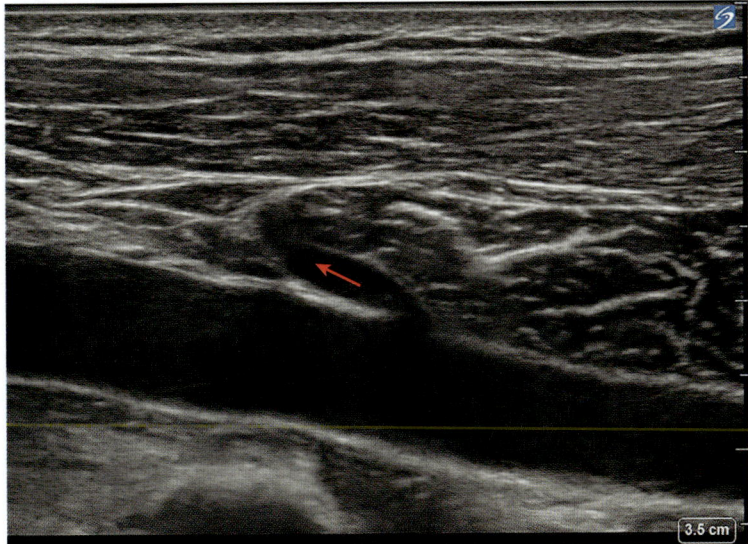

FIGURE 55.5 Long-axis view of the thoracoacromial artery *(red arrow)* wrapping around the corner of the pectoralis minor muscle. The lateral pectoral nerve runs with this recurrent artery as it forms the pectoral artery.

CHAPTER 56

Transversus Thoracis Muscular Plane Block

The transversus thoracis muscular (TTM) plane block is a parasternal approach to block the anterior branches of the intercostal nerves (T2 through T6). This block can be effective for surgeries and fractures near or at the sternum (median sternotomy, thymectomy, mediastinoscopy, pericardial window, etc.). This block also may be useful for sub-xiphoid incisions.

THE TRANSVERSUS THORACIS MUSCLE

The transversus thoracis muscle arises from the posterior surface of the lower third of the sternum. The muscle consists of four or five slips that pass laterally to the second through sixth costal cartilages.[1] The transversus thoracis muscle is smooth with uniform thickness (1 to 2 mm),[1] and this muscle is in continuity with the transversus abdominis muscle.[2]

INTERNAL MAMMARY VESSELS

The internal mammary vessels lie superficial to the transversus thoracis muscle. The internal mammary vessels are found within 20 mm of the lateral sternal border. Cranial to the level of the second or third rib, the vein is a single vessel that courses medial to the artery.[3] Caudal to the third rib, there are typically two veins, one medial and one lateral, flanking a single artery. The internal mammary veins have thin walls and are very sensitive to intrathoracic pressure. Although the block is shallow, due to the proximity of the internal mammary vessels, TTM is usually considered with similar precautions as for neuraxial blocks to reduce bleeding risks. Normal internal mammary (parasternal) lymph nodes are not visualized on ultrasound scans.[4,5]

SUGGESTED TECHNIQUE

ANATOMIC CONSIDERATIONS

TTM block can be performed at several intercostal interspaces. The second, third, and fourth intercostal spaces are sufficiently large for TTM block. TTM block at high thoracic intercostal interspaces (T1-2 or T2-3) usually have a single medial internal mammary vein. TTM block at lower thoracic intercostal interspaces (T3-4 or T4-5) can have underlying transversus thoracis muscle. The second rib articulates with the angle of the sternum and can be used for a bony reference landmark.

Liberal amounts of ultrasound gel can help even or level skin depressions between adjacent costal cartilages.

Examine the field for blood vessels with duplex power Doppler imaging prior to block. Use light touch with the transducer to establish the position of the internal mammary vein. It is important to identify the presence of a lateral lying internal mammary vein to reduce the chance of vascular puncture. If there is difficulty identifying the internal mammary vein(s), instruct the patient to take a deep breath in and hold it to increase the intrathoracic pressure and promote venous distention. Alternatively, if the patient is under general anesthesia, a Valsalva maneuver can be performed to distend the vein(s) (hold 30 cm water airway pressure for a few seconds while scanning).

There are recurrent intercostal branches that travel through the transversus thoracis compartment (these intercostal nerves head back away from midline). Local anesthetic also may travel between thoracic and abdominal compartments with the blood vessels. The internal mammary blood vessels can serve as tubular conduits to promote cephalo-caudal distribution of injected local anesthetic.

Inject about 10 to 15 mL of local anesthetic per side in normal sized adult patients.[6] Because of the proximity of the internal mammary veins to the central circulation, meticulous technique and avoidance of intravascular injection are required. Focal posterior displacement of the pleura is observed with transversus thoracic plane injection.[7]

ANATOMIC VARIATION

The sternalis muscle is an accessory muscle that lies over the pectoralis major and runs parallel to the sternum. This accessory muscle is observed in about 6% of normal subjects. Parasternal sonography is more difficult in the setting of chest wall deformity (e.g., pectus excavatum). A long, jointed xiphoid process causing an apparent mass in the epigastric region is an important normal variant.[8]

KEY POINTS

Transversus Thoracis Muscular Plane Block	The Essentials
Anatomy	One or two veins usually flank either side of the IMA.
	The TTM is about 1 to 2 mm in thickness.
	ICN branches travel adjacent to the mammary vessels.
Image orientation	The pectoralis major and internal intercostal muscle insert on the lateral edge of the sternum.
Positioning	Supine.
Operator	Standing on the side of the table.
Display	Across the table.
Transducer	High-frequency linear, 25–50 mm footprint
Initial depth setting	30 mm
Needle	21–25 gauge, 38–50 mm in length
Anatomic location	Begin by scanning the parasternal region in transverse view.
	Adjust the image to identify an intercostal interspace and the internal mammary vessels.
Approach	Transverse view, in-plane from lateral to medial.
	Place the needle tip between the internal intercostal and transversus thoracis muscles.
Sonographic assessment	Displacement of the pleura can be seen with injection.
	Injections can track in a cephalo-caudal fashion between intercostal interspaces (SAX slide or LAX view).
Anatomic variation	Some anatomic variation of the IMA and IMV position.
	Accessory sternalis muscle (about 6% of normal subjects).
	Pectus excavatum (and other chest wall deformities).
	Long, jointed xiphoid process.

ICN, Intercostal nerve; *IMA*, internal mammary artery; *IMV*, internal mammary vein; *LAX*, long axis; *SAX*, short axis; *TTM*, transversus thoracic muscle.

> **Clinical Pearls**
> - The transversus thoracis muscle arises from the lower third of the posterior surface of the sternum and xiphoid process. Similar to the innermost intercostal muscle, the transversus thoracis separates the intercostal nerves from the pleura.
> - The internal intercostal muscle has long course (without membranes) and inserts on the lateral aspect of the sternum. The pectoralis major covers the lateral edges of the sternum.
> - The internal mammary vessels and anterior intercostal nerves lie within the plane between the internal intercostal and transversus thoracis muscles.
> - The internal mammary blood vessels run approximately 1 cm lateral to the lateral border of the sternum, and the anterior branches of the intercostal nerves travel over the internal mammary artery.
> - Between the second and third ribs, the pleura may be visualized rather than the transversus thoracis muscle. The lower portions of the internal thoracic vessels are covered posteriorly by the transversus thoracis muscle.

References

1. Im JG, Webb WR, Rosen A, Gamsu G. Costal pleura: appearances at high-resolution CT. *Radiology.* 1989;171(1):125–131.
2. Baudoin YP, Hoch M, Protin XM, Otton BJ, Ginon B, Voiglio EJ. The superior epigastric artery does not pass through Larrey's space (trigonum sternocostale). *Surg Radiol Anat.* 2003;25(3–4):259–262.
3. Tuinder S, Dikmans R, Schipper RJ, et al. Anatomical evaluation of the internal mammary vessels based on magnetic resonance imaging (MRI). *J Plast Reconstr Aesthet Surg.* 2012;65(10):1363–1367.
4. Scatarige JC, Hamper UM, Sheth S, Allen HA 3rd. Parasternal sonography of the internal mammary vessels: technique, normal anatomy, and lymphadenopathy. *Radiology.* 1989;172(2):453–457.
5. Kuzo RS, Ben-Ami TE, Yousefzadeh DK, Ramirez JG. Internal mammary compartment: window to the mediastinum. *Radiology.* 1995;195(1):187–192.
6. Ueshima H, Hara E, Marui T, Otake H. The ultrasound-guided transversus thoracic muscle plane block is effective for the median sternotomy. *J Clin Anesth.* 2016;29:83.
7. Murata H, Hida K, Hara T. Transverse thoracic muscle plane block: tricks and tips to accomplish the block. *Reg Anesth Pain Med.* 2016;41(3):411–412.
8. Sanders RC, Knight RW. Radiological appearances of the xiphoid process presenting as an upper abdominal mass. *Radiology.* 1981;141(2):489–490.

TRANSVERSUS THORACIS MUSCULAR PLANE BLOCK 247

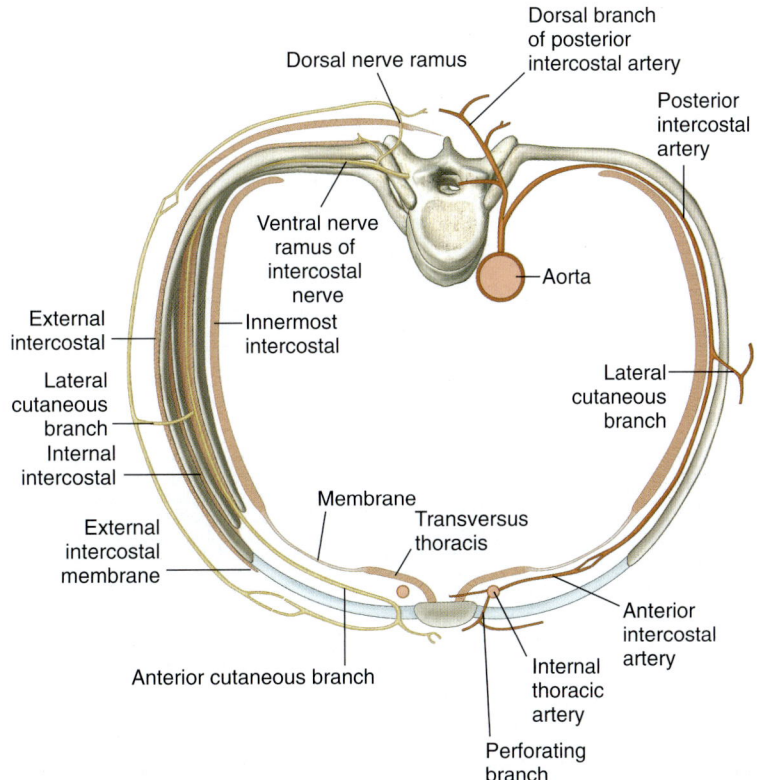

FIGURE 56.1 Drawing to show the course of the nerve and adjacent anatomy in the region of interest. Contents of an intercostal space.

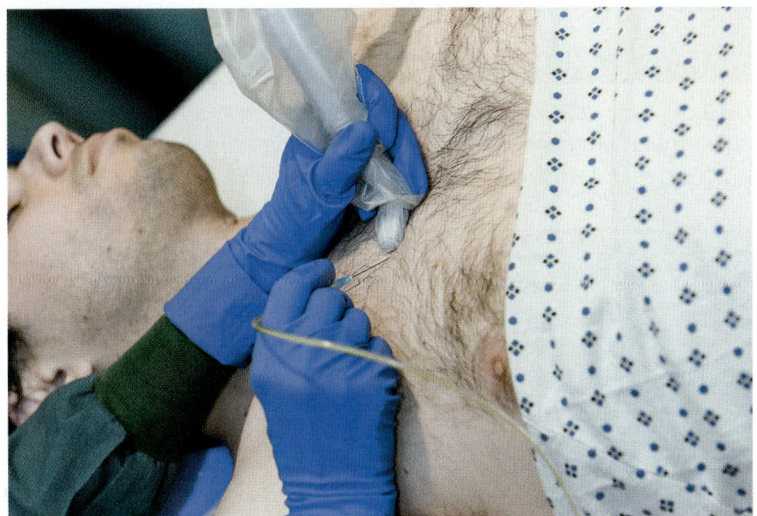

FIGURE 56.2 External photograph showing lateral to medial in-plane approach to transversus thoracis muscular plane block in the parasternal region.

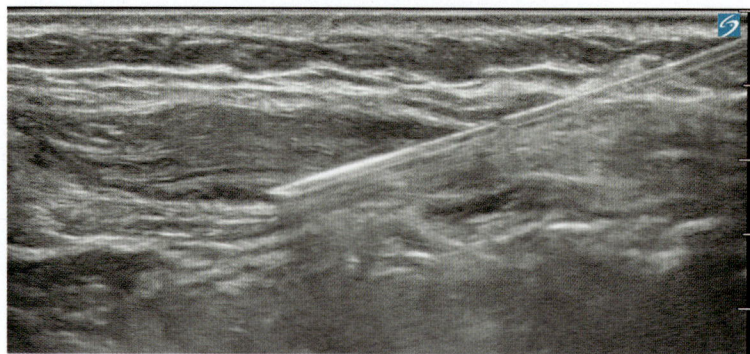

FIGURE 56.3 Sonogram showing in-plane approach transversus thoracis muscular plane block.

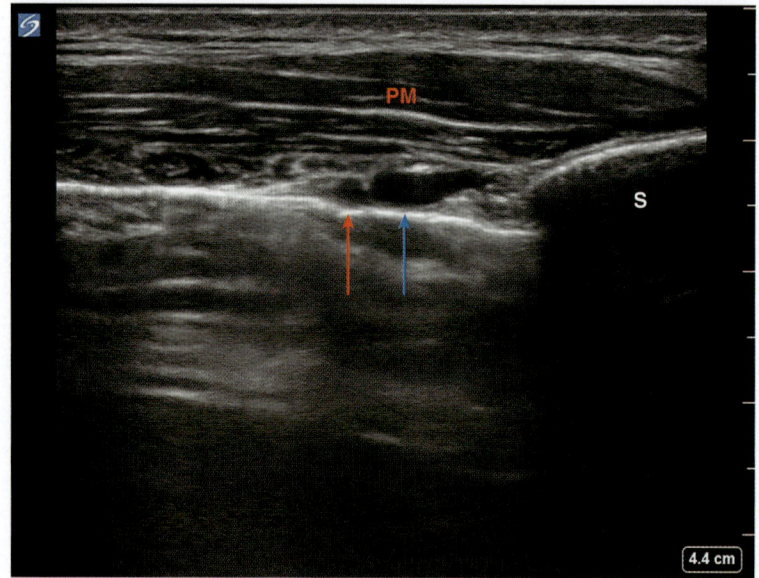

FIGURE 56.4 Short axis *(transverse)* view of the internal mammary artery *(red arrow)* and internal mammary vein *(blue arrow)* in the third intercostal interspace adjacent to the sternum (S) and pectoralis major (PM) muscle.

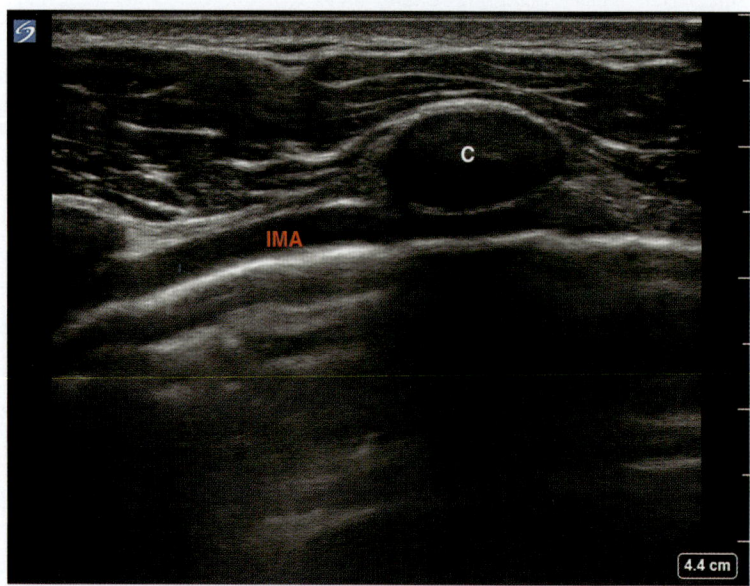

FIGURE 56.5 Long-axis (parasagittal) view of the internal mammary artery (IMA) as it travels under the costal cartilage (C).

Rectus Sheath Block

CHAPTER 57

See Video 57.1 on ExpertConsult.com.

The rectus abdominis is a vertical muscle of the anterior abdominal wall. The muscle is divided into compartments by the midline linea alba, paramedian linea semilunaris, and transverse fibrous bands.[1] Muscles of the lateral abdominal wall (the external oblique, internal oblique, and transversus abdominis) become aponeurotic as they approach the midline, and the rectus sheath consists of the rectus abdominis muscles surrounded by these aponeuroses.

Above the arcuate line, the transversalis fascia and the aponeuroses separate the rectus abdominis muscle from the abdominal cavity. Caudal to the arcuate line, the rectus abdominis muscle is in direct contact with the transversalis fascia. In this location, all three of the lateral abdominal wall muscles (external oblique, internal oblique, and transversus) have their aponeuroses pass anterior to the rectus abdominis muscle.[2]

Anterior cutaneous branches of the intercostal nerves enter the rectus sheath from the posterior and lateral sides.[3] Epigastric arteries and veins are sometimes identified within the rectus sheath, and the epigastric arteries are usually accompanied by two flanking veins. The anterior intercostal nerves can run alongside these vessels before rising to the surface through the rectus abdominis muscle. The nerves of the rectus sheath are too small to be directly imaged with ultrasound. A few emerging nerve fibers can bypass the rectus sheath as they travel toward the midline.

Rectus sheath block is useful as part of a combined anesthetic technique for outpatients.[4,5] The usual indication for this block is to provide pain relief after repair of umbilical or incisional hernias. It provides an excellent alternative to straight general anesthesia or epidural blocks for surgical procedures around the midline of the abdominal wall.

SUGGESTED TECHNIQUE

The rectus sheath block is usually performed after induction of general anesthesia for patient comfort and to reduce movement. The choice of ultrasound transducer is not critical to the success of the procedure. With the patient in the supine position, an in-plane approach from the lateral side of the patient is used, with the rectus abdominis muscle imaged in short-axis view (transverse); hand-on-needle provides excellent needle control. Tidal movement of the abdominal cavity with respiration or contraction of the abdominal wall muscles can make the procedure challenging.

Rectus sheath block is a plane block that does not rely on direct nerve imaging. The goal is to have the injected local anesthetic layer underneath the rectus abdominis muscle where the anterior intercostal nerves enter the rectus sheath. The transversalis fascia and aponeurosis of the transversus muscle form a double-layer appearance on ultrasound scans (the peritoneal stripe).[6] Therefore, the needle tip and injection should be placed between the rectus abdominis muscle and the double layer that constitutes the posterior aspect of the rectus sheath. To accomplish this view, the cephalocaudad placement of the transducer should be adjusted away from tendons to allow visualization of the double layer of the transversalis fascia.

Because the nerves enter the sheath from the lateral side, the lateral aspect of the rectus abdominis muscle is targeted. The lateral edge of the rectus sheath is a potentially safer approach because it is over the abdominal wall muscles rather than the abdominal cavity. Injection of a small volume of local anesthetic on pullback of the needle through the rectus abdominis muscle gives more complete distributions.

Because of the compartmental nature of the rectus abdominis muscle, two or four injections are usually performed for periumbilical surgery (right and left sides, and sometimes above and below the umbilicus). About 5 to 10 mL of local anesthetic is injected per side per compartment in adult patients. Because the tendinous inscriptions of the muscles are not complete posteriorly,[7,8] some communication between compartments is possible. If local anesthetic is observed to distribute between compartments, no further injection is necessary. The duration of rectus sheath blocks may not be as long as for transversus abdominis plane (TAP) blocks.[9]

The superior and inferior epigastric arteries anastomose through a vascular network. It is unlikely that large epigastric arteries will be found in the umbilical region because the contributing vessels course from above or below. Because of the lack of underlying bone, visible arterial pulsations are difficult to elicit with probe compression during rectus sheath blocks. Power Doppler can be useful during these procedures to confirm vascular identity.

In one study, 21% of rectus sheath injections guided by traditional loss-of-resistance techniques were intraperitoneal.[10] These intraperitoneal injections were detected by ultrasound imaging after initial needle placement. Although no complications were observed in this study, intraperitoneal injections are not clinically effective and presumably place patients at risk for injury.

KEY POINTS	
Rectus Sheath Block	**The Essentials**
Anatomy	The nerves of the rectus sheath enter the posterolateral side of the RA.
	The TA lies under the lateral aspect of the RA in the supraumbilical region.
	Epigastric arteries and veins usually lie deep within the midportion of the RA.
	Tendinous intersections divide adjacent rectus sheath compartments.
	These tendons are thought to be incomplete posteriorly.
	This should allow communication between adjacent compartments.
Positioning	Supine
Operator	Standing on the side of the patient
Display	Across the table
Transducer	High-frequency linear, 38- to 50-mm footprint
Initial depth setting	35–50 mm
Needle	20–21 gauge, 70–90 mm in length
Anatomic location	Begin by scanning the RA in transverse view.
	Slide transducer to midway between the tendinous intersections.
Approach	Transverse view of RA, in-plane from lateral to medial.
	Aim for the posterolateral corner of the RA.
	Place the needle tip between the RA and underlying fascial double layer.
	If necessary, scratch the needle tip against the fascial double layer.
	Bilateral injections are necessary for midline anesthesia.
Sonographic assessment	Desire side-to-side (medial-lateral) distribution over the double layer.
	"Swimming pool" or "smile" shaped appearance of distribution between RA and double layer.
	Desire cephalocaudad distribution between adjacent compartments.
	The "handlebar mustache" appearance of the longitudinal distribution between compartments.
Anatomic variation	Position of epigastric arteries and TA varies.

RA, Rectus abdominis muscle; *TA*, transversus abdominis muscle.

Clinical Pearls

- The extent to which the abdominal wall muscles underlie the lateral corner of the rectus abdominis muscle is variable. In some cases, there is no underlying muscle to separate the rectus from the abdominal cavity.
- The needle tip should be scratched against the double layer without actually puncturing it so as to place the tip between the rectus muscle and the double layer.
- A few milliliters of local anesthetic can be injected as the needle is removed to cover the path of nerves through the rectus muscle.
- The best way to perform rectus sheath blocks is to inject forward on one side and back for the contralateral side. In this fashion, the ultrasound display screen and operator remain in one position for bilateral injections.
- The fibers of the rectus abdominis course in a parallel direction with the muscle divided by transverse tendinous intersections.
- The nerves of the rectus sheath are too small (100 μm diameter) to be directly imaged with ultrasound.[3] Therefore, ultrasound-guided rectus sheath block relies on injecting between the rectus abdominis muscle and the underlying double layer of fascia at the point where the nerves are known to enter the rectus sheath.
- The rectus abdominis muscle is slightly narrower near its ends at the xiphoid process and pubic bone. The rectus sheath narrows at its cephalad and caudad ends as the linea semilunaris tapers toward the midline.
- Local anesthetic should be injected at the lateral edge of the rectus sheath for safe and effective rectus sheath blocks.[11]

References

1. Ali QM. Sonographic anatomy of the rectus sheath: an indication for new terminology and implications for rectus flaps. *Surg Radiol Anat*. 1993;15:349–353.
2. Monkhouse WS, Khalique A. Variations in the composition of the human rectus sheath: a study of the anterior abdominal wall. *J Anat*. 1986;145:61–66.
3. Rozen WM, Tran TM, Ashton MW, Barrington MJ, Ivanusic JJ, Taylor GI. Refining the course of the thoracolumbar nerves: a new understanding of the innervation of the anterior abdominal wall. *Clin Anat*. 2008;21:325–333.
4. Willschke H, Bösenberg A, Marhofer P, et al. Ultrasonography-guided rectus sheath block in paediatric anaesthesia: a new approach to an old technique. *Br J Anaesth*. 2006;97:244–249.
5. Sandeman DJ, Dilley AV. Ultrasound-guided rectus sheath block and catheter placement. *ANZ J Surg*. 2008;78:621–623.
6. Muradali D, Wilson S, Burns PN, Shapiro H, Hope-Simpson D. A specific sign of pneumoperitoneum on sonography: enhancement of the peritoneal stripe. *AJR Am J Roentgenol*. 1999;173(5):1257–1262.
7. Connell D, Ali K, Javid M, et al. Sonography and MRI of rectus abdominis muscle strain in elite tennis players. *AJR Am J Roentgenol*. 2006;187:1457–1461.
8. de Jose Maria B, Götzens V, Mabrok M. Ultrasound-guided umbilical nerve block in children: a brief description of a new approach. *Paediatr Anaesth*. 2007;17(1):44–50.
9. Murouchi T, Iwasaki S, Yamakage M. Chronological changes in ropivacaine concentration and analgesic effects between transversus abdominis plane block and rectus sheath block. *Reg Anesth Pain Med*. 2015;40(5):568–571.
10. Dolan J, Lucie P, Geary T, et al. The rectus sheath block: accuracy of local anesthetic placement by trainee anesthesiologists using loss of resistance or ultrasound guidance. *Reg Anesth Pain Med*. 2009;34:247–250.
11. Seidel R, Wree A, Schulze M. Does the approach influence the success rate for ultrasound-guided rectus sheath blocks? An anatomical case series. *Local Reg Anesth*. 2017;10:61–65.

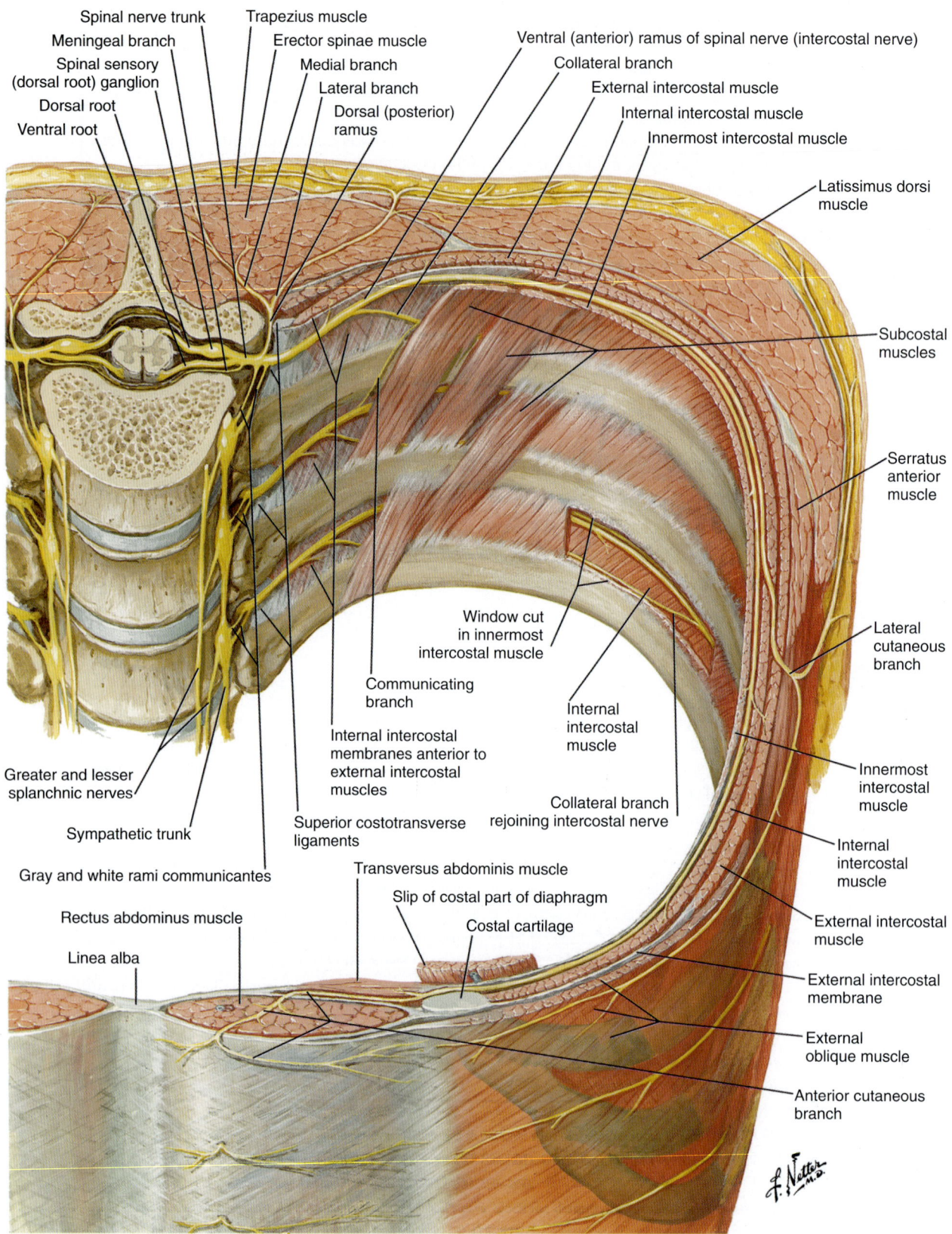

FIGURE 57.1 Thoracoabdominal nerves. Note the path of the anterior cutaneous branch of the intercostal nerve through the rectus abdominis muscle. (From netterimages.com, with permission.)

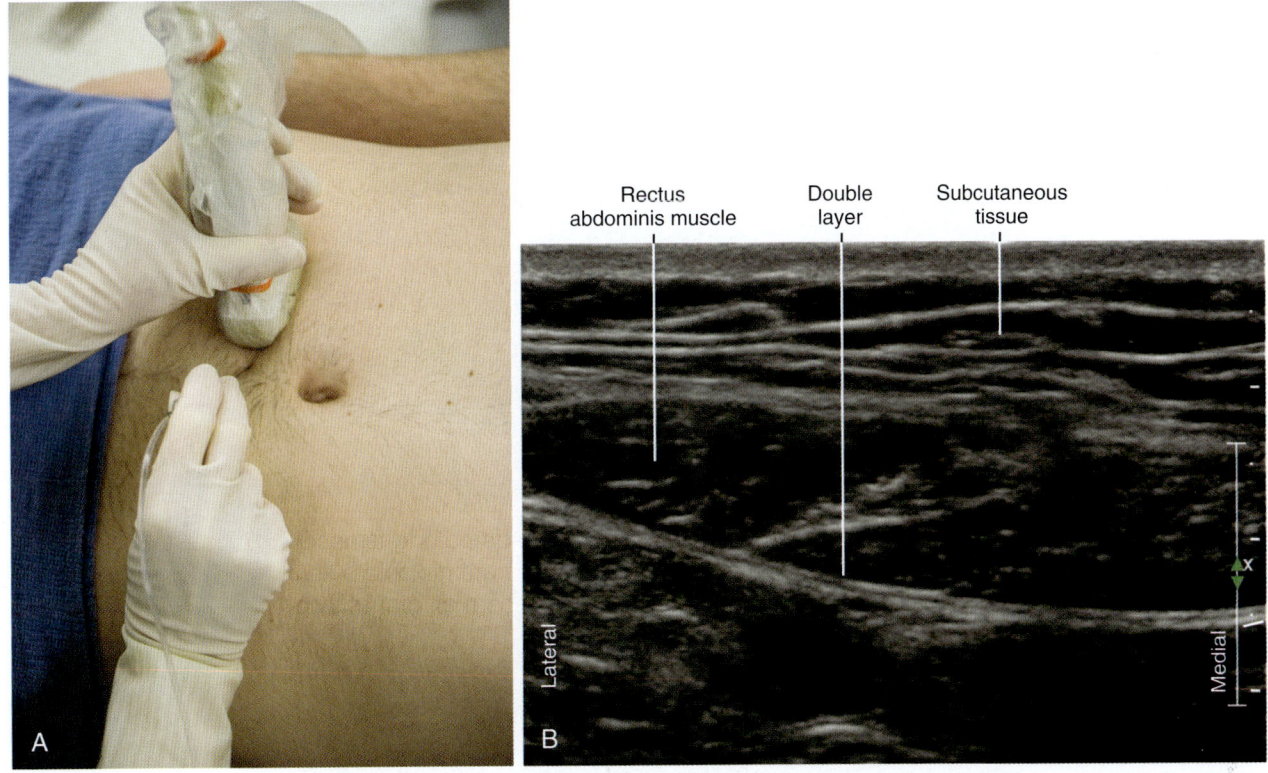

FIGURE 57.2 External photograph showing the approach to rectus sheath block in supine position. An in-plane approach from across the midline is shown (A). The corresponding sonogram in shown (B). The best way to perform rectus sheath blocks on both sides of the midline is to inject forward on one side compartment and back for the opposite side, with the screen and operator in one position.

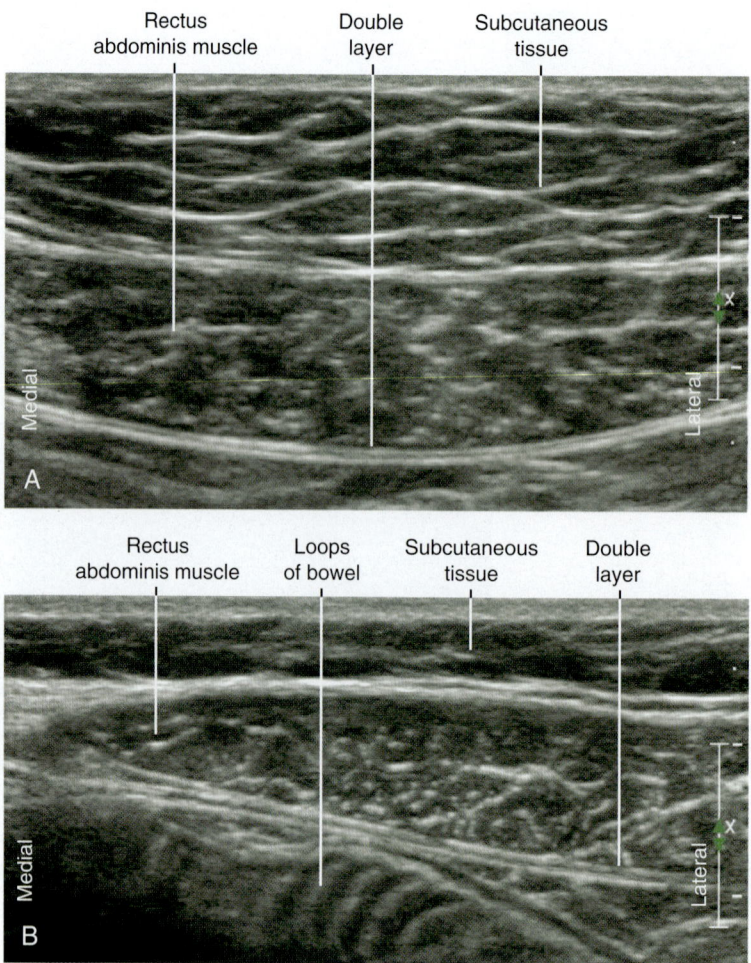

FIGURE 57.3 The double-layer sign indicates the presence of the aponeurosis of the transversus abdominis and transversalis fascia in transverse view (A). Closer to the midline, loops of bowel are visualized (B).

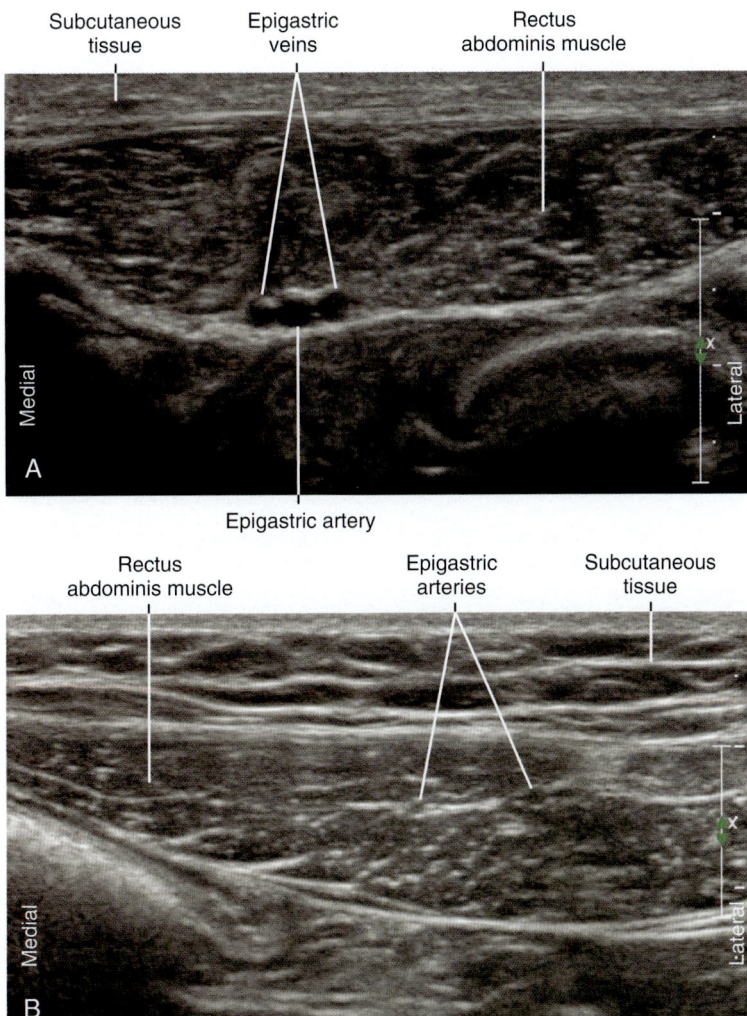

FIGURE 57.4 The epigastric arteries have variable position within the rectus sheath. In these examples from different patients, the arteries are seen either below (A) or within (B) the rectus sheath in transverse view.

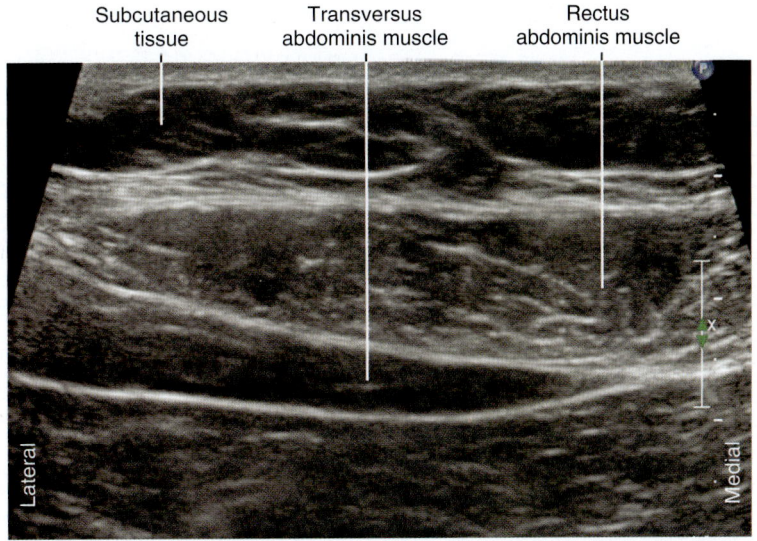

FIGURE 57.5 The transversus muscle on the lateral edge of the rectus abdominis in transverse view. The extent to which the abdominal wall muscles underlie the lateral corner of the rectus abdominis muscle is variable. In some cases, there is no underlying muscle to separate the rectus from the abdominal cavity.

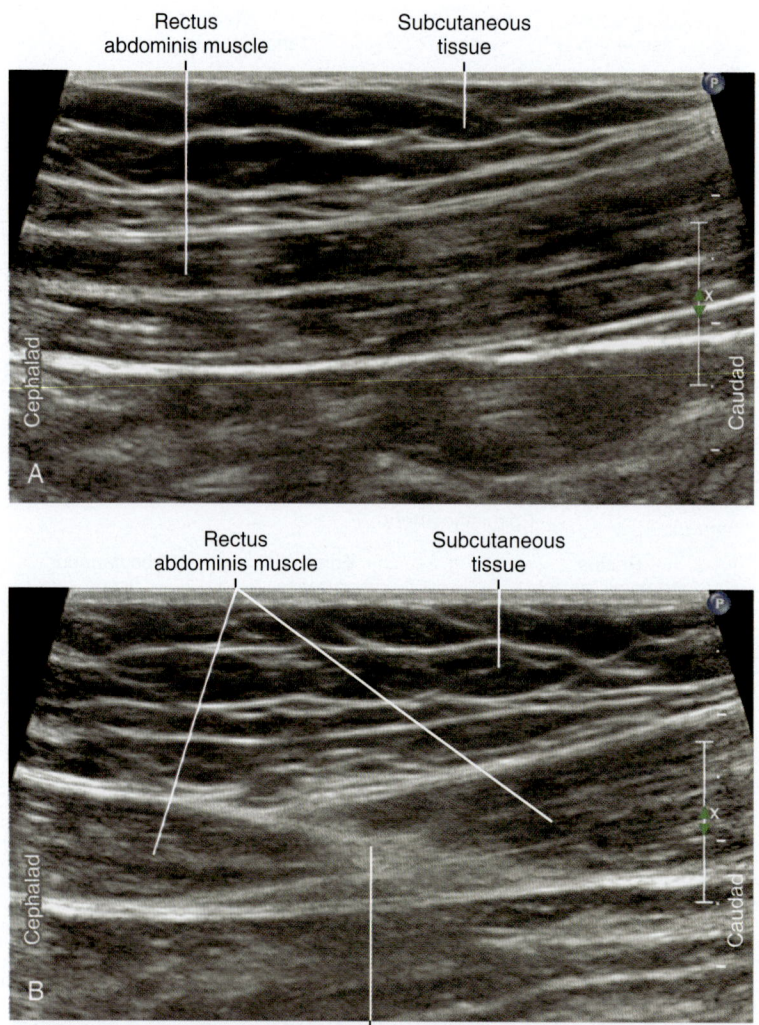

FIGURE 57.6 Longitudinal views of the rectus abdominis muscle within a single muscular compartment (A) and in separate rectus compartments (B). The fibers of the rectus abdominis course in a parallel direction, with the muscle divided by transverse tendinous intersections that are typically incomplete posteriorly.

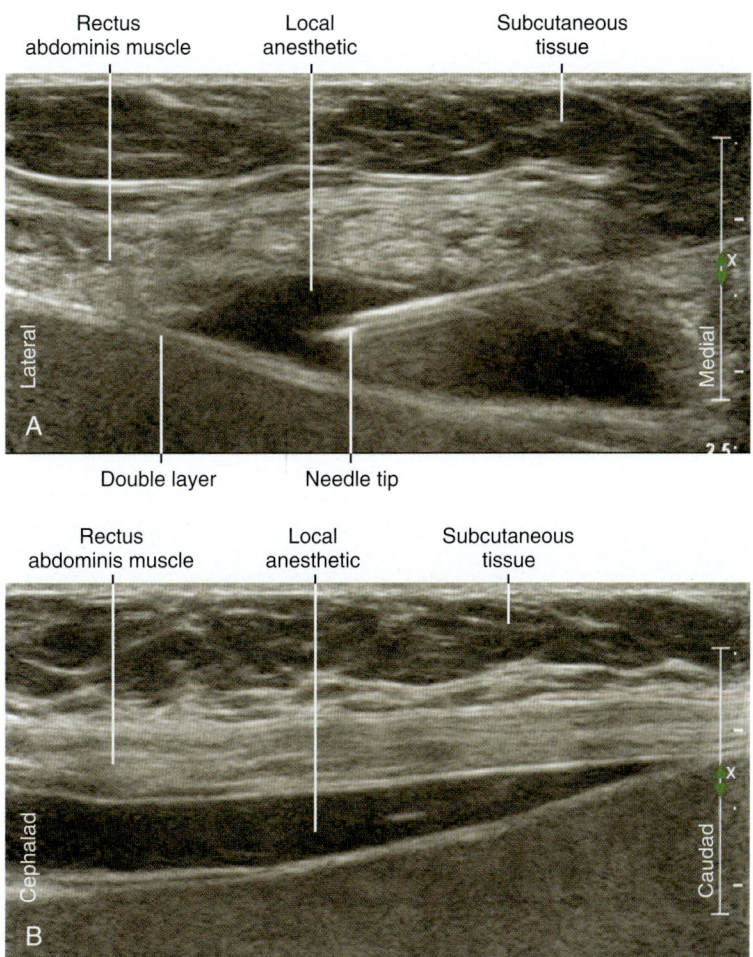

FIGURE 57.7 Image sequence showing rectus sheath block. An in-plane approach is demonstrated where the needle tip is placed between the rectus muscle and the double layer (A). Before injection, the needle tip is gently scratched against the double layer so as to place the tip between the rectus muscle and the double layer. Local anesthetic is seen to layer underneath the muscle, giving a swimming pool appearance of successful rectus sheath injection in transverse view. A few milliliters of local anesthetic can be injected as the needle is removed to cover the path of nerves through the rectus muscle. The corresponding longitudinal view is shown (B).

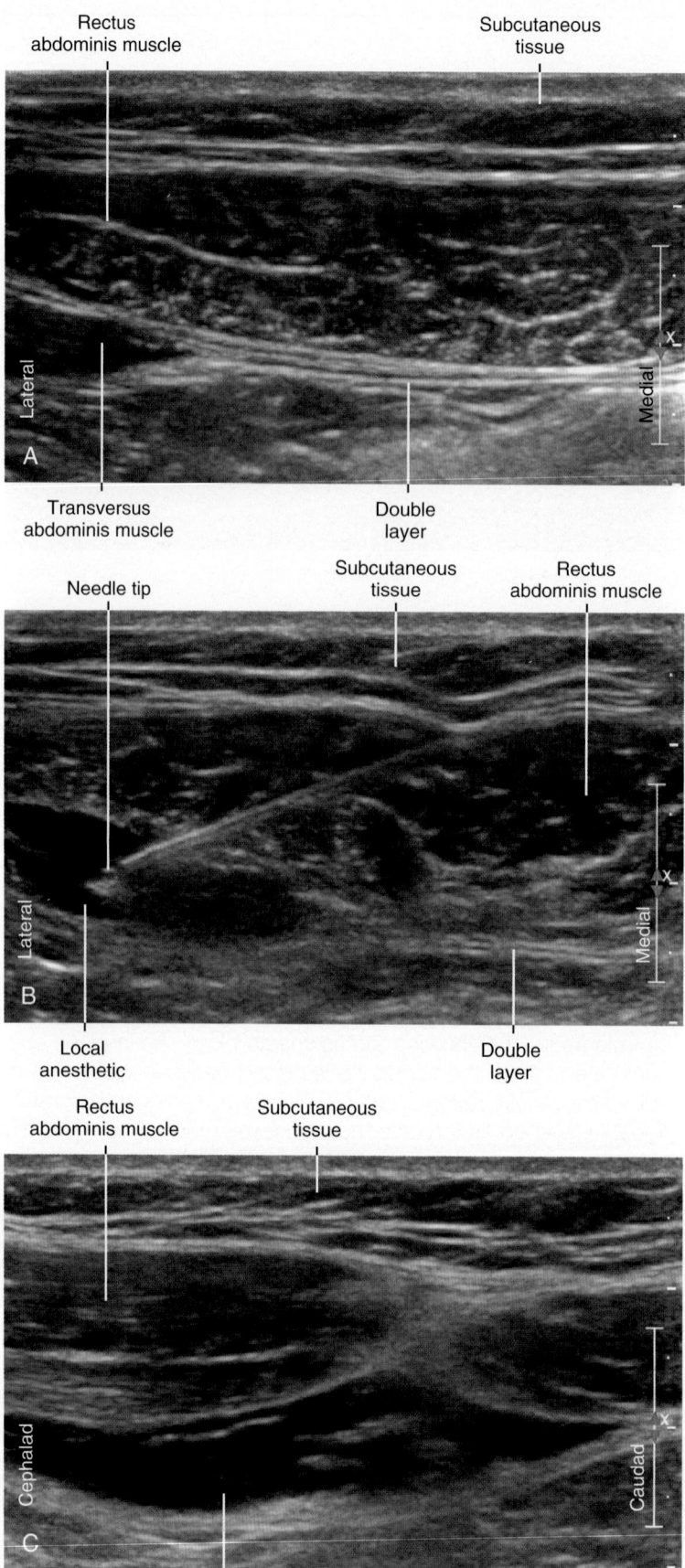

FIGURE 57.8 Image sequence showing rectus sheath block. Before needle tip placement, the double layer is identified (A). An in-plane approach is demonstrated where the needle tip and local anesthetic are placed between the rectus muscle and the double layer (B). After rectus sheath injection, longitudinal views can be used to assess the distribution (C). The "handlebar mustache" appearance verifies that local anesthetic has distributed to the adjacent compartment of the rectus abdominis muscle.

Ilioinguinal and Iliohypogastric Nerve Blocks

CHAPTER 58

Urs Eichenberger

See Video 57.1 on ExpertConsult.com.

The lower abdominal wall is primarily supplied by the subcostal, iliohypogastric (IH), ilioinguinal (IL), and genitofemoral nerves, the last three of which arise from the lumbar plexus. Blocks of the IL and IH nerves are often performed to provide postoperative pain relief from inguinal hernia repair in adults and children. In children, analgesia after inguinal hernia repair is often provided by either performing a caudal block or non-caudal regional analgesic techniques as IL and IH nerve blocks or wound infiltration in addition to general anesthesia. A recent systematic review and meta-analysis found caudal analgesia to be better but with significantly higher risk of motor block and urinary retention compared to the other techniques.[1] In adults, inguinal hernia repair is often performed under regional anesthesia as neuraxial block, paravertebral block (PVB), or local infiltration techniques alone. The authors of a recent systematic review and meta-analysis found PVB to decrease postoperative pain scores and analgesic requirements compared to transversus abdominis plane (TAP) blocks or inguinal nerve blocks. Furthermore, PVB was shown to have less severe side effects compared to general and neuraxial anesthesia.[2] Nevertheless, they concluded the choice between general anesthesia, neuraxial anesthesia, PVB and peripheral nerve blocks should be based on different factors. Because TAP blocks often fail to provide analgesia in the L1 distribution, IL and IH blocks may be of greater benefit for inguinal surgical procedures.[3]

Chronic postoperative pain after inguinal hernia repair is common, and the mechanisms of the pain generation are often unclear. The benefits of diagnostic blocks of the IL and IH nerves are controversial. One reason is that only very few chronic pain patients after inguinal hernia repair respond to these diagnostic pain blocks.[4] Another reason is that we were not able to selectively block the nerves in the past. We have now developed an ultrasound-guided technique to selectively target the IL and IH nerves in human cadavers.[5] Unfortunately, we could not show selective block of the nerves with this newly developed method in the subsequent volunteer study.[6]

The IH and IL nerves cross the anterior surface of the quadratus lumborum before piercing the transversus abdominis (TA) muscle. The quadratus lumborum (rather than the abdominal cavity) lies under the abdominal wall muscles between the costal margin and the pelvic brim when imaging posterior and lateral. Medially, the transversalis fascia separates the transversus muscle from the peritoneal cavity.

The IL and IH nerves emerge between the muscles of the abdominal wall. The longest-running course of the nerves is between the internal oblique and TAs. The IL nerve runs lateral, close to the iliac bone, and the IH nerve has a parallel course to the IL nerve, running cephalad (superior) and medial. Both nerves pierce the two more superficial muscles layers (internal and external oblique [EO]) more distally (caudal) at different and highly variable locations.[7] Of the three abdominal wall muscles (EO, internal oblique, and transversus), the internal oblique is usually the thickest.[8]

The deep (medial) circumflex artery is a recurrent branch of the external iliac artery. The deep circumflex artery pierces the transversus as it ascends the abdominal wall. Branches of the deep circumflex iliac artery (DCIA) often accompany the nerves.[9]

SUGGESTED TECHNIQUE

Nerve and muscle visibility are best about 5 cm cephalad and lateral to the anterior superior iliac spine (ASIS) and the pelvic brim.[5] In the classic location for IL block (2 cm medial and 2 cm superior to the anterior-superior iliac spine), the EO muscle is often aponeurotic; therefore, it is difficult to visualize this layer over the nerves. The first step is to obtain a view of the three abdominal wall muscles (EO, internal oblique, and transversus) at the previously mentioned location to identify the IL and IH nerves between the internal oblique and transversus abdominal muscles. Alternatively, the deep circumflex artery can be followed up from the external iliac artery until it meets one of the nerves. Because the IL nerve lies only a few mm medial to the iliac bone (iliac crest, IC), the lateral end of the transducer should always be in contact with the IC to avoid sliding too far medially and losing the possibility to visualize the IL nerve. About 10 mm more medial to the IL nerve, it is possible to see the IH nerve. About 1 to 2 cm more medial, a third neuronal structure, the subcostal nerve (SCN), is often visible.

Usually, the medial end of the transducer has to be slightly rotated cranial, pressed (especially in obese individuals) in direction of the vertebral column, and the transducer has to be slightly tilted caudal to obtain the best image of the nerves in short-axis (SAX) view. If the medial end of the transducer is not pressed in the direction of the vertebral column, the ultrasound beam cannot reach the IL nerve, because this nerve will be lying in the dorsal shadow of the IC.

One approach is to perform the block standing or sitting on the side to be blocked or across midline (across the table). The block needle usually approaches out-of-plane from caudal to cranial with SAX view of the nerves. An in-plane approach from lateral is often not possible (IC in the needle track), and from medial it is difficult to introduce the needle under the transducer, especially in obese patients (pressing the transducer end in direction vertebral column to visualize the ILN; see previous). The needle tip should be positioned between the internal oblique and transversus muscles. Local anesthetic should layer between these two muscles to block the targeted nerves.

KEY POINTS

Ilioinguinal and Iliohypogastric Nerve Block	The Essentials
Anatomy	The ILN and IHN lie between the IO and TA 5 cm cranial and slightly lateral to the ASIS.
	The ILN lies about 6 mm medial to the IC.
	The IHN lies about 10 mm medial to the ILN.
	The SCN lies about 2 cm medial of the IHN
	The IC has an inverted "U" appearance.
	The iliacus muscle lies under the TA at the IC.
	The DCIA is a recurrent branch of the external iliac artery.
	The ILN or IHN are often accompanied by the DCIA.
	The courses of the ILN and IHN parallel the inside of the pelvic brim.
	ILN and IHN are about 3 × 1.5 mm in diameter.
Image orientation	The ILH, ILH and SCN nerves lie medial to the IC.
Positioning	Supine
Operator	Standing or sitting at the side of the patient (either side)
Display	Across the table
Transducer	High-frequency linear, 38- to 50-mm footprint
Initial depth setting	25–30 mm
Needle	20–21 gauge, 50–70 mm in length

KEY POINTS—CONT'D

Ilioinguinal and Iliohypogastric Nerve Block — **The Essentials**

Anatomic location	Begin by placing the transducer above the IC.
	Look caudally and slightly lateral with the transducer (press the medial edge of the transducer in direction of the vertebral column) to image the ILN close to the IC.
	Rotate the transducer (medial edge slightly cranial) to obtain a SAX view of the nerves.
Approach	SAX view of ILN and IHN, out-of-plane from caudal to cranial. Place the needle tip between ILN and IHN near the base of the IC.
LA spread	The injection should layer between the IO and TA.
Anatomic variation	The ILN and IHN can be fused together (12%).
	The ILN and IHN cannot be visualized at the mentioned location, because they lie within the abdominal muscles (10%).

ASIS, Anterior superior iliac spine; *DCIA*, deep circumflex iliac artery; *EO*, external oblique; *IC*, iliac crest; *IHN*, iliohypogastric nerve; *ILN*, ilioinguinal nerve; *IO*, internal oblique muscle; *LA*, local anesthetic; *SAX*, short axis; *SCN*, subcostal nerve; *TA*, transversus abdominis muscle.

Clinical Pearls

- Ilioinguinal (IL) blocks are useful for pain relief after lower abdominal incisions (e.g., cesarean delivery, abdominal hysterectomy) and inguinal hernia repair.
- The course of the IL nerve (ILN) and deep circumflex iliac artery parallels the inside aspect of the pelvic brim.[9]
- The needle should be aimed at the corner of the neurovascular bundle, where the IL and IH nerves lie adjacent to the deep circumflex iliac artery. Power Doppler helps identify this small artery. In contrast to the artery, the nerves do not change colors with appropriate adjustment of the Doppler gain.
- The injection can be performed where the artery lies between the internal oblique and transversus muscle layers or as proximal as possible.
- The transversus abdominis muscle is thin; therefore, intraperitoneal placement of the needle tip can occur.
- The diameters of the IL and IH nerves are about 3 × 1.5 mm each. The two nerves usually lie about 10 mm apart from each other. The IL nerve lies about 6 mm from the iliac bone.
- One common anatomic variation in this region is fusion of the IL and IH nerves into a common trunk, occurring in about 12% of normal subjects.[8]
- The best imaging of these nerves is about 5 cm cranial and slightly posterior to the anterior-superior iliac spine. In this location, the two nerves consistently lie between the internal oblique and transversus abdominis muscles (90%).[8]
- The transducer should be slightly rotated (medial edge cranial), tilted slightly caudally, and pressed in direction of the vertebral column medially to image perpendicular to the course of the nerves and close enough to the bone that the iliac crest should be within the field of view. If the needle tip is sufficiently lateral, the iliacus or quadratus lumborum muscle, rather than the peritoneum, will lie under the transversus abdominis muscle.
- Because the cutaneous innervation of the inguinal nerves is highly variable, there are no accurate clinical tests of block assessment.

References

1. Shanthanna H, Singh B, Guyatt G. A systematic review and meta-analysis of caudal block as compared to noncaudal regional techniques for inguinal surgeries in children. *Biomed Res Int*. 2014;2014:890626.
2. Law LS, Tan M, Bai Y, Miller TE, Li YJ, Gan TJ. Paravertebral block for inguinal herniorrhaphy: a systematic review and meta-analysis of randomized controlled trials. *Anesth Analg*. 2015;121(2):556–569.
3. Fredrickson MJ, Paine C, Hamill J. Improved analgesia with the ilioinguinal block compared to the transversus abdominis plane block after pediatric inguinal surgery: a prospective randomized trial. *Paediatr Anaesth*. 2010;20:1022–1027.
4. Bischoff JM, Koscielniak-Nielsen ZJ, Kehlet H, Werner MU. Ultrasound-guided ilioinguinal/iliohypogastric nerve blocks for persistent inguinal postherniorrhaphy pain: a randomized, double-blind, placebo-controlled, crossover trial. *Anesth Analg*. 2012;114(6):1323–1329.
5. Eichenberger U, Greher M, Kirchmair L, Curatolo M, Moriggl B. Ultrasound-guided blocks of the ilioinguinal and iliohypogastric nerve: accuracy of a selective new technique confirmed by anatomical dissection. *Br J Anaesth*. 2006;97:238–243.
6. Schmutz M, Schumacher PM, Luyet C, Curatolo M, Eichenberger U. Ilioinguinal and iliohypogastric nerves cannot be selectively blocked by using ultrasound guidance: a volunteer study. *Br J Anaesth*. 2013;111(2):264–270.
7. Jamieson RW, Swigart LL, Anson BJ. Points of parietal perforation of the ilioinguinal and iliohypogastric nerves in relation to optimal sites for local anaesthesia. *Q Bull Northwest Univ Med Sch*. 1952;26:22–26.
8. Rankin G, Stokes M, Newham DJ. Abdominal muscle size and symmetry in normal subjects. *Muscle Nerve*. 2006;34:320–326.
9. Schlenz I, Burggasser G, Kuzbari R, Eichberger H, Gruber H, Holle J. External oblique abdominal muscle: a new look on its blood supply and innervation. *Anat Rec*. 1999;255:388–395.

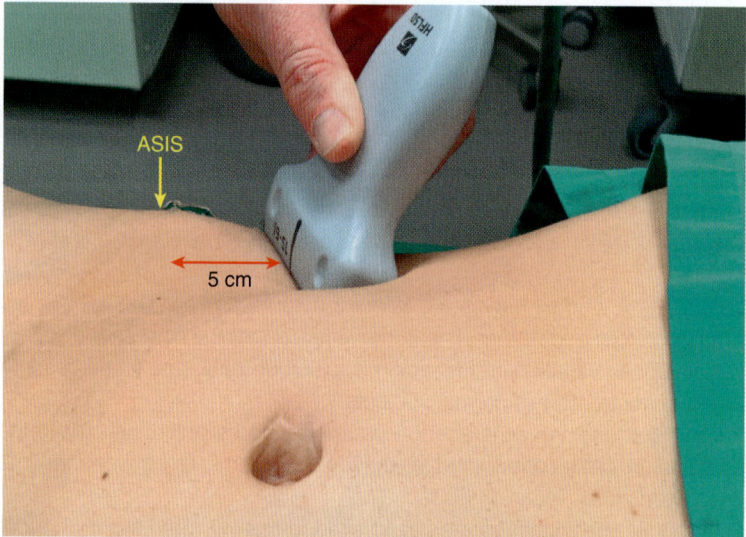

FIGURE 58.1 The transducer position to obtain the best visualization of the ilioinguinal and iliohypogastric nerves is about 5 cm cranial and slightly lateral to the anterior superior iliac spine (ASIS). To best view the nerves in short axis along their course (as shown in Fig. 58.6), the transducer must be tilted slightly caudally.

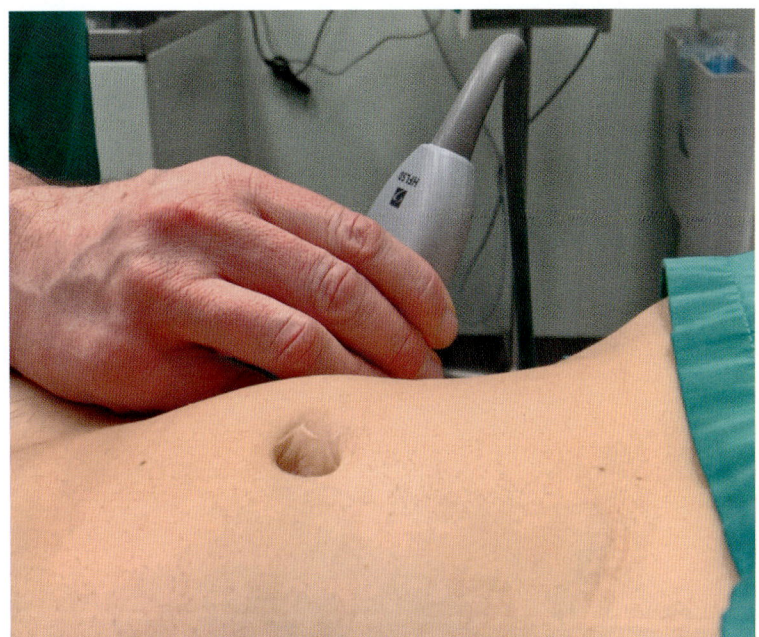

FIGURE 58.2 Transducer position from the opposite side. For right-handed physicians, it is best to pre-scan using the right hand and remain in contact with the patient to stabilize the transducer. This allows very small movements with the transducer (e.g., tilting, longitudinal sliding) to obtain the best possible image of the region. In the former images, the transducer is held differently to better show the transducer position in relation to the inguinal region.

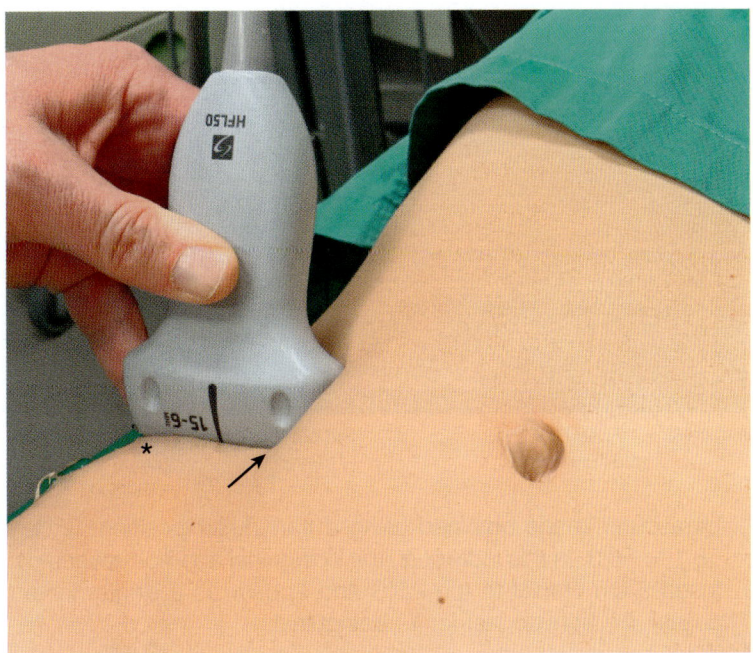

FIGURE 58.3 The lateral edge of the transducer must remain in contact with the iliac crest (*), and the abdominal wall is pressed dorsally with the medial edge *(arrow)* to obtain an image of the ilioinguinal nerve. This nerve runs very close (about 6 mm) to the inner face of the iliac bone and would be missed (in the bony shadow) if the ultrasound beam is directed from lateral to medial.

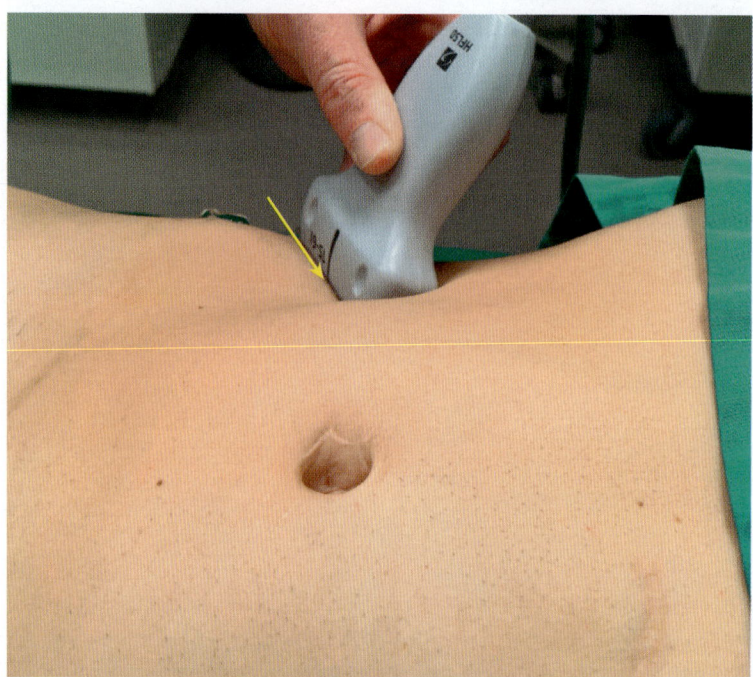

FIGURE 58.4 The best transducer position described in Fig. 58.3 has consequences for the puncture technique. The best puncture technique is an out-of-plane approach from caudal to cranial, as shown by the yellow arrow. In-line approaches from lateral to medial are inhibited by the iliac crest and from medial to lateral by the dorsally pressed transducer edge.

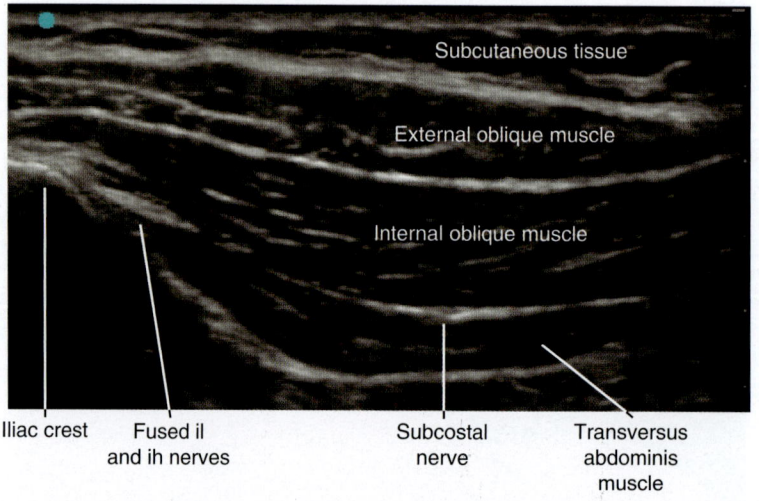

FIGURE 58.5 Ultrasound image obtained using a transducer position as described in Figs. 58.1 to 58.3. In this individual, the ilioinguinal and iliohypogastric nerves are still fused 5 cm cranial to the ASIS and appear as a single nerve (about 10% of cases). *IH*, Iliohypogastric; *IL*, ilioinguinal.

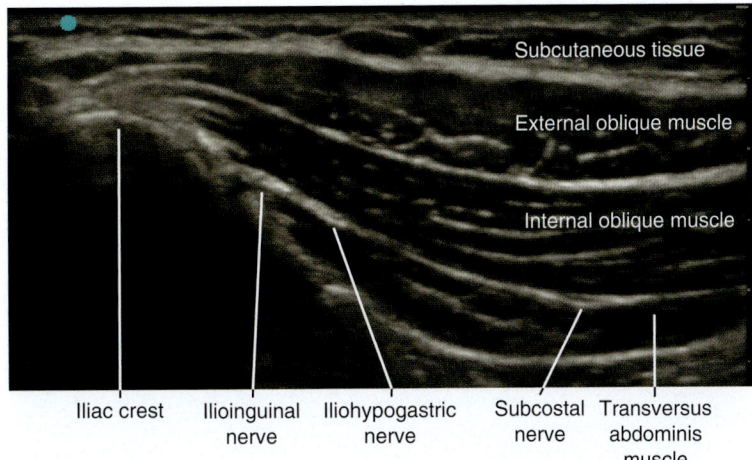

FIGURE 58.6 Transducer position slightly (2 cm) more caudal than in Fig. 5. The ilioinguinal and iliohypogastric nerves are divided. The distance between the two nerves is usually about 1 cm. The subcostal nerve is often mistaken for the IH nerve, especially if the medial edge of the transducer is not pressed against the abdominal wall; therefore, the (IL) nerve is in the shadow of the iliac crest. There is considerable distance between the IH and subcostal nerves.

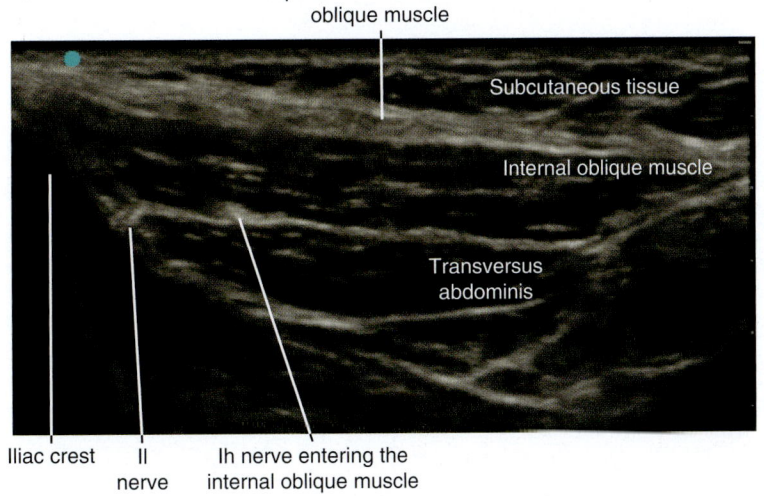

FIGURE 58.7 Transducer position now shown more caudal (3 to 4 cm) than in Fig. 58.6. The external oblique muscle is not visible (only its aponeurosis). The iliohypogastric nerve is entering the internal oblique muscle on its way more distal and superficial. Therefore, at this level, the nerves are often hardly visible by ultrasound imaging. *IH*, Iliohypogastric; *IL*, ilioinguinal.

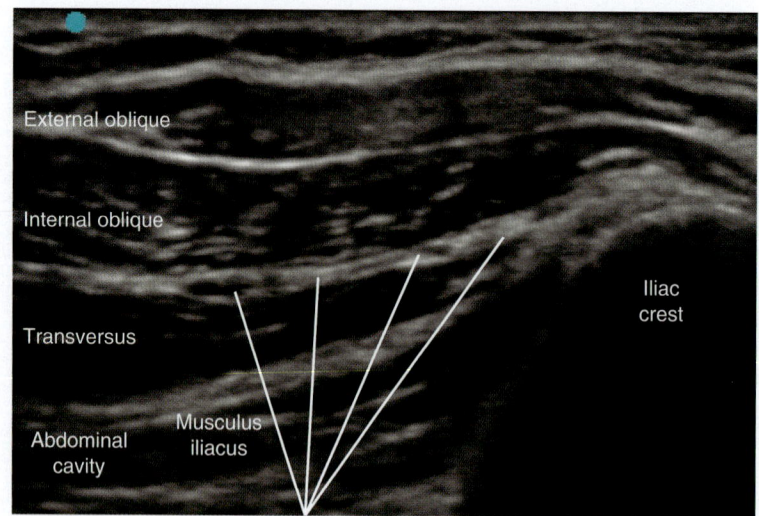

FIGURE 58.8 In some patients, the different nerves and vessels are difficult to demarcate from each other, as in this individual. The widely expanded neurovascular bundle is also seen.

Transversus Abdominis Plane Blocks

CHAPTER 59

Peter Hebbard

See Video 59.1, available on ExpertConsult.com.

ANATOMIC BACKGROUND

The key to using transversus abdominis plane (TAP) blocks for abdominal surgery analgesia is a thorough understanding of the anatomy.

The abdominal wall nerves from T7 to T9 emerge under the costal margin into the TAP and then penetrate the rectus abdominis muscle. Nerves T10 and T11 emerge from the end of the intercostal space, have a longer course within the plane, and then penetrate the rectus sheath and rectus abdominis muscle. The T12 and L1 nerves run from the anterior surface of quadratus lumborum muscle initially deep (inside) the transversus abdominis muscle. T12 penetrates to the TAP in a similar course to T11. However, the L1 nerves (ilioinguinal and iliohypogastric nerves) do not enter the TAP until they are superior to the anterior half of the iliac crest.[1] A continuous line from the xiphoid process to the iliac crest, just posterior to the anterior superior iliac spine (ASIS), is termed the **oblique subcostal line**, and it defines the anatomically optimal site for TAP block.[2]

As minimally invasive surgery has shown, a large part of the pain following abdominal organ surgery is derived from the incision (the area of analgesia covered by the TAP approaches). In a similar fashion to other nerve block techniques such as epidural and paravertebral blocks, it targets specific nerves that innervate the incision. The extent of block can be measured on the skin using sensory testing, and deficits in the block coverage are reflected in the areas of analgesia.

INDICATIONS AND CONTRAINDICATIONS FOR THE PROCEDURE

TAP blocks can be used for any surgery with pain derived from the abdominal wall. Very few complications have been reported after extensive worldwide experience. However, precautions should be taken regarding bleeding, infection, needle trauma to the abdominal structures, and local anesthetic toxicity. The only contraindications to TAP block are severe coagulopathy or the inability to adequately image and identify the target.

Clinical Pearls

- The oblique subcostal line is the neural plane along its entire length.
- Injections too far posterior will tend to miss L1 nerves.
- Transversus abdominis plane blocks do not block visceral or retro-peritoneal pain.

SUGGESTED TECHNIQUE

SUBCOSTAL TRANSVERSUS ABDOMINIS PLANE BLOCK

The optimal position for nerve block in the upper abdominal wall is close to the costal margin. This minimizes anatomical variation in penetration of the nerves into the rectus abdominis muscle. The nerves can penetrate the rectus abdominis relatively close to the costal margin, and an injection too far from the costal margin will not block them. The transversus abdominis muscle is always present deep to the rectus abdominis in this region. However, the muscle belly usually only extends a short distance from the costal margin. The target in this region is through the rectus sheath and superficial to transversus abdominis, as this is where the nerves emerge. As the nerves also penetrate the rectus sheath, a block above the sheath is also acceptable. This may be the only option if transversus abdominis is very small or deficient. Spread of local anesthetic can be achieved by volume or repositioning the needle. In this location, the layers split apart freely and a wide-spreading lens-shaped distribution of fluid is easy to make, either deep or superficial to the rectus sheath. Needle repositioning is done passing the needle tip along oblique subcostal line. This has the advantage of minimizing the volume of local anesthetic, and using minimal pressure with the ultrasound probe is essential. The needle can also be curved (bent) before insertion, which helps direct the tip parallel to the skin surface.

The superior epigastric arteries are sometimes imaged where they emerge into the TAP near the midline. These large arteries should be avoided. It has been suggested that the TAP has two compartments divided by the linea semilunaris at the edge of the rectus muscle. This is based on a lack of spread across the linea semilunaris in a contrast study.[3] The compartment superficial to the rectus sheath is distinct, and if the initial injection is made there, it will be contained at the edge of the rectus. However, free flow of fluid across the linea semilunaris is typical if the needle is immediately on the transversus abdominis muscle. Intermediate compartments also existing as an injection can be made with an obvious fascia layer observed between the fluid and both transversus and rectus abdominis. Regardless of the presence of compartments, a 20-mL injection of local anesthetic will only block less than half of the unilateral abdominal wall, and multiple needle positions are needed to make an extensive block.

The subcostal TAP zone continues lateral to the rectus abdominis muscle. This is called the lower subcostal zone, and injections around the end of the tenth rib produce block in the umbilical region. There is often a widening of the linea semilunaris in this area with fascia overlying the transversus abdominis muscle. The injection can still be placed immediately superficial to the transversus abdominis muscle.

Clinical Pearls

- Extend the block over the nerve supply to the incision.
- Keep close to the costal margin, superficial to the transversus muscle.
- Bend the needle into a curve before insertion.

ILIOINGUINAL TRANSVERSUS ABDOMINIS PLANE BLOCK

The oblique subcostal line continues across the anterolateral abdominal wall to reach the iliac crest in its anterior third. This is the position where the L1 nerves are lying within the TAP, very close to the iliac crest. The terminal branch of the deep circumflex iliac artery ascends in the abdominal wall near this location and is easily seen on imaging, often being mistaken for a nerve. To improve the chances of blocking the L1 nerves, the injectate should be placed so that it goes right next to the iliac crest. If needed, the needle should be redirected, as the nerves are usually within 1 to 2 cm of the bone. For cesarean section and inguinal hernia repairs, the injection should be placed just lateral to the ASIS imaged with the superior end of the probe pointing at about 45 degrees to the sagittal plane, toward the umbilicus. The transversus abdominis muscle in this view is imaged only in part deep to internal oblique, with the appearance of a crescent moon.

The curvilinear probe often produces better imaging of the fascia in this location due to the angle of the beam as well as a wide field of view and should be considered for all patients above a normal body mass index.

CONTINUOUS CATHETER TRANSVERSUS ABDOMINIS PLANE BLOCKS

Continuous nerve blocks can be performed within the TAP, and the oblique subcostal line is suitable for a catheter that can be passed along the TAP to allow local anesthetic to move along the line of the catheter. There is little evidence regarding the optimal technique, and multi-hole "soaker" catheters and end-hole catheters can be used. My preferred technique is to use a 15 to

20 cm Touhy needle and catheter set, and the longer needle is used for extensive incisions. The needle tip is passed into the TAP and then redirected along the oblique subcostal line, staying within the plane. This usually means entry through the rectus abdominis muscle. The entry and ending points of the block are determined by the location of the incision and surgery. Block of both sides can be performed by standing on one side of the patient. Standing on the patient's left, the blocks are conveniently done from superior to inferior while holding the needle in the right hand (Video 59.1). For blocks from inferior to superior, which may be needed to block right up to the xiphoid process, the operator can stand on the patient's right.

Using two catheters, it is important to observe overall safe dose limits of local anesthetic using postoperative continuous TAP catheters. My preferred regimen is to use up to 150 mg ropivacaine 0.25% to establish the blocks while hydro-dissecting via the needles. Bilateral injections of 20 mL ropivacaine 0.2% are made every 4 hours via a closed system and a pump (20 mg ropivacaine per hour). This can be increased to every 3 hours if needed.

PHARMACOKINETICS

A number of studies have measured the absorption of local anesthetic from the TAP following bolus injections. Plasma levels peak at 20 to 30 minutes, putting the absorption rate into the intermediate speed category, which is slower than paravertebral, intercostal, or interscalene areas and similar to axillary brachial plexus. In some instances, faster absorption has been documented, possibly from a greater proportion of intramuscular rather than interfascial deposition.

DISCUSSION AND COMMENTS

LATERAL TRANSVERSUS ABDOMINIS PLANE BLOCK

The original description of ultrasound-guided targeting of the TAP was of a position between the lowermost ribs and the iliac crest in the mid-axillary line. This corresponded to the suggested target area for the landmark-guided TAP block[4] that was being developed at the same time. The early literature on landmark-based TAP blocks suggested a lateral positioning of the injection with injection just above the iliac crest. Although this lateral approach has been shown to provide analgesia for lower abdominal surgery and is very simple to perform in many patients, we identified early in our experience that poor analgesia above the umbilicus was common, as was variable block of the inguinal region. Spread of fluid was measured in cadaveric dye studies and clinically showed that a single injection of 20 mL would only spread to 3 or 4 dermatomal levels. An interesting recent addition to our understanding of the block in this area has come from Stoving et al,[5] who carefully mapped the cutaneous block extent after lateral TAP block in volunteers. They demonstrated reliable block of the lateral cutaneous branches of T11 to L1. However, the block in the midline was limited with sparing of the L1 nerves. There was also a consistent limitation of the block in the mid-clavicular line that may represent an area of increased nerve anastomosis around the deep circumflex iliac artery.

The anatomical explanation of the L1 sparing is that these nerves are often deep to transversus abdominis muscle in the location of the block (often, the ilioinguinal nerve is positioned in the iliac fossa on the iliacus muscle). The lateral TAP block has no advantages over more anterior approaches. Unfortunately, it is the simplest and most studied TAP block technique. The variability in blocking the L1 nerves probably accounts for equivocal results in some studies, such as the surprising finding that while lateral TAP blocks are beneficial after cesarean section under spinal anesthesia[6] but confer no added benefit if intrathecal morphine is used.[7] Likewise, a study of single-injection lateral TAP block found no benefit at 2 or 24 hours after gynecological cancer surgery where most incisions were at or above the umbilicus.[8]

There have been few studies examining the effectiveness of extensive TAP blocks compared to other approaches. The Dual TAP as described by Borglum et al[3] is a combination of the upper subcostal TAP and the lateral TAP injections without manipulation of the needle. This approach has the advantage of simplicity, as passing the needle along the TAP takes extra time. Using 15 mL per injection, they showed a more extensive spread above T10 in volunteers than a single 30 mL lateral TAP injection. The subcostal oblique TAP block with catheters was compared to epidural analgesia for major upper abdominal surgery by Niraj et al,[9] with results favoring neither technique on pain scores and higher tramadol consumption in the TAP group. More recently, single-shot subcostal oblique TAP blocks were compared with subcostal oblique catheters by Yoshida[10] after midline laparotomy for gynecological malignancy. Morphine usage was reduced, particularly after 12 hours, as would be anticipated by the continued effect of local anesthetic in the infusion group. Upper subcostal TAP block with plain bupivacaine was compared to liposomal bupivacaine after donor nephrectomy by Hutchins et al[11] for a supra-umbilical midline incision. After comparable results in the first 24 hours, the liposomal bupivacaine group had better pain scores and lower opioid consumption than the plain bupivacaine group over the second 24 hours, which is consistent with the prolonged action of the liposomal bupivacaine in an effective location. As motor block is not a clinical problem in the abdominal wall, it may be a very useful site for ultra-long acting local anesthetics. Sometimes, the extent of motor block is visible as a distinct bulge in the abdominal wall muscles.

TRANSVERSUS ABDOMINIS PLANE BLOCK IN LAPAROSCOPIC SURGERY

Many studies have compared TAP block to a control without local anesthetic infiltration in the port sites, which is the logical alternative to a block technique. In this setting it may be effective, although it is not clear whether there is any improvement over port infiltration alone. There may be some advantage in TAP blocks in producing better relaxation of the abdominal wall for surgery as well as less pain from abdominal stretching. Arora et al in 2016[12] showed a clinically significant superiority of TAP blocks comparing a single lower subcostal TAP injection to port site infiltration for laparoscopic inguinal hernia repair, where a larger area of trauma to the abdominal wall is produced.

References

1. Jamieson RW, Swigart LL, Anson BJ. Points of parietal perforation of the ilioinguinal and iliohypogastric nerves in relation to optimal sites for local anaesthesia. *Q Bull Northwest Univ Med Sch*. 1952;26(1):22–26.
2. Hebbard PD, Barrington MJ, Vasey C. Ultrasound-guided continuous oblique subcostal transversus abdominis plane blockade: description of anatomy and clinical technique. *Reg Anesth Pain Med*. 2010;35(5):436–441.
3. Børglum J, Jensen K, Christensen AF, et al. Distribution patterns, dermatomal anesthesia, and ropivacaine serum concentrations after bilateral dual transversus abdominis plane block. *Reg Anesth Pain Med*. 2012;37(3):294–301.
4. McDonnell JG, O'Donnell BD, Farrell T, et al. Transversus abdominis plane block: a cadaveric and radiological evaluation. *Reg Anesth Pain Med*. 2007;32(5):399–404.
5. Støving K, Rothe C, Rosenstock CV, Aasvang EK, Lundstrøm LH, Lange KH. Cutaneous sensory block area, muscle-relaxing effect, and block duration of the transversus abdominis plane block: a randomized, blinded, and placebo-controlled study in healthy volunteers. *Reg Anesth Pain Med*. 2015;40(4):355–362.
6. Belavy D, Cowlishaw PJ, Howes M, Phillips F. Ultrasound-guided transversus abdominis plane block for analgesia after Caesarean delivery. *Br J Anaesth*. 2009;103(5):726–730.
7. McKeen DM, George RB, Boyd JC, Allen VM, Pink A. Transversus abdominis plane block does not improve early or late pain outcomes after Cesarean delivery: a randomized controlled trial. *Can J Anaesth*. 2014;61(7):631–640.
8. Griffiths JD, Barron FA, Grant S, Bjorksten AR, Hebbard P, Royse CF. Plasma ropivacaine concentrations after ultrasound-guided transversus abdominis plane block. *Br J Anaesth*. 2010;105(6):853–856.
9. Niraj G, Kelkar A, Jeyapalan I, et al. Comparison of analgesic efficacy of subcostal transversus abdominis plane blocks with epidural analgesia following upper abdominal surgery. *Anaesthesia*. 2011;66(6):465–471.
10. Yoshida T, Furutani K, Watanabe Y, Ohashi N, Baba H. Analgesic efficacy of bilateral continuous transversus abdominis plane blocks using an oblique subcostal approach in patients undergoing laparotomy for gynaecological cancer: a prospective, randomized, triple-blind, placebo-controlled study. *Br J Anaesth*. 2016;117(6):812–820.
11. Hutchins JL, Kesha R, Blanco F, Dunn T, Hochhalter R. Ultrasound-guided subcostal transversus abdominis plane blocks with liposomal bupivacaine vs. non-liposomal bupivacaine for postoperative pain control after laparoscopic hand-assisted donor nephrectomy: a prospective randomised observer-blinded study. *Anaesthesia*. 2016;71(8):930–937.
12. Arora S, Chhabra A, Subramaniam R, Arora MK, Misra MC, Bansal VK. Transversus abdominis plane block for laparoscopic inguinal hernia repair: a randomized trial. *J Clin Anesth*. 2016;33:357–364.

TRANSVERSUS ABDOMINIS PLANE BLOCKS

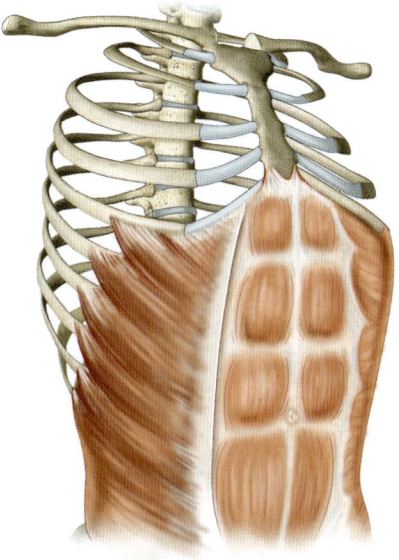

External oblique and rectus

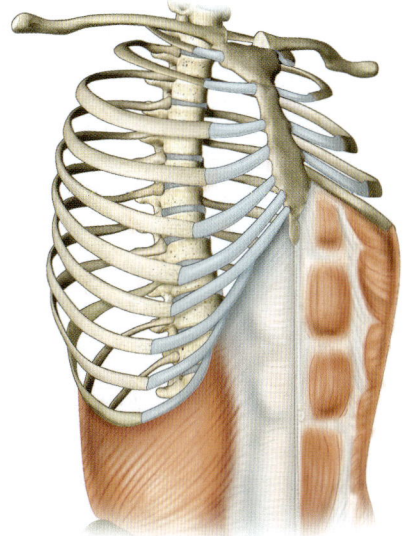

Internal oblique on right side

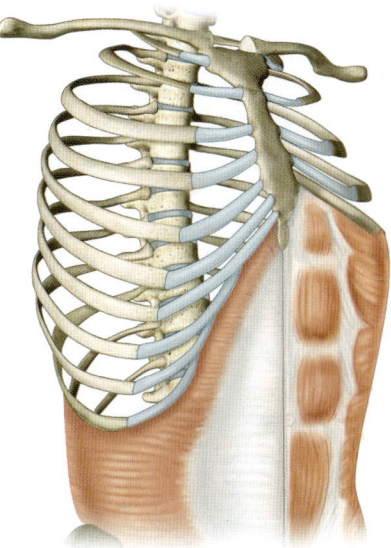

Transversus on right side

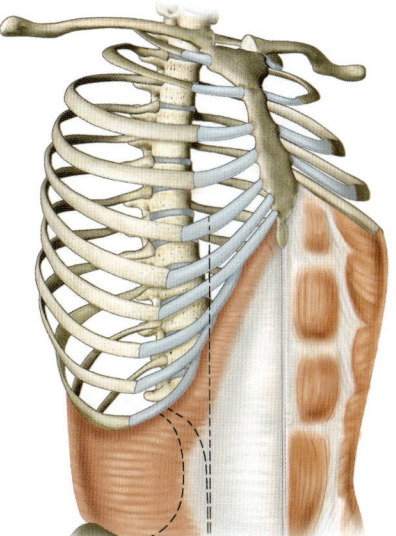

Summary of edges of muscle bellies

FIGURE 59.1 Anatomy of the transversus abdominis plane, edges of the muscles.

TRUNK BLOCKS

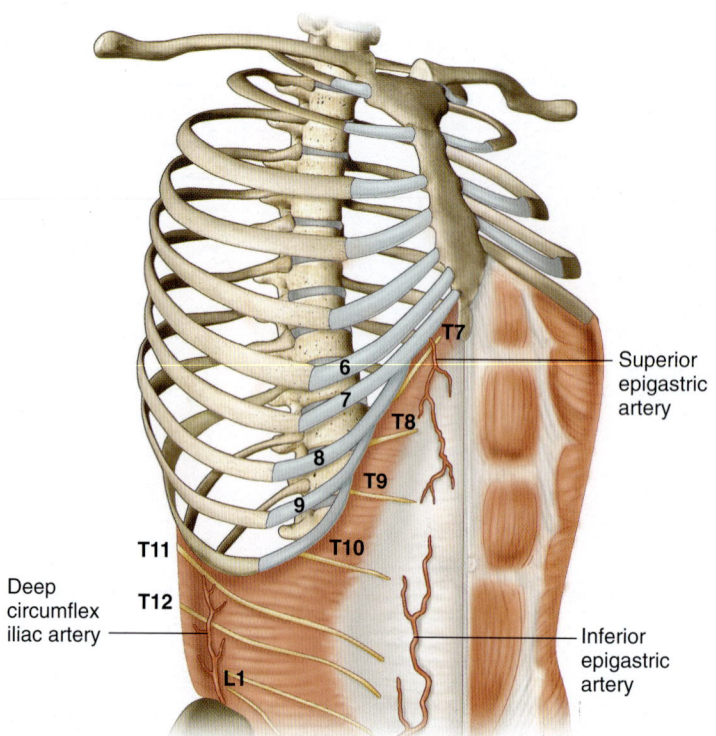

FIGURE 59.2 Anatomy of the transversus abdominis plane, arteries.

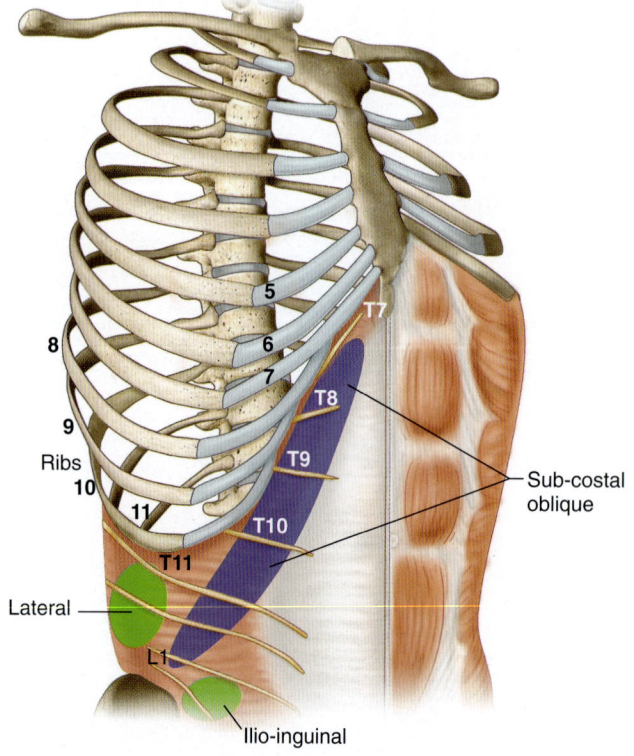

FIGURE 59.3 Transversus abdominis plane block zones.

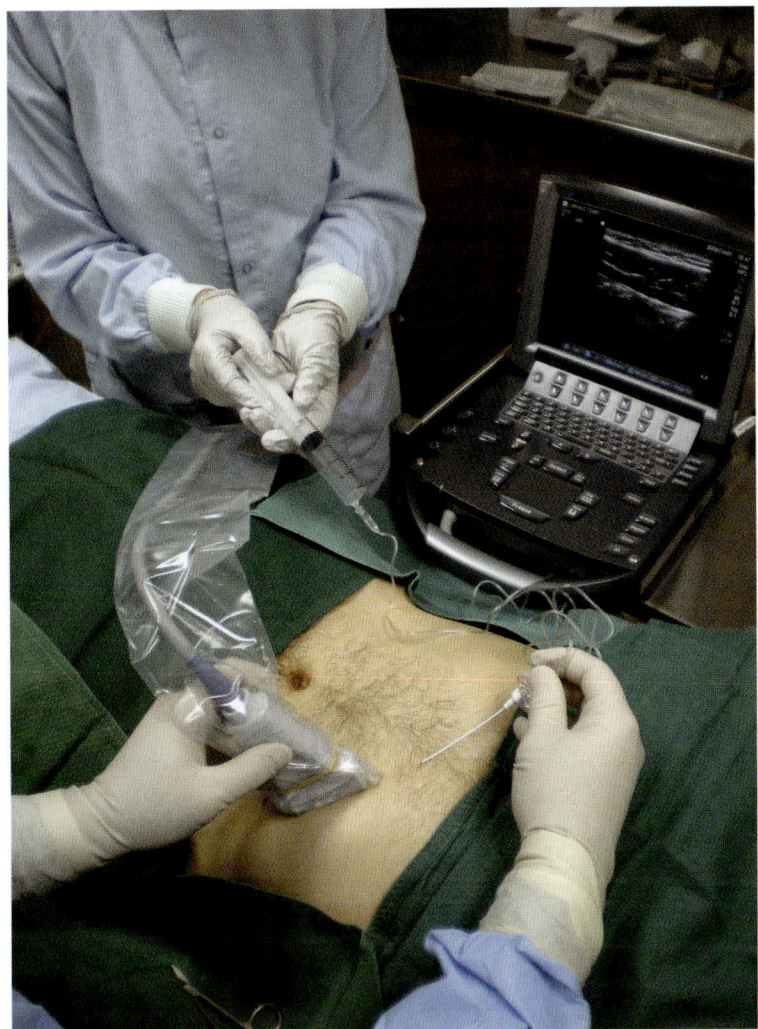

FIGURE 59.4 Photograph showing hand and needle position for subcostal oblique transversus abdominis plane.

274 TRUNK BLOCKS

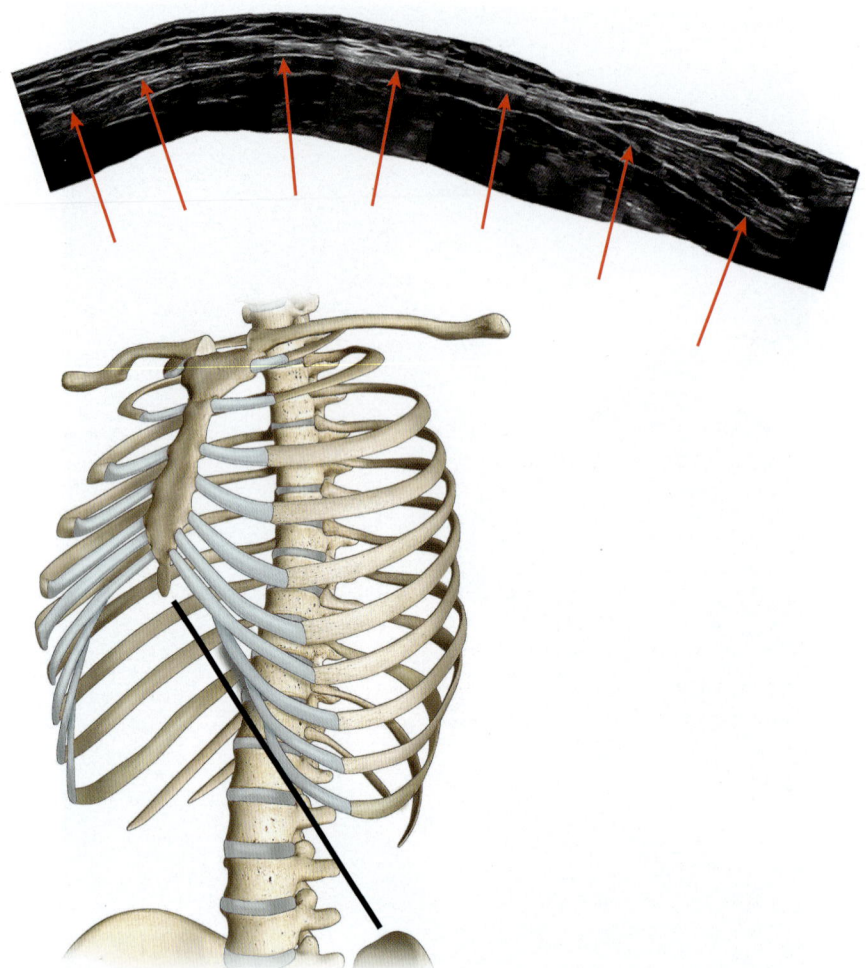

FIGURE 59.5 Composite ultrasound image along the oblique subcostal line.

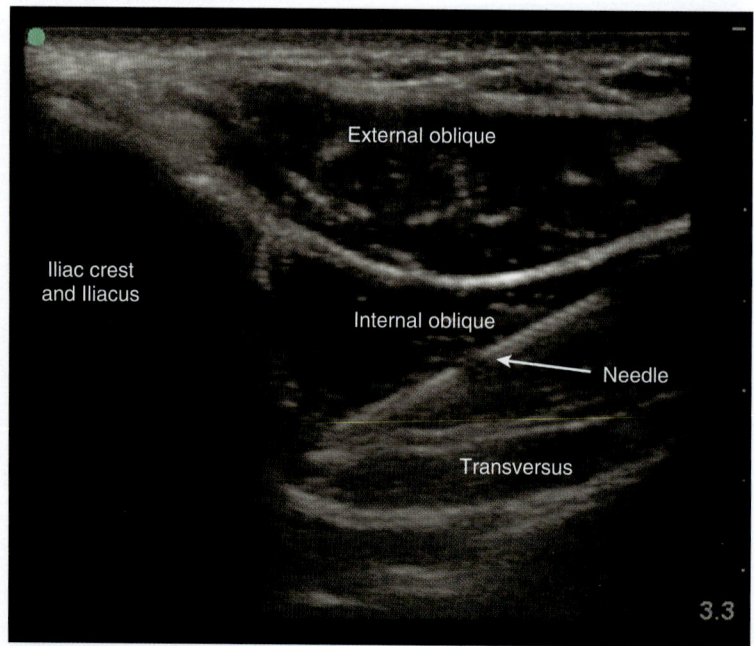

FIGURE 59.6 Ultrasound image for the ilioinguinal transversus abdominis plane block.

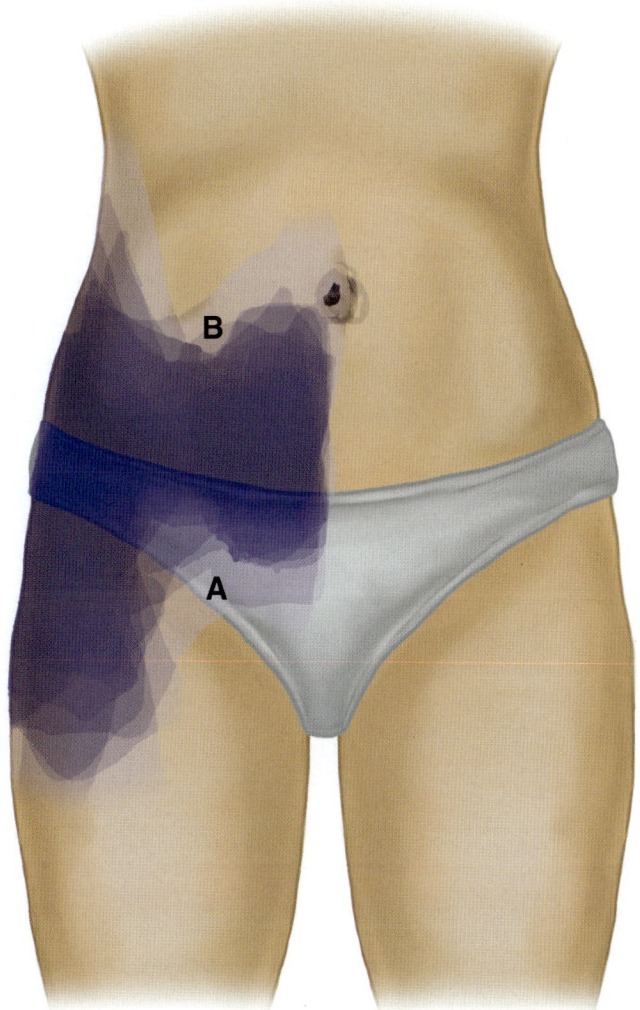

FIGURE 59.7 Composite image of the cutaneous block derived from the data of Støving et al. after a lateral transversus abdominis plane injection in 20 volunteers. Area A shows sparing in the inguinal region and less block along the deep circumflex iliac artery in area B.

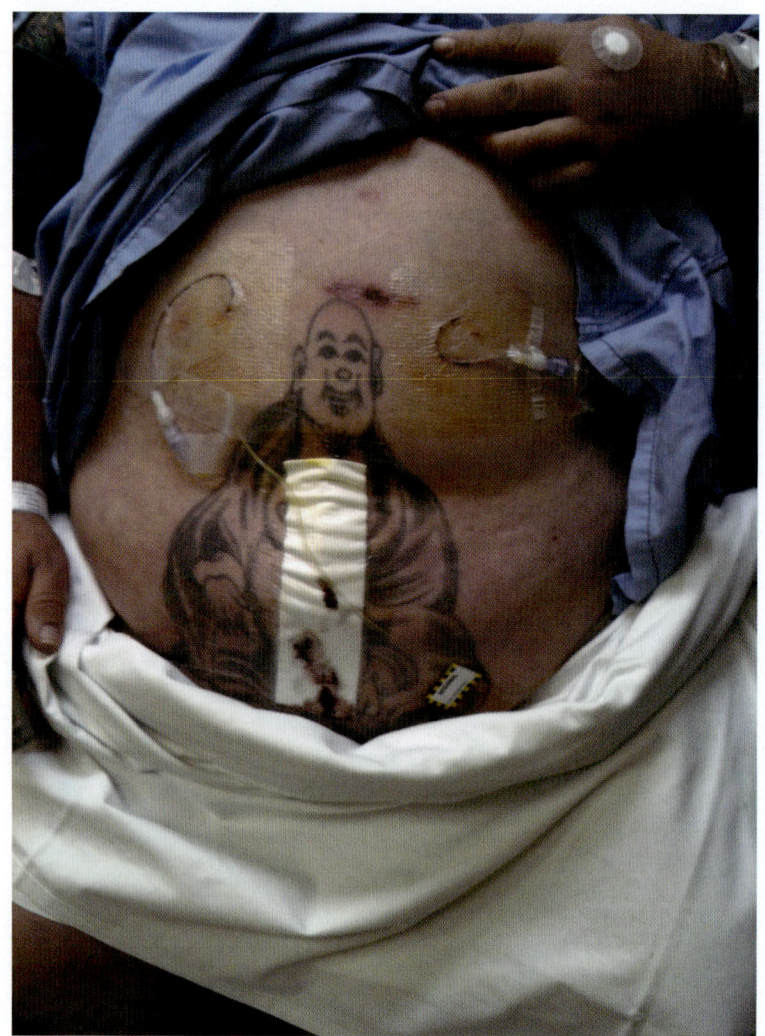

FIGURE 59.8 Bilateral subcostal oblique transversus abdominis plane catheters in a 140 kg postoperative patient. The superior extent of the motor block is shown by the loss of tone of the abdominal muscles inferior to the top of the dressing.

Quadratus Lumborum Blocks

CHAPTER 60

Hesham Elsharkawy

CLINICAL ANATOMY/SONOANATOMY

The quadratus lumborum (QL) is a posterior abdominal wall muscle that lies dorsolateral to the psoas major (PM) muscle. The QL muscle originates from the inner lip of the medial half of the iliac crest and inserts into the lower medial border of the last rib (usually the 12th rib). The medial border of the QL muscle attaches to the transverse processes of the lumbar vertebrae, and its lateral border is free and angled from craniomedial to caudolateral.

The QL muscle is separated from the surrounding muscles by thick fibrous thoracolumbar fascia (TLF). The transversalis fascia (TF) covers the transversus abdominis muscle and continues posteromedially, covering the anterior side of the investing fascia of both the QL and PM muscles.

The three-layer model of TLF comprises anterior, middle, and posterior layers. The QL muscle is located anterior to the middle layer, which is separated from the psoas by the anterior layer of the TF. The posterior and middle layers of the TLF fuse laterally to form the lateral raphe, which is the interwoven connective tissue where the transversus abdominis and internal oblique muscles take their origin (the posterior aponeurotic attachment). The middle layer of the TLF is multilayered (the intermuscular septum where muscles fuse) and medially attaches to the transverse processes of the vertebra.[1]

The subcostal and iliohypogastric nerves pass over the anterior surface of the QL muscle.

NOMENCLATURE AND POINTS OF INJECTION

Quadratus lumborum blocks (QLB) potentially block both the anterior and the lateral branches of the thoracoabdominal nerves. There is more than one approach described under the umbrella term of QLB (Table 60.1). The various QL blocks injection sites are illustrated in Fig. 60.6.

1-LATERAL QUADRATUS LUMBORUM (QLB1)

The needle can be directed from anterior to posterior toward the junction of the tapered transversus abdominis muscle and the QL muscle; local anesthetic will then be deposited in the lateral border of the QL muscle at the junction with the TF, superficial to the anterior layer of the TLF, and penetrate the aponeurotic attachment of the transversus abdominis muscle (the potential space medial to the abdominal wall muscles and anterolateral to the QL muscle). This block technique is coined QLB1.[2]

2-POSTERIOR QUADRATUS LUMBORUM (QLB2 BLOCK)

By advancing the needle more posteriorly, local anesthetic can be deposited posterior to the lateral edge of the QL muscle, between the QL muscle and posterior muscles (erector spinae, latissimus dorsi muscle, and serratus posterior inferior muscle) within the middle layer of the TLF in the anatomical location of the lumbar interfascial triangle.

Another possible variant for the posterior approach is directing the needle more medial on the posterior aspect of the QL muscle and observing local anesthetic spread toward the posterior medial aspect of the muscle through the intertransverse region. With this approach, the local anesthetic can gain access to the ventral rami between two transverse processes.[2]

TABLE 60.1 Main Features of Quadratus Lumborum Blocks

	QL Lateral (Type 1)	QL Posterior (Type 2)	QL Anterior (Transmuscular)
Clinical Indications	Abdominal surgery either above or below the umbilicus (any type of operation that requires intra-abdominal visceral pain coverage and abdominal wall incisions as high as T6)		
Dermatomes Covered	T6 to T12–L1; blocks the anterior and the lateral cutaneous branches of the nerves		
Lower Extremity Weakness	Not reported	Not reported	Potential
Spread to Lumbar Plexus	Not reported	Not reported	Potential
Potential Complications	Complications are related to the lack of anatomical understanding and needle expertise. It is possible to puncture intra-abdominal structures such as kidney, liver, and spleen. Bleeding		
Catheter Stability	Stable	Stable	Very stable
Injection Site	Lateral to QL muscle, anterolateral border of the QL muscle, at the junction with the transversalis fascia, within the anterior layer of the TLF, anterior to the posterior aponeurotic attachment of the transversus abdominis and internal oblique muscles	Posterior to the QL muscle, within the middle layer of the TLF	Anterior to the QL muscle, between the QL and the psoas major muscles, within the anterior layer of the TLF, close to the tip of the transverse process
Level of Difficulty	Intermediate	Intermediate	Advanced

QL, Quadratus lumborum; *TLF*, thoracolumbar fascia.

3-ANTERIOR QUADRATUS LUMBORUM (QLB3, OR TRANSMUSCULAR QLB, TRANSMUSCULAR QUADRATUS LUMBORUM BLOCK)

The needle can be advanced either from posterior through erector spinae muscle or anterior through the latissimus dorsi muscle and then through the QL muscle (transmuscular approach) to deposit the local anesthetic in the fascial plane between the fascial layers of the QL and PM muscles but posterior to the TF. In the three-layer model, the TLF will be between epimysium of the QL muscle and the anterior TLF.[3] A variety of needle trajectory can be used (anterior-to-posterior, posterior-to-anterior, or even caudal-to-cranial).[4]

PATIENT POSITIONING AND EQUIPMENT SELECTION

ULTRASOUND PROBE

Low-frequency (5 to 2 MHz) curved array ultrasound transducers can be used to provide a simultaneous adequate visualization of the three lateral abdominal wall muscle layers, the QL muscle, retroperitoneal space including the kidney, transverse processes, and the adjoining lumbar paravertebral area. High-frequency transducers more accurately depict the fascial planes and may suffice in some patients, particularly in children or small adults. The orientation marker can be directed laterally for a transverse scan and cranially for parasagittal scan.[3]

PATIENT POSITION

Lateral: The lateral decubitus position gives more exposure of the neuraxial structures and more stability in handling the ultrasound probe and needle, and patients are often more comfortable.

Supine: It is feasible to perform QL block in the supine position and lateral tilt of the torso with wedge under the lower flank, tilting the transducer probe posteromedially. The disadvantage of the supine position is impaired visualization of the lumbar paravertebral area.

Prone: The procedure can also be performed in the prone position with a pillow under the abdomen; however, positioning the patient can be logistically difficult, especially postoperatively after abdominal procedures.

Sitting: With the transmuscular approach and subcostal approaches, the patient can be positioned in the sitting position, which facilitates bilateral block procedure without patient repositioning.[3]

Clinical Pearls[5-8]

- The QL muscle attaches to the transverse processes, which are easier to identify.
- If the QL muscle is small and difficult to delineate, the ipsilateral hip joint is abducted and laterally flexed toward the same side of the block to contract the QL muscle (temporarily will thicken the QL muscle).
- While performing the block, especially with the subcostal approach, it is common to visualize the lower pole of the kidney and lower lobe of the liver and spleen. The QL muscle acts similar to a bed for the kidney, which helps identification of the QL muscle, but great caution should be taken to avoid any visceral injury.
- Apply color Doppler before insertion of the needle to detect the abdominal branches of the lumbar arteries on the posterior aspect of the quadratus lumborum muscle or any other vessels close to the transverse process or on the intended track of the needle.
- The tactile feedback (as pops) when encountering different fascial planes is not accurate in QL blocks due to the complexity of the anatomical planes, the multilayered components of the TLF muscle, and the approach angle. Therefore, visual confirmation using ultrasound and hydrodissection should be used.
- With the transmuscular quadratus lumborum block, the local anesthetic is deposited in the plane between the QL and psoas major muscle. Both during and after administration of the local anesthetic the transducer should be moved from the transverse to the longitudinal position. With the curvilinear probe in the longitudinal position, the local anesthetic can be seen to spread cephalad from the iliac crest to the 12th rib.
- We prefer to have the local anesthetic spread medially (toward the intervertebral foramen and closer to the paravertebral space) than directed anterolateral toward the IAP plane (Fig. 60.8).

ACKNOWLEDGMENTS

I acknowledge the contribution of Jeff Lorech to the images presented in this article. All images are taken with permission from the Cleveland Clinic art photography department.

References

1. Elsharkawy H. Quadratus lumborum block with paramedian sagittal oblique (subcostal) approach. *Anaesthesia.* 2016;71(2):241–242.
2. Willard FH, Vleeming A, Schuenke MD, Danneels L, Schleip R. The thoracolumbar fascia: anatomy, function and clinical considerations. *J Anat.* 2012;221:507–536.
3. Adhikary SD, El Boghdadly K, Nasralah Z, et al. A radiologic and anatomic assessment of injectate spread following transmuscular quadratus lumborum block in cadavers. *Anaesthesia.* 2017;72:73–79.
4. El-Boghdadly K, Elsharkawy H, Short A, Chin KJ. Quadratus lumborum block nomenclature and anatomical considerations. *Reg Anesth Pain Med.* 2016;41(4):548–549.

5. Blanco R, Ansari T, Girgis E. Quadratus lumborum block for postoperative pain after caesarean section: a randomised controlled trial. *Eur J Anaesthesiol.* 2015;32:1–7.
6. Blanco R, Ansari T, Riad W, Shetty N. Quadratus lumborum block versus transversus abdominis plane block for postoperative pain after cesarean delivery, a randomized controlled trial. *Reg Anesth Pain Med.* 2016;41:757–762.
7. Hebbard PD. Transversalis fascia plane block, a novel ultrasound-guided abdominal wall nerve block. *Can J Anaesth.* 2009;56:618–620.
8. Elsharkawy H. Ultrasound-guided quadratus lumborum block: how do i do it? American Society of Regional Anesthesia and Pain Medicine Newsletter, November; 2015:36–42.

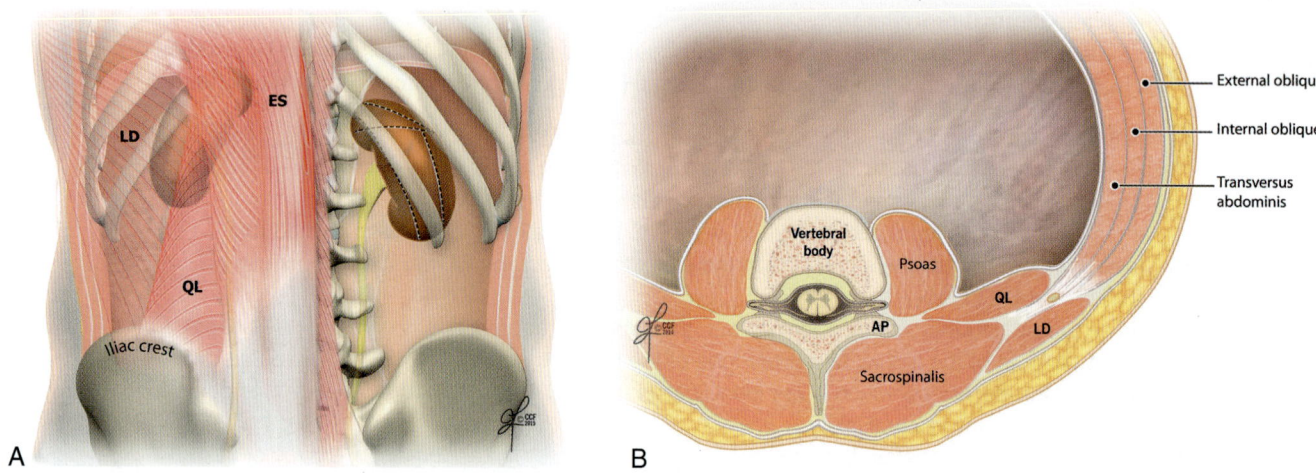

FIGURE 60.1 The Quadratus lumborum muscle in two views, A: QL muscle from the back covered by the erector spinae and latissimus dorsi muscles. B: QL muscle cross section showing the surrounding muscles. *AP*, Articulate process; *ES*, Erector Spinae; *LD*, Latissimus Dorsi; *QL*, Quadratus Lumborum. (Reprinted with permission, Cleveland Clinic Center for Medical Art & Photography © 2017. All Rights Reserved.)

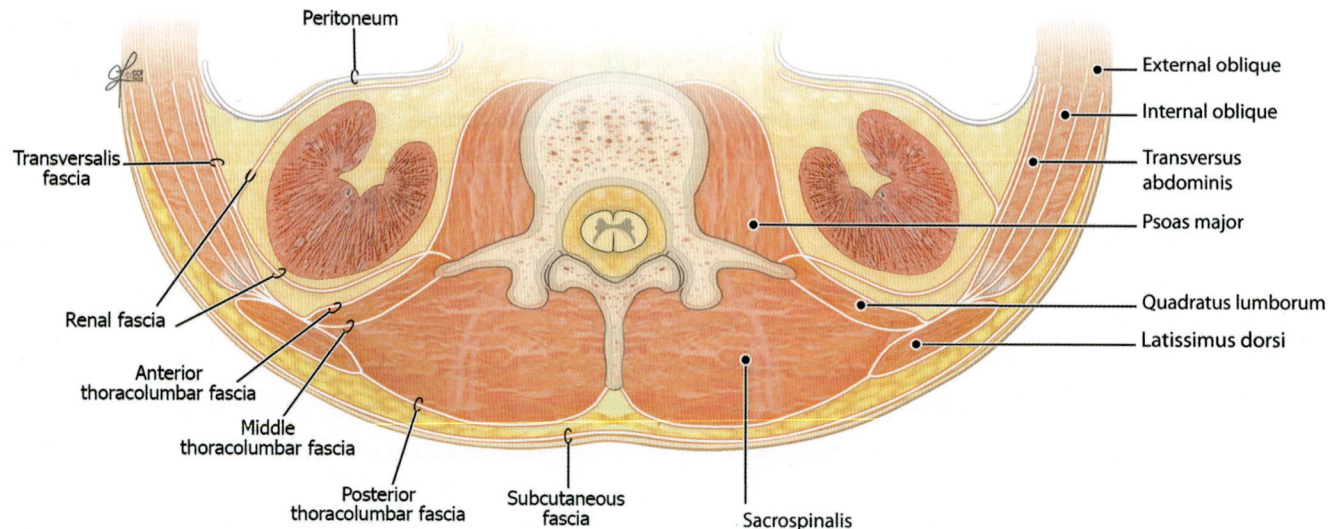

FIGURE 60.2 A cross section and sagittal with the different layers of the thoracolumbar fascia, renal fascia, and the anatomy relations of the of the quadratus lumborum muscle. (Reprinted with permission, Cleveland Clinic Center for Medical Art & Photography © 2017. All Rights Reserved.)

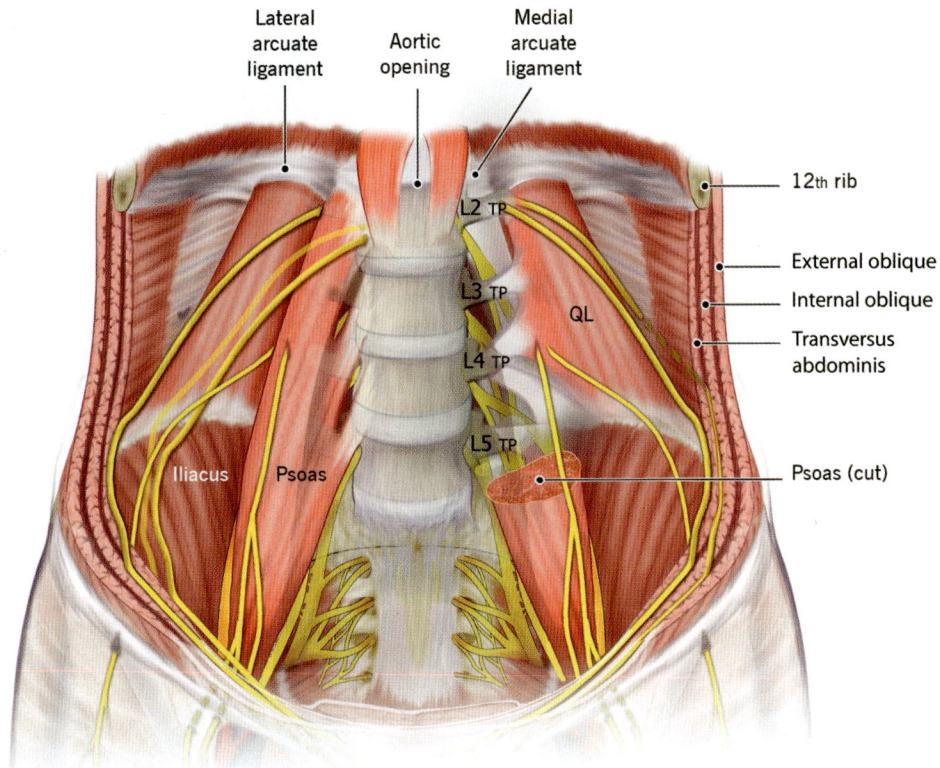

FIGURE 60.3 Quadratus lumborum (QL) muscle from the front; on the left side, the Psoas muscle cut showing the ventral rami of the spinal nerve roots pass in front of QL. (Reprinted with permission, Cleveland Clinic Center for Medical Art & Photography © 2017. All Rights Reserved.)

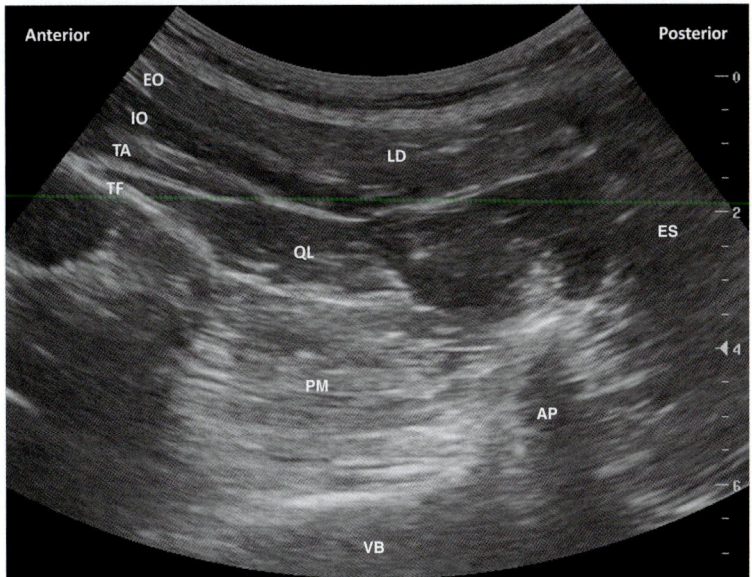

FIGURE 60.4 Ultrasound image of the lateral abdominal wall. *AP*, Articular process; *EO*, external oblique; *ES*, Erector-Spinae; *IO*, internal oblique; *LD*, latissimus dorsi; *QL*, quadrates lumborum; *TA*; transversus abdominis; *TF*, transversalis fascia; *TP*, transverse process. (Reprinted with permission, Cleveland Clinic Center for Medical Art & Photography © 2017. All Rights Reserved.)

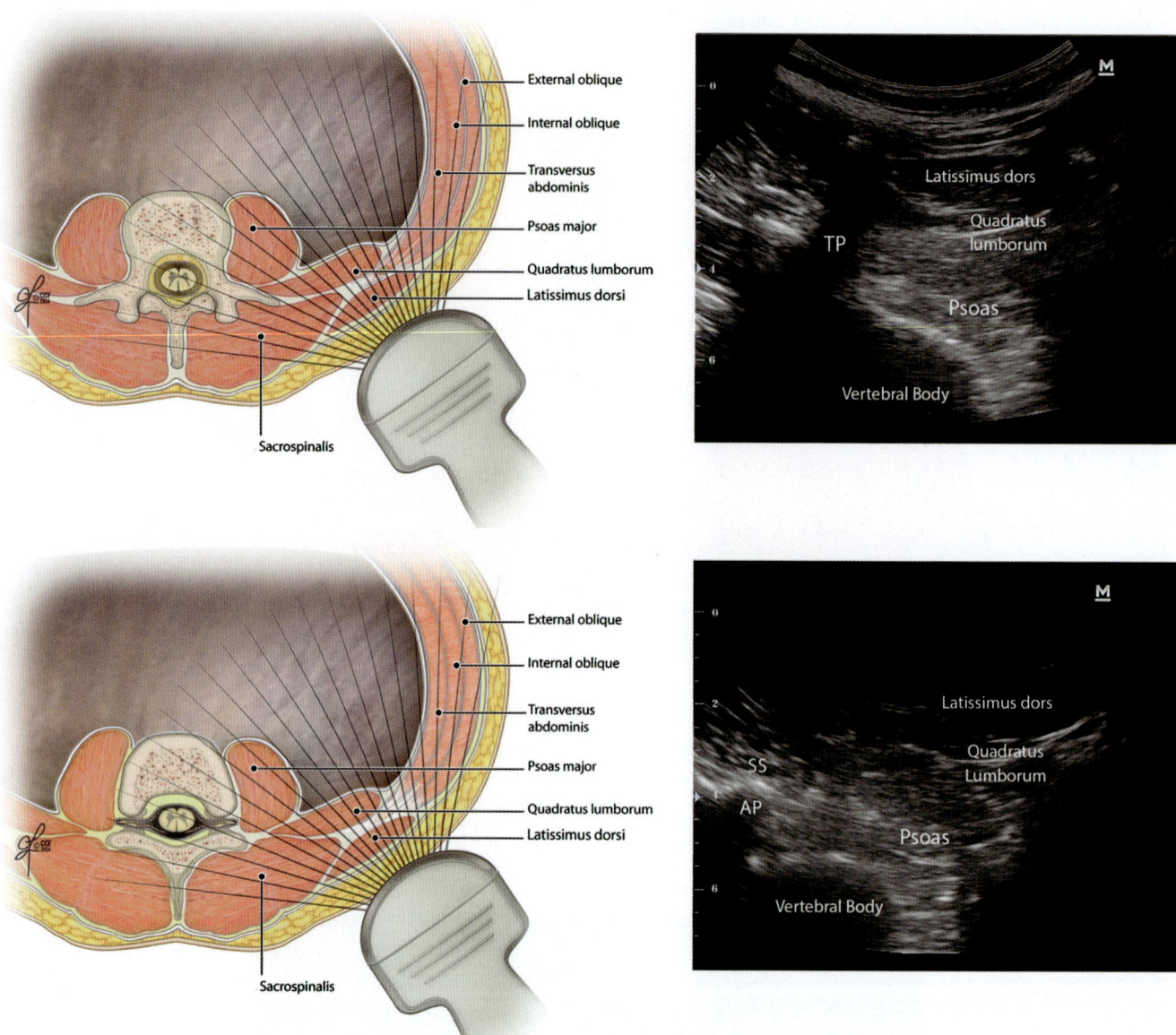

FIGURE 60.5 Scanning technique to identify QL, psoas and ES muscles at the level of transverse process (top left, Transverse process view) and between two transverse processes (bottom left, inter-transverse process view) with correlating ultrasound images on the right. *AP*, Articular process; *IF*, inter-vertebral foramen; *QL*, Quadrates lumborum; *SS*, sacrospinalis; *TP*, transverse process. (Reprinted with permission, Cleveland Clinic Center for Medical Art & Photography © 2017. All Rights Reserved.)

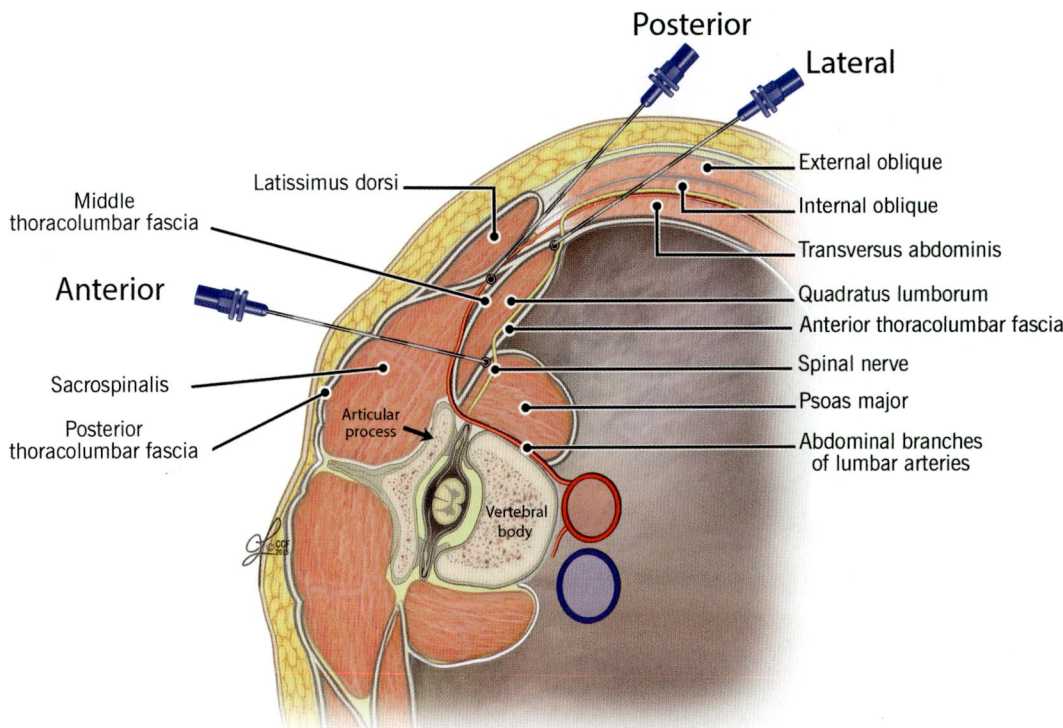

FIGURE 60.6 Nomenclature and trajectory of needle for all three approaches to quadratus lumborum block (QLB1, QLB2, and QLB3). (Reprinted with permission, Cleveland Clinic Center for Medical Art & Photography © 2017. All Rights Reserved.)

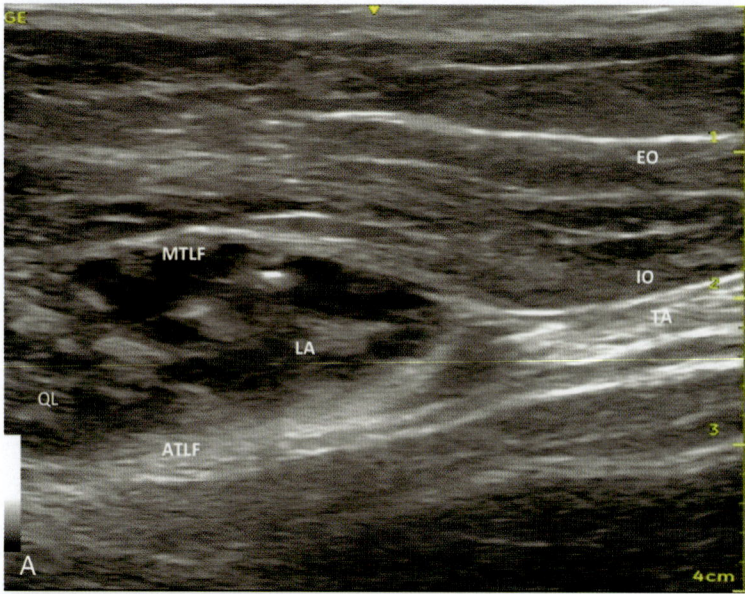
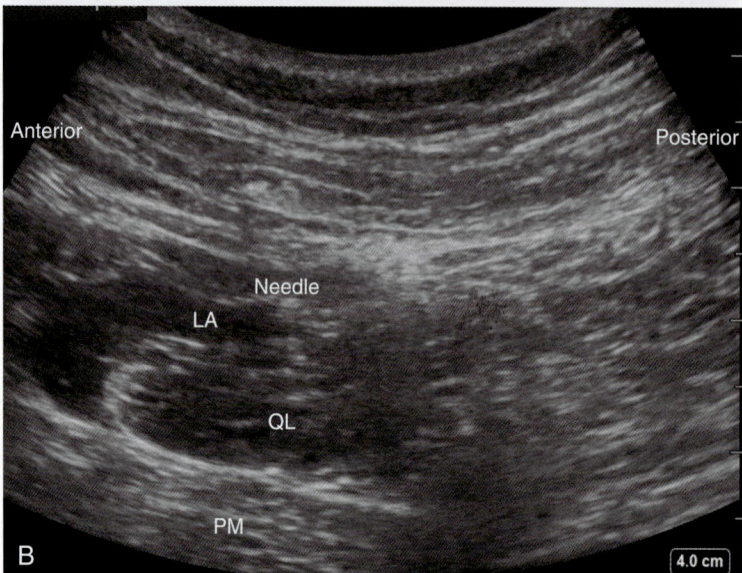
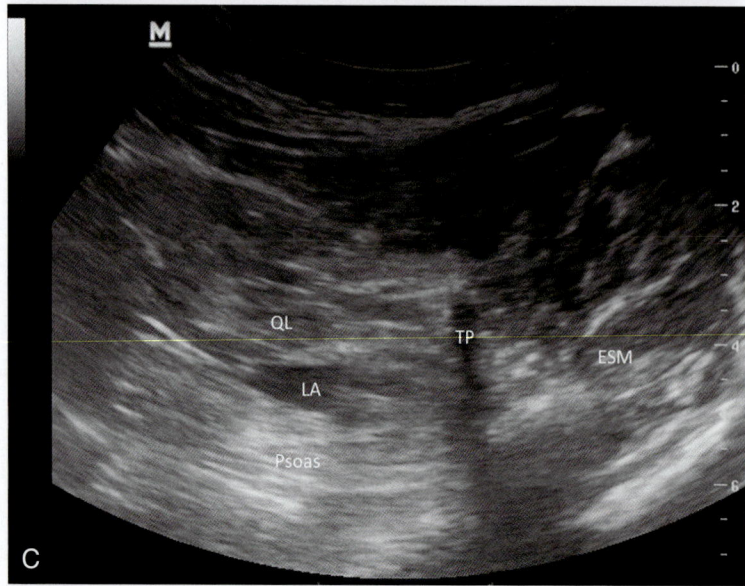

FIGURE 60.7 Ultrasound image illustrates the trajectory of needle and medication spread in the approach of lateral QL block 1 (Panel A), posterior QL block 2 (Panel B), and transmuscular anterior QL block (Panel C). *ATLF*, Anterior thoracolumbar fascia; *EO*, external oblique; *ESM*, erector spinae muscle; *IO*, internal oblique; *LA*, local anesthetic; *MTLF*, middle thoracolumbar fascia; *PM*, psoas major; *QL*, quadratus lumborum; *TA*, transversus abdominis; *TP*, transverse process. (Reprinted with permission, Cleveland Clinic Center for Medical Art & Photography © 2017. All Rights Reserved.)

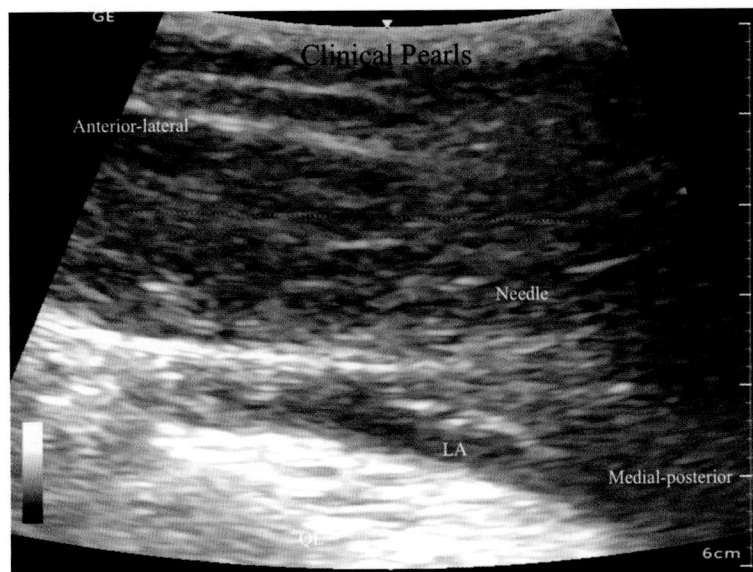

FIGURE 60.8 The injected local anesthetic separates the QL and LD muscles indicating local anesthetic spread posteromedial. *ES*, Erector spinae muscle; *LD*, latissimus dorsi muscle; *PM*, psoas major muscle; *QL*, Quadratus lumborum muscle. (Reprinted with permission, Cleveland Clinic Center for Medical Art & Photography © 2017. All Rights Reserved.)

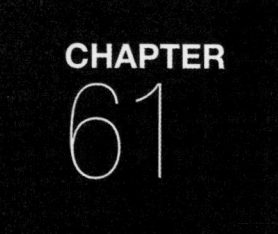

Thoracic Paravertebral Block

Manoj Kumar Karmakar

 See Video 61.1 on ExpertConsult.com.

INTRODUCTION

Thoracic paravertebral block (TPVB) is the technique of injecting local anesthetic alongside the thoracic vertebra close to where the spinal nerves emerge from the intervertebral foramina.[1] This produces ipsilateral somatic and sympathetic nerve blockade in multiple contiguous thoracic dermatomes (segmental thoracic anesthesia) both above and below the site of injection.[1,2] It is effective in treating acute and chronic pain of unilateral origin from the chest and abdomen.[1] Bilateral TPVB also has been described.[1] Recently there has been an increase in interest in the use of ultrasound to assist or guide TPVB in real time.[3] This chapter briefly describes the basic principles of TPVB, the sonoanatomy of the thoracic paravertebral space (TPVS), and the technique of ultrasound-guided (USG) TPVB.

GROSS ANATOMY

The TPVS is a wedge-shaped space that lies on either side of the vertebral column (Fig. 61.1).[1] It is wider on the left than on the right,[1] and the parietal pleura forms the anterolateral boundary. The base is formed by the vertebral body, intervertebral disc, and contents of the intervertebral foramen (see Fig. 61.1).[1] The superior costotransverse ligament (SCTL) forms the posterior wall of the TPVS. This ligament extends from the lower border of the transverse process above to the upper border of the transverse process below (Figs. 61.2 and 61.3), and the intertransverse ligament also is interposed between two transverse processes (see Figs. 61.2–61.4). The SCTL is continuous laterally with the internal intercostal membrane, which is the medial extension of the internal intercostal muscle medial to the angle of the rib (see Fig. 61.4). The apex of the TPVS is continuous with the intercostal space lateral to the tips of the transverse processes (see Fig. 61.4).[1] Interposed between the parietal pleura anteriorly and the SCTL posteriorly is the fibroelastic *endothoracic fascia* (see Figs. 61.1 and 61.4),[4–6] which is the deep fascia of the thorax that lines the internal aspect of the thoracic cage (Fig. 61.5).[5,6] In the paravertebral location, the endothoracic fascia is loosely applied to the ribs (see Fig. 61.5) and fuses medially with the periosteum at the midpoint of the vertebral body (see Fig. 61.1).[1] There is an intervening layer of loose areolar connective tissue, "the subserous fascia,"[1] between the parietal pleura and the endothoracic fascia (see Figs. 61.1 and 61.2). The endothoracic fascia thus divides the TPVS into two potential fascial compartments, the anterior *extrapleural paravertebral compartment* and the posterior *subendothoracic paravertebral compartment* (see Figs. 61.1 and 61.2).[1] The TPVS contains fatty tissue[1] that line the intercostal (spinal) nerve, the dorsal ramus, intercostal vessels, rami communicantes, and sympathetic chain (see Figs. 61.1 and 61.2).[1] The spinal nerves in the TPVS are segmented into small bundles lying freely among the fat and devoid of a fascial sheath, which make them susceptible to local anesthetic blockade.[7] The intercostal nerves and vessels are located behind the endothoracic fascia, while the sympathetic trunk is located anterior to it in the TPVS (see Fig. 61.5).[1,8]

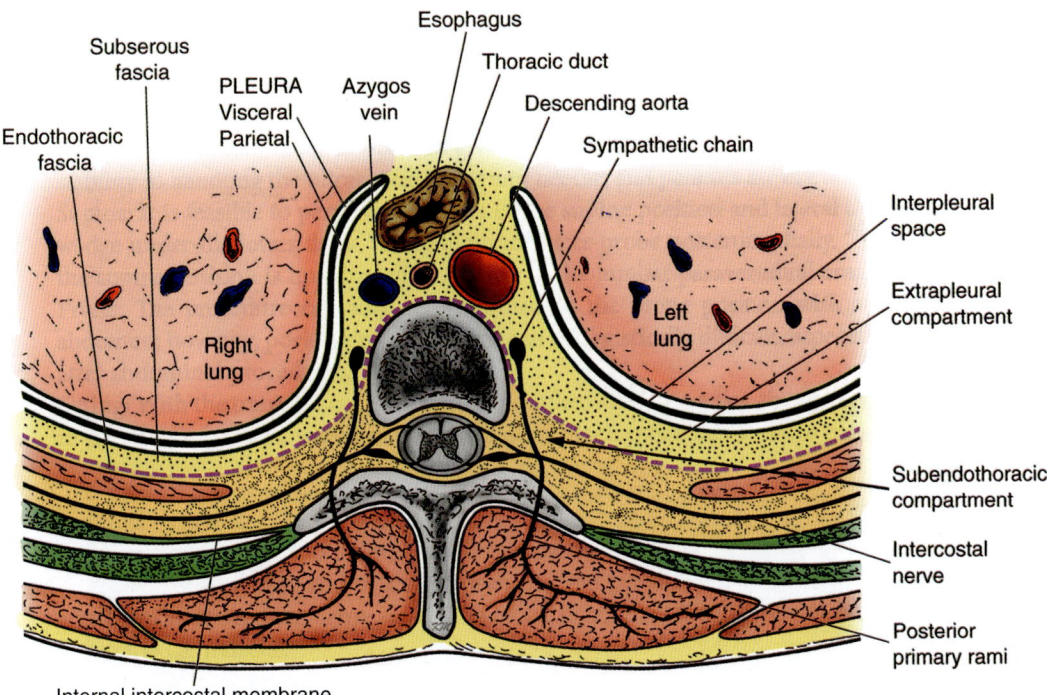

FIGURE 61.1 Transverse anatomy of the thoracic paravertebral space.

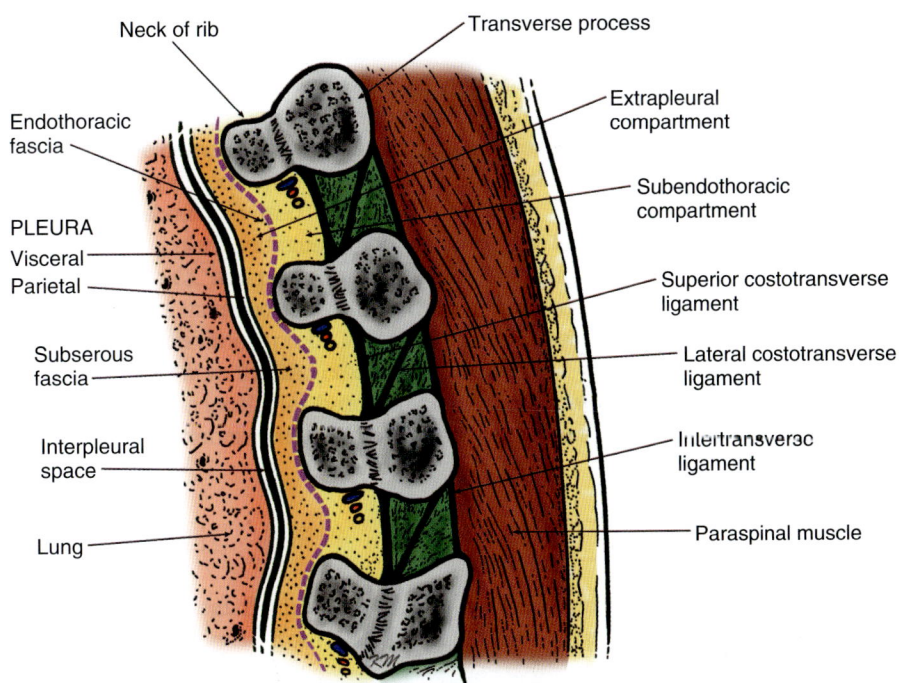

FIGURE 61.2 Sagittal anatomy of the thoracic paravertebral space.

COMMUNICATIONS OF THE THORACIC PARAVERTEBRAL SPACE

The TPVS is continuous with the epidural space medially via the intervertebral foramen,[9–11] the intercostal space laterally,[1,7,9,10] and the contralateral TPVS via the epidural and prevertebral space.[1] The cranial extension of the TPVS is still not defined, but we have observed direct paravertebral

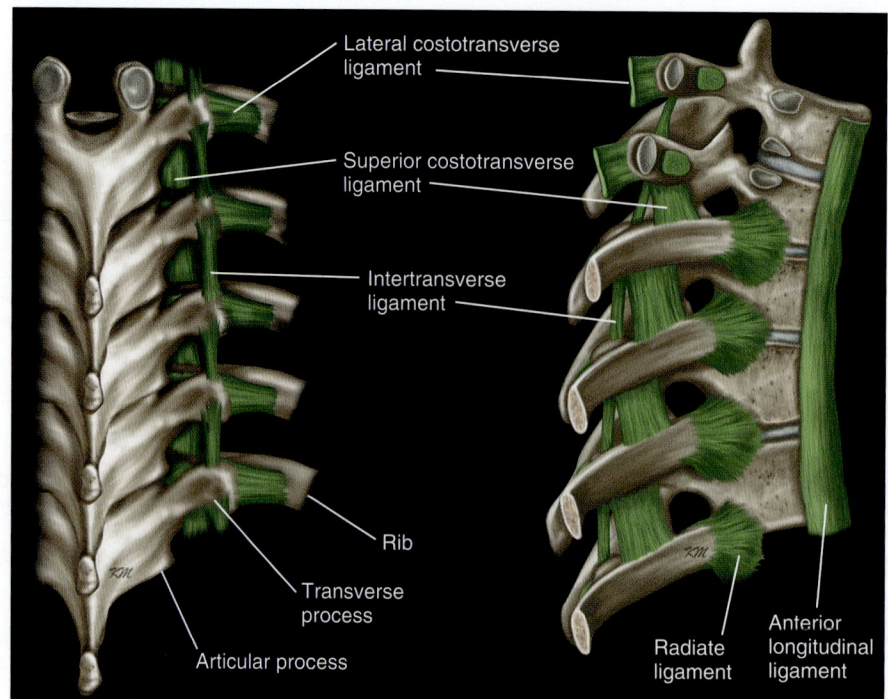

FIGURE 61.3 Ligaments attached to the transverse process of the thoracic vertebra.

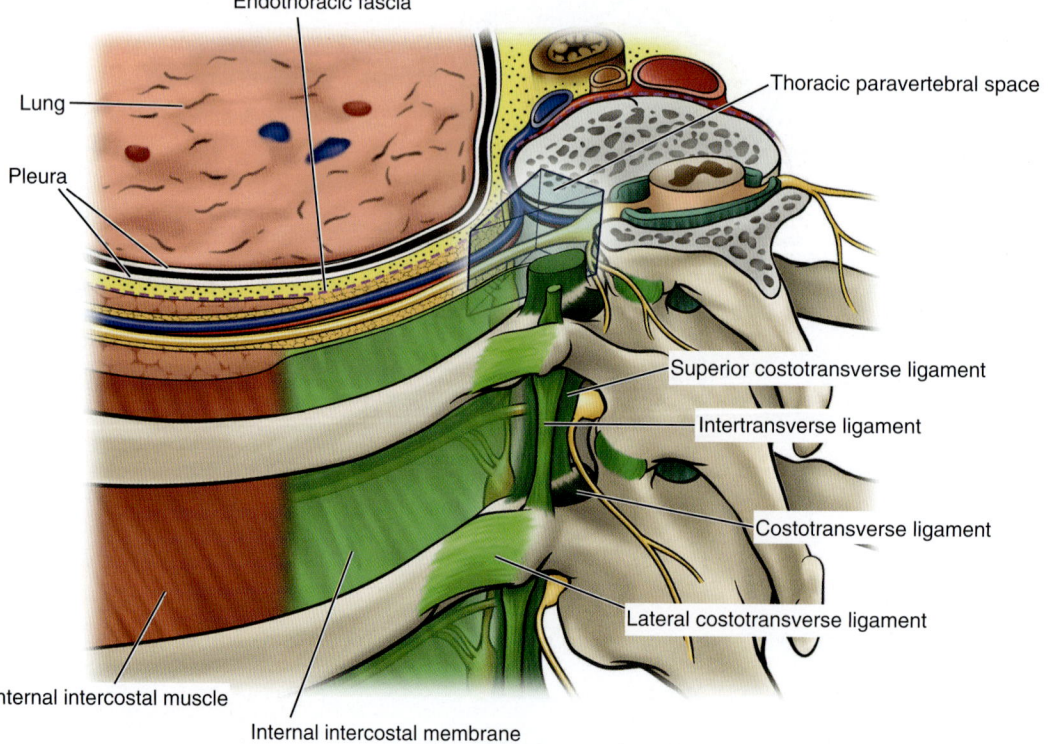

FIGURE 61.4 Anatomy of the thoracic paravertebral region showing the various paravertebral ligaments and their anatomical relationship to the thoracic paravertebral space.

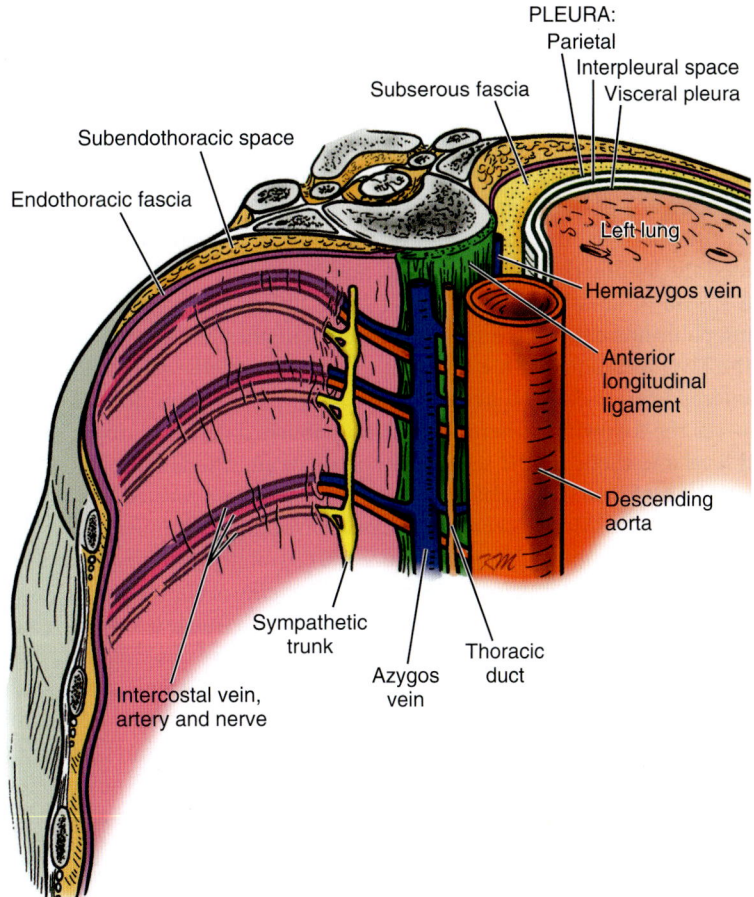

FIGURE 61.5 The endothoracic fascia and its anatomical relationship to the thoracic paravertebral space. Note the fascial compartments and the location of the neurovascular structures in relation to the endothoracic fascia.

spread of radio-opaque contrast medium from the thoracic to the cervical region, indicating that there is a direct continuity between the thoracic and cervical paravertebral regions. Ipsilateral Horner's syndrome after thoracic paravertebral injections also has been reported.[11,12] The anatomic pathway for the spread of an injectate from the thoracic to the cervical paravertebral space is still not clear. The endothoracic fascia is continuous superiorly with the scalene or Sibson fascia[4] and attached to the medial border of the first rib in front and the transverse process of the seventh cervical vertebra behind.[4] Therefore, an injection posterior to the endothoracic fascia in the subendothoracic paravertebral compartment of the upper thoracic region is unlikely to spread cranially via the paravertebral space because of the attachment of the endothoracic fascia to the transverse process. However, we believe that an injection anterior to the endothoracic fascia in the extrapleural paravertebral compartment may spread to the cervical paravertebral region via the subserous layer of loose areolar connective tissue, which also provides the connective tissue investment for the mediastinal structures,[4] and is continuous with the connective tissue investing the neurovascular structures in the root of the neck.

The caudal boundary of the TPVS is formed by the origin of the psoas major muscle,[13] and spread through the TPVS to the lumbar region is thought to be unlikely.[13] Ipsilateral lumbar spinal nerves are occasionally involved after a lower thoracic paravertebral injection.[2,14] Saito and colleagues have demonstrated ipsilateral thoracolumbar spread of colored dye in cadavers.[15] We also have reported ipsilateral thoracolumbar anesthesia and radiological spread of contrast below the diaphragm.[16] These observations challenge the concept of lumbar nerve root sparing following TPVB.[13] The exact mechanism for the ipsilateral thoracolumbar spread of local anesthetic or contrast medium is not clear, but it is suggested that it occurs via the subendothoracic fascial compartment[16] to the retroperitoneal space where the ilioinguinal and iliohypogastric nerves are located.[16]

MECHANISM OF BLOCKADE

A thoracic paravertebral injection may remain localized to the space injected or it may spread to the contiguous paravertebral spaces above and below,[6,9,10] the intercostal space laterally,[9–11] the epidural space medially[9,11] or a combination of these to affect ipsilateral somatic[2,14] and sympathetic nerves,[2] including the posterior primary ramus in multiple contiguous thoracic dermatomes.[1] The majority of the published data describing spread or distribution of anesthesia after TPVB have implemented the landmark based technique, and currently there is a paucity of data describing segmental spread of anesthesia in vivo after USG TPVB. Therefore caution must be exercised interpreting published data on the segmental spread of anesthesia after a TPVB, since it may not apply to the USG technique with a different direction of needle advancement (landmark based TPVB—anteroposterior directed needle—and USG TPVB—lateral to medial for the intercostal approach—see the following). There also are no published data describing the effects of volume or dose of local anesthetic on the segmental spread of anesthesia after USG TPVB.

Eason and Wyatt found that at least four intercostal spaces are covered by a single 15-mL injection of 0.375% bupivacaine.[17] More recently, 15 mL of bupivacaine 0.5% injected into the TPVS has been shown to produce mean unilateral somatic block over 5 (range 1 to 9) dermatomes and sympathetic block over 8 (range 6 to 10) dermatomes.[2] Similarly, 1.5 mg/kg of bupivacaine 0.5% produced sensory loss at the level of injection with a mean superior spread of 1.4 (range 0 to 4) dermatomes and a mean inferior spread of 2.8 (range 0 to 7) dermatomes.[14] We also have observed a median ipsilateral loss of sensation to cold (ice) of 5 dermatomes (range 3 to 11 dermatomes) after a single paravertebral injection of 1.5 mg/kg (0.3 mL/kg) of 0.5% bupivacaine with epinephrine 1:200,000 in patients with multiple fractured ribs.[12] The median distribution of sensory loss in our cohort of patients was 1.5 dermatomes (range, 1 to 3 dermatomes) above and 2.5 dermatomes (range, 0 to 9 dermatomes) below the level of injection.[12] In children, 0.25 (SD 0.12) mL/kg of contrast medium injected into the TPVS produces radiological spread over 5.7 (SD 1.6) segments.[18]

Cumulative evidence therefore suggests that a single-injection TPVB produces ipsilateral segmental thoracic anesthesia,[1,2,12,19] but the dermatomal distribution of sensory blockade is unpredictable and variable.[1,2,12,19] The reason for this variability is not clear, but anatomical and physical factors have been hypothesized.[1,2,19] Factors such as age, gender, height, weight, injectate volume or the dose of bupivacaine, previous posterolateral thoracotomy, or the spread of a radio-opaque contrast medium does not appear to affect the distribution of sensory blockade after a single-injection TPVB.[19] Paravertebral injections performed at 2-week intervals in the same patient also produces different degrees of sensory blockade.[19] Thoracic paravertebral anesthesia does not appear to be gravity dependent, but there is a tendency for preferential caudal spread of somatic[2,13,20] and sympathetic blockade.[2]

Naja and colleagues[21] recently studied the spread of a radiopaque contrast medium in the TPVS using chest radiographs after locating the TPVS using nerve stimulation.[21] They defined the needle tip to be dorsal to the endothoracic fascia when the motor response was elicited at 2.5 mA and ventral to it (and presumably close to the spinal nerve) when the motor response was elicited at ≤0.5 mA.[21] Naja and colleagues[21] clearly demonstrated an association between an injection at two different locations within the TPVS or after identifying the TPVS using two different current thresholds and the pattern of spread of contrast.[21] They concluded that an injection ventral to the endothoracic fascia, with a low nerve stimulating current (≤0.5 mA), more frequently results in a longitudinal and multisegmental spread of contrast, whereas an injection dorsal to the endothoracic fascia, with a high nerve-stimulating current (2.5 mA), results in a cloud-like and limited segmental spread of the contrast.[21] The interpretation of the results of this study[21] has been questioned,[22] because with the methodology described, it is not possible to determine with certainty where the injections were made relative to the endothoracic fascia. While Naja and colleagues described the spinal nerves as ventral to the endothoracic fascia,[21] published literature suggests that they are located dorsal to the endothoracic fascia and in the subendothoracic paravertebral compartment (see Figs. 61.1 and 61.5).[1,5]

There is controversy about epidural spread and its contribution to the extension of TPVB. Radio-opaque contrast medium infused through an extrapleural paravertebral catheter placed intraoperatively under direct vision remains confined to the paravertebral space.[23] In contrast, varying degrees of epidural spread has been shown to occur after 70% of percutaneous paravertebral injections.[11] These injections are mostly unilateral, and the volume involved is considered too small to produce clinically significant epidural block.[24] Cadaveric dissection also confirms that only a small proportion of the injectate enters the epidural space[10] and remains confined to the side of injection. The vertebral attachment of the endothoracic fascia attenuates prevertebral spread[25] and may influence epidural spread after an extrapleural paravertebral compartment injection. Clinically, sensory anesthesia is predominantly ipsilateral and greater after epidural spread than after only paravertebral spread.[11] Therefore, current evidence suggests that ipsilateral epidural spread of discrete amounts of local anesthetic occurs after thoracic paravertebral injection and contributes to the extension of TPVB.

Bilateral symmetrical anesthesia is described[11,12,26] and may be due to extensive epidural spread,[11] inadvertent intrathecal injection into the dural sleeve,[1] or inadvertent epidural injection via a catheter that was intended for the paravertebral space.[12] Bilateral symmetrical anesthesia may also occur more commonly with the median injection technique or the use of large volumes of injectate (>25 mL).[1] Segmental contralateral anesthesia adjacent to the site of injection has been shown to occur in 1.1% of paravertebral injections[24] and may be due to either prevertebral[6,27] or epidural[28] spread to the contralateral TPVS. We also have observed mean segmental contralateral anesthesia of 2.5 (1.5) dermatomes in 20% of patients after a single-injection TPVB. More recently, we have reported contralateral anesthesia over 9 (7 to 11) dermatomes in 35% of patients after a multiple-injection TPVB that was used for surgical anesthesia during percutaneous radiofrequency ablation of liver tumors.[29]

The exact mechanism for prevertebral spread is not clear, but we have proposed that it occurs through the "extrapleural compartment" of the TPVS via the subserous layer of connective tissue.[6] It is also not known if there are differences in the incidence of contralateral anesthesia between a single-injection and a multiple-injection TPVB, but our experience (described previously) suggests that it may be more common after a multiple-injection technique.[29] Bilateral sympathetic blockade may also occur in the absence of bilateral sensory blockade due to prevertebral spread[6] to the contralateral sympathetic chain, which is more anteriorly placed in the TPVS and more susceptible to local anesthetic agents. This may be one explanation for bilateral Horner's syndrome reported after unilateral TPVB.[11]

Ipsilateral lumbar spinal nerves also are occasionally involved after a lower thoracic paravertebral injection.[2,14] This has also been our experience,[16] and we have also observed ipsilateral radiological spread of contrast below the diaphragm.[16] Saito and colleagues have shown in a group of volunteers that single-injection TPVB at T11 using 22 mL of local anesthetic produced mean loss of sensation to pin-prick of 6 (8 to 13) segment and extended from T5 to L5 segments.[30] Saito and colleagues have also demonstrated ipsilateral thoracolumbar spread of colored dye in cadavers.[15] These observations challenge the concept of lumbar nerve root sparing following TPVB.[13]

THORACIC PARAVERTEBRAL BLOCK—ANATOMICAL LANDMARK BASED TECHNIQUES

There are several different techniques for TPVB, and it can be performed with the patient in the sitting, lateral decubitus (with the side to be blocked uppermost), or prone position.[1] The two most commonly used techniques for TPVB involve eliciting "loss of resistance"[17] or advancing the block needle by a fixed predetermined distance[31] after the transverse process is located. At the appropriate dermatome and under strict aseptic precautions, a 22-G Tuohy needle (for a single-shot injection) or an 18 or 16-G Tuohy needle (if a catheter is to be inserted) is introduced 2.5 cm lateral to the highest point of the spinous process and advanced perpendicular to the skin in all planes until the transverse process is contacted. For safety, it is imperative to locate the transverse process before the needle is advanced any further to avoid deep needle insertion and possible inadvertent pleural puncture. Once the transverse process is located, the needle is withdrawn to the subcutaneous tissue and readvanced in a cephalad direction to pass through the space between the two transverse processes until loss of resistance is elicited as the needle traverses the SCTL, usually within 1.5 to 2 cm from the transverse process. Occasionally, a subtle pop may be felt. Unlike epidural space localization, the loss of resistance felt as the needle enters the TPVS is subjective and indefinite,[17,32] and is usually a small change in resistance rather than a definite give. It is the author's experience that the loss of resistance is best appreciated if one uses a glass syringe filled with air. Luyet et al.[33] have recently demonstrated the presence of a gap between the medial and lateral portions of the SCTL in cadavers, which they propose is a possible reason for not being able to elicit a loss of resistance in all cases.[33]

Alternatively, for landmark based TPVB, the block needle may also be advance by a fixed predetermined distance (1 to 2 cm) once the needle is walked off the transverse process without eliciting loss of resistance.[31] This variation has been used effectively with few complications such as pneumothorax.[31] Other techniques that have been used to perform TPVB include "the medial approach," "pressure measurement technique," "paravertebral-peridural block," "fluoroscopy guidance," and "paravertebral catheter placement under direct vision at thoracotomy."[1]

ULTRASOUND-GUIDED THORACIC PARAVERTEBRAL BLOCK

There has recently been increased interest in the use of ultrasound for peripheral nerve blocks including TPVB.[3,34–41] However, data on the use of ultrasound for TPVB are limited with only a few publications in the literature.[3,34–41]

Pusch and colleagues[41] used ultrasound to measure the distance from the skin to the transverse process and pleura in women who were scheduled to receive a single-shot TPVB at T4 for breast surgery and found a good correlation between needle insertion depth from the skin to the transverse process and that measured using ultrasound.[41] They also found a strong correlation between ultrasound-measured distance from the skin to the parietal pleura and the distance from the skin to the paravertebral space measured after needle placement.[41] Hara and colleagues[37] were the first group to describe USG TPVB (single-shot), which they successfully performed in 25 women undergoing breast surgery.[37] They performed a sagittal scan over the paravertebral area at the T4 level and were able to delineate the transverse processes, the ligaments (intertransverse and costotransverse ligaments), and the pleura; they were also able to measure the distance from the skin to these structures before block placement.[37] The block needle was inserted, under ultrasound guidance, in the short axis of the ultrasound beam (out-of-plane technique) until it contacted the transverse process. Loss of resistance to saline was then elicited by advancing the needle above the transverse process, without ultrasound guidance, and the spread of the local anesthetic injection was visualized in real time using ultrasound.[37] Hara and colleagues report observing turbulence at the level of the injection in all cases and forward displacement of the parietal pleura in four (16%) cases.[37] Since all injections resulted in successful block, these sonographic changes may be considered as objective evidence of a correct paravertebral injection during USG TPVB. Another interesting observation that Hara and colleagues made in their cohort of patients was that while they were able to delineate the parietal pleura at the T4 level in all their patients, it was not possible to do so at the T1 level in any patient.[37] The exact reason for this difference is not clear, but it may relate to the greater depth to the paravertebral space in the upper thoracic region compared to the mid-thoracic region[42] and the use of high-frequency ultrasound, which lacks penetration and thus lacks the ability to visualize structures at a depth such as the pleura. Future research should investigate if low-frequency ultrasound, which penetrates deeper into tissues, can circumvent this problem in the upper thoracic region.

Luyet and colleagues[39] performed a cadaver study in which they investigated the feasibility of performing USG TPVB and catheter placement.[39] The authors performed a sagittal scan of the paravertebral region at the mid-thoracic level (T4 to T8) using low-frequency ultrasound (2 to 5 MHz).[39] They could delineate the underlying paravertebral anatomy (transverse process, costotransverse ligament and pleura) and observed that the best views of the paravertebral anatomy were obtained with the transducer tilted slightly obliquely, that is, with the upper part of the transducer directed slightly medially in the sagittal axis.[39] An 18-G Tuohy needle was then inserted in the plane of the ultrasound beam (in-plane technique) and advanced under ultrasound guidance to the TPVS. Correct position of the needle in the paravertebral space was confirmed by injecting saline and observing distension of the paravertebral space,[39] similar to that reported by Hara and colleagues.[37] A catheter was then inserted through the Tuohy needle, and 10 mL of a dilute contrast medium was injected via the catheter, after which axial computed tomography (CT) scans of the thoracic spine was performed. The catheter itself could not be visualized, and various types of contrast spread were noted on the CT scans: paravertebral, epidural (only), intercostal, prevertebral, and pleural.[39] The incidence of pleural puncture (5%) with the ultrasound (US) technique described[39] appears to be higher than that reported after landmark-based techniques (pleural puncture 1.1%).[24] However, this was a cadaver study, and the results may not translate into clinical practice. Further clinical research evaluating the technique of USG paravertebral catheter placement as described by Luyet and colleagues[39] is warranted.

Shibata and colleagues,[34] Ben-Ari and colleagues,[35] and Renes and colleagues[40] describe an intercostal approach to the paravertebral space. While there are minor differences in the three approaches,[34,35,40] it essentially involves performing a transverse scan of the paravertebral region using a high-frequency linear[34,35] or a low-frequency curved array[40] transducer at the desired level and advancing the block needle from a lateral to medial direction in the plane of the ultrasound beam[34,35,40] until the tip of the block needle is confirmed to be in the apex of the TPVS.[34,35,40] On a transverse sonogram, the apex of the TPVS is identified as a wedge-shaped hypoechoic space between the hyperechoic parietal pleura anteriorly and the internal intercostal membrane posteriorly and is continuous laterally with the posterior intercostal space.[34] Therefore, local anesthetic injected into the posterior intercostal space can spread medially to the TPVS. A correct injection is confirmed by observing anterior displacement of the parietal pleura and widening of the apex of the TPVS.[35,40] Shibata and colleagues[34] suggest that since the block needle is inserted tangential to the pleura, this technique should reduce the risk of pleural puncture. However, since the block needle is advanced in the direction of the intervertebral foramen, there is need for larger clinical trials to determine the incidence of complications after a TPVB since complications appear to be more common with medially directed needle.

O'Riain and colleagues[43] in a cadaver and clinical study describe an in-plane technique of performing USG TPVB. A high-frequency linear transducer (10 to 5 MHz) was positioned at a point 2.5 cm lateral to the tip of the spinous process in the longitudinal axis, producing a paramedian sagittal scan of the TPVS.[43] The authors describe the contiguous transverse processes as two dark lines.[43] The parietal pleura was deep to the transverse process and also seen as a hyperechoic structure that moved with respiration.[43] The SCTL was less well defined, but it was seen as a collection of linear echogenic bands interspersed with hypoechoic areas between two contiguous transverse processes.[43] The TPVS was seen as a hypoechoic space between the SCTL and the parietal pleura.[43] For the block, the midpoint of the transducer was positioned midway between two contiguous transverse processes, and a Tuohy needle (18-G) was inserted in-plane and in a cephalad orientation until it traversed the SCTL.[43] Saline was injected to confirm needle position by demonstrating anterior displacement of the parietal pleura and to facilitate catheter placement.[43] The authors comment that it was difficult to track the tip of the advancing needle, which they attribute to the acute angle of needle insertion.[43] Nevertheless, they were able to successfully place a paravertebral catheter in 8 of the 10 attempts in the cadavers, and all patients in the clinical study ($n = 9$) had evidence of thoracic wall anesthesia and provided postoperative analgesia.[43]

Marhofer and colleagues[36] have described a lateral USG TPVB in a cohort of 20 patients undergoing breast cancer surgery under light general anesthesia.[36] They performed a transverse scan of the thoracic paravertebral region using a high-frequency (15 to 6 MHz) linear array transducer at the T3 and T6 vertebral level. They were able to identify the internal intercostal membrane, transverse process, and pleura in all cases. A 22-G facette tip needle was inserted in real time using an out-of-plane technique.[36] Once the tip of the needle was in the paravertebral space, between the internal intercostal membrane and the pleura, local anesthetic was injected, which resulted in anterior displacement of the pleura.[36]

SONOANATOMY RELEVANT FOR THORACIC PARAVERTEBRAL BLOCK

BASIC CONSIDERATIONS

An ultrasound scan for TPVB can be performed in the transverse (axial scan) or longitudinal (sagittal scan) axis and with the patient in the sitting, lateral decubitus, or prone position. The prone position is preferable in patients presenting for a chronic pain procedure when fluoroscopy may also be used in conjunction with ultrasound imaging. Currently, there are no data demonstrating an optimal axis for the scan or the intervention. It is often a matter of individual preference and experience. The transducer used for the ultrasound scan depends on the body habitus of the patient. High-frequency ultrasound provides better resolution than low-frequency ultrasound, but its penetration is poor. Moreover, if an operator has to scan at a depth using high-frequency ultrasound, then the field of view is compromised. Under such circumstances, it may be preferable to use a low-frequency ultrasound transducer (2 to 5 MHz) with a divergent beam and a wide field of view. Published data suggests that a high-frequency linear transducer (13 to 6 MHz) is most frequently used for scanning the thoracic paravertebral region.[34–37] This may be because the transverse process, costotransverse ligament, and the pleura in the mid-thoracic region are located at a relatively shallow depth and lend to ideal conditions for imaging with a high-frequency linear array transducer. We have been using a low-frequency curved array transducer (2 to 5 MHz) to perform the transverse scan of the thoracic paravertebral region and guide the block needle with high success rates (details below).

TRANSVERSE SCAN OF THE THORACIC PARAVERTEBRAL REGION

For a transverse scan of the thoracic paravertebral region, a high-frequency linear array transducer is positioned lateral to the thoracic spinous process at the target level with the orientation marker directed laterally (Fig. 61.6). On a transverse sonogram, the paraspinal muscles are clearly delineated and lie superficial to the transverse process (Figs. 61.7 and 61.8). The transverse process is seen as a hyperechoic structure, anterior to which there is a dark acoustic shadow that completely obscures the TPVS (see Figs. 61.7 and 61.8).

Lateral to the transverse process, the hyperechoic pleura moves with respiration and exhibits the typical "lung sliding,"[44] which is the sonographic appearance of the pleural surfaces moving relative to each other within the thorax. Comet tail artifacts, which are reverberation artifacts, also may be seen deep to the pleura and within the lung tissue and are often synchronous with respiration.[44] A hypoechoic space also is seen between the parietal pleura and the internal intercostal membrane (see Fig. 61.7), which is the medial extension of the internal intercostal muscle and is continuous medially with the SCTL (see Fig. 61.4). This hypoechoic space represents the medial limit of the posterior intercostal space or the apex of the TPVS (see Fig. 61.4), and the two spaces communicate with each other (see Fig. 61.7).

Local anesthetic injected medially into the TPVS can often be seen to spread laterally to distend the posterior intercostal space, or vice versa, that is, local anesthetic injected laterally into the

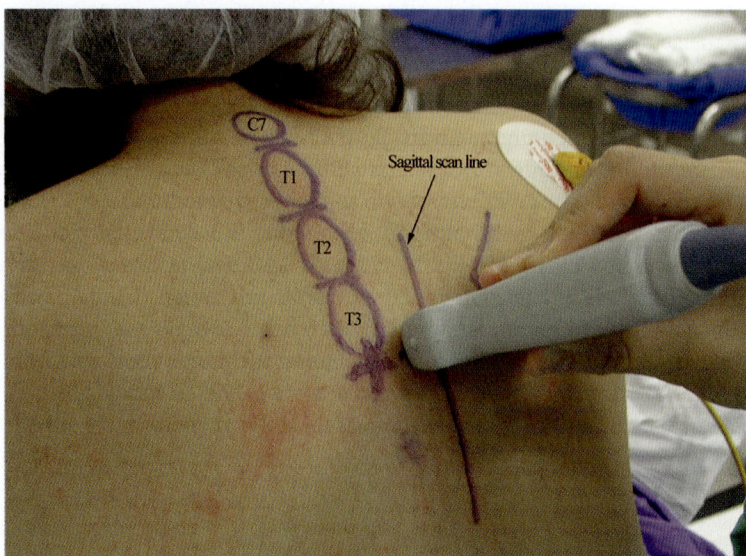

FIGURE 61.6 Transverse ultrasound scan of the thoracic paravertebral region with the patient in the sitting position. Note the position of the ultrasound transducer relative to the spine.

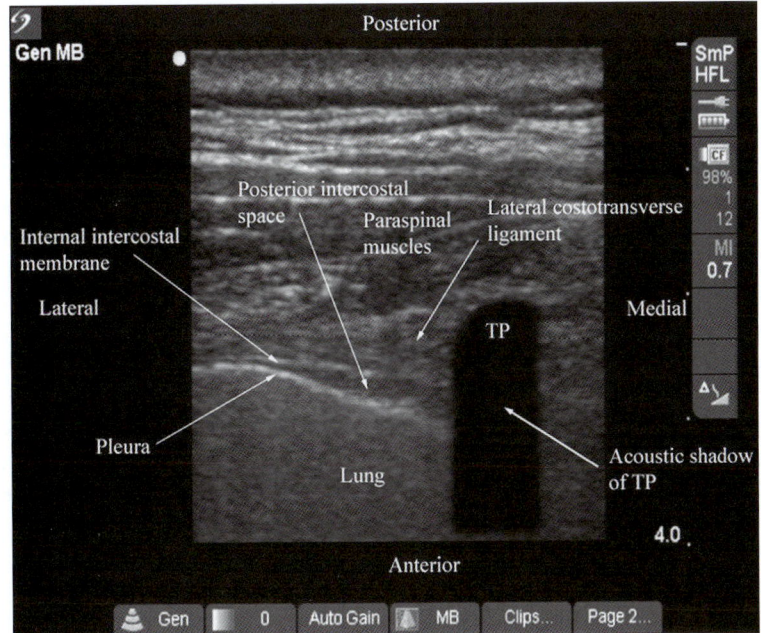

FIGURE 61.7 Transverse sonogram of the thoracic paravertebral region with the ultrasound beam being insonated over the transverse process. Note how the acoustic shadow of the transverse process *(TP)* obscures the thoracic paravertebral space (TPVS). The hypoechoic space between the parietal pleura and the lateral costotransverse ligament and internal intercostal membrane laterally represents the apex of the TPVS or the medial limit of the posterior intercostal space.

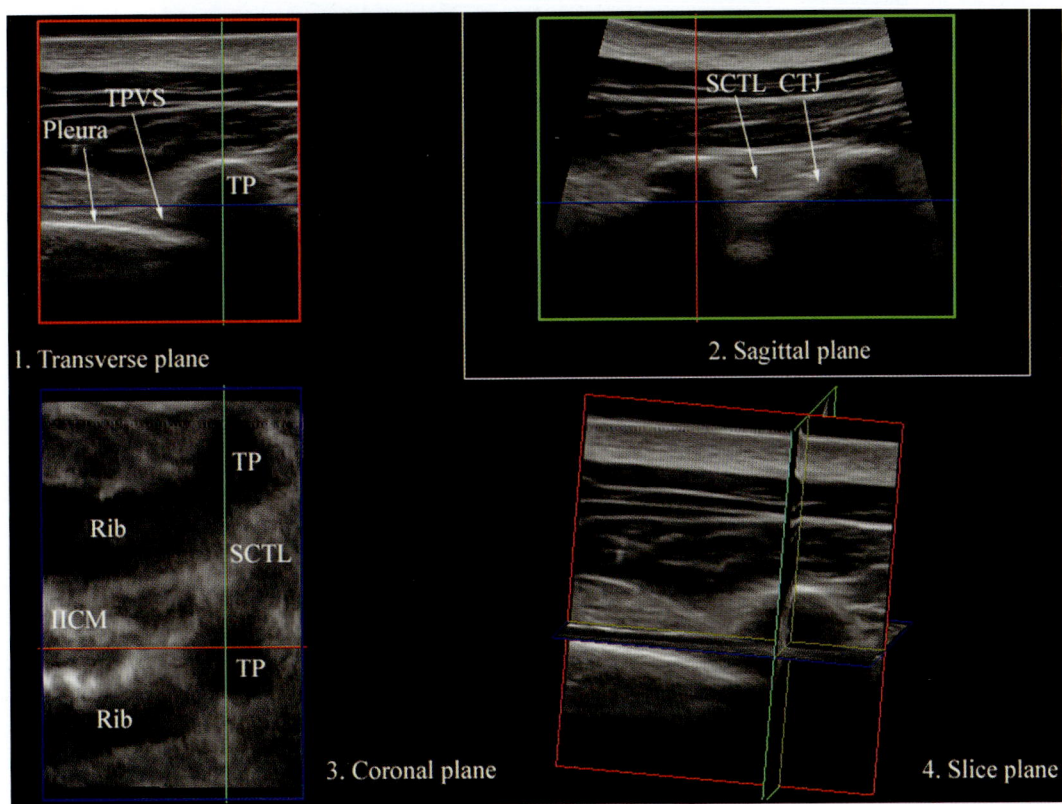

FIGURE 61.8 A multiplanar three-dimensional ultrasound view of the thoracic paravertebral region with the reference marker or "marker dot" placed over the transverse process *(TP)*. Note how the three slice planes (*red*—transverse, *green*—sagittal, and *blue*—coronal) have been obtained and how the superior costotransverse ligament *(SCTL)* is continuous with the internal intercostal membrane *(IICM)* laterally in the coronal plane. *CTJ,* Costotransverse junction; *TPVS,* thoracic paravertebral space.

posterior intercostal space can spread medially to the paravertebral space. The latter is the anatomical basis for the intercostal approach for USG TPVB (see below, *technique 3*).[34,35] The SCTL that forms the posterior border of the TPVS is also visible, and it blends laterally with the internal intercostal membrane, which forms the posterior border of the posterior intercostal space (see Figs. 61.7 and 61.8). The communication between the TPVS and the posterior intercostal space also is clearly seen (see Figs. 61.7 and 61.8).

We have recently evaluated the use a low-frequency (2 to 5 MHz) curved array transducer to perform a transverse scan of the thoracic paravertebral region and USG TPVB (*data to be published*). To the best of our knowledge, there are limited published data describing the use of a low-frequency ultrasound transducer for USG TPVB, and there are no published data describing the detailed sonoanatomy of the thoracic paravertebral region using a low-frequency curved array transducer. Our preliminary experience is that satisfactory ultrasound images of the paravertebral region are obtained using a low-frequency transducer. The wide field of view produced by the divergent ultrasound beam is an added advantage when compared to the narrow rectangular field of view produced by a linear array transducer during USG TPVB. Using a curved array transducer, the transverse scan can be performed with the ultrasound beam being insonated at four different contiguous locations (Fig. 61.9): (1) midline over the spinous process, (2) at the level of the rib and costotransverse articulation, (3) at the level of the transverse process, and (4) at the level of the articular process.

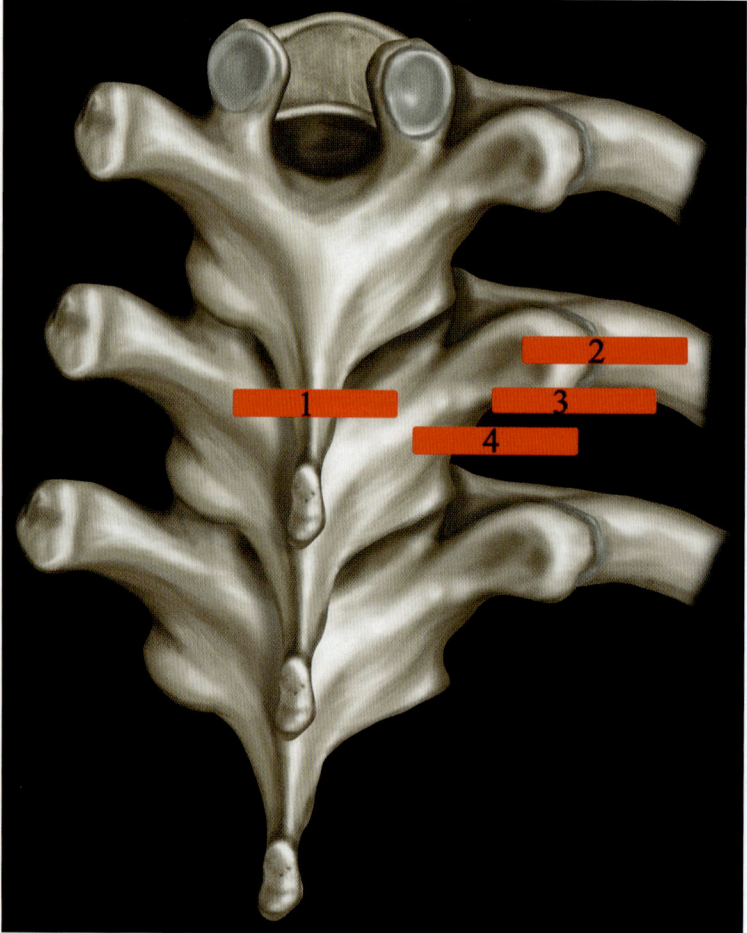

FIGURE 61.9 The thoracic spine and the various sites at which the transverse scans are performed using a low-frequency curved array transducer. Position 1—midline over the spinous process, position 2—at the level of the transverse process and rib, position 3—at the level of the transverse process, and position 4—at the level of the inferior articular process.

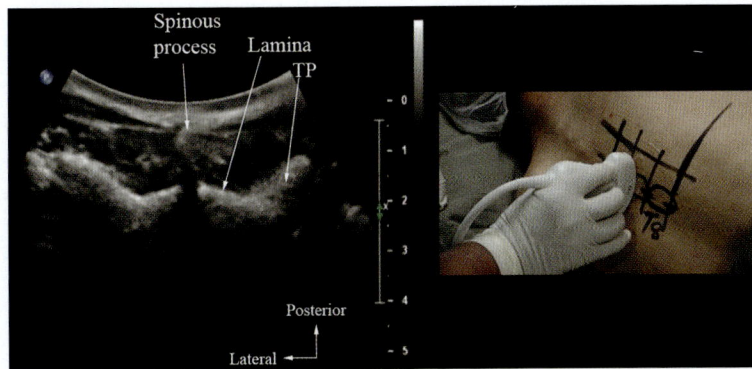

FIGURE 61.10 Midline transverse scan of the thoracic spine using a low-frequency curved array transducer with the ultrasound beam being insonated over the spinous process (position 1). Note the hyperechoic spinous process (SP) with its acoustic shadow in the midline. The hyperechoic lamina and the posteriorly directed transverse process *(TP)* are seen laterally on either side of the midline. The acoustic shadow of the SP, TP and the lamina completely obscure the spinal canal and the paravertebral space. The hyperechoic pleura is visible lateral to the TP.

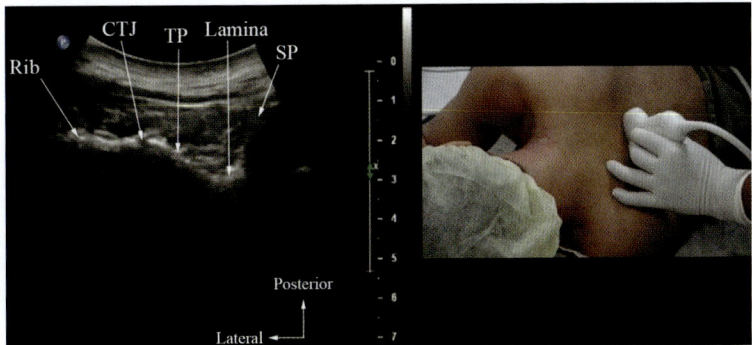

FIGURE 61.11 Paramedian transverse scan of the right thoracic paravertebral region using a curved array transducer and with the ultrasound beam being insonated over the transverse process *(TP)* and rib (position 2). Note the large acoustic shadow produced by the lamina, transverse process and rib, the posteriorly directed TP, and the costotransverse junction *(CTJ)*. *SP*, Spinous process.

Each of these four ultrasound scan windows produces a very distinct sonogram reflecting the different osseous and musculoskeletal structures that are visualized in the sonograms. On a transverse sonogram in the midline (**position 1**), the spinous process is visualized as an echogenic dot with a corresponding acoustic shadow anteriorly (Fig. 61.10). Due to the steep caudal angulation of the spinous process in the mid-thoracic region (see Fig. 61.9), the spinous process that is visualized on the sonogram caused from the vertebra is higher than the visualizations caused by the transverse, lamina, and the articular processes. Since the spinous process and transverse process cast a large acoustic shadow, visualization of the paravertebral anatomy is limited with this ultrasound scan window.

With the transducer positioned slightly laterally (**position 2**, see Fig. 61.9), the echogenic outlines of the lamina, transverse process, and the rib with their corresponding acoustic shadows are clearly delineated (Figs. 61.11 and 61.12). However, unlike the transverse process of the lumbar vertebra, which are more or less at right angles to the vertebral body, the transverse processes in the thoracic spine are directed posteriorly (Figs. 61.13 and 61.14), and this posterior angulation can be clearly delineated in the transverse sonogram (see Fig. 61.12). Once the transverse process, costotransverse articulation, and the rib are identified, one can gently slide the transducer caudally until the acoustic shadow of the rib is no longer visualized (**position 3**, see Fig. 61.9) and the echogenic outline of the lamina and transverse process with their acoustic shadow are seen (Fig.

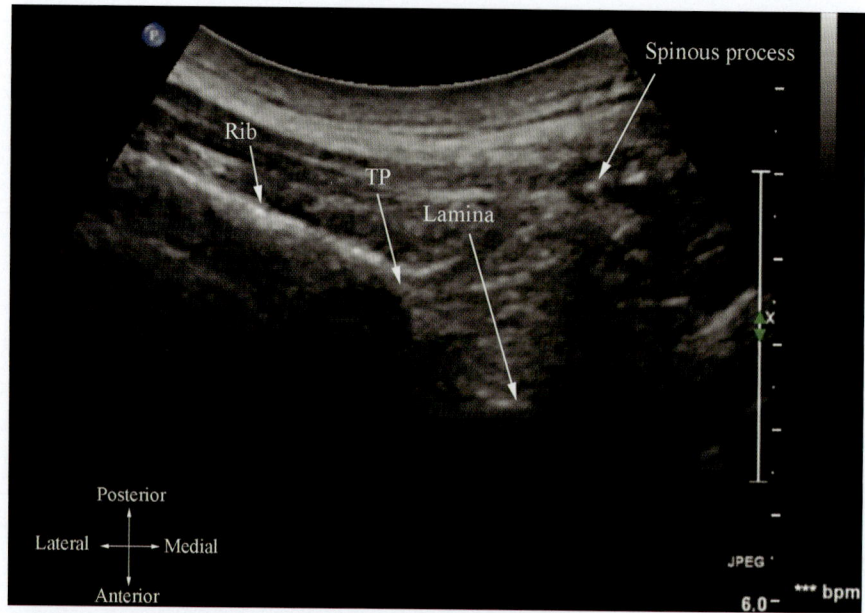

FIGURE 61.12 Paramedian transverse scan (zoomed view) of the right thoracic paravertebral region using a low-frequency curved array transducer with the ultrasound beam being insonated over the transverse process *(TP)* and the rib (position 2). Note how the acoustic shadow of the TP and rib completely obscures the underlying paravertebral anatomy.

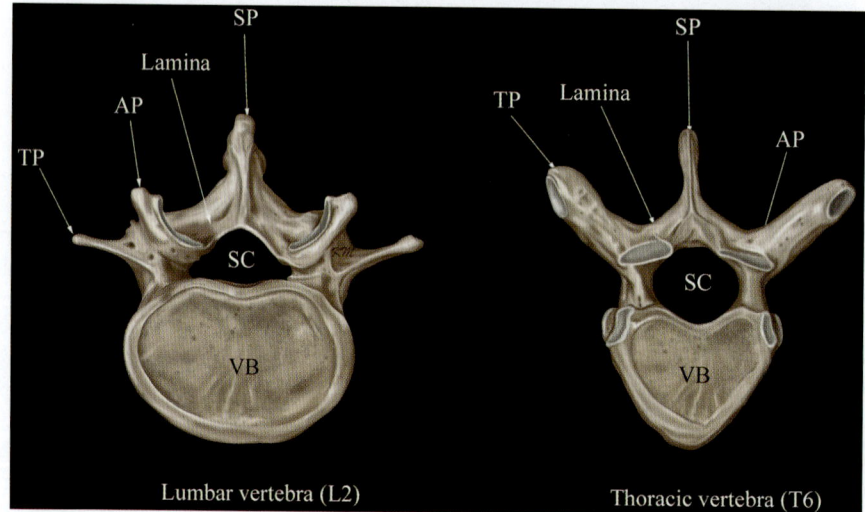

FIGURE 61.13 Figure showing the differences in the size, shape, and orientation of the transverse process *(TP)* of a thoracic and lumbar vertebra. Note how the TP of a thoracic vertebra is directed posteriorly. *AP,* Articular process; *SC,* spinal canal; *SP,* spinous process; *VB,* vertebral body.

61.15). Lateral to the transverse process, the echogenic pleura and lung is visualized anteriorly, the thick echogenic SCTL is visualized posteriorly, and the hypoechoic apical part of the paravertebral space is interposed between the two (Fig. 61.16). Finally, if one now slides or gently tilts the transducer slightly caudally (**position 4**, see Fig. 61.9), the ultrasound beam is insonated at the level of the inferior articular process (Figs. 61.17–61.20). The acoustic shadow of the lamina and transverse process disappears, and the echogenic inferior articular process (Fig. 61.21) with its acoustic shadow is now seen medially (Fig. 61.22). As in the scan at the level of the transverse process (see Fig. 61.16), the SCTL, parietal pleura, lung, and the apical part of the paravertebral space are also clearly delineated. However, the area of the acoustic shadow at the level of the articular process is significantly less than that at the level of the transverse process (see Fig. 61.22).

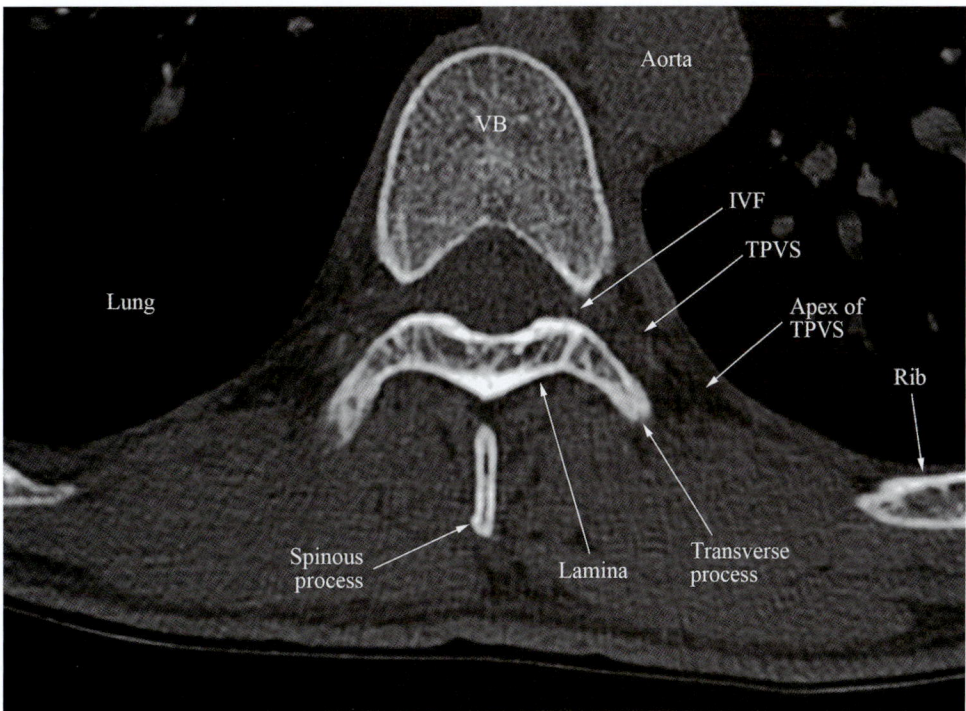

FIGURE 61.14 Transverse CT of the thoracic spine showing the anatomical relationship of the vertebral body *(VB)* and transverse process to the thoracic paravertebral space *(TPVS)*. *IVF*, Intervertebral foramen.

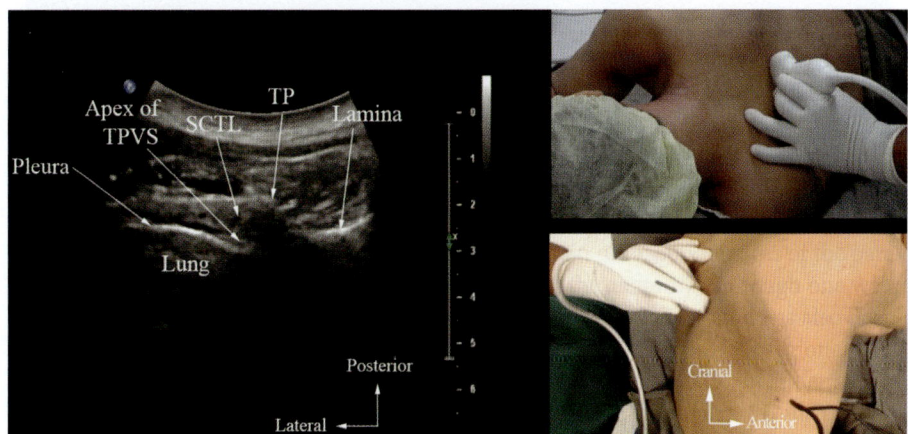

FIGURE 61.15 Paramedian transverse scan of the right thoracic paravertebral region using a low-frequency curved array transducer with the ultrasound beam being insonated at the level of the transverse process *(TP*, position 3). Inset images illustrate the position and orientation of the ultrasound transducer. *SCTL*, Superior costotransverse ligament; *TPVS*, thoracic paravertebral space.

This may make the transverse ultrasound scan window at the level of the articular process more suitable for ultrasound imaging during an USG TPVB. Currently there are no published data describing the use of a transverse scan at the level of the articular process for USG TPVB. We have successfully performed over the last 4 to 5 years a few thousand individual paravertebral injections using this approach and with no major complications. Consequently, it is our ultrasound scan window of choice for USG TPVB.

SAGITTAL SCAN OF THE THORACIC PARAVERTEBRAL REGION

Published data on sagittal sonography of the thoracic paravertebral region in the clinical setting are limited and have been described with the use of a high-frequency linear array transducer.[37,43]

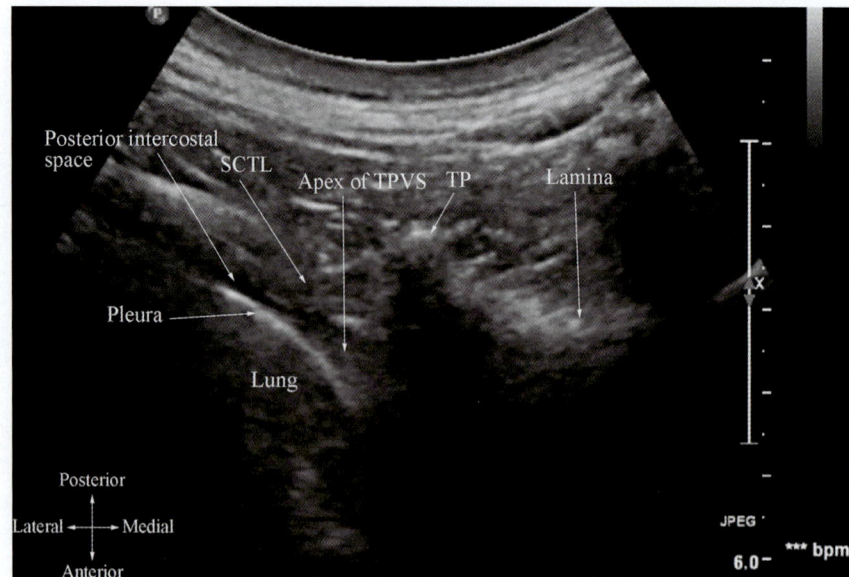

FIGURE 61.16 Paramedian transverse sonogram of the right thoracic paravertebral region (zoomed view) from the level of the transverse process (*TP*, position 3). Note the hyperechoic TP and its acoustic shadow. The apex of the thoracic paravertebral space *(TPVS)*, parietal pleura, and the superior costotransverse ligament *(SCTL)* are seen lateral to the TP.

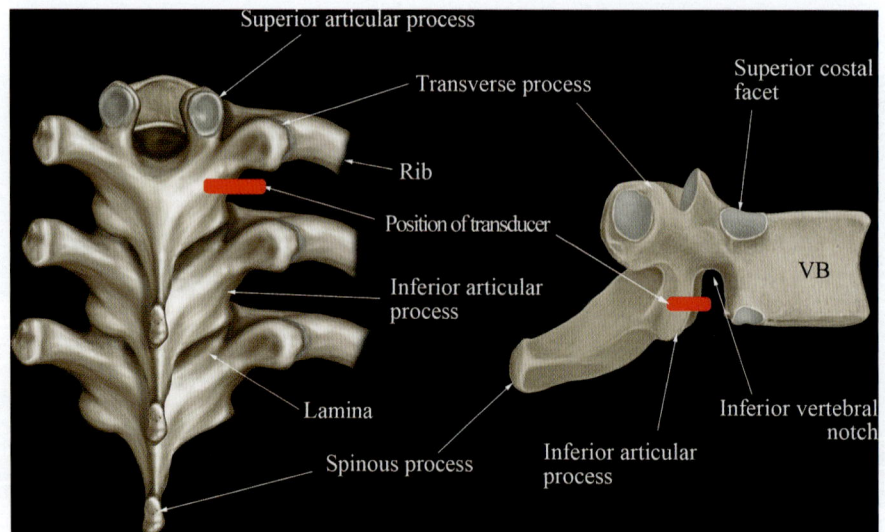

FIGURE 61.17 The osseous structures that are insonated during a transverse ultrasound scan of the thoracic paravertebral region through the inter-transverse space and at the level of the inferior articular process. Note the relationship of the inferior articular process to the inferior vertebral notch and the intervertebral foramen. *VB*, Vertebral body.

During a sagittal scan of the thoracic paravertebral region, the ultrasound transducer is positioned 2 to 3 cm lateral to the midline (paramedian) with its orientation marker directed cranially (Fig. 61.23). On a sagittal sonogram, the transverse processes are seen as hyperechoeic and rounded structures deep to the paraspinal muscles, and they cast an acoustic shadow anteriorly (Fig. 61.24). Between the acoustic shadows of two adjacent transverse processes there is an acoustic window produced by reflections from the SCTL and intertransverse ligaments, the paravertebral space and its contents, the parietal pleura, and lung tissue (in a posterior to anterior direction) (see Fig. 61.24).

We have observed that the pleura and the paravertebral space are not clearly delineated in a true sagittal scan (see Fig. 61.24), which may be due to the loss of spatial resolution at the depth

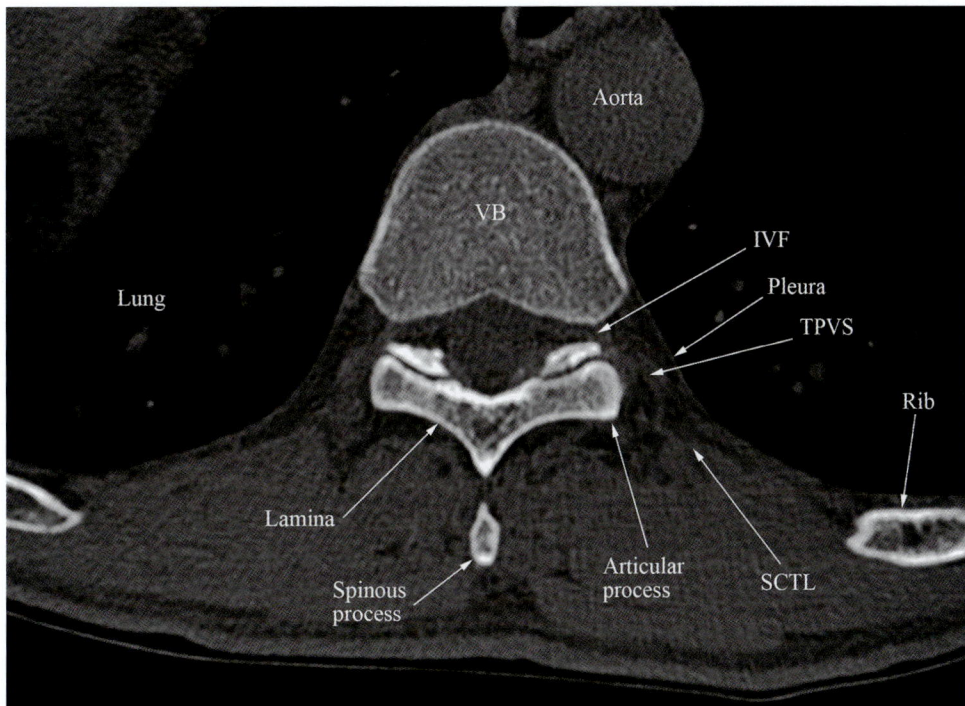

FIGURE 61.18 Transverse computed tomography of the thoracic spine showing the anatomical relationship of the inferior articular process of the vertebra to the intervertebral foramen and the thoracic paravertebral space (TPVS). *IVF*, Intervertebral foramen; *SCTL*, superior costotransverse ligament; *VB*, vertebral body.

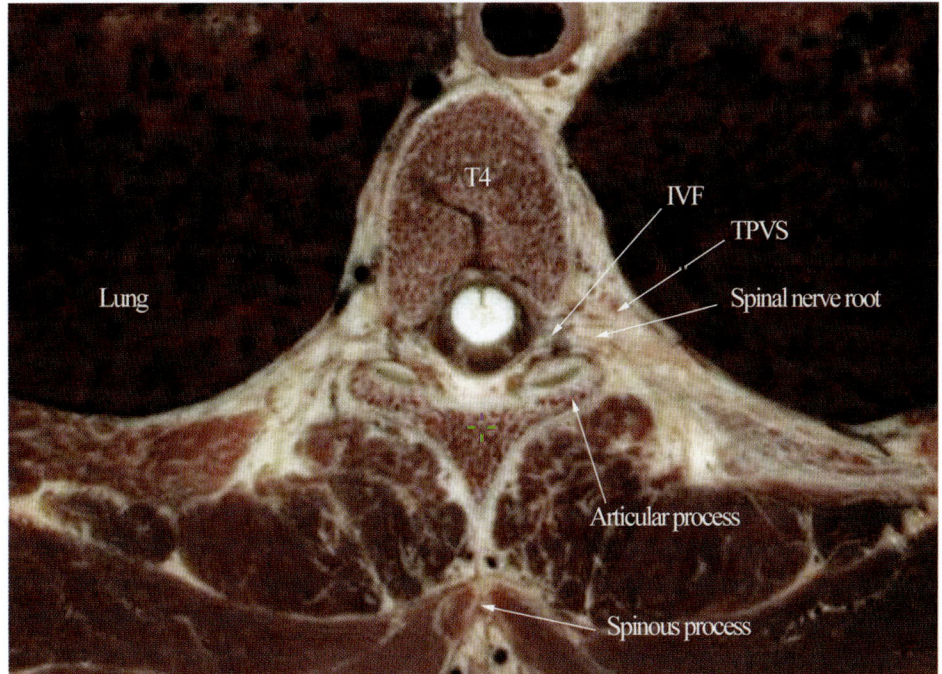

FIGURE 61.19 Cross-sectional cadaver anatomic section of the thoracic spine through the T4 vertebral body and inferior articular process of the vertebra corresponding to the level at which the transverse scan is performed at the level of the articular process (position 4 in Fig. 61.9). Note the position of the intervertebral foramen (*IVF*) relative to the inferior articular process and the spinal nerve root as it exits the IVF. *TPVS*, Thoracic paravertebral space.

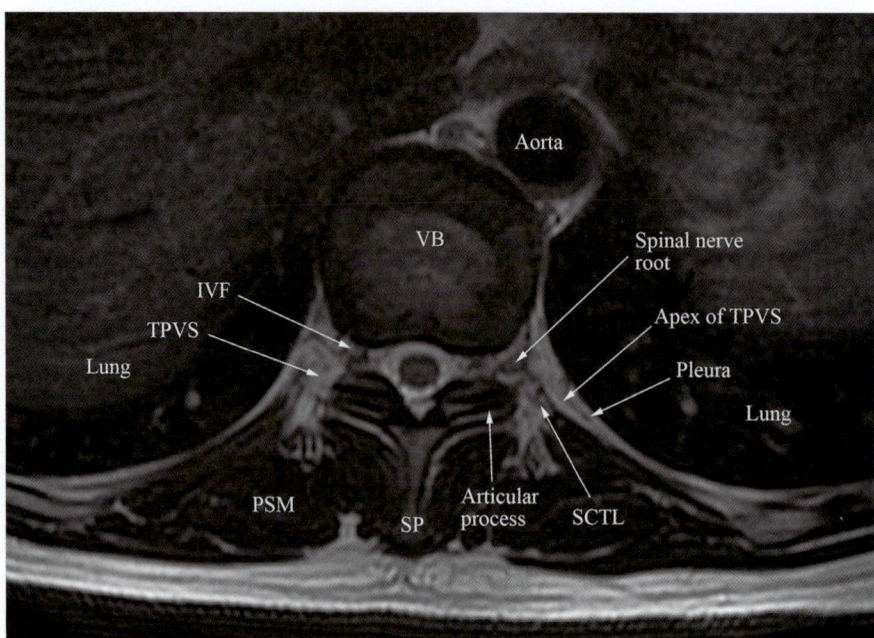

FIGURE 61.20 Transverse T1-weighted magnetic resonance imaging (MRI) of the thoracic spine showing the anatomical relationship of the inferior articular process of the vertebra to the intervertebral foramen *(IVF)* and the thoracic paravertebral space *(TPVS)*. Note the spinal nerve root as it exits the IVF. *PSM*, Paraspinal muscles; *SCTL*, superior costotransverse ligament; *SP*, spinous process; *VB*, vertebral body.

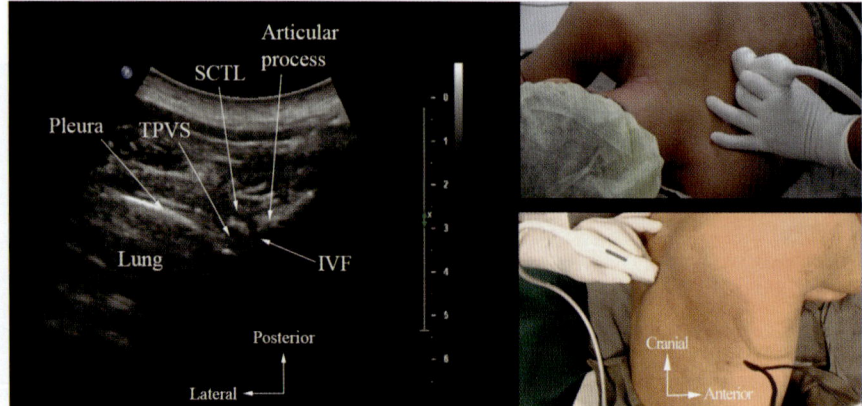

FIGURE 61.21 Paramedian transverse scan of the right thoracic paravertebral region using a low-frequency curved array transducer with the ultrasound beam being insonated through the intertransverse space, that is, between two adjoining thoracic transverse processes, and at the level of the articular process (position 4). Inset images illustrate the position and orientation of the ultrasound transducer. *IVF*, Intervertebral foramen; *SCTL*, Superior costotransverse ligament; *TPVS*, thoracic paravertebral space.

or due to "anisotropy," because the ultrasound beam is not at right angles to the pleura due to its anteromedial reflection close to the vertebral bodies (see Fig. 61.1). It is also our observation that the ultrasound visibility of the transverse process, SCTL, TPVS, and the pleura are better when the ultrasound beam is insonated with a slightly outward tilt (oblique axis) (Fig. 61.25). We believe this is due to the ultrasound beam being at right angles to the pleura, which reduces anisotropy.

It is difficult to define an optimal angle of lateral tilt for the paramedian sagittal oblique scan, but in clinical practice, we recommend that one should gently tilt the transducer outward (laterally)

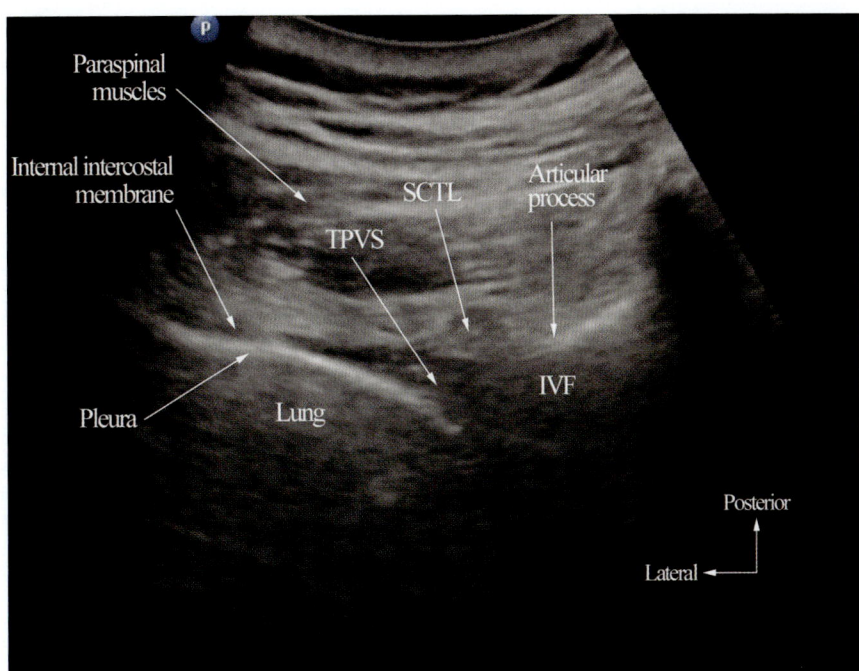

FIGURE 61.22 Paramedian transverse sonogram of the right thoracic paravertebral region (zoomed view) with the ultrasound beam being insonated through the intertransverse space, that is, between two adjoining thoracic transverse processes, and at the level of the articular process (position 4). Note the hyperechoic inferior articular process and its acoustic shadow medially, which obscures the underlying intervertebral foramen *(IVF)*. As with the paramedian transverse scan at position 3 (refer to Fig. 61.16), the apex of the thoracic paravertebral space *(TPVS)*, parietal pleura, and the superior costotransverse ligament *(SCTL)* are visualized laterally, but the area of the acoustic shadow is minimal in this ultrasound scan window.

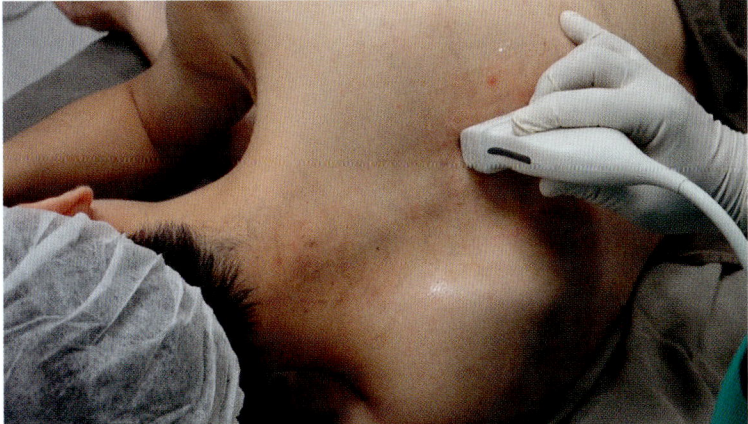

FIGURE 61.23 The position of the patient (lateral) and how the ultrasound transducer is oriented during a paramedian sagittal scan of the thoracic paravertebral region.

until the parietal pleura is clearly visualized (see Fig. 61.25). A pitfall of the lateral tilt maneuver is that one may see the same result if the ultrasound transducer is inadvertently manipulated or tilted too far laterally so that it is now insonating the rib and the posterior intercostal space (Fig. 61.26) instead of the transverse process and the apical part of the paravertebral space. The clinical implication is that one may unknowingly perform a posterior intercostal injection instead of a paravertebral injection and, depending on the approach used, the potential for pleural puncture

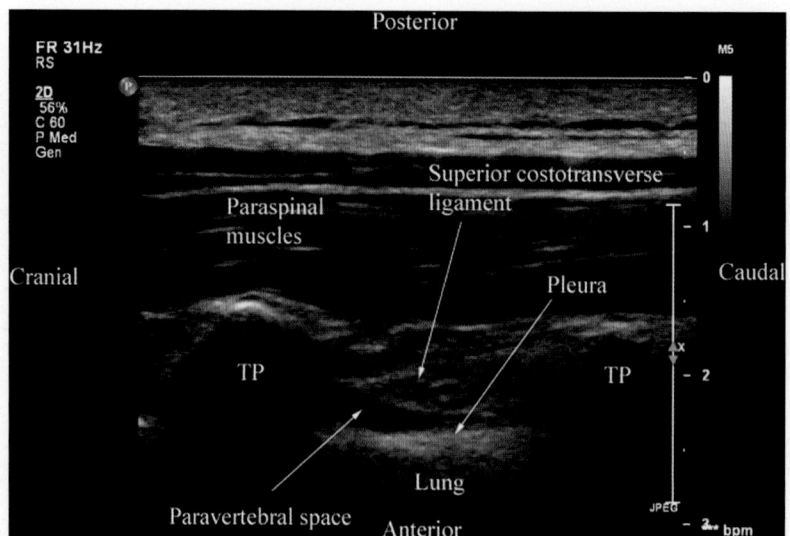

FIGURE 61.24 Paramedian sagittal sonogram of the thoracic paravertebral region. Note that although the superior costotransverse ligament, pleura, and the thoracic paravertebral space are visible, they are not clearly delineated (compare with Fig. 61.25 from the same patient). *TP*, Transverse process.

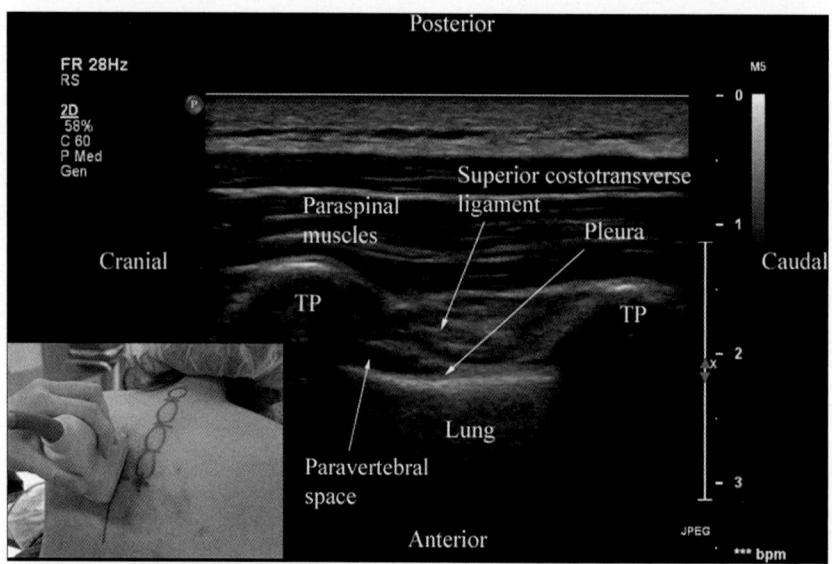

FIGURE 61.25 Paramedian sagittal oblique sonogram of the thoracic paravertebral region. The picture in the inset shows how the ultrasound transducer is tilted slightly laterally (outward) during the scan. Note the pleura, superior costotransverse ligament, and the paravertebral space are now clearly delineated (same patient as in Fig. 61.24). *TP*, Transverse process.

may be greater with the intercostal injection. Also, segmental spread of anesthesia is limited with an intercostal injection. Therefore, there is a "transition zone" (Fig. 61.27) between the rib, costotransverse junction, and the transverse process where one may misinterpret the identity of the osseous structure being visualized in the sagittal sonogram. This subtle difference in anatomy can be easily recognized in multiplanar three-dimensional (3D) images of the paravertebral region (see Figs. 61.8, 61.28, and 61.29). A sagittal slice display more clearly demonstrates the change in the sonographic pattern of the various osseous structures in the paravertebral region (see Fig. 61.29). Therefore, while performing an USG TPVB using the sagittal ultrasound scan window, it is important to differentiate the transverse process from the rib in the sagittal sonogram of the thoracic paravertebral region (see Fig. 61.27).

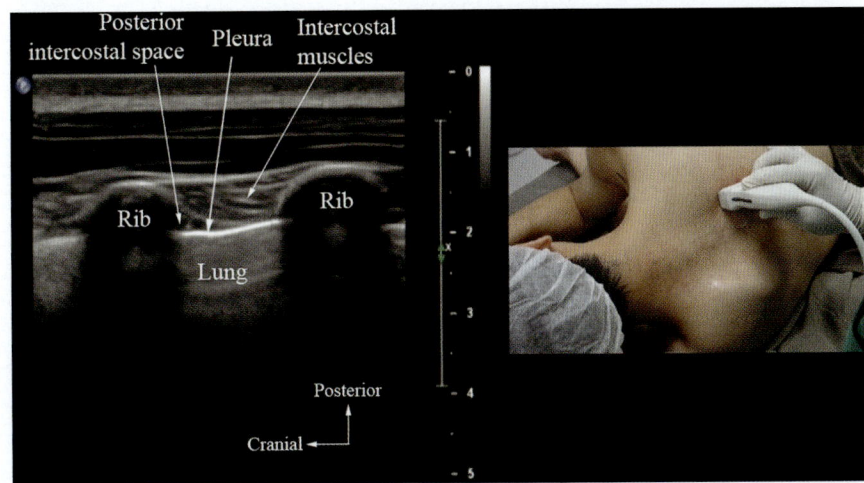

FIGURE 61.26 Paramedian sagittal oblique scan of the right mid-thoracic paravertebral region, using a high-frequency linear transducer, whereby the ribs instead of the transverse processes are being insonated. Note the pleura is also very clearly delineated in this sonogram.

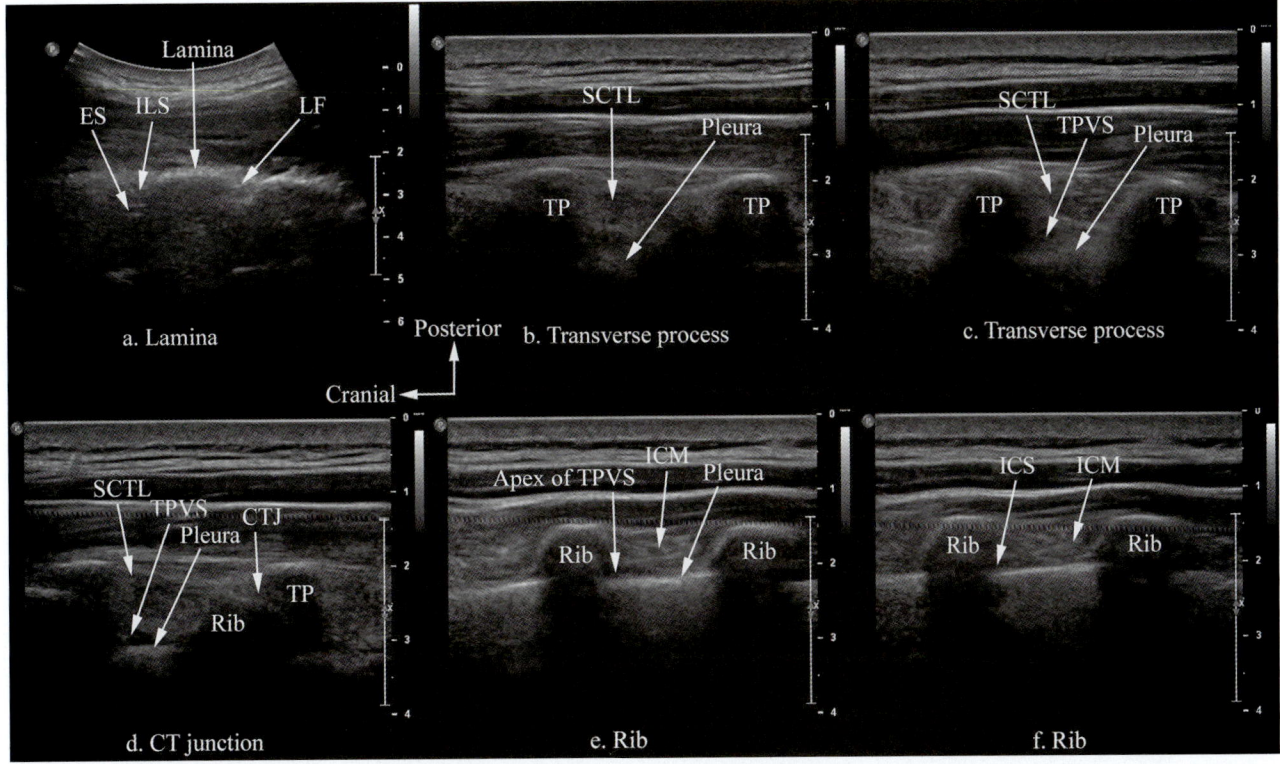

FIGURE 61.27 A sequence of sagittal sonograms of the thoracic paravertebral region (from the same subject), showing the transition of the anatomy from the level of the lamina to the ribs. Note the difference in the sonographic appearance of the lamina, transverse process (TP), and the ribs. Also note the relative depths at which each osseous structure is located. The articulation of the rib with the transverse process at the costotransverse junction (CTJ) is also clearly delineated in (D). The pleura is not clearly visualized at the level of the TP's, but it is at the level of the ribs. *ES*, Epidural space; *ICM*, intercostal muscles; *ICS*, intercostal space; *ILS*, interlaminar space; *LF*, ligamentum flavum; *SCTL*, superior costotransverse ligament; *TPVS*, thoracic paravertebral space.

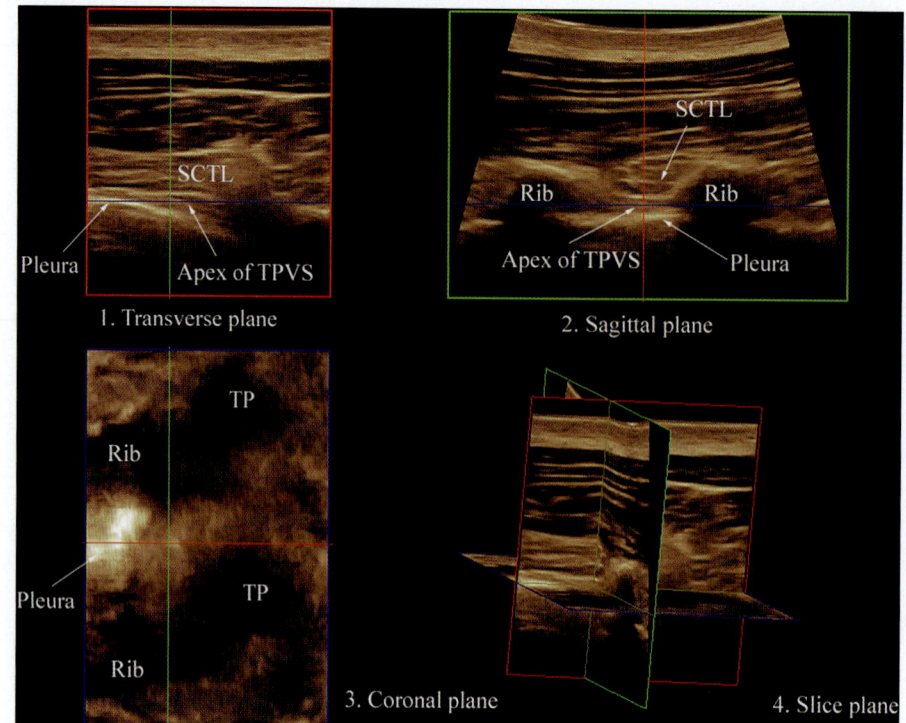

FIGURE 61.28 A multiplanar 3D ultrasound image of the thoracic paravertebral region in color (sepia tone) with the reference marker or "marker dot" placed over the apex of the thoracic paravertebral space *(TPVS)*. Note the hyperechoic pleura in the coronal plane. *SCTL,* Superior costotransverse ligament; *TP,* transverse process.

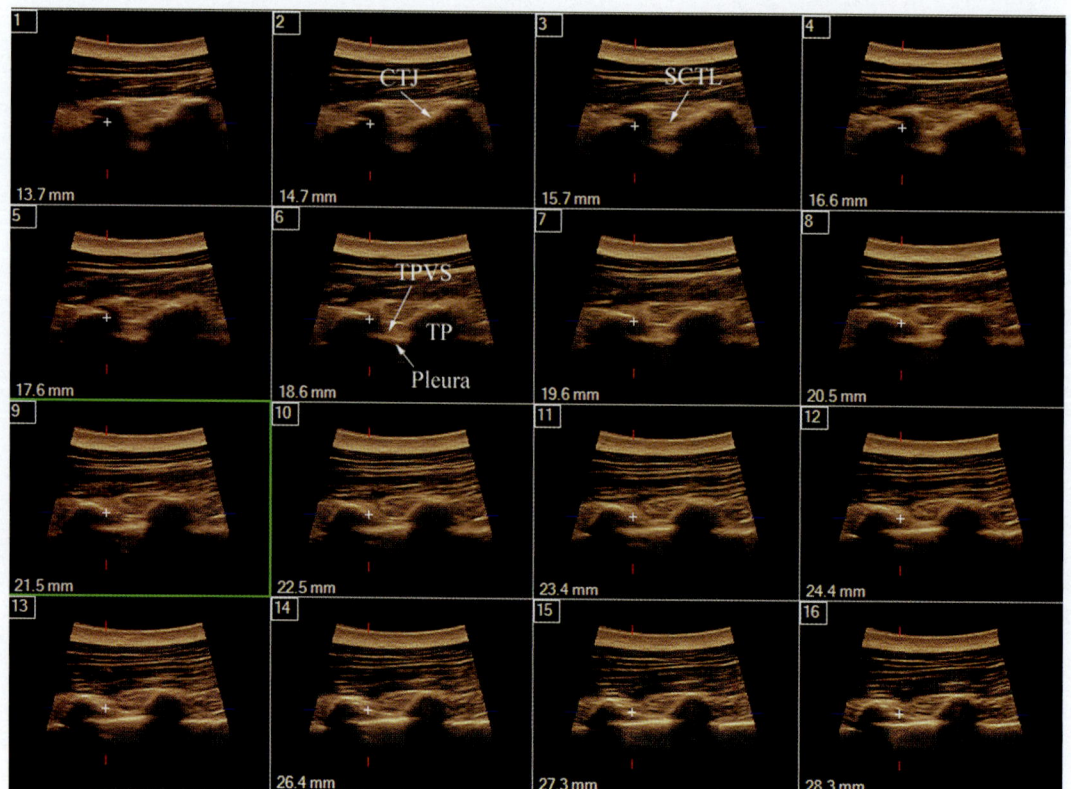

FIGURE 61.29 A sagittal iSlice display of the thoracic paravertebral region in color (sepia tone). In this figure, 16 contiguous sagittal cuts of the acquired paravertebral volume that are 1 mm apart are displayed. *CTJ,* Costotransverse junction; *SCTL,* superior costotransverse ligament; *TP,* transverse process; *TPVS,* thoracic paravertebral space.

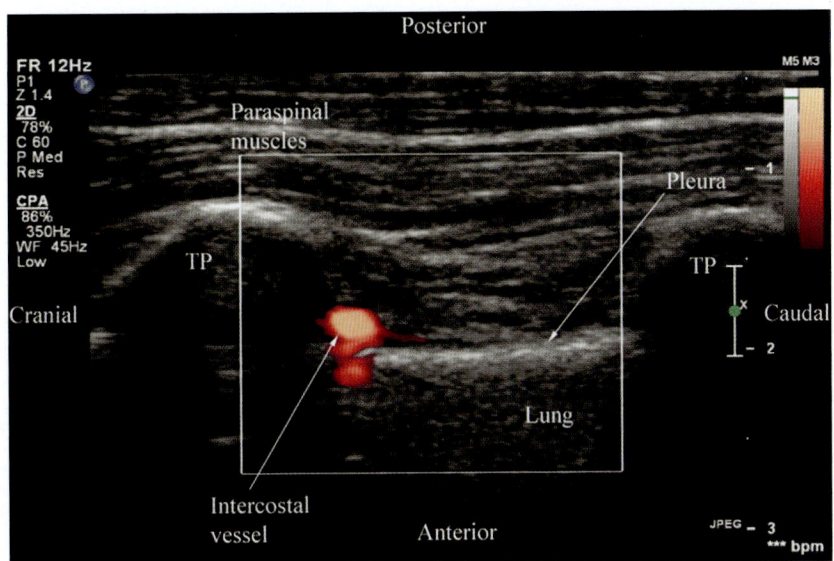

FIGURE 61.30 Paramedian sagittal oblique sonogram of the thoracic paravertebral region showing the Power Doppler signal from the intercostal artery in the paravertebral space. *TP*, Transverse process.

The intercostal vessels also are readily visualized close to the inferior border of the transverse process in a paramedian sagittal oblique scan using color or power Doppler ultrasound (Fig. 61.30), but we have not been able to delineate the intercostal nerves with current ultrasound technology.

THREE DIMENSIONAL SONOANATOMY OF THE THORACIC PARAVERTEBRAL REGION

As described, it is possible to obtain high-resolution 2D ultrasound images of the paravertebral anatomy in the transverse[34,35,37,40] and sagittal[37,43] axis. However, this requires the operator to rotate the ultrasound transducer through 90 degrees. 3D ultrasound imaging technology is currently available and allows one to simultaneously visualize the anatomy of a volume or area of interest in the transverse, sagittal, and coronal planes without having to move or rotate the transducer. Using traditional 2D ultrasound, it is not possible to obtain ultrasound images of the paravertebral anatomy in the coronal axis. The coronal view presents the anatomy as though one were looking down on to the surface being imaged, analogous to a "birds-eye view" and has also been referred to as the "plan view." The potential utility of the coronal view during USG regional anesthesia is not clear, but has been used to visualize the spread of a local anesthetic on either side of a nerve during peripheral nerve blockade. It is also feasible to perform volumetric 3D ultrasound imaging of the thoracic paravertebral region and study the acquired data set in various 3D formats.[45]

In a multiplanar view of the thoracic paravertebral volume (anatomy) it is possible to simultaneously visualize the transverse (x-axis), sagittal (y-axis), and coronal (z-axis) images of the paravertebral anatomy (see Figs. 61.8 and 61.28). Moreover, when the reference point or the "marker dot," a point where all the three orthogonal planes intersect, is moved in any of the 2D images of the multiplanar display, it automatically updates its position in the other 2D images. This allows one to navigate through or electronically dissect through the paravertebral volume, which in our experience helps in better understanding the 3D anatomy of the paravertebral region. In addition, by using the "marker dot," it is also possible to visualize a specific point or anatomical structure in all the three planes simultaneously. This feature facilitates validation of the sonographic appearance of a given anatomical structure in the paravertebral region and to exclude artifacts. The anatomical information obtained in a 3D ultrasound image is also more detailed than that seen in a 2D ultrasound. Structures such as the costotransverse junction (Fig. 61.8) and surfaces (faces) of the paravertebral volume (Fig. 61.31), which are otherwise not visualized using 2D ultrasound imaging, are clearly delineated using 3D ultrasound. One is also able to display and study the acquired data set similar to a computerized tomogram in a slice display (see Figs. 61.29 and 61.32). Overall,

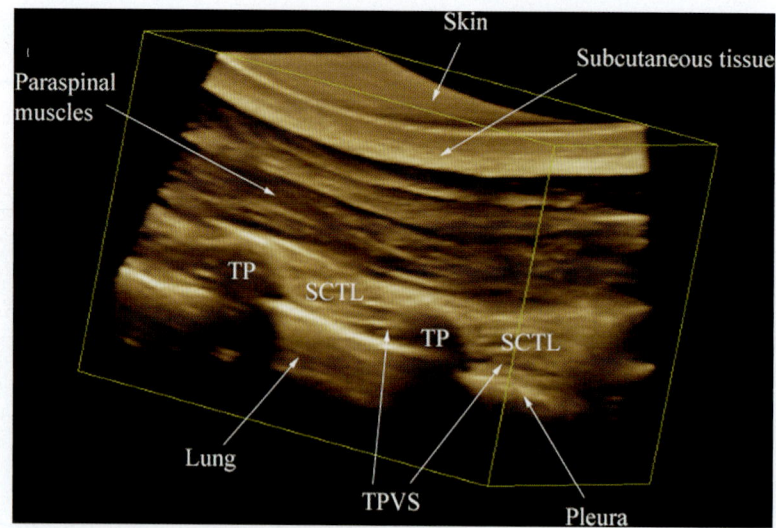

FIGURE 61.31 A rendered three-dimensional ultrasound image of the thoracic paravertebral region. The acquired paravertebral volume has been rendered such that the sagittal anatomy is being visualized from the lateral (intercostal space) side. Note the apical part of the thoracic paravertebral space *(TPVS)* is clearly delineated between the superior costotransverse ligament *(SCTL)* and the parietal pleura. *TP*, Transverse process.

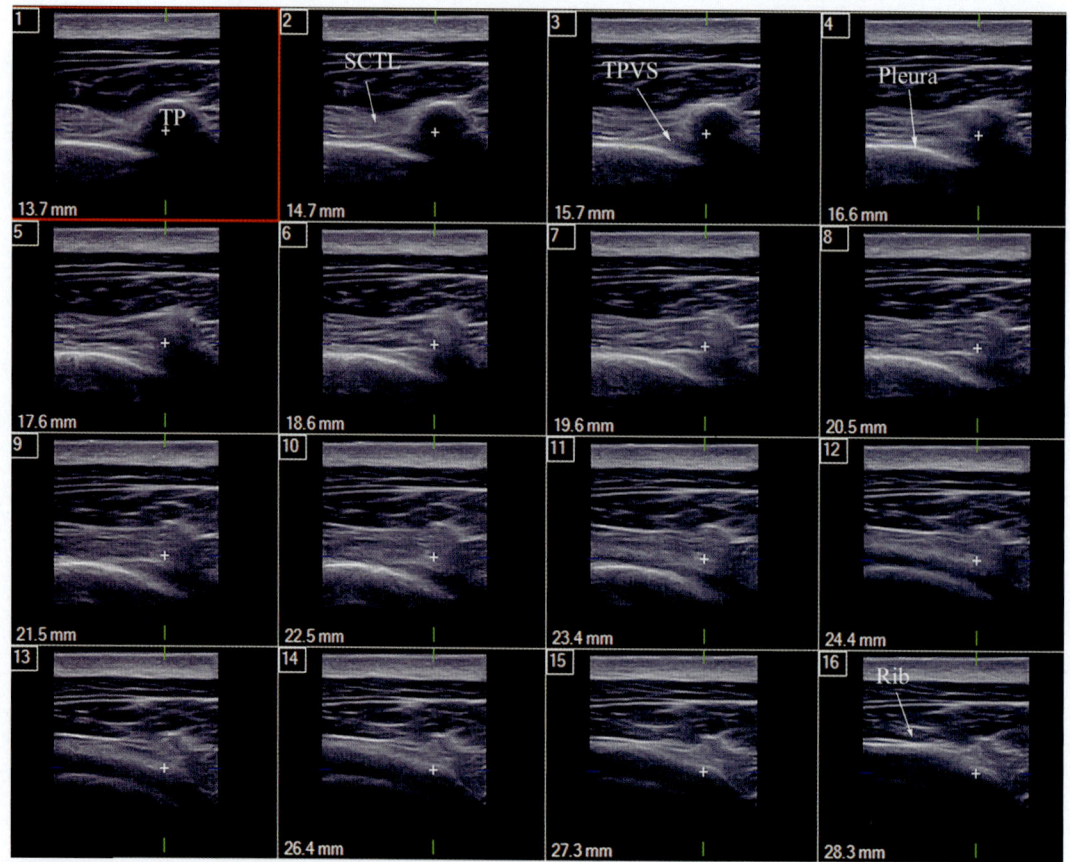

FIGURE 61.32 A transverse iSlice display of the thoracic paravertebral region in color *(blue tone)*. In this figure, 16 contiguous transverse cuts of the acquired paravertebral volume that are 1 mm apart are displayed. *SCTL*, Superior costotransverse ligament; *TP*, transverse process; *TPVS*, thoracic paravertebral space.

it is our opinion that volumetric 3D US imaging allows the anesthesiologist to develop a better spatial awareness of the paravertebral anatomy.

A current limitation of the most methods used to generate 3D images of the paravertebral anatomy is that most methods are retrospective rather than in real time. Real-time 3D imaging (also called 4D imaging), is possible today but is limited by the lack of ability of computers in the ultrasound systems to process the large volume of data. Consequently, the screen refresh rate of most 3D US systems is slower than the 2D US systems, resulting in visible pauses in the 4D image and making them unsuitable for real-time needle guidance. The integrated mechanical transducers are also bulky due to the moving parts within the casing of the transducer and thus cumbersome to handle if used for real-time needle guidance.

Smaller 2D array 3D ultrasound transducers are currently available. Such transducers have no moving mechanical parts, the ultrasound beam is electronically steered, and the transducers are also ergonomically much easier to handle. However, they operate between 2 and 6 MHz, are phased array transducers, and produce a small pyramidal shaped volume that is ideal for cardiac but not musculoskeletal imaging. Nevertheless, such transducers have been used for imaging and needle guidance in regional anesthesia. In our opinion, the quality of the 3D ultrasound images produced by the 2D array transducers in previous reports have been poor. In contrast, the high-frequency 3D 4D volume linear array transducers operate between 13 to 18 MHz, which is ideal for musculoskeletal ultrasound imaging, and produce high-resolution 3D images, as shown in Figs. 61.8, 61.28, 61.29, 61.31, and 61.32. Therefore, we believe that the role of the currently available 3D ultrasound technology in regional anesthesia will be limited to previewing and studying the anatomy of a volume of interest. In contrast, it may also be useful for visualizing the distribution and extent of spread of a local anesthetic after a paravertebral block. Offline measurements of distance, area, and volume can also be done retrospectively using the acquired data set. Future research to determine the utility of 3D ultrasound imaging for TPVB is warranted.

TECHNIQUES OF ULTRASOUND-GUIDED THORACIC PARAVERTEBRAL BLOCK

Several different techniques have been described for USG TPVB in the literature,[46] but there are no data or consensus on the most effective or safest approach for USG TPVB. Therefore, until more safety data is available, it is difficult to recommend any one technique. There are pros and cons of each approach, and they are highlighted in the following section. Overall, USG TPVB can be performed using any one of the following three different approaches described.

Transverse Scan With Short-Axis Needle Insertion (Technique 1)

In this technique, a transverse scan of the thoracic paravertebral region is performed at the desired level and at the level of the transverse process, and the block needle inserted in the short axis of the ultrasound beam (Fig. 61.33). During the scout scan, the depth to the transverse process and pleura are determined. The direction of needle insertion with this approach is similar to that with a surface anatomical landmarks based TPVB. Since the needle is inserted in the short axis, it is visualized only as a bright spot and needle tracking can be very challenging. The aim of this approach is to guide the needle to the transverse process (TP). Once the TP is contacted, the needle is withdrawn slightly and readvanced by a predetermined distance of 1.5 cm so as to pass under the transverse process into the TPVS. Alternatively, the needle can be inserted laterally into the apex of the TPVS.[36] After negative aspiration for blood or cerebrospinal fluid, the calculated dose of local anesthetic is injected in aliquots. Following the injection, it is common to see widening of the apex of the TPVS and anterior displacement of the pleura by the local anesthetic (see Fig. 61.33). The local anesthetic may also spread to the posterior intercostal space laterally. Widening of the contiguous paravertebral spaces by the injected local anesthetic can also be visualized on a sagittal scan after the injection.

Paramedian Sagittal Scan With in-Plane Needle Insertion (Technique 2)

In this approach, a paramedian sagittal oblique scan is performed as described in technique 1 (see Fig. 61.25), and the block needle is inserted in the plane of the ultrasound beam (Fig. 61.34). It is our experience that although the block needle is inserted in the plane of the ultrasound

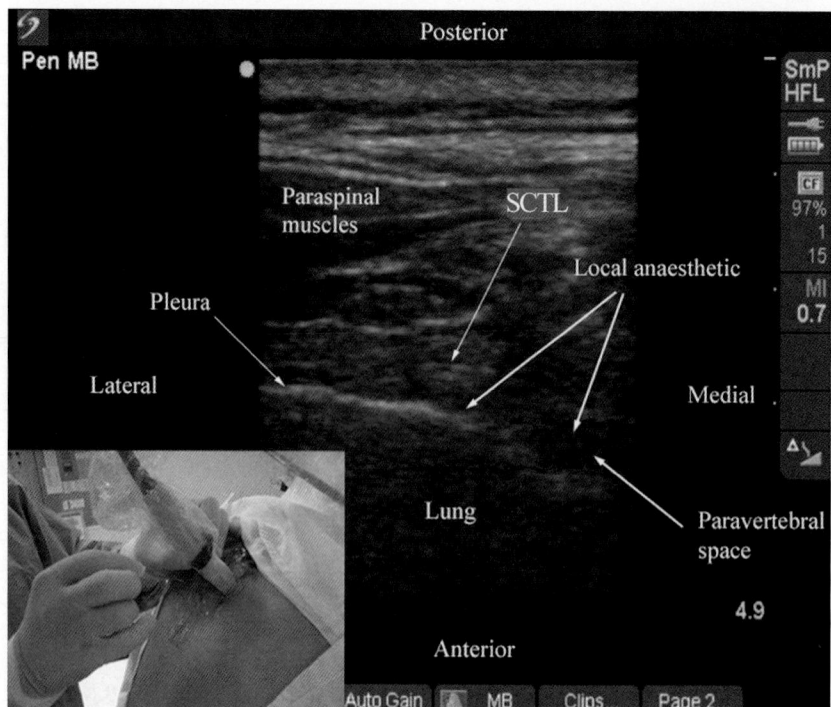

FIGURE 61.33 Ultrasound-guided thoracic paravertebral block using a transverse scan in which the block needle is inserted in the short axis of the ultrasound plane (technique 1). Note the widening of the paravertebral space and anterior displacement of the pleura by the local anesthetic on the transverse sonogram. The local anesthetic is also seen to spread to the posterior intercostal space laterally. The picture in the inset shows the orientation of the transducer and the direction in which the needle is inserted. *SCTL*, Superior costotransverse ligament.

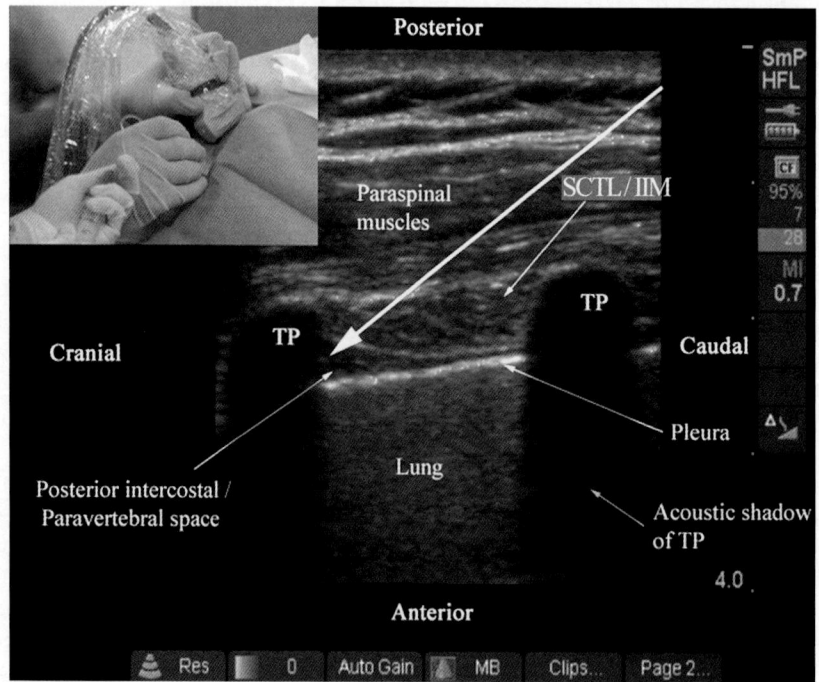

FIGURE 61.34 Ultrasound-guided thoracic paravertebral block using a paramedian sagittal oblique scan (technique 2). The long white arrow represents the direction in which the needle is inserted, and the picture in the inset shows how the block needle is inserted in the long axis of the ultrasound plane. Visualizing the block needle with this approach can be very challenging. The picture in the inset shows how the transducer is oriented and the direction in which the needle is inserted. *IIM*, Internal intercostal membrane; *SCL*, superior costotransverse ligament; *TP*, transverse process.

beam, it is often quite challenging to visualize the needle with this approach. This is in agreement with what O'Riain and colleagues have previously reported.[43] This may be because the block needle is often inserted at an acute angle, and the ultrasound beam is also insonated with a slight oblique (outward) tilt for optimal visibility of the TPVS. We therefore do not use this approach, but if one were to elect to use this technique, then the author recommends advancing the block needle under ultrasound guidance to deliberately contact the lower border of the TP after which the needle is slightly withdrawn and readvanced to pass under the lower border of the TP. A test bolus of normal saline (2 to 3 mL) is then injected, and sonographic evidence (pleural displacement) is sought to ensure that the tip of the needle is in the TPVS (Fig. 61.35). A calculated dose of local anesthetic is then injected in small aliquots. Following the injection, it is common to see anterior displacement of the pleura, widening of the paravertebral space, and an increased echogenicity of the pleura (see Fig. 61.35), which are objective signs of a correct injection into the TPVS. We have also observed, in real time, spread of the injected local anesthetic to the contiguous paravertebral spaces (see Fig. 61.35), confirming previous reports that the contiguous TPVS's communicate with each other.[1]

Intercostal Approach to the Thoracic Paravertebral Space (Technique 3)

In this approach, a transverse scan is performed as described earlier (Fig. 61.8), and the block needle is inserted in the plane of the ultrasound beam from a lateral to medial direction (Figs. 61.36 and 61.37) until the tip of the block needle is seen to lie in the posterior intercostal space or the apex of the TPVS. A test bolus of normal saline (2 to 3 mL) is then injected, and sonographic evidence is sought to ensure that the tip of the needle is in the apical part of the TPVS. A calculated dose of local anesthetic is then slowly injected in small aliquots. It is common to see widening of the paravertebral space and anterior displacement of the parietal pleura during the injection (see Fig. 61.36). Compared with the previous techniques, the block needle is best visualized with this approach because it is inserted in the plane of the ultrasound beam. However, since the needle is inserted from a lateral to medial direction (i.e., toward the intervertebral

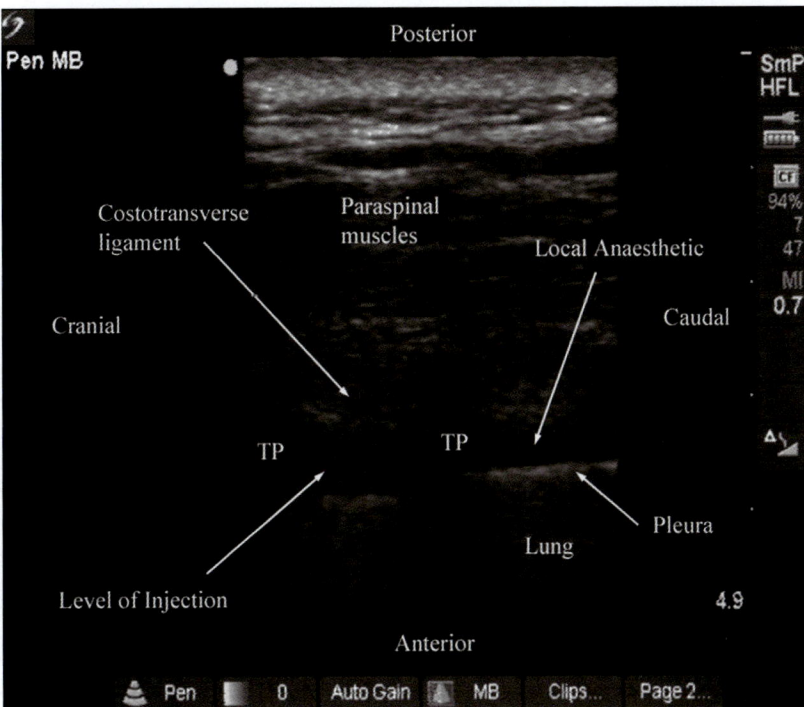

FIGURE 61.35 Paramedian sagittal oblique sonogram of the TPVS after local anesthetic injection (technique 2). Note the widening of the paravertebral space and displacement of the parietal pleura. The local anesthetic is also seen to have spread to the contiguous paravertebral space from the level of injection. *TP*, Transverse process.

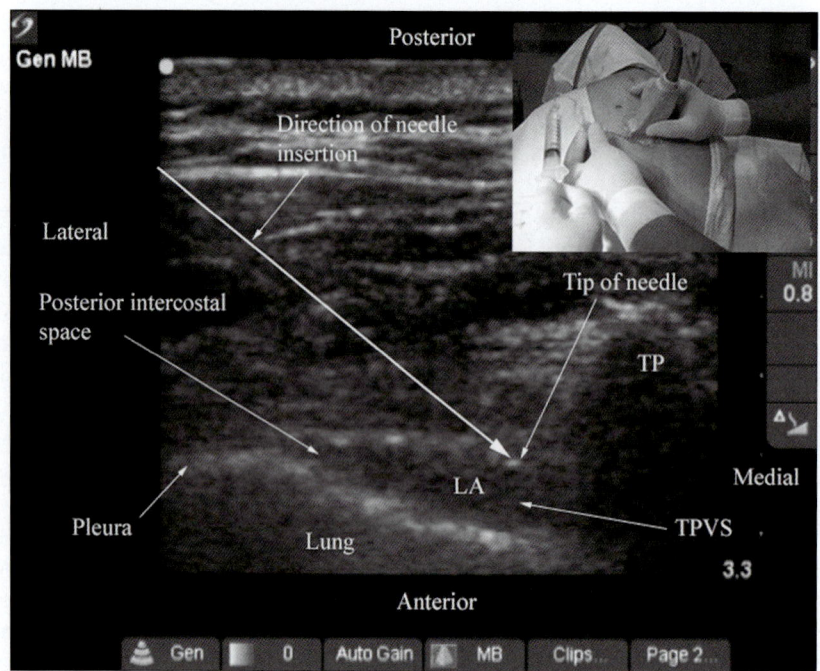

FIGURE 61.36 Transverse sonogram of the thoracic paravertebral space *(TPVS)* after the local anesthetic injection (technique 3; at the level of the transverse process *[TP]*). Note the widening of the paravertebral space, anterior displacement of the pleura, and spread of local anesthetic *(LA)* to the posterior intercostal space laterally. The long white arrow represents the direction in which the block needle is inserted. The picture in the inset shows how the block needle is inserted in the plane of the ultrasound beam from a lateral to medial direction.

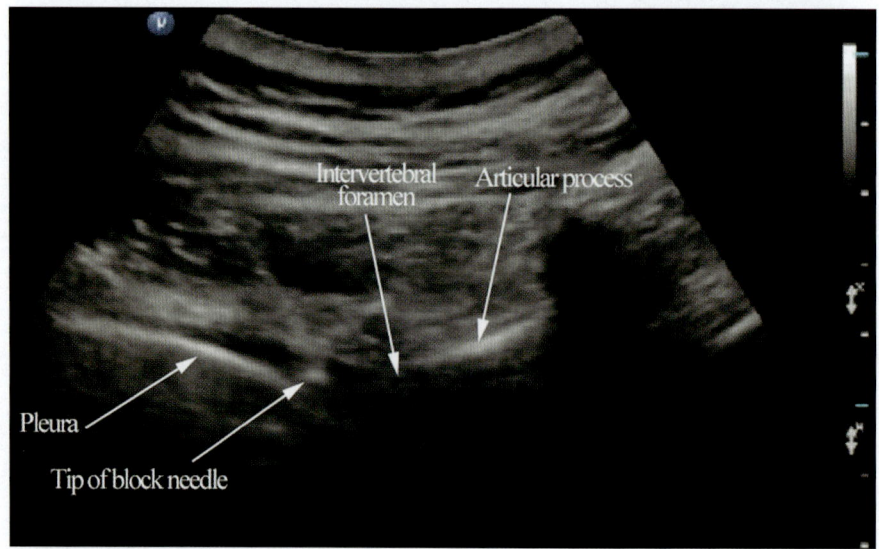

FIGURE 61.37 Ultrasound-guided thoracic paravertebral block with an in-plane needle insertion using the transverse ultrasound scan window at the level of the articular process (technique 3).

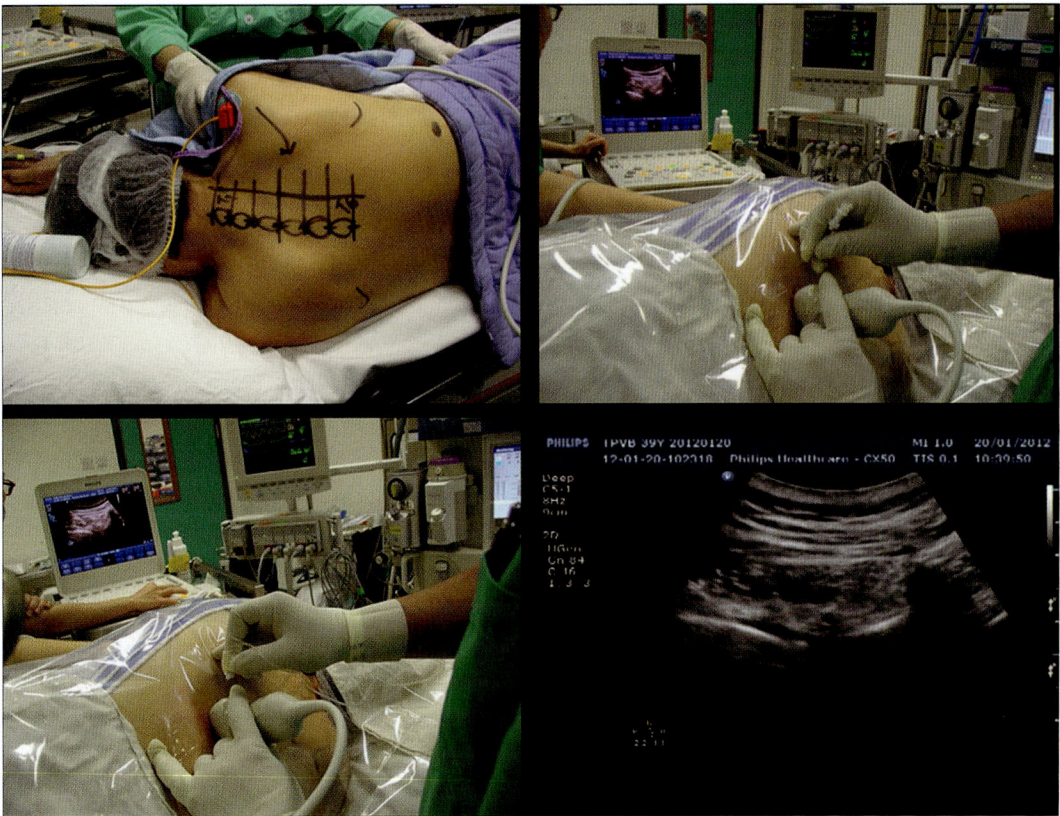

FIGURE 61.38 Ultrasound-guided multilevel thoracic paravertebral block (T1–T6) for surgical anesthesia during major breast cancer surgery. The figure also shows the ergonomics used for block placement.

foramen), it may predispose to a higher incidence of epidural spread or central neuraxial complications.

We have modified this approach, and instead of performing the ultrasound scan and injection at the level of the transverse process, as described by Shibata and colleagues,[34] the procedure is performed at the level of the inferior articular process (see Figs. 61.17–61.22). Without the transverse process in the path of the advancing block needle, we believe this approach allows visualization of a greater part of the paravertebral space and offers less bony obstruction (see Fig. 61.22). However, one must note that the intervertebral foramen is located immediately anterior to the inferior articular process. Therefore, one must avoid inserting the block needle too deep or performing the local anesthetic injection adjacent to articular process. It is yet to be seen how the intercostal approach to the paravertebral space compares in regard to epidural spread and central neuraxial complications when compared to the traditional method of performing TPVB. Our preliminary experience with the modified approach described above and for several thousand individual paravertebral injections over the last 5 to 6 years has been very encouraging, and we have not experienced any major neuraxial complications. We are now routinely using USG multilevel TPVB in conjunction with light sedation for surgical anesthesia during major breast cancer surgery (Fig. 61.38).

CONCLUSION

It is currently possible to accurately image parts of the TPVS. Being able to delineate the relevant anatomy of the TPVS before and during a TPVB in real-time may offer several advantages, and it appears to be a promising alternative to the traditional landmark based techniques for TPVB. Using ultrasound, one is able to preview the paravertebral anatomy prior to block placement and determine the depth to the transverse process and pleura. The latter defines the maximum safe depth for needle insertion and may help reduce the incidence of pleural puncture. Ultrasound guidance during TPVB also allows the block needle to be advanced accurately to the TPVS and visualize the distribution of the local anesthetic during the injection in real time. This may translate into improved technical outcomes, higher success rates, and reduced needle-related complications. However, although there are many different techniques of performing USG TPVB, an optimal axis for ultrasound imaging and needle insertion needs to be established, because visualization of the block needle during an USG TPVB can be challenging. Ultrasound is also an excellent teaching tool for demonstrating the anatomy relevant for TPVB and has the potential to improve the learning curve of this technique. Currently there are limited outcome data after USG TPVB, and future research to establish its role in clinical practice is warranted.

ACKNOWLEDGMENTS

The cadaver anatomical sections are courtesy of the Visible Human Server at École Polytechnique Fédérale de Lausanne, Visible Human Visualization Software (http://visiblehuman.epfl.ch), and Gold Standard Multimedia (www.gsm.org). The figures were reproduced with kind permission from www.aic.cuhk.edu.hk/usgraweb.

References

1. Karmakar MK. Thoracic paravertebral block. *Anesthesiology*. 2001;95:771–780.
2. Cheema SP, Ilsley D, Richardson J, Sabanathan S. A thermographic study of paravertebral analgesia. *Anaesthesia*. 1995;50:118–121.
3. Karmakar MK. Ultrasound-guided thoracic paravertebral block. *Tech Reg Anesth Pain Manag*. 2009;13:142–149.
4. Dugan DJ, Samson PC. Surgical significance of the endothoracic fascia. The anatomic basis for empyemectomy and other extrapleural technics. *Am J Surg*. 1975;130:151–158.
5. Karmakar MK, Chung DC. Variability of a thoracic paravertebral block. Are we ignoring the endothoracic fascia? *Reg Anesth Pain Med*. 2000;25(3):325–327.
6. Karmakar MK, Kwok WH, Kew J. Thoracic paravertebral block: radiological evidence of contralateral spread anterior to the vertebral bodies. *Br J Anaesth*. 2000;84(2):263–265.
7. Nunn JF, Slavin G. Posterior intercostal nerve block for pain relief after cholecystectomy. Anatomical basis and efficacy. *Br J Anaesth*. 1980;52:253–260.
8. Pernkopf E. Thorax, abdomen and extremities. In: Ferner H, ed. *Atlas of topographical and applied human anatomy*. 2nd ed. Baltimore: Urban and Schwarzenberg; 1980:127–129.
9. Conacher ID, Kokri M. Postoperative paravertebral blocks for thoracic surgery. A radiological appraisal. *Br J Anaesth*. 1987;59:155–161.
10. Conacher ID. Resin injection of thoracic paravertebral spaces. *Br J Anaesth*. 1988;61:657–661.
11. Purcell-Jones G, Pither CE, Justins DM. Paravertebral somatic nerve block: a clinical, radiographic, and computed tomography study in chronic pain patients. *Anesth Analg*. 1989;68:32–39.
12. Karmakar MK, Critchley LA, Ho AM, Gin T, Lee TW, Yim AP. Continuous thoracic paravertebral infusion of bupivacaine for pain management in patients with multiple fractured ribs. *Chest*. 2003;123:424–431.
13. Lönnqvist PA, Hildingsson U. The caudal boundary of the thoracic paravertebral space. A study in human cadavers. *Anaesthesia*. 1992;47:1051–1052.
14. Richardson J, Jones J, Atkinson R. The effect of thoracic paravertebral blockade on intercostal somatosensory evoked potentials. *Anesth Analg*. 1998;87:373–376.
15. Saito T, Den S, Tanuma K, Tanuma Y, Carney E, Carlsson C. Anatomical bases for paravertebral anesthetic block: fluid communication between the thoracic and lumbar paravertebral regions. *Surg Radiol Anat*. 1999;21:359–363.
16. Karmakar MK, Gin T, Ho AM. Ipsilateral thoraco-lumbar anaesthesia and paravertebral spread after low thoracic paravertebral injection. *Br J Anaesth*. 2001;87:312–316.
17. Eason MJ, Wyatt R. Paravertebral thoracic block-a reappraisal. *Anaesthesia*. 1979;34:638–642.
18. Lönnqvist PA, Hesser U. Radiological and clinical distribution of thoracic paravertebral blockade in infants and children. *Paediatr Anaesth*. 1993;3:83–87.
19. Cheema S, Richardson J, McGurgan P. Factors affecting the spread of bupivacaine in the adult thoracic paravertebral space. *Anaesthesia*. 2003;58:684–687.

20. Naja ZM, El-Rajab M, Al-Tannir MA, et al. Thoracic paravertebral block: influence of the number of injections. *Reg Anesth Pain Med*. 2006;31:196–201.
21. Naja MZ, Ziade MF, El RM, El TK, Lonnqvist PA. Varying anatomical injection points within the thoracic paravertebral space: effect on spread of solution and nerve blockade. *Anaesthesia*. 2004;59:459–463.
22. Lang SA, Saito T. Thoracic paravertebral nerve block, nerve stimulator guidance and the endothoracic fascia. *Anaesthesia*. 2005;60:930–931.
23. Eng J, Sabanathan S. Continuous paravertebral block for postthoracotomy analgesia in children. *J Pediatr Surg*. 1992;27:556–557.
24. Lönnqvist PA, MacKenzie J, Soni AK, Conacher ID. Paravertebral blockade. Failure rate and complications. *Anaesthesia*. 1995;50:813–815.
25. Moore DC, Bush WH, Scurlock JE. Intercostal nerve block: a roentgenographic anatomic study of technique and absorption in humans. *Anesth Analg*. 1980;59:815–825.
26. Pusch F, Freitag H, Weinstabl C, Obwegeser R, Huber E, Wildling E. Single-injection paravertebral block compared to general anaesthesia in breast surgery. *Acta Anaesthesiol Scand*. 1999;43:770–774.
27. Karmakar MK, Chui PT, Joynt GM, Ho AM. Thoracic paravertebral block for management of pain associated with multiple fractured ribs in patients with concomitant lumbar spinal trauma. *Reg Anesth Pain Med*. 2001;26:169–173.
28. MacIntosh R, Bryce-Smith R. *Local analgesia and abdominal surgery*. 2nd ed. Edinburgh, Scotland: E&S Livingstone; 1962:26–32.
29. Cheung N, Karmakar M. Right thoracic paravertebral anaesthesia for percutaneous radiofrequency ablation of liver tumours. *Br J Radiol*. 2011;84:785–789.
30. Saito T, Den S, Cheema SP, et al. A single-injection, multi-segmental paravertebral block-extension of somatosensory and sympathetic block in volunteers. *Acta Anaesthesiol Scand*. 2001;45:30–33.
31. Greengrass R, O'Brien F, Lyerly K, et al. Paravertebral block for breast cancer surgery. *Can J Anaesth*. 1996;43:858–861.
32. Richardson J, Cheema SP, Hawkins J, Sabanathan S. Thoracic paravertebral space location. A new method using pressure measurement. *Anaesthesia*. 1996;51:137–139.
33. Luyet C, Herrmann G, Ross S, Vogt A, Greif R, Moriggl B, et al. Ultrasound-guided thoracic paravertebral puncture and placement of catheters in human cadavers: where do catheters go? *Br J Anaesth*. 2011;106:246–254.
34. Shibata Y, Nishiwaki K. Ultrasound-guided intercostal approach to thoracic paravertebral block. *Anesth Analg*. 2009;109:996–997.
35. Ben-Ari A, Moreno M, Chelly JE, Bigeleisen PE. Ultrasound-guided paravertebral block using an intercostal approach. *Anesth Analg*. 2009;109:1691–1694.
36. Marhofer P, Kettner SC, Hajbok L, Dubsky P, Fleischmann E. Lateral ultrasound-guided paravertebral blockade: an anatomical-based description of a new technique. *Br J Anaesth*. 2010;105:526–532.
37. Hara K, Sakura S, Nomura T, Saito Y. Ultrasound guided thoracic paravertebral block in breast surgery. *Anaesthesia*. 2009;64:223–225.
38. Cowie B, McGlade D, Ivanusic J, Barrington MJ. Ultrasound-guided thoracic paravertebral blockade: a cadaveric study. *Anesth Analg*. 2010;110:1735–1739.
39. Luyet C, Eichenberger U, Greif R, Vogt A, Szucs FZ, Moriggl B. Ultrasound-guided paravertebral puncture and placement of catheters in human cadavers: an imaging study. *Br J Anaesth*. 2009;102:534–539.
40. Renes SH, Bruhn J, Gielen MJ, Scheffer GJ, van Geffen GJ. In-plane ultrasound-guided thoracic paravertebral block: a preliminary report of 36 cases with radiologic confirmation of catheter position. *Reg Anesth Pain Med*. 2010;35:212–216.
41. Pusch F, Wildling E, Klimscha W, Weinstabl C. Sonographic measurement of needle insertion depth in paravertebral blocks in women. *Br J Anaesth*. 2000;85(6):841–843.
42. Naja MZ, Gustafsson AC, Ziade MF, et al. Distance between the skin and the thoracic paravertebral space. *Anaesthesia*. 2005;60:680–684.
43. O'Riain SC, Donnell BO, Cuffe T, Harmon DC, Fraher JP, Shorten G. Thoracic paravertebral block using real-time ultrasound guidance. *Anesth Analg*. 2010;110:248–251.
44. Lichtenstein DA, Menu Y. A bedside ultrasound sign ruling out pneumothorax in the critically ill. Lung sliding. *Chest*. 1995;108:1345–1348.
45. Karmakar MK, Li X, Li J, Hadzic A. Volumetric three-dimensional ultrasound imaging of the anatomy relevant for thoracic paravertebral block. *Anesth Analg*. 2012;115(5):1246–1250.
46. Krediet AC, Moayeri N, van Geffen GJ, et al. Different approaches to ultrasound-guided thoracic paravertebral block: an illustrated review. *Anesthesiology*. 2015;123:459–474.

CHAPTER 62

Pudendal Nerve Block in Children

L. Stephen Long

INTRODUCTION

The pudendal nerve is the major paired nerve of the perineum. It supplies sensation to the genitalia and perineal skin, and motor innervation to the external anal and external urethral sphincters. It is a branch of the sacral plexus (S2 through S4). With ultrasound, the nerve is most easily visualized in the pudendal canal, where it travels with the pudendal artery and vein.[1]

For adults, pudendal blocks are used to provide analgesia for procedures involving the perineal area, to treat pelvic pain associated with conditions such as interstitial cystitis, and to diagnose and treat pudendal neuralgia.[2,3]

In pediatrics, pudendal blocks compete with caudal blocks when perineal analgesia is needed. Compared to caudal blocks, pudendal blocks offer several advantages for pediatric patients. First, the analgesia lasts for up to 24 hours, whereas caudal analgesia typically dissipates after 6 hours. Second, pudendal blocks target the perineum, and there is no blockade of the lower extremities. Third, the blocks can be successfully performed in pediatric patients of any age.

Pudendal nerve blocks have been shown to be superior to caudal blocks for hypospadias surgery in children, providing superior analgesia of longer duration.[4,5] Additional indications include but are not limited to circumcisions and the array of genitoplastic procedures.

Pudendal nerve blocks carry a small risk of infection and nerve or vascular injury. Theoretically, such complications have the potential to lead to more serious problems, such as impotence.[6]

SUGGESTED TECHNIQUE

With the table in Trendelenburg, place the patient in the lithotomy position with a towel or blanket under the hips, to rotate the pelvis anteriorly. Palpate the ischial tuberosity and place a low-frequency curved transducer in transverse orientation over the tuberosity. Move the transducer posteriorly until the lesser sciatic notch is visualized as a curved hyperechoic line (an inverted "U" shape). Continue to move the transducer posteriorly until the ischial spine appears as a flat hyperechoic line. Medial to the ischial spine are the superficial sacrotuberous ligament (STL) and deeper sacrospinous ligament (SSL). The pudendal canal is between the STL and SSL, adjacent to the ischial spine. Locate the pudendal artery with visible pulsations. The pudendal nerve is usually located medial to the artery. In the medial to lateral direction, in-plane with the probe, insert a 50- to 100-mm, short-bevel, 22-gauge needle. Advance the needle until it penetrates the STL. Aspirate for blood before injecting approximately 0.1 mL/kg of bupivacaine 0.25% or ropivacaine 0.25% without epinephrine around the nerve.

DISCUSSION AND COMMENTS

The pudendal block has distinct advantages over the caudal blocks for urologic procedures in children. It has been shown to provide superior analgesia of a longer duration for hypospadias repair. The caudal block, however, is a familiar and simple procedure for many anesthesiologists, and therefore performing the pudendal block may require more time and effort. Nonetheless, the benefit of pudendal blocks for older children undergoing painful urologic procedures is clear.

Clinical Pearls

- Pudendal blocks last significantly longer than caudal blocks do.
- Pudendal blocks target the perineal area only, leaving the lower extremities unaffected.
- Pudendal blocks can be performed in children of any age.
- Have an assistant help position the patient in lithotomy.
- The skin entry point for the block needle is typically located at the 3- and 9-o'clock position a few centimeters lateral to the anus.
- A pop will be felt when the needle penetrates the STL. If a second pop is felt, the needle may have been advanced too deep and through the SSL.

References

1. Bendtsen TF, Parras T, Moriggl B, et al. Ultrasound-guided pudendal nerve block at the entrance of the pudendal (Alcock) canal: description of anatomy and clinical technique. *Reg Anesth Pain Med.* 2016;41:140–145.
2. Lean LL, Hegarty D, Harmon D. Analgesic effect of bilateral ultrasound-guided pudendal nerve blocks in management of interstitial cystitis. *J Anesth.* 2012;26(1):128–129.
3. Aissaoui Y, Bruyere R, Mustapha H, Bry D, Kamili ND, Miller C. A randomized controlled trial of pudendal nerve block for pain relief after episiotomy. *Anesth Analg.* 2008;107:625–629.
4. Naja ZM, Ziade FM, Kamel R, El-Kayali S, Daoud N, El-Rajab MA. The effectiveness of pudendal nerve block versus caudal block anesthesia for hypospadias in children. *Anesth Analg.* 2013;117:1401–1407.
5. Kendigelen P, Tutuncu AC, Emre S, Altindas F, Kaya G. Pudendal versus caudal block in children undergoing hypospadias surgery. *Reg Anesth Pain Med.* 2016;41:1–6.
6. Rosen MP, Greenfield AJ, Walker TG, et al. Arteriogenic impotence: findings in 195 impotent men examined with selective internal pudendal angiography. *Radiology.* 1990;174:1043–1048.

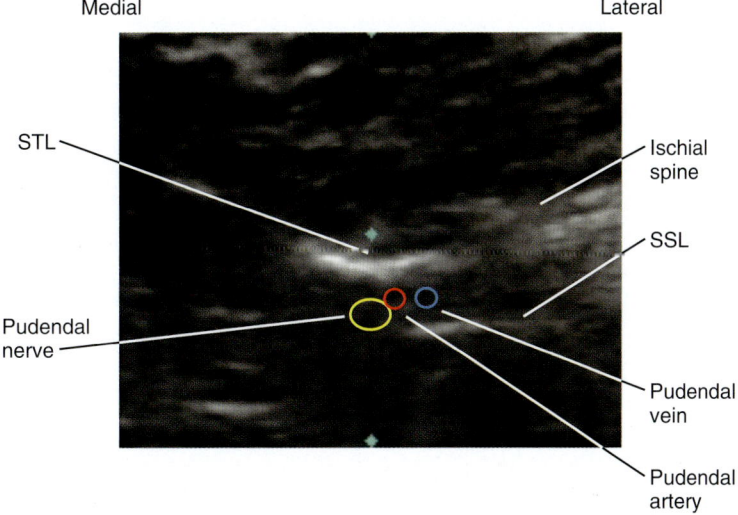

FIGURE 62.1 Relationship of the ischial spine, sacrotuberous ligament (STL), sacrospinous ligament (SSL), and pudendal neurovascular bundle in a 7-year-old, 30.5-kg patient undergoing bilateral pudendal nerve blocks for hypospadius repair. Each *diamond marking* represents 1 cm of depth. For enhancement, the superficial 2 cm of the image, which shows subcutaneous tissue, have been cropped.

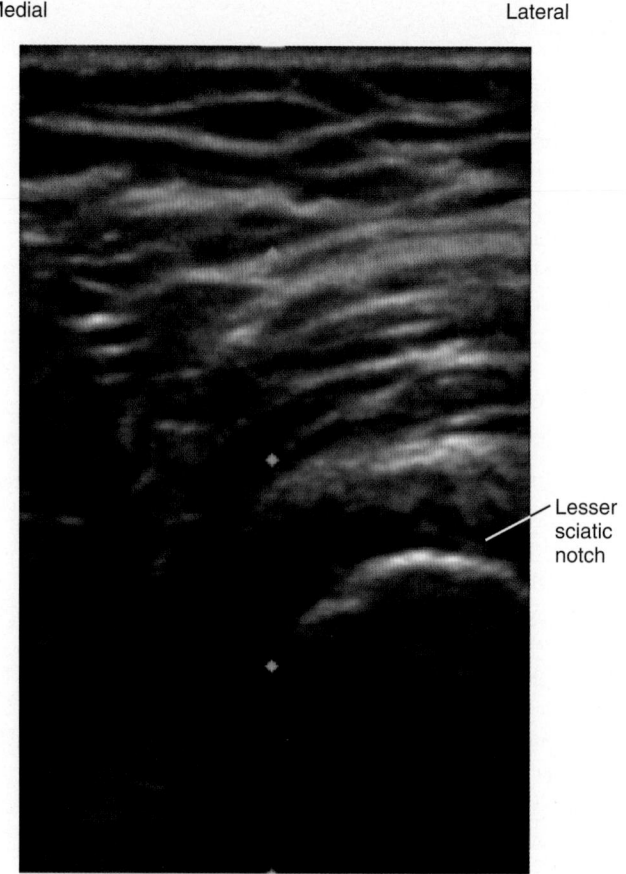

FIGURE 62.2 The lesser sciatic notch appears as a hyperechoic inverted "U." Each *diamond marking* represents 1 cm of depth. The image is not cropped.

Neuraxial Block

CHAPTER 63

See Video 63.1 on ExpertConsult.com.

INTRODUCTION

In many patients, epidural and spinal blocks are routine procedures guided by loss of resistance and confirmation of free flow of cerebrospinal fluid, respectively. However, in patients with obesity or advanced age, these neuraxial blocks can be more challenging and may benefit from imaging guidance. Ultrasound can estimate the location and level of spinous interspaces. There also is evidence that ultrasound guidance improves the learning curve and reduces epidural failure rates of residents in training.[1,2] Ultrasound imaging has been reported as useful for guiding neuraxial anesthetics in patients with prior surgical instrumentation or scoliosis. However, there remain current limitations to the use of ultrasound technology to guide neuraxial blocks.

Neuraxial imaging with ultrasound can be difficult because of the depth of the structures of interest and the surrounding bone. The narrow acoustic window makes online approaches (imaging during needle placement) inherently challenging. Simultaneous ultrasound imaging and needle placement for neuraxial procedures is difficult in adult patients. Online approaches to neuraxial procedures are more commonly used in pediatric patients. Most practitioners use the offline technique (skin markings prior to needle insertion) when using ultrasound to guide neuraxial blocks in adults. With the offline technique, the needle follows the same angle that is used for optimal visualization of the neuraxial structures.[3]

Selection of the correct interspace is important to the success of the subarachnoid block. The interspace selected for injection of spinal anesthetic drugs affects the resultant distribution. The failure rate at lower lumbar interspaces can be as high as 7%.[4,5] These failures probably relate to the site of the injection with respect to the peak of the lumbosacral curve. One of the potential benefits of ultrasound is to help establish the correct interspace for neuraxial block, especially in challenging patients with scoliosis or obesity (Class I recommendation).[6]

The accuracy of ultrasonography in correctly identifying lumbar interspace levels is in the 71% to 76% range for patients undergoing magnetic resonance imaging to evaluate the lumbar spine. The ability to estimate the interspace level is especially complex in patients with transitional vertebrae. These anomalies include lumbarization of the sacral spine (an unfused first sacral vertebra) and sacralization of the lumbar spine (fusion of L5 with the sacrum). The number of ribs also can vary, making estimation of level relative to the thoracic vertebrae challenging. Although ultrasound has limited ability to assess the interspace level, assessment by palpation is more inaccurate.

Longitudinal paramedian imaging planes provide the best visualization of neuraxial structures.[7] With these views, the width of the acoustic window (the intervertebral space) is largest relative to the shadowing of the corresponding vertebral bone. Several authors have described the epidural space and adjacent bone as having a sawtooth configuration in this parasagittal view. The "saw sign" of longitudinal paramedian views inclines toward the skin surface in the caudal direction.

Midline transverse imaging planes are often used for offline markings for midline approaches for lumbar epidurals and spinals. This transverse view has been described as having a "flying bat" or "cat ears" appearance. In this view the articular processes (the rounded mammillary processes) of the facet joints form the ears of the bat and indicate the widest part of the interlaminar space. Although transverse imaging planes most closely resemble midline approaches, this view is limited by overhanging bone of the spinous processes and shadowing by the interspinous ligaments. Transverse imaging planes have been shown to be effective at lumbar interspaces for marking the needle insertion point and estimating needle depth to loss of resistance. However, these views are not helpful at midthoracic levels because of the narrower acoustic windows across the midline produced by the steep inclination of the spinous processes. In addition, the thoracic region lacks prominent articular processes that can serve as sonographic landmarks. It can be difficult to obtain symmetric midline transverse views of the neuraxis (in particular, the rounded articular processes) in patients with scoliosis due to rotation of the spine.

Ultrasound is an accurate imaging modality for depiction of the dura mater. The dura appears highly echogenic on ultrasound scans, defined by a single- or double-layer hyperechoic signal. It can be difficult to resolve the echo signals of the ligamentum flavum and posterior dura, and therefore this signal is sometimes referred to as the posterior complex (Table 63.1). The anterior complex consists of the anterior dura, posterior longitudinal ligament, and vertebral body. This produces a wider hyperechoic band that is deeper and parallel to the first band (the equals sign). Because the subarachnoid space contains few endogenous scatterers of ultrasound, it appears echo free on ultrasound scans (Table 63.2).

SUGGESTED TECHNIQUE FOR OFFLINE LUMBAR EPIDURAL CATHETER PLACEMENT

Use a low-frequency curved array (center frequency near 4 MHz) to obtain the best midline transverse view of the lumbar epidural space. The best transverse view is one in which the articular processes are prominent and symmetrically displayed on the screen. The probe slides in a cephalocaudal fashion to obtain an interlaminar view (so that no spinous process is seen within the field of imaging). The probe is then tilted to enhance imaging of the articular processes, with some rotation to make the articular processes symmetric on the display. Sliding in a medial-lateral fashion may be necessary to center the articular processes on the display. If the transducer is significantly rotated, then some repositioning of the patient may be necessary. Similarly, flexion of the lumbar spine can improve visibility and access to lumbar interspaces. The depth to the epidural space is then measured (this is most accurately done using the readout from a cursor scrolled over the anterior aspect of the posterior echo complex). The tilt (inclination) of the transducer is also noted (which is usually around 15 degrees cephalad in the lumbar region).

Mark the interspace with crosshairs on the skin using indelible ink. The intersection of the crosshairs can be marked by firmly indenting the skin with a needle hub. Mark the patient in the same position as for the interventional procedure. Changes in patient positioning reduce the accuracy of the markings.

Check or verify the level by moving the probe down to the sacrum and counting back up to the marked interspace using a longitudinal paramedian view. If this interspace is deemed too high or low, the adjacent spaces can be scanned and marked.

TABLE 63.1 Anatomic Structures That Comprise the Posterior and Anterior Echo Complexes as Seen in Longitudinal Paramedian View of the Neuraxis (the "Equals Sign")

Ultrasound Image	Structure
Posterior complex	Ligamentum flavum
	Posterior epidural space
	Posterior dura
Anterior complex	Anterior dura
	Anterior epidural space
	Posterior longitudinal ligament
	Vertebral body

These two echo complexes appear as parallel hyperechoic bands on ultrasound scans. The equals sign is not truly symmetric because the anterior echo complex is wider than the posterior echo complex (which appears more similar to a straight line). In the thoracic region the interspaces are smaller, and therefore the equals sign is not as long in its cephalocaudad dimension in comparison with the lumbar region. The equals sign indicates that the spinal canal and hypoechoic subarachnoid space are correctly imaged because this is not seen with offaxis views. Structures are listed from posterior to anterior.

TABLE 63.2 Measurements Potentially Useful for Guiding Offline Approaches to Neuraxial Blocks

Anatomic Structure	Measurement and Comments	View	Approximate Value	Variation	Significance
Depth of posterior epidural space	From skin to anterior aspect of posterior echo complex	Transverse midline	5 cm	Depends on body size and girth	Correlates with needle depth for loss of resistance
	No transducer compression in obese subjects	Longitudinal paramedian		Deeper at lower lumbar interspaces	
AP width of subarachnoid space	From anterior aspect of posterior echo complex to posterior aspect of anterior echo complex	Longitudinal paramedian	1.4 cm	Smaller at lower lumbar interspaces	Does not correlate with extent of SAB block
				Wider (1–2 mm) in sitting position	May correlate with extent of SAB block after epidural fluid bolus injection (untested). Hydrostatic forces cause distention of subarachnoid space.
ML interspace distance	ML width of anterior echo complex	Transverse midline		Wider at lower lumbar interspaces	May correlate with ease of LOR or SAB technique (untested)
AP width of posterior epidural space	Must resolve ligamentum flavum and posterior dura echoes (doublet)	Longitudinal paramedian	0.5 cm	Widest in midline and tapers laterally	May correlate with ease of LOR technique (untested)
Interspace length	Cephalocaudal length of posterior or anterior echo complex	Longitudinal paramedian		Narrower at thoracic interspaces	May correlate with ease of LOR technique (untested)
Inclination of lamina	Along surface of the lamina	Longitudinal paramedian	15 degrees	Steeper angle at thoracic interspaces	May correlate with angle of needle insertion for LOR (untested)
	Also can use a line from the cephalad end of the vertebral body echo through the center of the ligamentum flavum				Difficult to estimate because of the large range of possible angles

Approximate values shown are for average-sized adults in the lumbar region.
AP, Anteroposterior; *LOR*, loss of resistance; *ML*, mediolateral; *SAB*, subarachnoid block.
From Grau T, Leipold RW, Horter J, Conradi R, Martin E, Motsch J. The lumbar epidural space in pregnancy: visualization by ultrasonography. *Br J Anaesth*. 2001;86:798–804; Grau T, Leipold RW, Conradi R, Martin E. Ultrasound control for presumed difficult epidural puncture. *Acta Anaesthesiol Scand*. 2001;45:766–771; Arzola C, Balki M, Carvalho JC. The antero-posterior diameter of the lumbar dural sac does not predict sensory levels of spinal anesthesia for cesarean delivery. *Can J Anaesth*. 2007;54 (8):620–625; Hirasawa Y, Bashir WA, Smith FW, Magnusson ML, Pope MH, Takahashi K. Postural changes of the dural sac in the lumbar spines of asymptomatic individuals using positional stand-up magnetic resonance imaging. *Spine*. 2007;32:E136–E140; Borges BC, Wieczorek P, Balki M, Carvalho JC. Sonoanatomy of the lumbar spine of pregnant women at term. *Reg Anesth Pain Med*. 2009;34(6):581–585; Salman A, Arzola C, Tharmaratnam U, Balki M. Ultrasound imaging of the thoracic spine in paramedian sagittal oblique plane: the correlation between estimated and actual depth to the epidural space. *Reg Anesth Pain Med*. 2011;36(6):542–547.

Remove all the gel with dry gauze and then proceed with lumbar epidural catheter placement by testing for loss of resistance in the usual sterile fashion. The noted depth can be off by as much as 0.5 to 1 cm (Table 63.3). If unsuccessful on the first attempt, try redirecting the needle in a cephalocaudal fashion. This is suggested because the greatest uncertainty with the offline technique is the tilt (inclination) of the transducer.

COMMENTS

SKIN MARKINGS

Use a liberal amount of gel for neuraxial imaging. This has two advantages. First, skin contact for acoustic coupling will be improved, especially for thin patients where the imaging surface is not flat. Second, the gel imprint of the transducer when it is removed facilitates subsequent skin markings.[8] Firmly press the needle hub against the skin and gently turn it back and forth to make a skin indentation. This mark will not be removed with skin prep.

Offline skin markings for neuraxial block are not as accurate in obese patients because of the deep target structures. In addition, poor image quality may be a factor in some cases. Elderly patients are particularly difficult to image for neuraxial block because the interspaces are small and the soft tissue structures calcify, which will scatter sound waves and compromise imaging quality. There are conditions such as ankylosing spondylitis that can resemble aging in terms of ultrasound imaging. Although ligaments readily calcify with aging, the adjacent muscles are relatively spared. This is a reason why longitudinal paramedian views are preferred for elderly patients.

LEVEL ESTIMATION

The best way to count interspaces is using the anterior dural complexes (to avoid mistakenly counting changes in the bony contours as posterior dural complexes). The transverse processes of the lower lumbar spine (L4 and L5) are short and stout to allow greater mobility of the lumbar spine near the sacrum. The L5 to S1 interspace is short in its cephalocaudal dimension.

HIGH-RESOLUTION ULTRASOUND IMAGING OF THE NEURAXIS

On occasion, high-resolution ultrasound imaging can resolve a doublet within the posterior dural complex (the ligamentum flavum and posterior dura separately). The ligamentum flavum and posterior dura run nearly parallel to each other, with a small angle between them because the posterior epidural space is slightly wider at the cephalad end of an interspace.

The amount of fat in the posterior epidural space is related to age and body weight. Epidural fat decreases with age[9] and increases with obesity.[10] The amount of epidural fat also varies according to spinal location, being lowest in the cervical spine and highest in the lumbosacral spinal region.[11]

TABLE 63.3 Reasons for Discrepancies Between Offline Estimates of Epidural Space Depth and Needle Depth for Loss of Resistance	
Offline Markings	**Reasons for Discrepancies in Depth Estimates**
	Probe compression
	Local anesthetic skin wheal
	Needle trajectory
	Needle advancement (soft tissue elastic properties)

Offline estimates of the depth of the epidural space are reasonably accurate because the skin mobility is limited and the underlying tissue (primarily bone and ligaments) is relatively firm compared with other body regions. However, there are several reasons why these depth estimates differ from those obtained from needle depths at loss of resistance.

The spinal cord and cauda equina have characteristic cardiac pulsations that are sometimes evident on ultrasound scans in adult patients.[12] The spinal cord pulses posteriorly and caudally due to blood flow in the anterior spinal artery.[13]

OUTCOMES

Studies have suggested that ultrasound guidance reduces needle passes for neuraxial procedures.[14] No study has shown a reduction in the chance of dural puncture when ultrasound guidance is used for epidural placement (but no study has been adequately powered to detect such a difference in this relatively uncommon event).

Clinical Pearls

- The spinous processes give a long triangular shadow down the midline on transverse views using a curved array transducer. If this shadow is seen, the probe position must be adjusted in the cephalocaudal direction.
- There are many sacral morphologies, but usually the hyperechoic sacral line can be used as a reference for establishing the lumbar level. The sacrum shadow is continuous so there is no underlying equals sign.
- Probe compression in obese subjects can lead to underestimation of the distance to the epidural space.
- Because there is a strong concordance in their measurements, longitudinal paramedian views can be used to check the distances to the epidural space if transverse views are not adequate.
- Avoid epidural attempts at interspaces where the posterior echo complex is incomplete or missing (with good visualization of the articular processes). Although this may relate to acoustic shadowing by the spinous processes or interspinous ligaments, these interspaces may have a midline gap in the ligamentum flavum and may be at higher risk of dural puncture.
- Ultrasound imaging can be used to help decide when an extra-long needle is necessary for epidurals or spinals. If the posterior epidural space echo is more than 8 cm from the skin (or the spinous process deeper than 4 cm), a longer needle is chosen (more than 9 cm in length).
- Ultrasound imaging accelerates and improves the learning curve for epidural catheter placement.

References

1. Grau T, Bartusseck E, Conradi R, Martin E, Motsch J. Ultrasound imaging improves learning curves in obstetric epidural anesthesia: a preliminary study. *Can J Anaesth*. 2003;50(10):1047–1050.
2. Vallejo MC, Phelps AL, Singh S, Orebaugh SL, Sah N. Ultrasound decreases the failed labor epidural rate in resident trainees. *Int J Obstet Anesth*. 2010;19(4):373–378.
3. Kessler J, Moriggl B, Grau T. Ultrasound-guided regional anesthesia: learning with an optimized cadaver model. *Surg Radiol Anat*. 2014;36(4):383–392.
4. Munhall RJ, Sukhani R, Winnie AP. Incidence and etiology of failed spinal anesthetics in a university hospital: a prospective study. *Anesth Analg*. 1988;67:843–848.
5. Tarkkila PJ. Incidence and causes of failed spinal anesthetics in a university hospital: a prospective study. *Reg Anesth*. 1991;16:48–51.
6. Neal JM, Barrington MJ, Brull R, et al. The Second ASRA Practice Advisory on Neurologic Complications Associated With Regional Anesthesia and Pain Medicine: Executive Summary 2015. *Reg Anesth Pain Med*. 2015;40(5):401–430.
7. Grau T, Leipold RW, Horter J, et al. Paramedian access to the epidural space: the optimum window for ultrasound imaging. *J Clin Anesth*. 2001A;13:213–217.
8. Manickam BP, McDonald A. Surface marking technique to locate needle insertion point of ultrasound-guided neuraxial block. *Br J Anaesth*. 2016;116(4):568–569.
9. Igarashi T, Hirabayashi Y, Shimizu R, Saitoh K, Fukuda H, Mitsuhata H. The lumbar extradural structure changes with increasing age. *Br J Anaesth*. 1997;78:149–152.

10. Wu HT, Schweitzer ME, Parker L. Is epidural fat associated with body habitus? *J Comput Assist Tomogr*. 2005;29:99–102.
11. Narouze S, Benzon HT, Provenzano DA, et al. Interventional spine and pain procedures in patients on antiplatelet and anticoagulant medications. *Reg Anesth Pain Med*. 2015;40:182–212.
12. McLeod AJ, Baxter JS, Ameri G, et al. Detection and visualization of dural pulsation for spine needle interventions. *Int J Comput Assist Radiol Surg*. 2015;10(6):947–958.
13. Rubin JM, Dohrmann GJ. The spine and spinal cord during neurosurgical operations: real-time ultrasonography. *Radiology*. 1985;155(1):197–200.
14. Kallidaikurichi Srinivasan K, Iohom G, Loughnane F, Lee PJ. Conventional landmark-guided midline versus preprocedure ultrasound-guided paramedian techniques in spinal anesthesia. *Anesth Analg*. 2015;121(4):1089–1096.

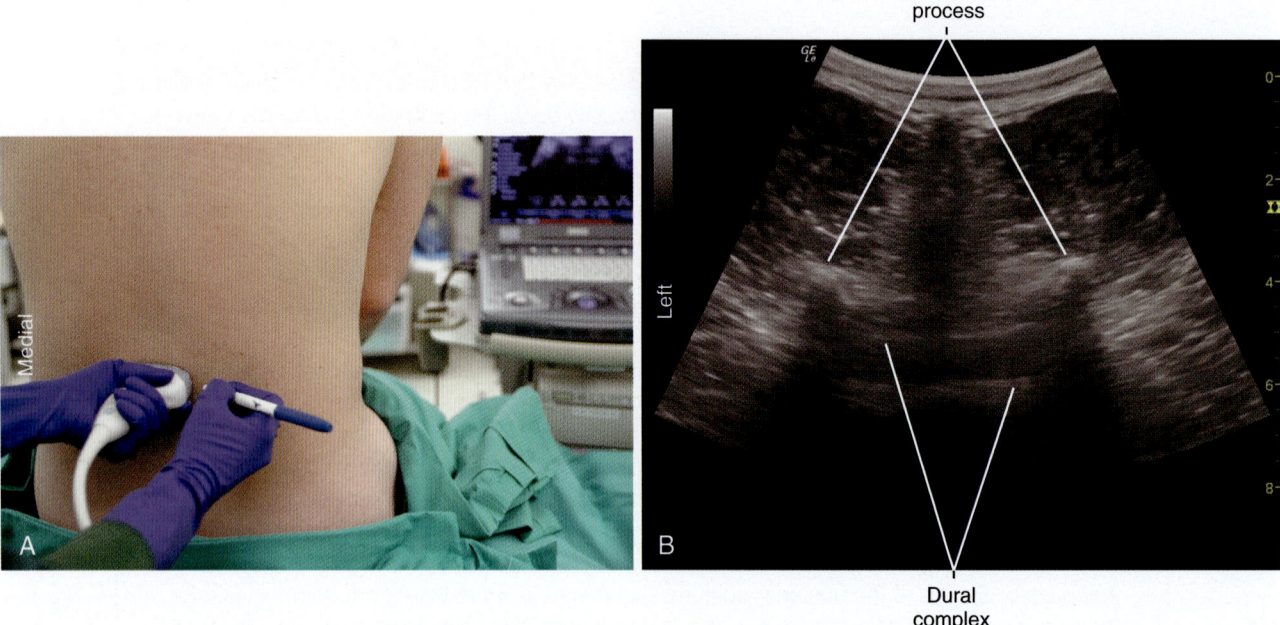

FIGURE 63.1 External photograph showing transducer position for transverse midline view of the neuraxis and offline technique (A). Corresponding sonogram (B). This transverse midline sonogram demonstrates the acoustic shadows of the articular processes.

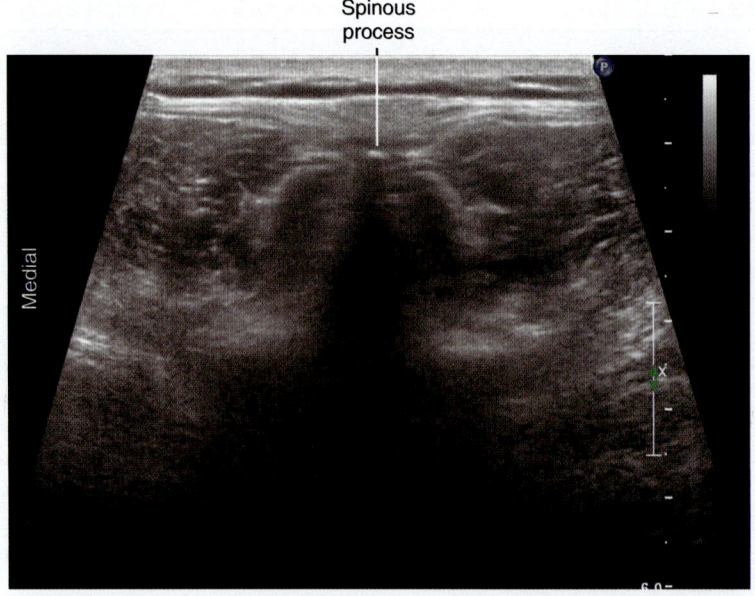

FIGURE 63.2 If the probe is moved away from an interspace, a spinous process is viewed and produces a triangular acoustic shadow (transverse midline view).

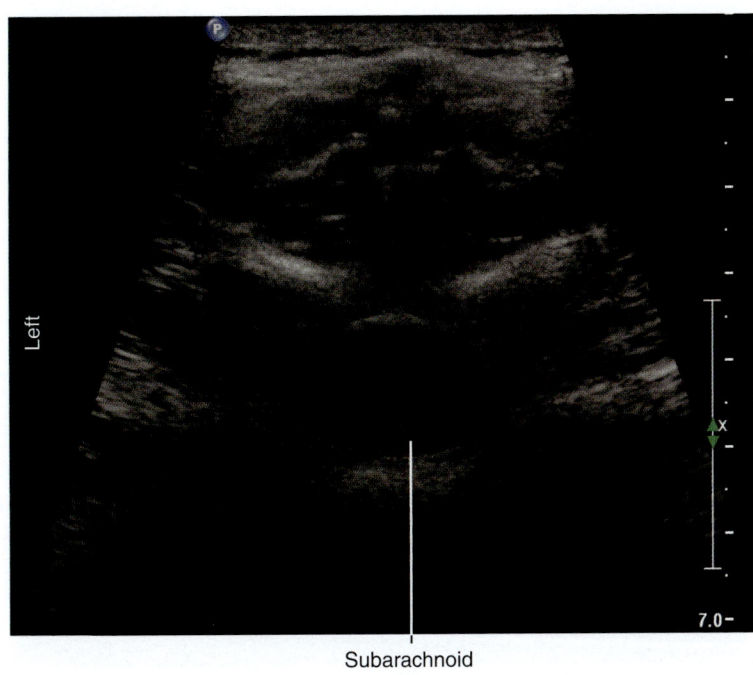

FIGURE 63.3 At higher levels (high lumbar or low thoracic interspaces), the roundedness of the subarachnoid space and dural echoes can be appreciated on transverse midline view of the interspace.

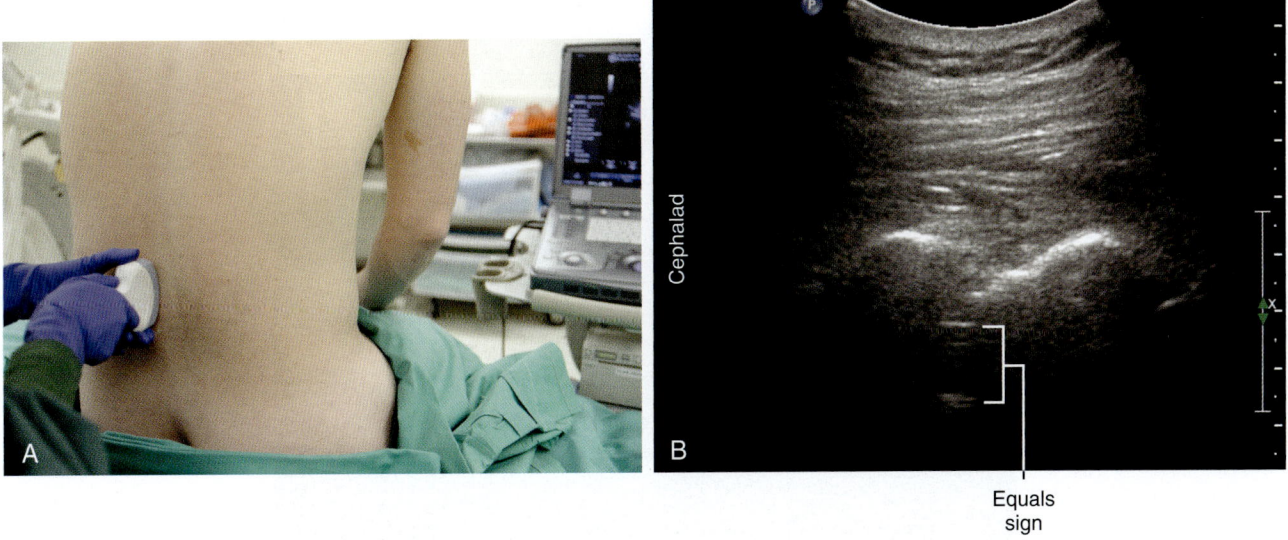

FIGURE 63.4 External photograph showing transducer position for longitudinal paramedian view of the neuraxis and offline technique (A). Corresponding sonogram demonstrates the "saw sign" (B). The saw sign represents the base of the lamina and articular processes of the lumbar vertebrae (the teeth of the saw) and the interspaces (the spaces between the teeth). To obtain this view, the transducer is placed 2 to 3 cm off midline and tilted to the center of the spinal canal. The "equals" sign of the posterior and anterior dural echo complexes is evident. With a curved transducer, the anterior complex is slightly longer than the posterior complex in longitudinal paramedian view because of the beam angles.

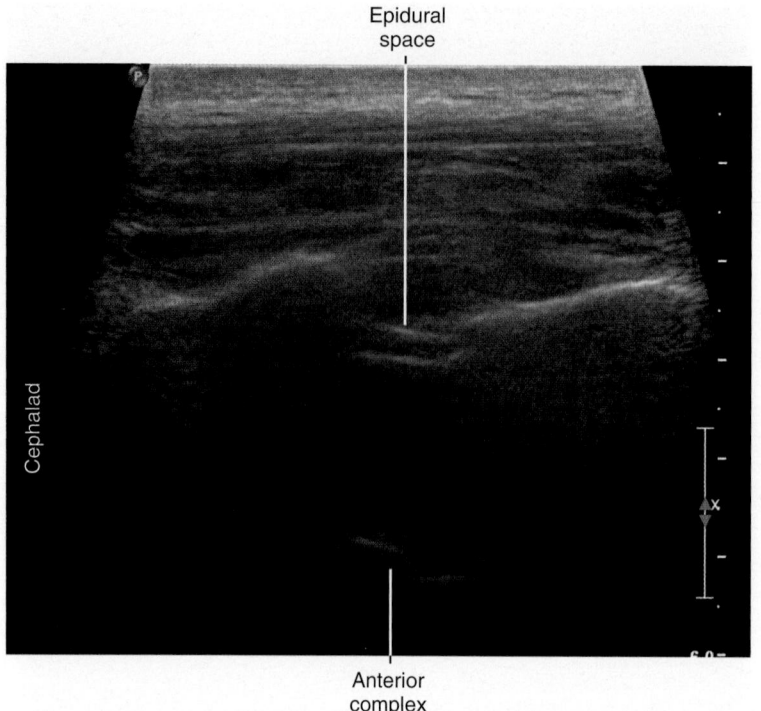

FIGURE 63.5 In some subjects, the echoes from the ligamentum flavum and posterior dura (the posterior complex) can be resolved into a doublet of separate echoes, indicating direct imaging of the posterior epidural space in longitudinal paramedian view.

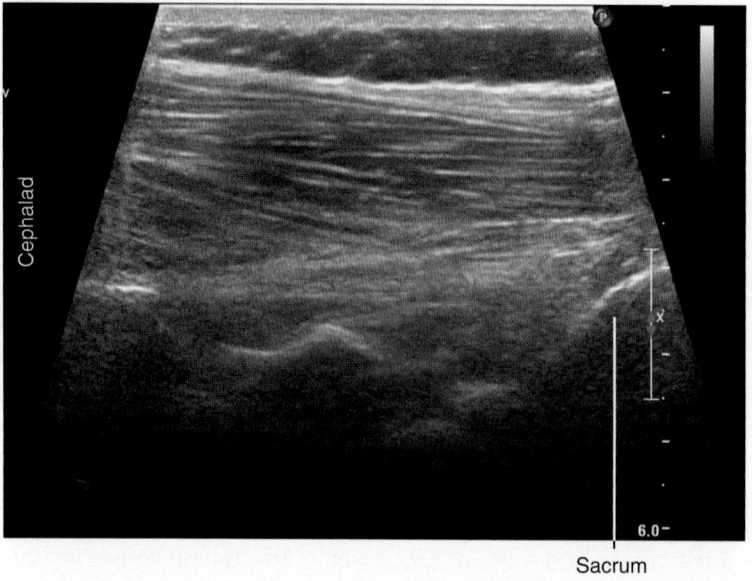

FIGURE 63.6 Longitudinal paramedian view at the lower lumbar interspaces. The acoustic window shows the spinal canal. The hyperechoic linear echoes of the sacrum can be identified and, by inference, the L5 to S1 interspace.

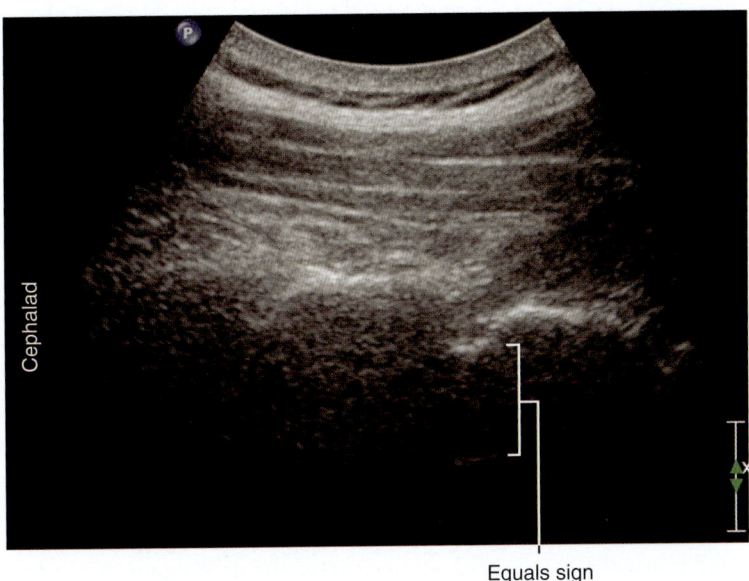

FIGURE 63.7 Longitudinal paramedian views of the thoracic spine reveal smaller interspaces for epidural catheter placement.

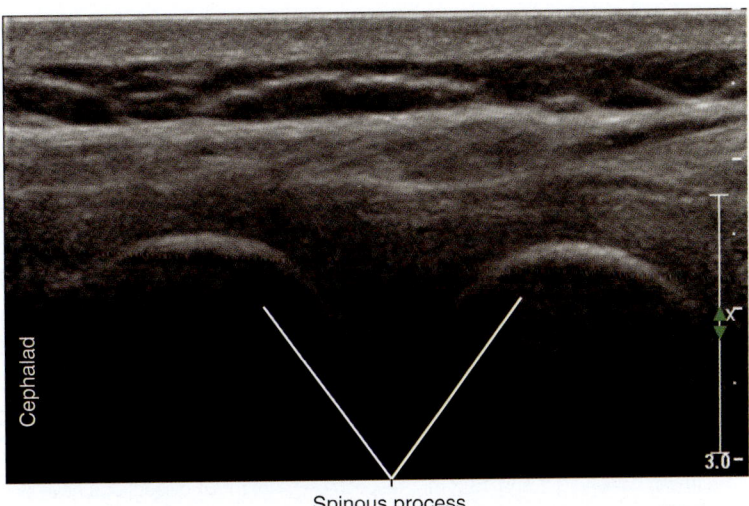

FIGURE 63.8 Midline longitudinal view demonstrating the spinous processes and interspace. This view can be useful in obese subjects for offline markings to help guide midline approaches to neuraxial blocks.

Caudal Epidural Block

The caudal epidural space can be accessed through the sacrococcygeal ligament that covers the sacral hiatus. This procedure is normally performed by placing a needle or catheter through the sacrococcygeal ligament for injection of local anesthetic drugs. The caudal approach is usually the most superficial access to the epidural space. Unlike subarachnoid blocks, caudal blocks are relatively easy to perform in the prone position. Caudal blocks provide anesthesia for genitourinary and anorectal surgical procedures.

The sacral hiatus is the caudal termination of the sacral canal. The volume of the epidural space within the sacral canal is highly variable, with estimates ranging from 10 to 26 mL in adults (Table 64.1). Because the sacral canal volume varies, the dose required to achieve a given level

TABLE 64.1 Normal Adult Values for Caudal Epidural Block

Measurement	Estimate	Range	Method	N	Reference
Sacrococcygeal ligament width	11 mm	2–18 mm	US (Transverse View)	339	Kim et al., 2016
Sacral canal diameter	7 mm	1–15 mm	US (Longitudinal View)	339	Kim et al., 2016
Tip of dural sac	S2	S1–S3	Anatomic Dissection	1227	Trotter, 1947
Distance between dural sac and sacral hiatus	61 mm	34–80 mm	MRI	37	Crighton et al., 1997
Angle of approach	58 degrees	40–74 degrees	MRI	37	Crighton et al., 1997
Sacral volume	14 mL	10–27 mL	MRI	37	Crighton et al., 1997

Sacrococcygeal ligament width = the transverse distance between the inner borders of the sacral cornua. Other reports of the intercornual distance have been measured between the peaks of the cornua and are therefore larger estimates (12 mm; Aggarwal et al., 2009).
Sacral canal diameter = antero-posterior diameter of the sacral hiatus. Values of 2 mm of less have been associated with failure of caudal anesthesia.
Tip of dural sac = the median level of the position. A range of values has been measured with both myelography and MRI (dural sacs as low-lying as S4 have been reported in normal subjects).
Distance between the dural sac and sacral hiatus has been reported to be as low as 16 mm in other reports (Trotter, 1947).
Angle of approach = angle of the sacral canal. Average estimates in children are approximately 21 degrees (range 10 to 38 degrees; Park et al., 2006).
Sacral volume = volume of the caudal epidural space. Note that sacral canal volume was significantly smaller in females than in males (mean values 13.2 and 16.5 mL, respectively). Anatomic dissections have yielded a broader range of volume estimates (12 to 65 mL; Trotter, 1947).
US, Ultrasound; MRI, magnetic resonance imaging; N, number of observations.
Table references:
Kim DH, Park JH, Lee SC. Ultrasonographic evaluation of anatomic variations in the sacral hiatus: implications for caudal epidural injections. *Spine (Phila Pa 1976)*. 2016 Jul 1;41(13):E759–E763. PMID: 27340767.
Trotter M. Variations of the sacral canal; their significance in the administration of caudal analgesia. *Curr Res Anesth Analg*. 1947 Sep–Oct;26(5):192–202. PMID: 20262465.
Crighton IM, Barry BP, Hobbs GJ. A study of the anatomy of the caudal space using magnetic resonance imaging. *Br J Anaesth*. 1997;78:391–395. PMID: 9135359.
Park JH, Koo BN, Kim JY, Cho JE, Kim WO, Kil HK. Determination of the optimal angle for needle insertion during caudal block in children using ultrasound imaging. *Anaesthesia*. 2006;61:946–949. PMID: 16978308.
Aggarwal A, Aggarwal A, Harjeet, Sahni D. Morphometry of sacral hiatus and its clinical relevance in caudal epidural block. *Surg Radiol Anat*. 2009 Dec;31(10):793–800. PMID: 19578805.

of caudal epidural block varies from individual to individual. The S5 and coccygeal nerves normally exit the sacral canal through the sacral hiatus. The sacral and coccygeal cornua (horns) articulate to form an arch-like structure.

In adults, the dural sac of the subarachnoid space usually ends between the S1 and S2 sacral segments, although there is variation in the position of the caudal termination of the dural sac. The distance between the dural sac and sacrococcygeal ligament has been reported to range from 34 mm to 80 mm.

Variations in sacral anatomy are relatively common. A number of conditions can make caudal block difficult, including narrowing or complete absence of the sacral hiatus. These conditions occur in 3% to 6% of anatomic specimens. The sacral cornua are prominent (>3 mm of bony prominence on each side) in only 21% of adult sacrums; therefore, assessment by palpation can be problematic.

The sacral epidural space is highly vascular. Inadvertent intravenous injection is relatively common during caudal block, occurring in about 5% to 10% of these procedures.

Ultrasound can be used to guide caudal blocks in pediatric and adult patients. Sonography can determine the location and size of the sacral hiatus for needle tip placement. In addition, ultrasound can be used to image the distribution after caudal epidural injection. However, in adults, the bone of the sacrum prevents ultrasound imaging of most of the sacral canal. One concern is that acoustic shadowing from the overlying bone can prevent detection of intravascular injection during caudal blocks. Ultrasound imaging may be of particular utility in guiding caudal injections in patients with spinal dysraphism.

SUGGESTED TECHNIQUE

Caudal block with ultrasound is optimally performed in prone position with sterile transducer cover and skin preparation. The wide variety of transducer selections for caudal block depends on patient size. In thin adult patients, a 5- to 10-MHz small-footprint "hockey-stick" transducer is appropriate. Average-sized adults image well with a standard linear transducer for the procedure. For obese patients, a lower-frequency curvilinear array is optimal.

The sacral hiatus is easiest to image in transverse view over the midline. The sacral cornua appear as two inverted "U"–shaped hyperechoic structures. The sacrococcygeal ligament and base of the sacrum appear as two parallel bandlike structures between the cornua. The sacral hiatus lies between these two hyperechoic bands.

A 21-gauge, 5- to 7-cm echogenic needle can be used for in-plane caudal block through the sacral hiatus. Two common approaches are the longitudinal in-plane approach and transverse out-of-plane approach.

There is a characteristic tent and recoil when the sacrococcygeal ligament is punctured by the block needle (the ligament is 2 mm to 3 mm thick). This is more likely to be detected with ultrasound imaging than by tactile sense. As the needle punctures the sacrococcygeal ligament, the needle tip disappears because of acoustic shadowing from the overlying bone.

Ultrasound imaging can be used to assess the injection distribution for caudal block. Some investigators have favored a transverse view to assess the test injection distribution. With the probe in transverse position, it is possible to observe bilateral spread. Anterior displacement of the posterior dura occurs in more than 90% of caudal epidural injections. Turbulence of the injection, as manifested by a mosaic pattern on color Doppler, also indicates successful injection. Longitudinal paramedian view can be advantageous for assessing the level of injection in adults with the sacrum in the field as a reference point.

Clinical Pearls

- Caudal block is the most commonly performed regional anesthesia technique in pediatric patients undergoing surgical procedures. Although there appear to be benefits of ultrasound guidance for adults, complications rates are no different in children.[1]

Clinical Pearls—cont'd

- The transducer must be tilted to enhance echoes from the sacrococcygeal ligament because it exhibits a high degree of anisotropy. For this same reason, it is difficult to visualize the sacrococcygeal ligament along its entire length.
- Perform the caudal block where there is the widest separation gap between the anterior and posterior surfaces of the sacral canal (the largest step-off).
- The optimal angle for needle insertion, defined by the base of the sacrum and the skin surface, varies but is about 21 degrees in children.[2]
- In adults, the angle of the sacral canal varies with gender. This angle is about 20 degrees in men and 30 to 45 degrees in women.
- Because the sacrococcygeal ligament is thick (2 mm to 3 mm in adults),[1] the needle should be advanced slightly after visible and tactile sense of tent and recoil so that the entire bevel opening is within the caudal epidural space.
- Do not advance the needle more than 2.0 cm into the sacral canal to avoid dural puncture in adults (this distance is even smaller in children).
- Injection in the caudal epidural space is usually easily detected (distention of the space, displacement of the dura, findings on color Doppler, etc.).[3] The sacrococcygeal ligament should rise or bow with injection as the caudal epidural space distends.
- Aspirate to help rule out intravascular needle tip placement. Aspirate frequently because the caudal epidural space is highly vascular.
- Of the ultrasound tests, turbulence is more sensitive than color flow Doppler (95.0% vs. 78.8%).[4] In this pediatric study, the caudal space was identified while scanning a few centimeters above the point of needle insertion.
- After injection, fluid will undergo redistribution within the caudal epidural space over about 15 to 20 minutes.[5]
- The lateral aspect of the foot is reliably innervated by S1 for cutaneous assessment of the upper extent of sacral caudal block.
- Several ultrasound parameters have been associated with difficulty of caudal epidural block, including a canal diameter (anteroposterior) of less than 2 mm or a transverse width of less than 5 mm.[6-8]
- Even in pediatric patients, the sacral cornua are not always palpable.[9] Although sacral anomalies can be identified with ultrasound imaging (e.g., spina bifida occulta, sacral agenesis, cord tethering), these conditions are not common.[9]
- Total spinal anesthesia and postdural puncture headache are possible after dural puncture in the caudal region. Ultrasound guidance has been suggested to help further reduce the chance of these relatively uncommon complications.[10]

References

1. Suresh S, Long J, Birmingham PK, De Oliveira GS Jr. Are caudal blocks for pain control safe in children? An analysis of 18,650 caudal blocks from the Pediatric Regional Anesthesia Network (PRAN) database. *Anesth Analg.* 2015;120(1):151–156. PMID: 25393589.
2. Park JH, Koo BN, Kim JY, Cho JE, Kim WO, Kil HK. Determination of the optimal angle for needle insertion during caudal block in children using ultrasound imaging. *Anaesthesia.* 2006;61:946–949. PMID: 16978308.
3. Tsui B, Leipoldt C, Desai S. Color flow Doppler ultrasonography can distinguish caudal epidural injection from intrathecal injection. *Anesth Analg.* 2013;116(6):1376–1379. PMID: 23558836.
4. Raghunathan K, Schwartz D, Connelly NR. Determining the accuracy of caudal needle placement in children: a comparison of the swoosh test and ultrasonography. *Paediatr Anaesth.* 2008;18(7):606–612. PMID: 18616491.
5. Lundblad M, Eksborg S, Lönnqvist PA. Secondary spread of caudal block as assessed by ultrasonography. *Br J Anaesth.* 2012;108(4):675–681. PMID: 22315327.
6. Chen CP, Wong AM, Hsu CC, Tsai WC, Chang CN, Lin SC, et al. Ultrasound as a screening tool for proceeding with caudal epidural injections. *Arch Phys Med Rehabil.* 2010;91(3):358–363. PMID: 20298824.
7. Park GY, Kwon DR, Cho HK. Anatomic differences in the sacral hiatus during caudal epidural injection using ultrasound guidance. *J Ultrasound Med.* 2015;34(12):2143–2148. PMID: 26491092.

8. Kim DH, Park JH, Lee SC. Ultrasonographic evaluation of anatomic variations in the sacral hiatus: implications for caudal epidural injections. *Spine*. 2016;41(13):E759–E763. PMID: 27340767.
9. Mirjalili SA, Taghavi K, Frawley G, Craw S. Should we abandon landmark-based technique for caudal anesthesia in neonates and infants? *Paediatr Anaesth*. 2015;25(5):511–516. PMID: 25597342.
10. Lee HJ, Min JY, Kim HI, Byon HJ. Measuring the depth of the caudal epidural space to prevent dural sac puncture during caudal block in children. *Paediatr Anaesth*. 2017;27:540–544. PMID: 28332251.

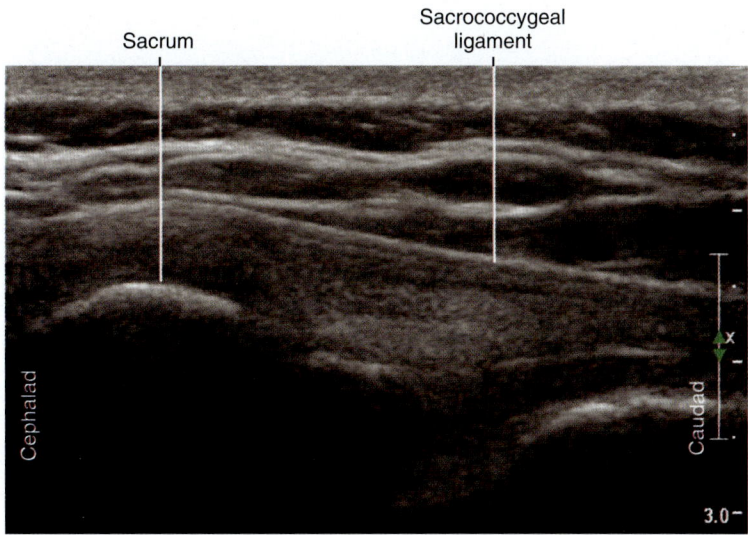

FIGURE 64.1 Longitudinal in-plane approach to caudal epidural block. Sonogram obtained before needle placement. In this sonogram, the sacrococcygeal ligament can be seen overlying the sacral hiatus.

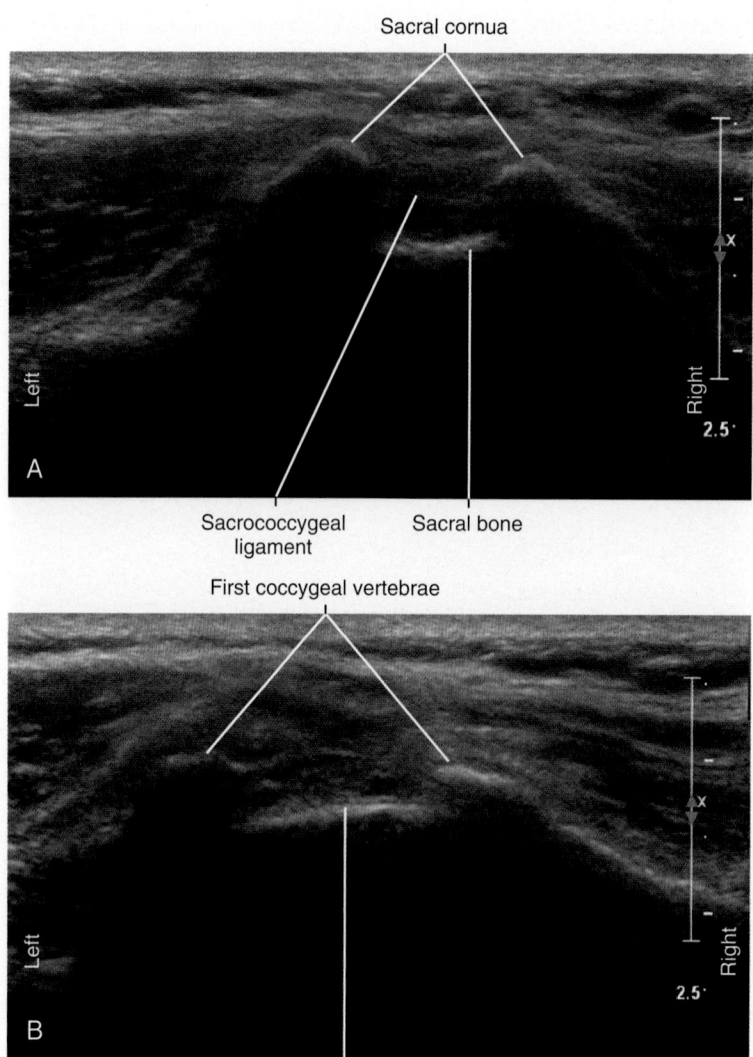

FIGURE 64.2 Transverse view of the sacral cornua (A). These bones appear as inverted "U" shapes in transverse view with acoustic shadowing. The hyperechoic lines between the cornua are the sacrococcygeal ligament and underlying sacral bone, with the sacral hiatus lying between these two structures. More distally, the caudal epidural space narrows as the transverse processes of the first coccygeal vertebra come into view (B). This indicates the transducer is caudal to the sacral hiatus.

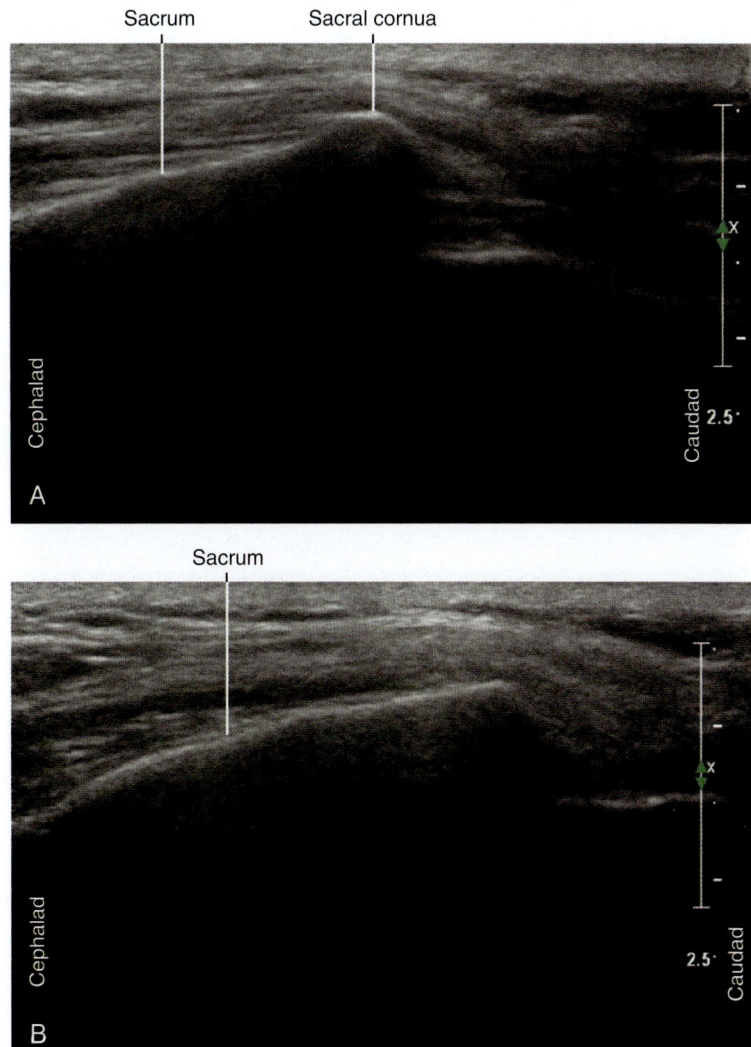

FIGURE 64.3 Longitudinal view of the sacrum demonstrating the presence (A) or absence (B) of the sacral cornua in the imaging plane.

TRUNK BLOCKS

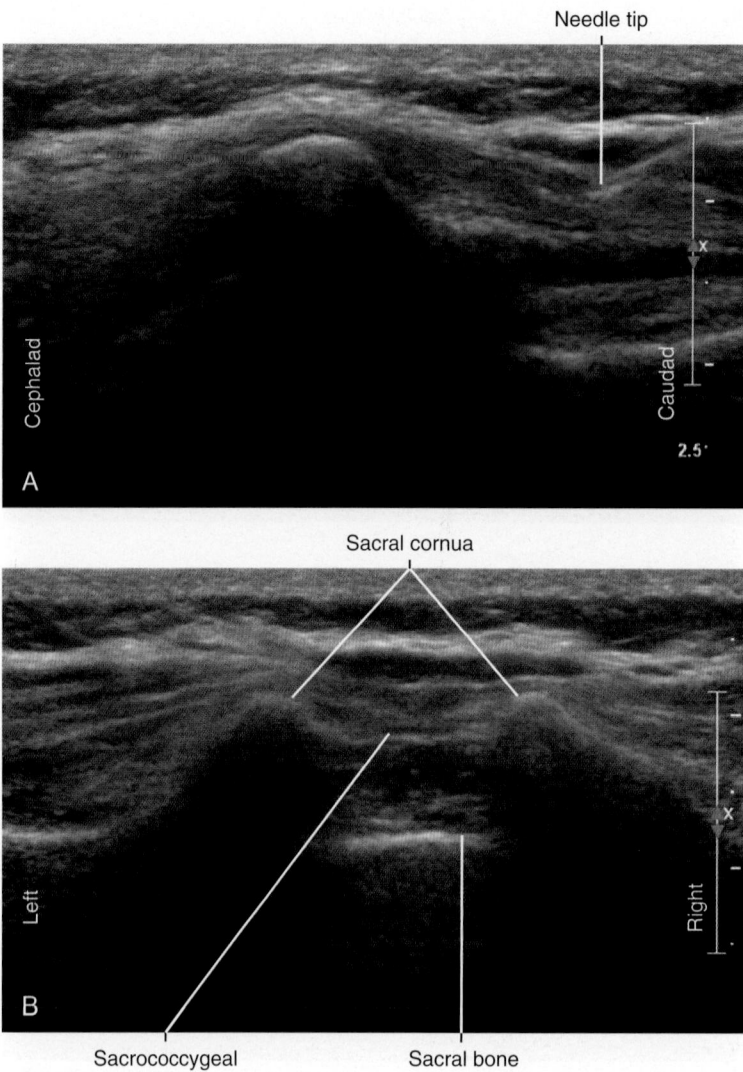

FIGURE 64.4 Longitudinal in-plane approach to caudal epidural block (A). The corresponding transverse view is shown (B).

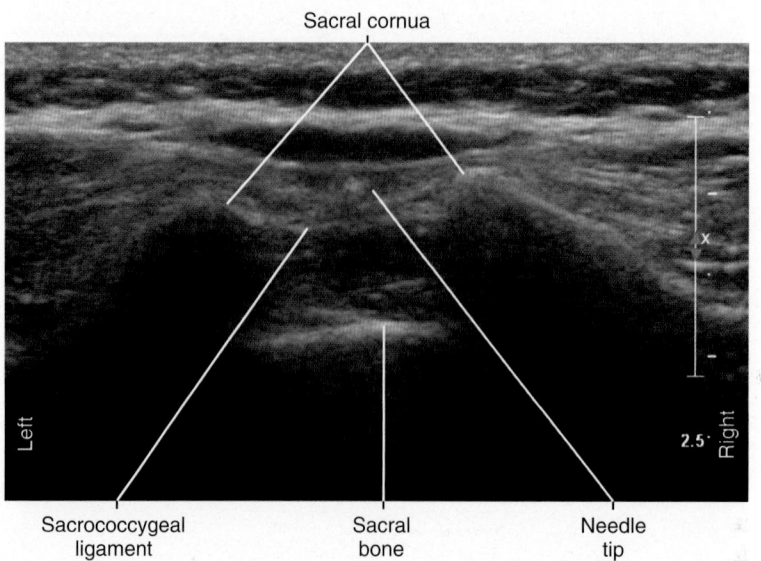

FIGURE 64.5 Transverse out-of-plane approach to caudal epidural block. The needle tip crosses the plane of imaging as an echogenic dot.

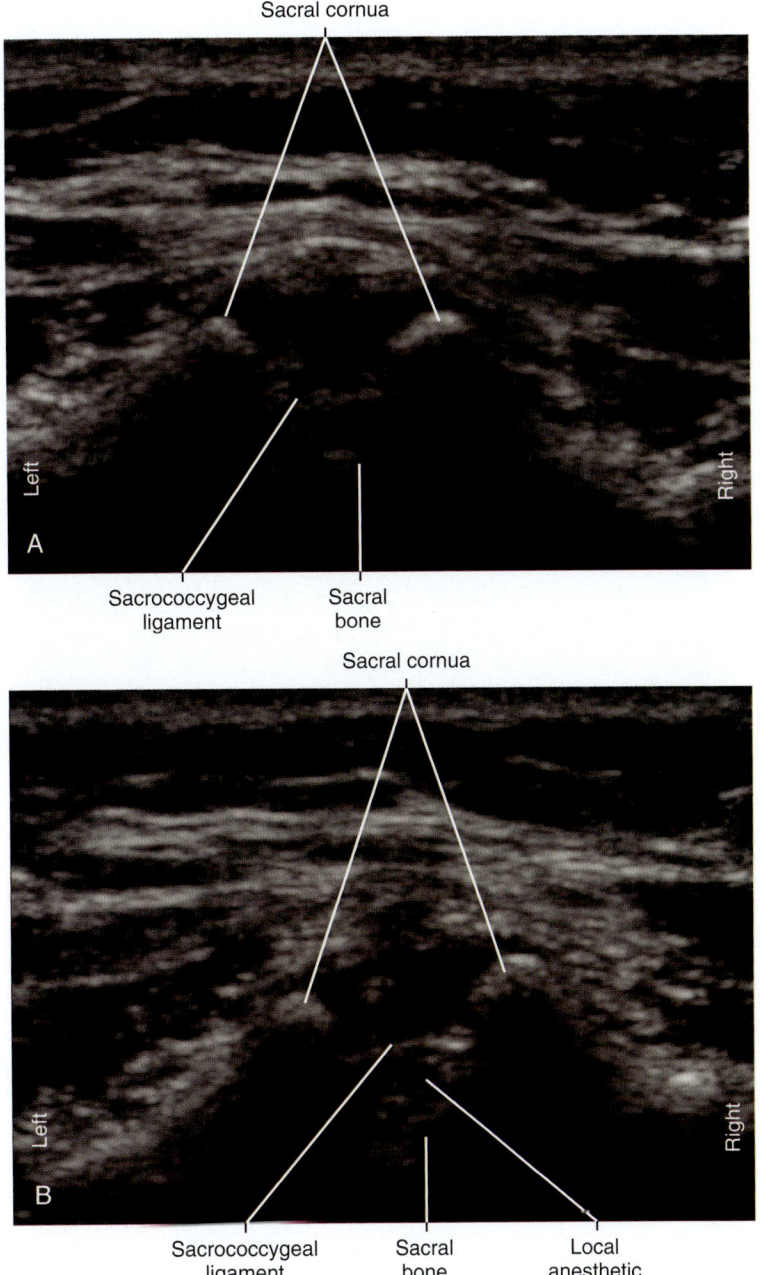

FIGURE 64.6 Pediatric caudal epidural guided by ultrasound. These transverse sonograms show the sacral cornua and caudal epidural space before (A) and after (B) injection of local anesthetic. The injection of local anesthetic distributes throughout the caudal epidural space and tents the sacrococcygeal ligament.

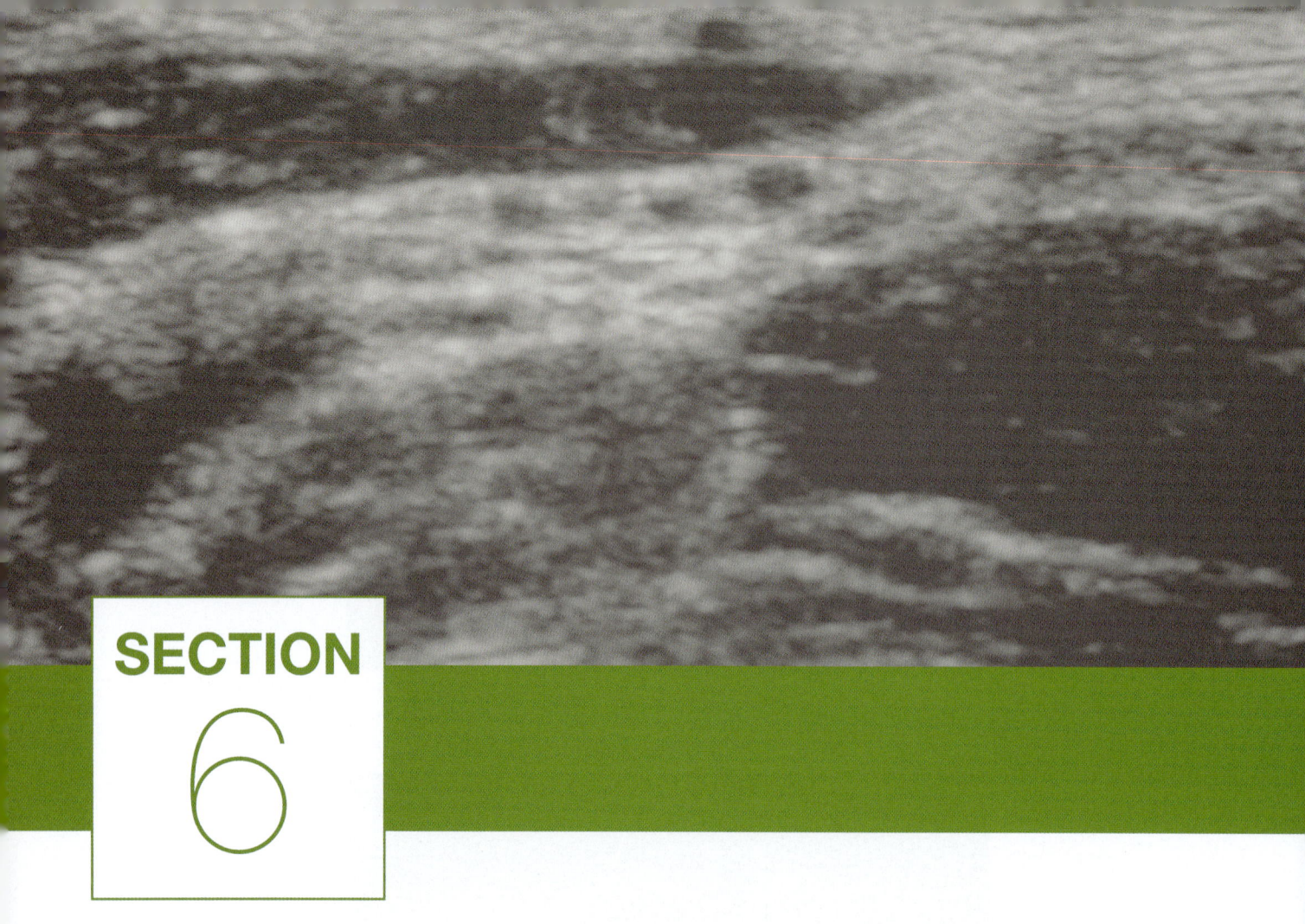

SECTION 6

Head and Neck Blocks

CHAPTER 65

Supraorbital Nerve Block

The supraorbital nerve (SON) is a branch of the ophthalmic division of the trigeminal nerve (V1). This nerve travels through the supraorbital foramen or notch to provide sensory innervation to the upper eyelid and forehead. After leaving the orbit, the SON lies deep to (or within) the periorbital muscles (orbicularis oculi, corrugator supercilii and frontalis). The SON does not emerge from the foramen/notch as a single discrete nerve, but rather as a collection of branches that are bundled together.

The dividing line between the SON territory and the greater occipital nerve territory is typically at the vertex of the head. In some cases, SON innervation can extend as far posteriorly as the lambdoid suture. The medial and lateral extent of the SON distribution is limited by the supratrochlear and zygomaticotemporal nerve territories, respectively.

SON blocks are used to provide local anesthesia of the forehead or treat supraorbital neuralgia manifest as frontal headaches. These blocks can be used for a variety of neurosurgical procedures.[1] In cases of supraorbital neuralgia, a Tinel sign can sometimes be elicited over the SON at the supraorbital notch.

Potential advantages of ultrasound guidance for SON block include less local anesthetic volume, fewer arterial punctures, and less periorbital swelling. If lower volumes are used, it may be possible to reduce block of adjacent nerves (such as the temporal branch of the facial nerve). More complete blocks (i.e., more extensive medial and lateral coverage, and deeper periosteal fibers of the frontal bone) also are possible.[2] Because the exit point of the SON is not constant, ultrasound imaging is a useful tool to guide these regional blocks. Ultrasound is a highly effective tool for identifying features of supraorbital foramen morphology and associated pathology.[3,4]

SUGGESTED TECHNIQUE

The supraorbital foramen/notch is approximately 2.5 cm from the midline (range 2 to 3.5 cm), slightly medial to the midpupillary line.[5,6] This exit point is usually 1 to 2 mm superior to the orbital rim but may be as much as 2 cm for accessory foramina.[7] The supraorbital foramen/notch is located at the lower border of the corrugator supercilii muscle, where medial and lateral branches of the SON diverge from each other. The supraorbital artery and nerve run together into the frontalis muscle, the artery superficial to the nerve.[2]

SON block can be done awake or asleep (there is a low risk of paresthesia and nerve injury).
The operator and machine remain in one location for bilateral SON block.
Povidone-iodine is typically used for skin prep before SON block (avoid chlorhexidine contamination of the eyes).
Light touch with the transducer is necessary because the supraorbital artery is superficial and therefore easily compressed against the adjacent bone.
For supraorbital block, use an in-plane approach from either side.
Limit the injection volume to less than 3 mL per side to reduce periorbital swelling.
The block can be performed either above or below the eyebrow (which can be pushed up or down with the transducer).

COMMENTS

INCOMPLETE BLOCK

Potential causes of failed or incomplete SON blocks include duplicate foramina, superior/high foramina, and injection not sufficiently deep to cover the periosteal branches. Identification of the main foramen/notch does not entirely rule out the possibility of a high foramen because duplication is possible. Scan the region 1 to 2 cm above the main foramen/notch to help rule out this possibility.

HEMATOMA AND SWELLING

Puncture of the supraorbital artery can lead to significant swelling from hemorrhage into the loose connective tissue of the upper eyelid. If inadvertent arterial puncture occurs, hold firm pressure against the orbital ridge with gauze for 5 minutes. Puncture of the supraorbital artery can theoretically lead to SON impingement.

MOTOR BLOCK OF FACIAL MUSCLES

Motor block of facial muscles innervated by the temporal branch of the facial nerve is possible. This can occur transiently after local anesthetic injection, and expectant management with reassurance are generally sufficient. If inability to close the eyelid occurs, use a transparent eye shield to protect the cornea.

KEY POINTS

Supraorbital Nerve Block	The Essentials
Anatomy	The supraorbital foramen/notch and artery are about 1 mm in diameter.
Image orientation	Arbitrary.
Positioning	Supine
Operator	Standing on the side of the table
Display	Across the table
Transducer	High-frequency linear, 23- to 38-mm footprint
Initial depth setting	20 mm
Needle	25 gauge, 38 mm in length
Anatomic location	Begin by scanning the orbital rim 2.5 cm from the midline
Approach	SAX view of SON, in-plane from either side
	Place the needle tip adjacent to or underneath the SOA for injection
Sonographic assessment	Injection should track centrally along the SOA towards the foramen/notch
Anatomic variation	Supraorbital foramen or notch (about equal incidence)
	Accessory supraorbital foramina, including superior foramina

SOA, Supraorbital artery; *SAX*, short axis; *SON*, supraorbital nerve.

Clinical Pearls

- The ideal needle path is adjacent to or between the supraorbital artery and nerve so that the injection will separate these two anatomic structures.
- Power Doppler can be used to help locate the position of the supraorbital artery.
- The periorbital muscles of facial expression are very thin and difficult to distinguish on ultrasound scans (only 1 or 2 mm thick).

> **Clinical Pearls—cont'd**
> - For operations near the midline, perform bilateral blocks.
> - The supraorbital nerve and artery are intertwined along their courses with a variety of exit patterns from the orbit.[8]

References

1. Watson R, Leslie K. Nerve blocks versus subcutaneous infiltration for stereotactic frame placement. *Anesth Analg.* 2001;92(2):424–427. PMID: 11159245.
2. Malet T, Braun M, Fyad JP, George JL. Anatomic study of the distal supraorbital nerve. *Surg Radiol Anat.* 1997;19(6):377–384. PMID: 9479712.
3. Garg RK, Lee KS, Kohn SC, Baskaya MK, Afifi AM. Can sonography distinguish a supraorbital notch from a foramen? *J Ultrasound Med.* 2015;34(11):2089–2091. PMID: 26432823.
4. Tijssen C, Schoemaker K, Visser L. Supraorbital neuralgia caused by nerve entrapment visualized on ultrasonography. *Headache.* 2013;53(2):376–377. PMID: 23094662.
5. Andersen NB, Bovim G, Sjaastad O. The frontotemporal peripheral nerves. Topographic variations of the supraorbital, supratrochlear and auriculotemporal nerves and their possible clinical significance. *Surg Radiol Anat.* 2001;23(2):97–104. PMID: 11462869.
6. Christensen KN, Lachman N, Pawlina W, Baum CL. Cutaneous depth of the supraorbital nerve: a cadaveric anatomic study with clinical applications to dermatology. *Dermatol Surg.* 2014;40(12):1342–1348. PMID: 25357169.
7. Beer GM, Putz R, Mager K, Schumacher M, Keil W. Variations of the frontal exit of the supraorbital nerve: an anatomic study. *Plast Reconstr Surg.* 1998;102(2):334–341. PMID: 9703067.
8. Berchtold V, Stofferin H, Moriggl B, Brenner E, Pauzenberger R, Konschake M. The supraorbital region revisited: an anatomic exploration of the neurovascular bundle with regard to frontal migraine headache. *J Plast Reconstr Aesthet Surg.* 2017;70:1171–1180. PMID: 28712884

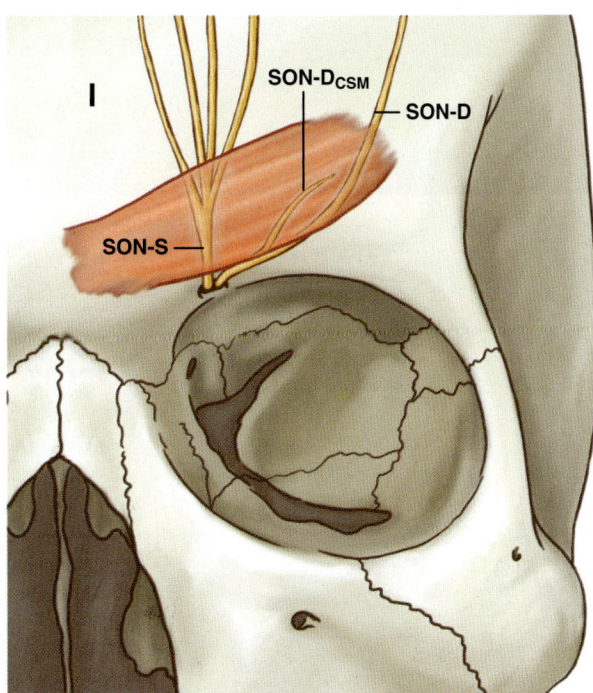

FIGURE 65.1 Course of the supraorbital nerve deep to the corrugator muscle. Supraorbital nerve branching pattern. Type I supraorbital nerve branching pattern, the most common type. *SON-S*, Superficial division of the supraorbital nerve; *SON-D*, deep division of the supraorbital nerve; $SON-D_{CSM}$, branch from the deep division of the supraorbital nerve. (Redrawn from Janis JE, Ghavami A, Lemmon JA, Leedy JE, Guyuron B. The anatomy of the corrugator supercilii muscle: part II. Supraorbital nerve branching patterns. *Plast Reconstr Surg.* 2008 Jan;121(1):233–240. PMID: 18176226.)

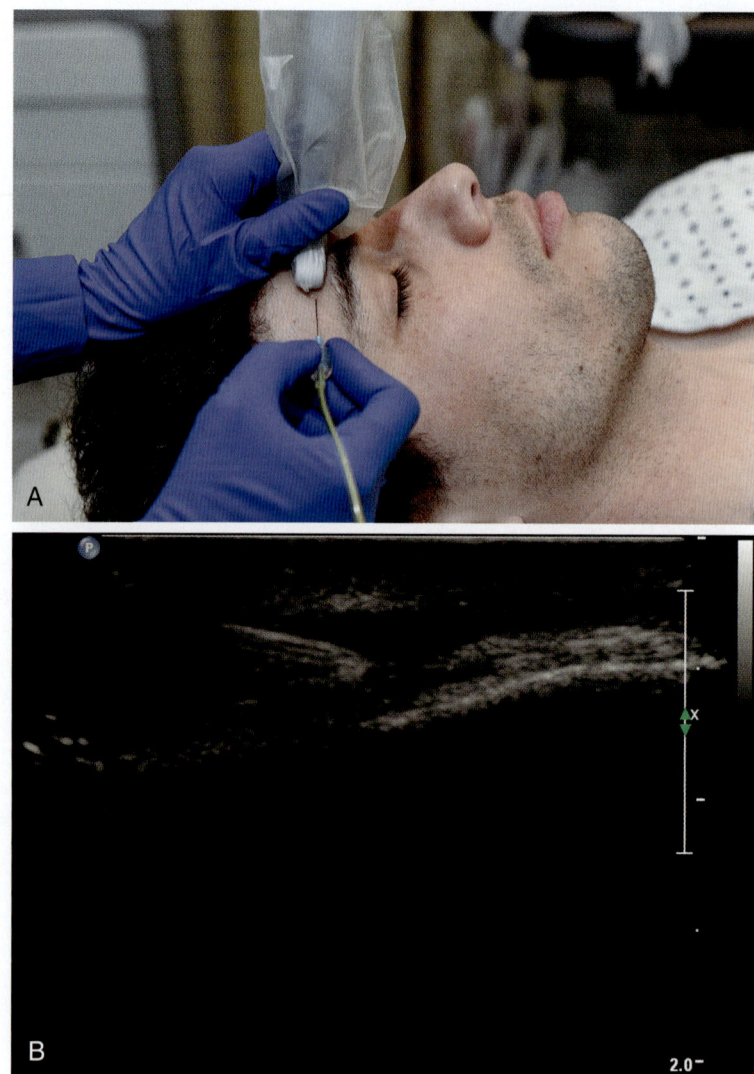

FIGURE 65.2 External photograph showing in-plane approach to supraorbital nerve block (A). Corresponding sonogram (B).

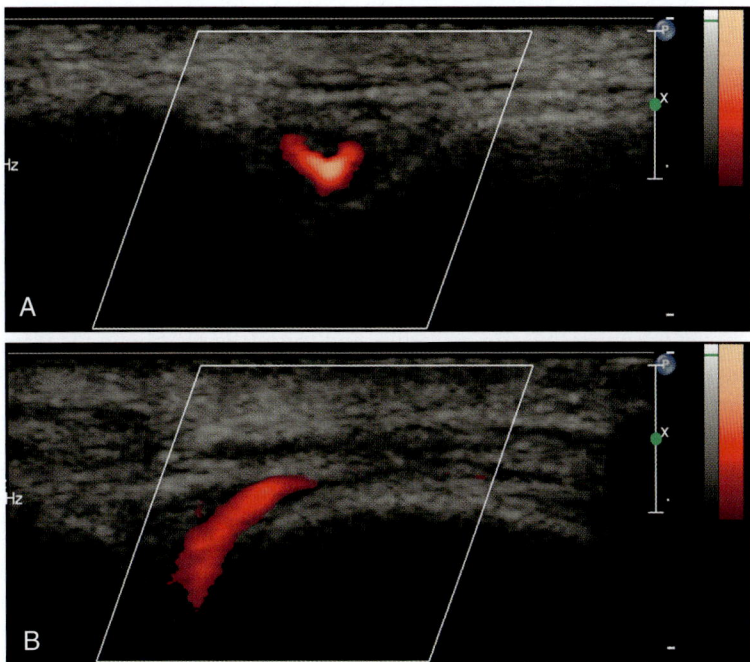

FIGURE 65.3 The supraorbital foramen with power Doppler of the supraorbital artery (short-axis (A) and long-axis (B) views of the supraorbital artery at the supraorbital foramen).

CHAPTER 66

Mental Nerve Block

The mental nerve is a branch of the inferior alveolar nerve from the third division of the trigeminal nerve. The inferior alveolar nerve enters the mandibular foramen to travel within the mandibular canal and form the mental nerve. At its exit from the mental foramen on the buccal side of the mandible, the mental nerve is divided into several branches. The mental nerve emerges from the mental foramen to supply the chin, lower lip, and teeth (the distribution is primarily medial to the position of the mental foramen). The border territories include the infraorbital (V2), buccal (V3), and transverse cervical (C2, C3) nerves.

The mental nerve also provides innervation to the lower incisors. The mandibular canal usually continues after the mental foramen as a smaller incisive canal containing an anterior extension of the neurovascular bundle. When no well-defined (corticalized) incisive mandibular canal exists, the incisive bundle traverses the marrow spaces (without any bony canal).

The mental foramen usually lies below the corner of the lip (the chelion), below the second mandibular premolar tooth, and about halfway between the tooth cusp and the inferior border of the mandible.[1,2] However, the position of the foramen relative to the mandible varies with age. Elderly patients who are edentulous have decay of the alveolar ridge. This brings the mental foramen closer to the upper border of the mandible. A severely resorbed alveolar ridge can make identification of the mental foramen even more difficult to palpate.

SUGGESTED TECHNIQUE

Ultrasound imaging can establish foramen location and morphology for optimal approach. With proper needle positioning within the canal, more extensive block can result.

Most mental foramina are oval in shape (average vertical and horizontal diameters of 1.7 and 2.5 mm, respectively).[2,3] The presence of multiple mental foramina is relatively rare, being observed in about 2% of cases.[4,5]

For this block, the operator stands near the head of the bed and faces across the table. The block is performed in supine position with the head turned to the opposite side and stabilized with a foam doughnut. A narrow linear transducer is used (hockey stick, 20 to 25 mm footprint, rectangular or trapezoidal formatted image).

It is important to direct the needle to enter the mental foramen easily. Rotate the transducer until the long axis and lowest rim of the foramen is identified. This is usually when the transducer is aligned with the mandibular canal or the oblique line of the body of the mandible.

Approach the mental foramen from posterior and slightly superior at 45 degrees with respect to the skin surface. The block needle is advanced well into the mental canal ($\approx$ 6 mm) for successful block and to achieve anesthesia of the lower incisors. Limit the total local anesthetic volume to less than 6 mL (about 2 mL should be sufficient if injected within the canal). Hold pressure over the site with the transducer while injecting to promote retrograde flow of local anesthetic into the mandibular canal. The block needle passes through the platysma and depressor anguli oris muscles on the approach to the canal. Care is taken not to puncture the facial artery, which lies on the posterior side of the foramen.

KEY POINTS

Mental Nerve Block	The Essentials
Anatomy	The MTN exits the mental foramen, with nearby facial artery.
	The MF is about 2.5 mm in diameter.
Positioning	Supine
Operator	Standing at the side of the patient
	Display across the table
Transducer	High-frequency linear, 23- to 38-mm footprint
Initial depth setting	20 mm
Needle	25 gauge, 38 mm in length
Anatomic location	Halfway between the upper and lower borders of mandible near the corner of the mouth.
	The MF lies approximately 2.5 cm from the midline.
Approach	Transverse view of MF, in-plane from lateral to medial
	Place the needle tip into the MF.
Sonographic assessment	Injection distribution observed within the MF
Anatomic variation	Multiple foramina (2%)
	Accessory foramina usually lie within 1 cm of the primary foramen.

MF, Mental foramen; *MTN*, mental nerve.

Clinical Pearls

- Advance the block needle 6 mm into the mental canal for successful block.
- Local anesthetic injected within the mental foramen tracks centrally along the inferior alveolar nerve within the mandibular canal.
- Use a 25-gauge, 38-mm needle for placement in the mental canal.
- Facial hair can make imaging for mental canal block challenging.
- The alveolar ridge of the mandible decays with age and loss of dentition. Therefore, the relative position of the mental foramen with respect to the mandible varies with age and state of dentition (bone resorption).
- The facial artery and vein lie close to the mental foramen.
- Bilateral mental nerve blocks are often needed for lower incisor, lip, and chin surgery.

References

1. Laher AE, Wells M, Motara F, et al. Finding the mental foramen. *Surg Radiol Anat.* 2016;38(4):469–476.
2. Laher AE, Mahomed Z. The ultrasonographic determination of the position of the mental foramen and its relation to hard tissue landmarks. *Acta Med Acad.* 2016;45(1):51–60.
3. Møystad A, Bjørnland T, Friedland B, Donoff RB. Ultrasonographic pilot study of mental foramen size, with and without postoperative neurosensory dysfunction. *Oral Surg Oral Med Oral Pathol Oral Radiol.* 2015;120(2):275–280.
4. Voljevica A, Talović E, Hasanović A. Morphological and morphometric analysis of the shape, position, number and size of mental foramen on human mandibles. *Acta Med Acad.* 2015;44(1):31–38.
5. Agthong S, Huanmanop T, Chentanez V. Anatomical variations of the supraorbital, infraorbital, and mental foramina related to gender and side. *J Oral Maxillofac Surg.* 2005;63:800–804.

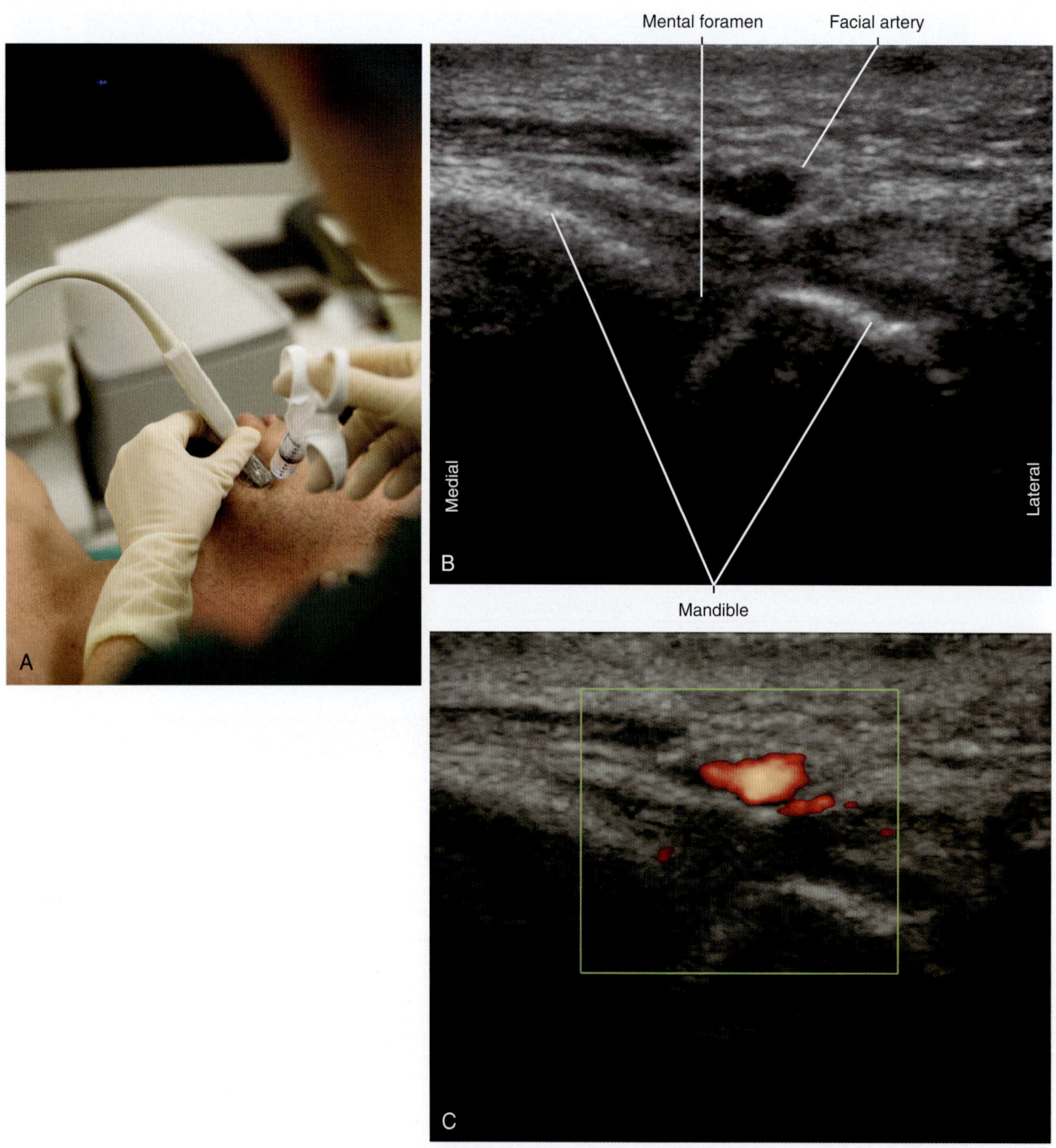

FIGURE 66.1 External photograph showing an approach to mental nerve block. An in-plane approach from the posterior aspect of the mandible is shown (A). The corresponding sonogram of the mental foramen is shown (B). Power Doppler verifies the presence of a blood vessel lying over the foramen (C).

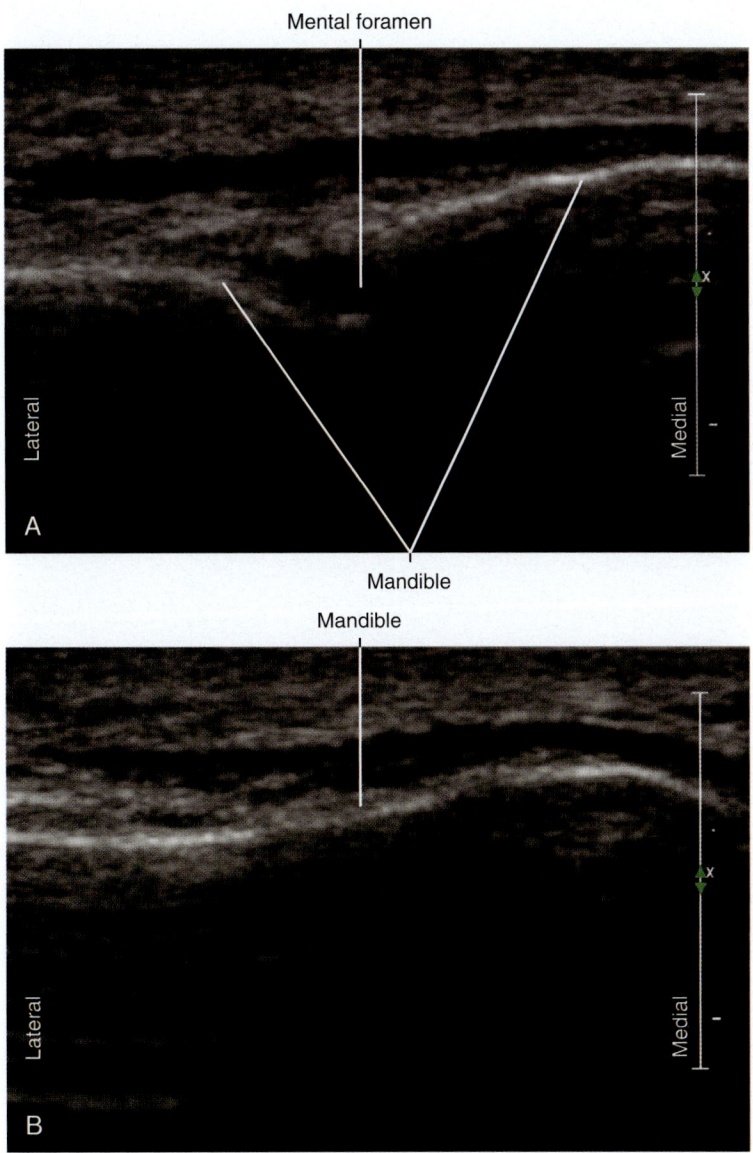

FIGURE 66.2 Ultrasound image of the mental foramen (A) contrasted with the smooth bony contour of the mandible (B).

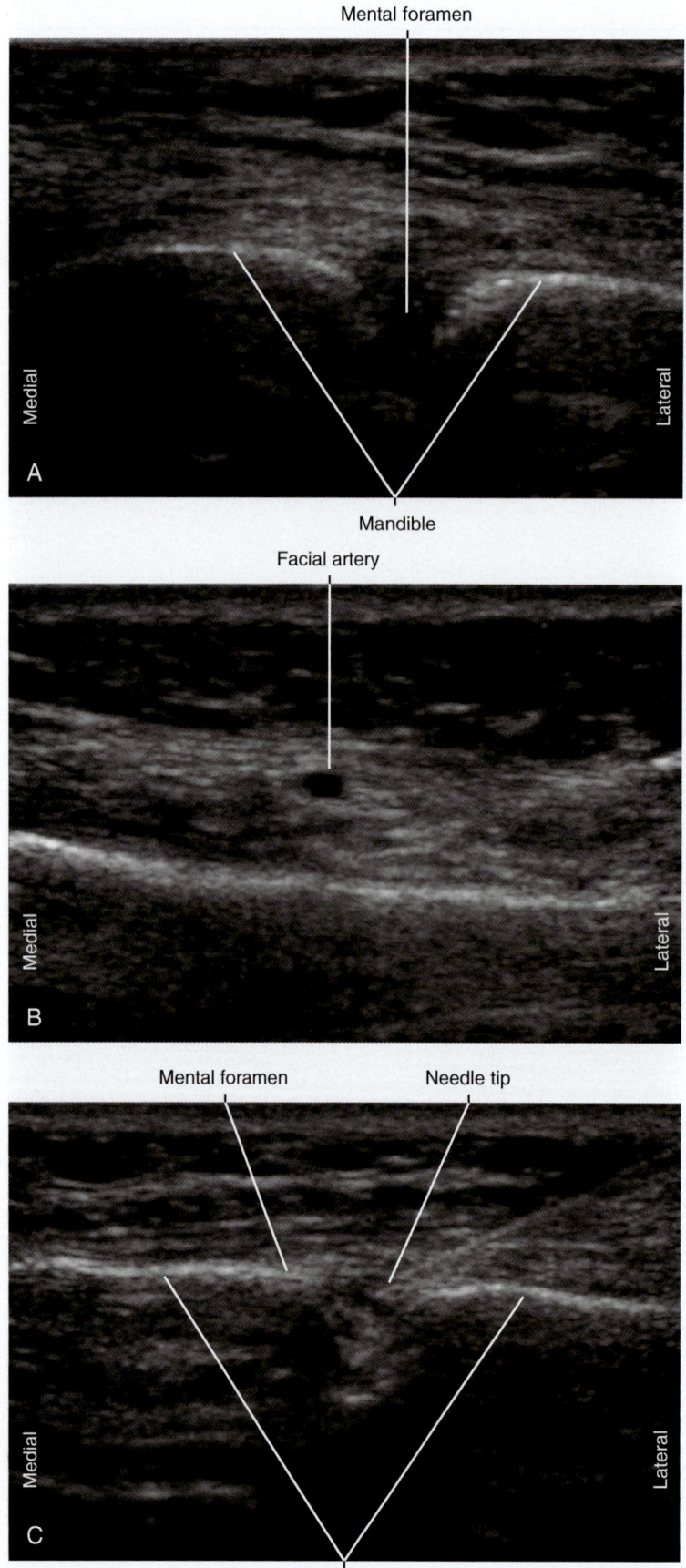

FIGURE 66.3 Image sequence showing mental nerve block in the mental foramen. The mental foramen is first identified and then the angle of approach is planned (A). The facial artery is identified posterior to the mental foramen (B). The block needle is placed within the mental foramen for injection of local anesthetic (C).

Superior Laryngeal Nerve Block

CHAPTER 67

The superior laryngeal nerve is a branch of the vagus nerve (cranial nerve X). At some variable point in the neck, it divides into internal and external branches. The internal branch provides sensory innervation of the larynx above the vocal cords, while the external branch innervates the cricothyroid muscle, which is an adductor tensor of the vocal cords. Both these branches are difficult to identify.[1]

The superior laryngeal nerve lies in close proximity to the superior laryngeal artery. The internal branch of the superior laryngeal nerve lies on average 2.4 mm inferior to the greater horn of the hyoid bone.[2] The hyoid bone is "U" shaped in transverse scans of the neck. The internal branch enters the larynx through an aperture (ostium) in the thyrohyoid membrane together with the superior laryngeal artery and vein. This branch arborizes as it pierces the thyrohyoid membrane. The mucosa of the larynx contains a dense concentration of sensory receptors that are involved in airway reflexes.[3]

Traditional superior laryngeal block is guided by palpation of the hyoid bone. However, palpation can be difficult when edema or hematoma exist, as commonly observed after fracture of the mandible.[4]

Block of the superior laryngeal nerve is sometimes used to facilitate awake fiberoptic intubation, transesophageal echocardiography, or upper endoscopy. Superior laryngeal block may prevent laryngospasm.

SUGGESTED TECHNIQUE

A hockey-stick transducer with a small footprint can be used for imaging. A 25- or 27-gauge, 1.25-inch hypodermic needle can be used for this block. The patient is instructed not to swallow because this causes substantial movement of the hyoid bone. The nerve is superficial, so an out-of-plane approach can be used to guide infiltration inferior to the hyoid bone. Make the injection close to the tip of the greater horn of the hyoid bone where the superior laryngeal nerve divides into its internal and external branches (near the posterolateral border of the hyoid bone).

Acoustic standoff can be used to improve imaging of the superficial nerve. It addition, the conforming gel dissipates the transducer pressure over a larger area. This improves patient tolerance of transducer placement over a sensitive area of the neck. Do not apply pressure on the carotid sinus with the transducer. A small curved transducer can be used for light touch for during scanning and easily matches the contours of the neck.[5]

Clinical Pearls

- The external branch of the superior laryngeal nerve lies near the superior pole of the thyroid gland. It can be difficult to identify, even with direct surgical dissection and nerve stimulation.
- The internal branch of the superior laryngeal nerve lies immediately inferior and deep to the greater cornu of the hyoid bone. This branch is about 2 mm in diameter in this location. The internal branch travels 7 mm before piercing the thyrohyoid membrane to supply sensory innervation to the larynx above the vocal cords.
- The superior laryngeal nerve lies superior and medial to the superior laryngeal artery. The superior laryngeal nerve descends to join the superior laryngeal artery below the greater cornu (inferior horn) of the hyoid bone. Ultrasound can be used to guide injection of local anesthetic above the superior laryngeal artery.

Continued

> ### Clinical Pearls—cont'd
>
> - One concern is that aspiration may occur at any time throughout the duration of superior laryngeal nerve block.[6] This block is best performed in patients who are NPO (nothing per mouth, nil per os).
> - Block assessment is performed by testing phonation (the external motor branch of the superior laryngeal nerve to the cricothyroid muscle) or by fiberoptic examination. If the external superior laryngeal nerve is blocked, the vocal cords will not be closed during fiberoptic intubation.

References

1. Friedman M, LoSavio P, Ibrahim H. Superior laryngeal nerve identification and preservation in thyroidectomy. *Arch Otolaryngol Head Neck Surg.* 2002;128(3):296–303.
2. Furlan JC. Anatomical study applied to anesthetic block technique of the superior laryngeal nerve. *Acta Anaesthesiol Scand.* 2002;46:199–202.
3. Sanders I, Mu L. Anatomy of the human internal superior laryngeal nerve. *Anat Rec.* 1998;252(4):646–656.
4. Gotta AW, Sullivan CA. Anaesthesia of the upper airway using topical anaesthetic and superior laryngeal nerve block. *Br J Anaesth.* 1981;53(10):1055–1058.
5. Krause M, Khatibi B, Sztain JF, Rahman P, Shapiro AB, Sandhu NS. Ultrasound-guided airway blocks using a curvilinear probe. *J Clin Anesth.* 2016;33:408–412.
6. McLoughlin AL. Superior laryngeal nerve block as a supplement to total intravenous anesthesia for rigid laser bronchoscopy in a patient with myasthenic syndrome: risk of aspiration? *Anesth Analg.* 1993;76:903–904.

SUPERIOR LARYNGEAL NERVE BLOCK

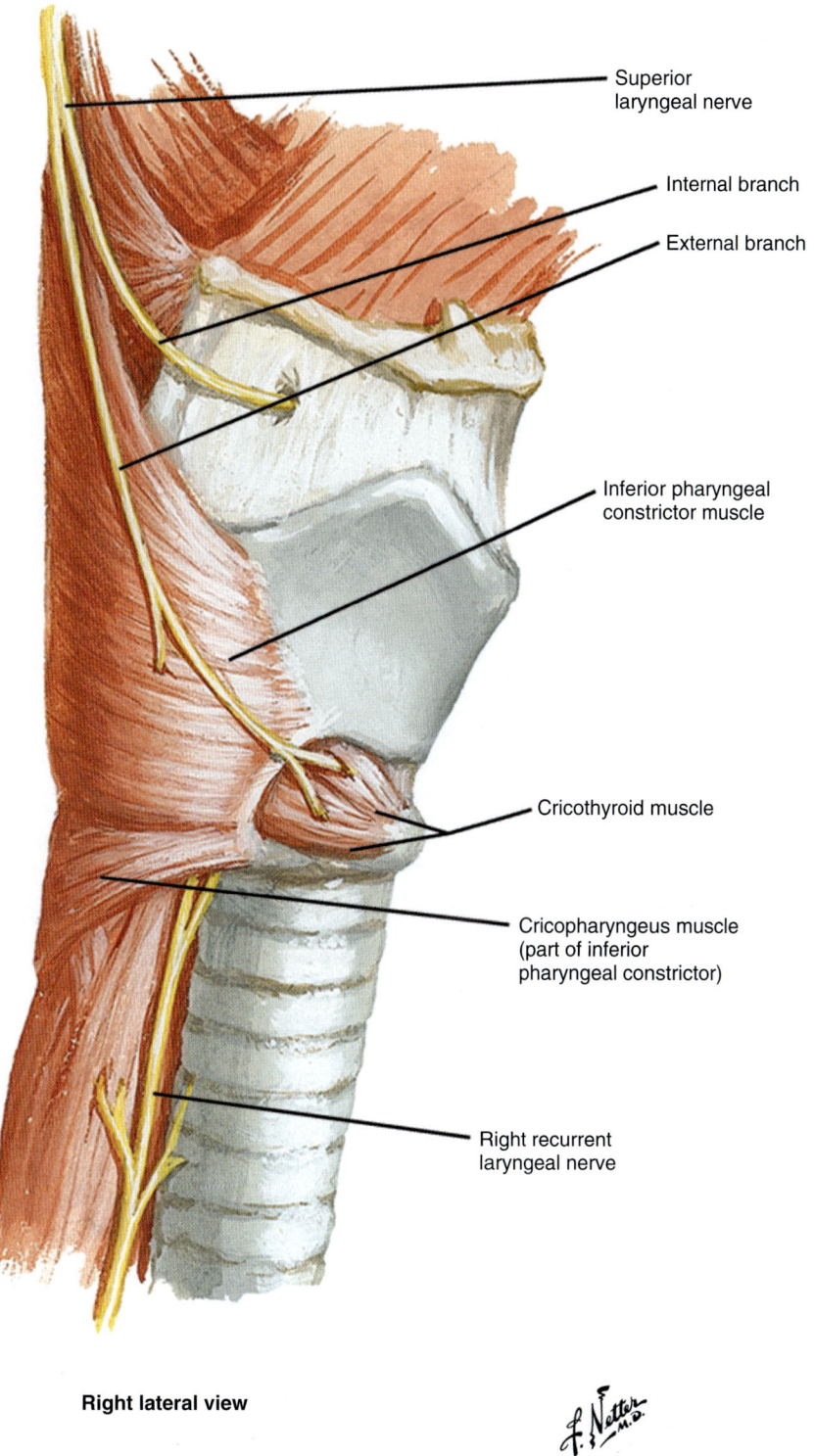

Right lateral view

FIGURE 67.1 Nerves of the larynx. (From netterimages.com, with permission.)

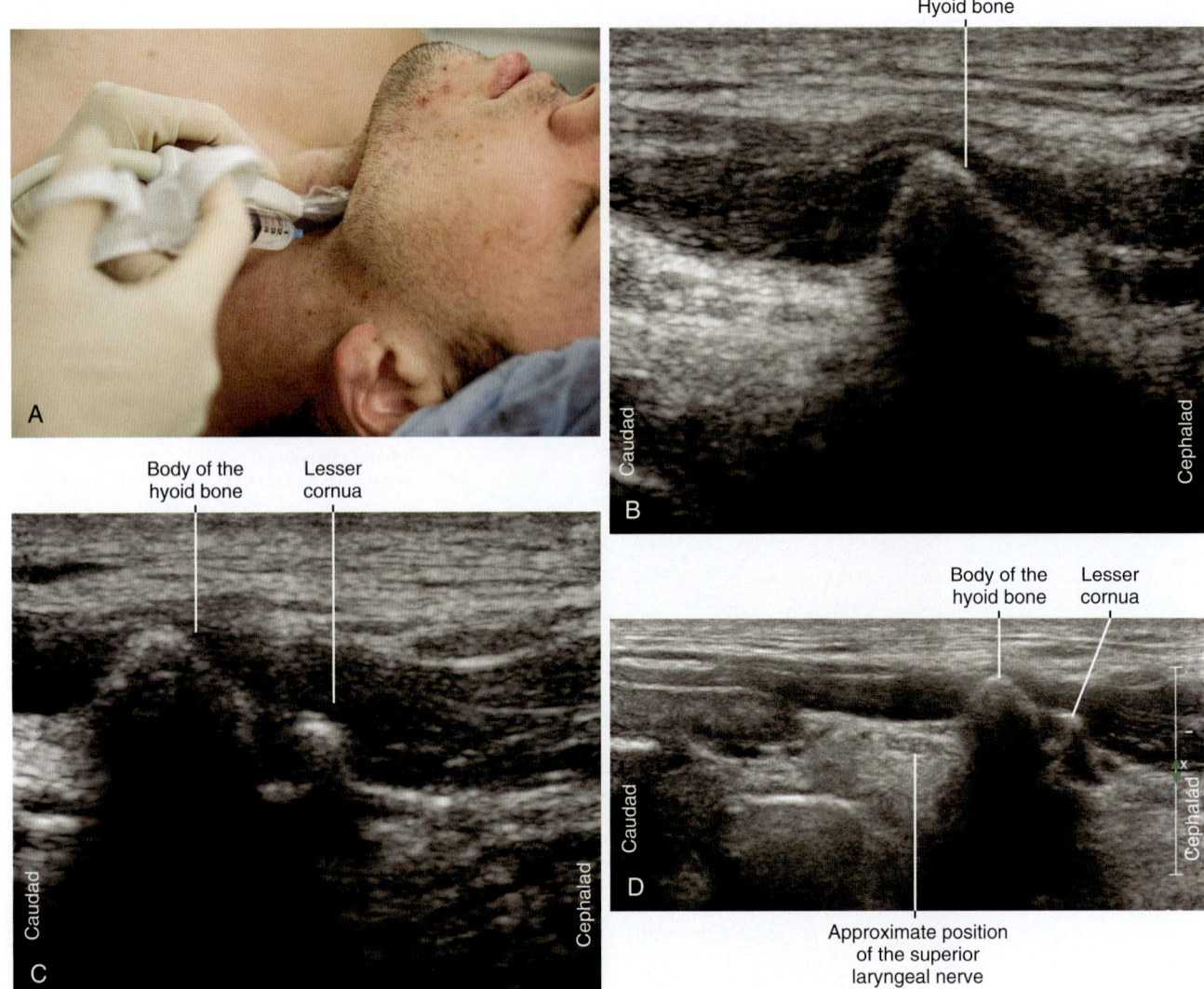

FIGURE 67.2 External photograph showing an approach to superior laryngeal nerve block with ultrasound imaging. An out-of-plane approach from the lateral aspect of the neck is shown (A). Corresponding sonograms for a short-axis view of the hyoid bone (B), at the level of the lesser cornua (C), and view with a broad linear probe (D). The hyoid bone can give a triangular acoustic shadow when viewed in short axis that can help identify its location. The hyoid bone has two horns, the lesser (superior) cornua and the greater (inferior) cornua. The superior cornua of the hyoid bone is highly echogenic. Despite its name, the greater (longer) horn of the hyoid bone is difficult to image because the hyoid bone narrows substantially in the posterior direction.

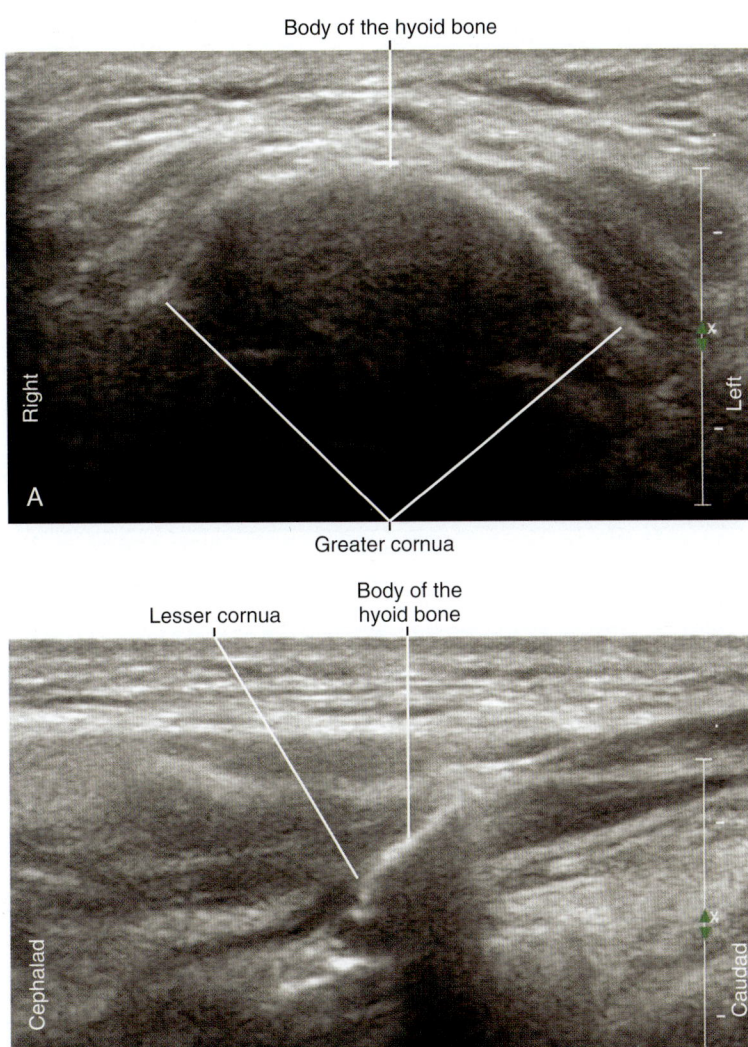

FIGURE 67.3 Long-axis view of the hyoid bone (A) shown with a sloping short-axis view of the lesser cornua (B). The hyoid is a small U-shaped bone as seen in this long-axis view. The internal branch of the superior laryngeal nerve lies immediately inferior and deep to the greater cornua of the hyoid bone.

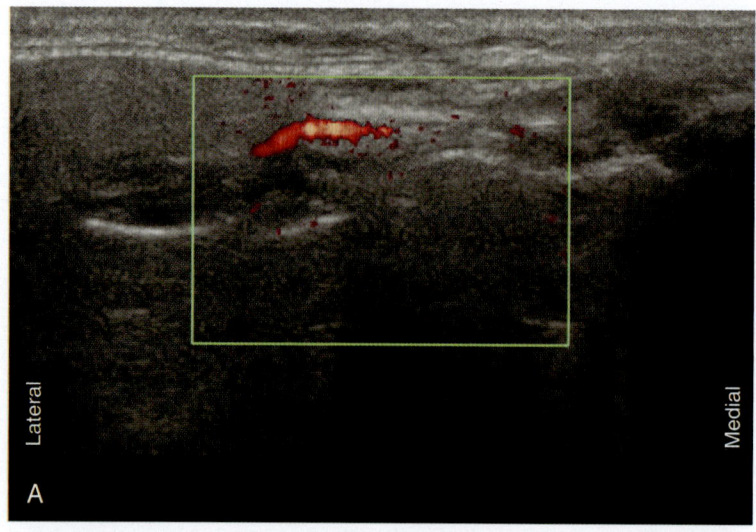
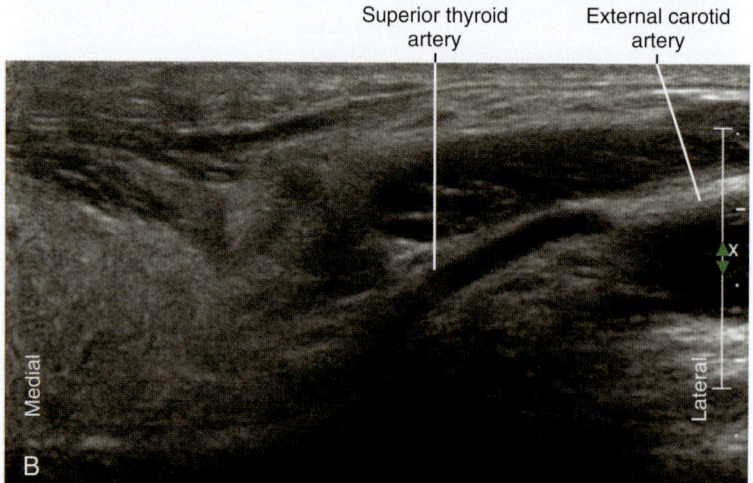

FIGURE 67.4 Power Doppler imaging of the superior laryngeal artery as it descends into the larynx (A). The superior laryngeal nerve lies superior to the superior laryngeal artery. Sonogram showing the origin of the superior thyroid artery from the external carotid (B). The superior thyroid artery is the first branch of the external carotid artery, and it gives rise to the superior laryngeal artery.

Transtracheal Block

CHAPTER 68

Transtracheal block provides topical anesthesia of small branches of the recurrent laryngeal nerve that lines the tracheal lumen below the vocal cords. Because transtracheal injection usually elicits a strong cough reflex, local anesthetic also will distribute over the walls of the larynx and pharynx in the territory of the superior laryngeal nerve. This injection can improve conditions for awake fiberoptic intubation and upper endoscopy.

The distance from the skin to the cricothyroid membrane is highly variable. Moreover, palpation assessment of the cricothyroid membrane is frequently inaccurate.[1] Ultrasound guidance is particularly useful for transtracheal injections in obese subjects with poorly palpable landmarks.

Ultrasound can be used to refine transtracheal injection (performed through the cricothyroid membrane, not between the first and second tracheal rings, etc.). The goal is to guide needle placement through the cricothyroid membrane and not puncture the cricoid cartilage, adjacent tracheal rings, or esophagus. Ultrasound imaging can be used to verify that the thyroid gland isthmus and blood vessels are not within the field of view.

IDENTIFICATION OF THE CRICOTHYROID MEMBRANE

The cricothyroid membrane forms a shallow flattened hyperechoic band. The cricoid cartilage is larger and shallower than the tracheal rings. The cricoid cartilage is 2 to 4 mm thick and is draped over the sides of the infraglottic air column.

There is discontinuity in the surface of the air column, with the cricothyroid membrane being the shallowest part of the air surface. The surface of the air column bends at the junction of the first tracheal ring and the cricoid cartilage (the point of inflection is best appreciated in longitudinal view).

SUGGESTED TECHNIQUE

The patient is in supine position (level bed, headrest, shoulder role if possible). Maximum possible extension of the head will open the cricothyroid membrane and thereby improve exposure when cervical spine precautions are not necessary.

The operator can stand at the side or head of the bed. A small footprint transducer is generally favored (25 mm footprint, linear or curved). A transverse view of the trachea and cricoid cartilage is obtained by locating the interspace between the cricoid cartilage and thyroid cartilage. Optimize the image for transtracheal injection (maximize the distance between the medial edges of the cricoid cartilage).

A short 25-gauge needle will help avoid trauma to the opposite side of the tracheal wall and underlying structures such as the esophagus. The ideal needle length is to the center of the trachea. An out-of-plane approach from cephalad to caudad can be used.

Use a syringe containing the exact dose of local anesthetic to be given. A 5-mL syringe with 4 mL of 2 or 4% lidocaine can be used for laryngotracheal anesthesia.

Puncture the cricothyroid membrane in the range of midline (from 11 o'clock to 1 o'clock in the transverse plane). Tent and recoil of the cricothyroid membrane can be observed as the needle tip enters the tracheal lumen.

Coughing should occur with transtracheal injection (if not, instruct the patient to cough to promote distribution). The onset of lidocaine topical analgesia is within 1 to 5 minutes; the duration is variable.

In patients at risk for cervical spine injury transtracheal injection is possible with a hard collar in place (with a narrow linear transducer through the cutout region of the hard collar).

ANATOMIC VARIATION

These anatomic structures can lie over the airway: accessory thyroid tissue, accessory infrahyoid muscle(s), prominent veins (anterior jugular and inferior thyroid).

KEY POINTS

Transtracheal Block	The Essentials
Anatomy	The cricothyroid membrane is a hyperechoic line between the thyroid cartilage and the cricoid cartilage (the "airline").
Image orientation	The medial edges of the cricoid cartilage are usually in the field of view.
Positioning	Supine position (headrest and shoulder role if possible).
Operator	Standing on the side or head of bed.
Display	Across the table.
Transducer	High-frequency.
	Small footprint (23–25 mm, linear or curved).
Initial depth setting	30 mm
Needle	25 gauge, 10–38 mm in length
Anatomic location	Scan between the thyroid cartilage and cricoid cartilage for rapid identification of the cricothyroid membrane.
Approach	Transverse view of the cricothyroid membrane, out-of-plane from the cephalad side.
	Place the needle tip through the cricothyroid membrane (sometimes tent and recoil of the membrane is observed).
Sonographic assessment	It is not possible to image the needle tip when it is within the air column.
Anatomic variation	Accessory veins, muscle, and thyroid tissue are possible.

Clinical Pearls

- The anterior neck region is particularly sensitive to transducer compression, particularly near the trachea, thyroid cartilage, and hyoid bone.
- The median cricothyroid ligament is composed of firm connective tissue.
- The inferior thyroid vein travels down the midline and drains the thyroid gland with increased caliber lower in the neck.
- Some practitioners favor a small curved transducer that maintains excellent contact with the contours of the neck with minimal pressure.[4]
- The cricothyroid membrane can be rapidly identified in transverse view using the "TACA" technique (sequential identification of the Thyroid cartilage-Airline-Cricoid cartilage-Airline), where airline refers to the hyperechoic line from the air-tissue border just inside of the cricoid membrane, which is often observed together with reverberation artifacts.[5]

References

1. Elliott DS, Baker PA, Scott MR, Birch CW, Thompson JM. Accuracy of surface landmark identification for cannula cricothyroidotomy. *Anaesthesia*. 2010;65(9):889–894. PMID: 20645953.
2. Tsui B, Ip V, Walji A. Airway sonography in live models and cadavers. *J Ultrasound Med*. 2013;32(6):1049–1058. PMID: 23716527.
3. Or DY, Karmakar MK, Lam GC, Hui JW, Li JW, Chen PP. Multiplanar 3D ultrasound imaging to assess the anatomy of the upper airway and measure the subglottic and tracheal diameters in adults. *Br J Radiol*. 2013;86(1030):20130253. PMID: 23966375.
4. Krause M, Khatibi B, Sztain JF, Rahman P, Shapiro AB, Sandhu NS. Ultrasound-guided airway blocks using a curvilinear probe. *J Clin Anesth*. 2016;33:408–412. PMID: 27555201.
5. Kristensen MS, Teoh WH, Rudolph SS. Ultrasonographic identification of the cricothyroid membrane: best evidence, techniques, and clinical impact. *Br J Anaesth*. 2016;117(suppl 1):i39–i48. PMID: 27432055.

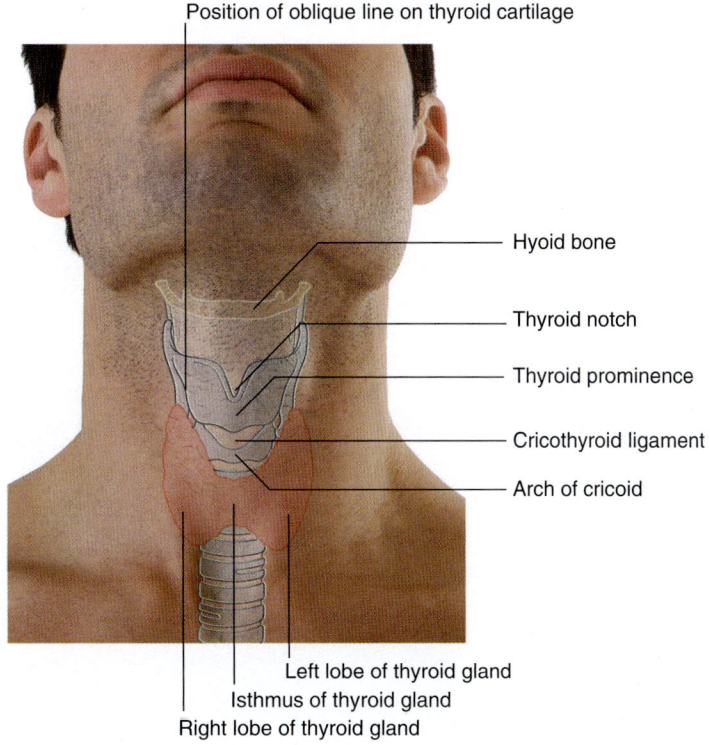

FIGURE 68.1 Anterior view of the neck. (From Drake RL, Vogl W, Mitchell AWM. *Gray's anatomy for students*. Philadelphia: Churchill Livingstone; 2004.)

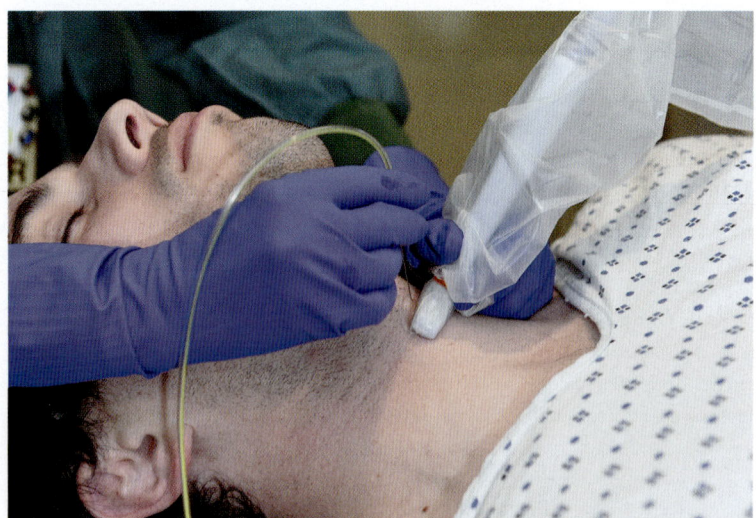

FIGURE 68.2 External photograph showing out-of-plane approach to transtracheal injection.

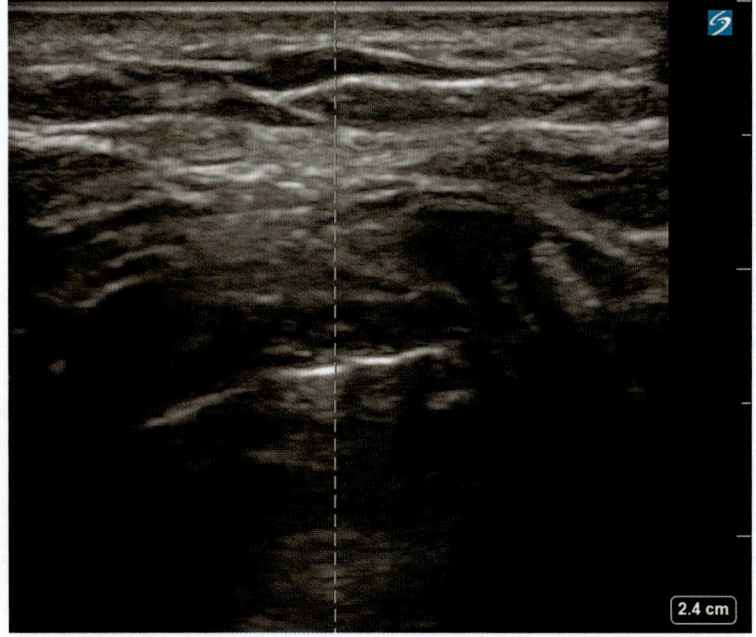

FIGURE 68.3 The "devil's horns" appearance of the cricoid cartilage and cricothyroid membrane in transverse view. The cricoid cartilage will appear incomplete anteriorly (discontinuity) in transverse view when the transducer is slid cephalad from a more complete view of the cricoid cartilage. Although the cricoid cartilage is a complete ring, it may appear incomplete anteriorly in transverse view due to its shape. The cricothyroid membrane is nearly flat to the skin surface and not as smooth and round as a tracheal ring. A dashed center line is used to guide the out-of-plane injection. Note the distance to the cricothyroid membrane is highly variable and depends on body habitus.

Greater Occipital Nerve Block

Manfred Greher

CHAPTER 69

The greater occipital nerve (GON) is the sensory branch of the primary dorsal ramus of C2 with possible contribution from the C3 dorsal ramus. It emerges between C1 and C2 below the posterior arch of the atlas and the lamina of the axis. Curling around the inferior border of the obliquus capitis inferior muscle (OCIM) first, it courses cephalad from lateral to medial and constantly passes on top of the OCIM below the semispinalis capitis muscle (SSCM) across the roof of the suboccipital triangle. After penetrating the medial head of the SSCM, it pierces the trapezius muscle (TM) and invariably the splenius capitis muscle (SCM) before reaching the subcutaneous tissue at the superior nuchal line medial to the occipital artery as it further ascends with the artery. Dividing into branches, the GON innervates the posterior hemicranial part of the scalp to the vertex.

The OCIM, which connects the spinous process of C2 with the transverse process of C1 and therefore runs from medio-caudal to latero-cranial, is the landmark muscle for GON blocks, as the nerve's anatomical relationship is constant and reliable relative to the muscle. At C2, the GON lies constantly on top of the OCIM, while the lamina of C2 is located below the OCIM. The vertebral artery can be found at the lateral border of the lamina deep and anterior to the OCIM.

The ultrasound-guided technique to selectively block the GON at the level of C2 has first been described in a cadaveric study in 2010.[1]

GON blocks are indicated in occipital neuralgia and different types of headaches such as cervicogenic headache, cluster type headache, post-dural puncture headache, or migraine and can be performed unilaterally or bilaterally.[2,3]

SUGGESTED TECHNIQUE

The patient is placed in a lateral decubitus position with the side to block on top for a unilateral GON block. To compensate for cervical lordosis, the head and neck are flexed with a pillow to support the head to avoid any tilting and to ensure a straight cervical spine for orientation.

The first step is to identify the external occipital protuberance with a high-frequency linear transducer in a transverse image orientation. From this starting point, the transducer should be moved caudally in the midline over the arch of the atlas to locate the spinous process of C2, which is always bifid and shows two distinct tubercles. Sliding the transducer down the neck in this fashion, C2 can be clearly distinguished from C3, because C2 forms the uppermost bifid spinous process.

The OCIM is then identified by moving the probe laterally and slightly rotating the lateral end of the probe cranially. The transducer should be placed exactly parallel to the OCIM, which attaches medially to the spinous process of C2 and laterally to the transverse process of C1. Sometimes, the vertebral artery, lateral and deep to the OCIM, can be visualized in Color Flow- or Power-Doppler.

After identifying the GON, which lies on top of the OCIM, the ultrasound-guided injection is performed with a sharp 25-gauge needle attached to a line extension and a 5-mL syringe of local anesthetic, out-of-plane from caudal to cranial or in-plane from lateral to medial. Careful aspiration and incremental injection helps avoid intravascular application, because the nerve is sometimes accompanied by small vessels. If the local anesthetic is placed in the right layer between the OCIM and the SSCM, 2 to 3 mL is sufficient to surround and block the GON.

The procedure may be repeated on the contralateral side if necessary. In these bilateral injections, sitting position of the patient can be advantageous.

DISCUSSION AND COMMENTS

Recent clinical studies have proven the technical feasibility and efficacy of this ultrasound-guided procedure.[4,5] Several advantages compared to the classical block site medial to the occipital artery at the level of the superior nuchal line include improved sonographic visibility, injection central to possible nerve entrapment or branching and distant to the occipital artery, as well as increased diagnostic selectivity with lower amounts of local anesthetic.

The other two nerves innervating occipital skin areas are the lesser occipital nerve (LON) and the third occipital nerve (TON). The LON is one of the four branches of the cervical plexus and ascends from the ventral roots of C2 and C3 behind the posterior border of the sternocleidomastoid muscle to innervate an area lateral to the GON. The TON originates from the dorsal ramus of C3, and crosses and supplies the C2/3 zygapophyseal joint, which is the only facet joint in the body exclusively innervated by a single nerve. The TON finally provides sensory innervation to the occipital skin area medial and caudal to the GON.

KEY POINTS

Greater Occipital Nerve Block	The Essentials
Anatomy	The GON is located on top of the OCIM at the level of C2.
Image orientation	The GON lies lateral to the C2 spinous process and medial to the vertebral artery.
Positioning	Lateral decubitus with the side to block on top or sitting both with the head and neck flexed
Operator	Sitting or standing behind the patient
Display	Across the table
Transducer	High-frequency linear, 23- to 38-mm footprint
Initial depth setting	30 mm
Needle	25 gauge, 38 mm in length
Anatomic location	Begin with a midline transverse view of the external occipital protuberance.
	Slide the transducer caudally over the arch of the atlas to localize the bifid spinous process of C2.
	Move the probe laterally and rotate the lateral end more cranially to visualize the transverse process of C1.
	Identify the GON on top of the OCIM.
Approach	Longitudinal view of OCIM, out-of-plane or in-plane from lateral to medial
Sonographic assessment	Injection distribution observed between the OCIM and the SSCM around the GON
Anatomic variation	Small veins and arteries close to the GON

GON, Greater occipital nerve; *OCIM*, obliquus capitis inferior muscle; *SSCM*, semispinalis capitis muscle.

Clinical Pearls

- The GON arises from the C2 dorsal ramus and can best be blocked under ultrasound guidance on the surface of the OCIM in different types of occipital headaches.
- With a probe position exactly parallel to the OCIM, this muscle characteristically appears rather hypoechoic (dark) and streaky (parallel linear echoes).

Clinical Pearls—cont'd

- The GON always lies on the surface of the OCIM with a monofascicular appearance and an average diameter of 4 × 2 mm.
- With more experience, placing the transducer between the mastoid process and the estimated position of the C2 spinous process shortens the procedure and allows visualizing both the OCIM and the GON more rapidly in many cases.
- Bilateral GON blocks can sometimes cause temporary dizziness and vertigo, which should be discussed with the patient before the procedure.

References

1. Greher M, Moriggl B, Curatolo M, et al. Sonographic visualization and ultrasound—guided blockade of the greater occipital nerve: a comparison of two selective techniques confirmed by anatomical dissection. *Br J Anaesth*. 2010;104:637–642.
2. Afridi SK, Shields KG, Bhola R, et al. Greater occipital nerve injection in primary headache syndromes–prolonged effects from a single injection. *Pain*. 2006;122:126–129.
3. Naja Z, Al-Tannir M, El-Rajab M, et al. Nerve stimulator-guided occipital nerve blockade for postdural puncture headache. *Pain Pract*. 2009;9:51–58.
4. Pingree MJ, Sole JS, O'Brien TG, et al. Clinical efficacy of an ultrasound-guided greater occipital nerve block at the level of C2. *Reg Anesth Pain Med*. 2017;42:99–104.
5. Zipfel J, Kastler A, Tatu L, et al. Ultrasound-guided intermediate site greater occipital nerve infiltration: a technical feasibility study. *Pain Physician*. 2016;19:E1027–E1034.

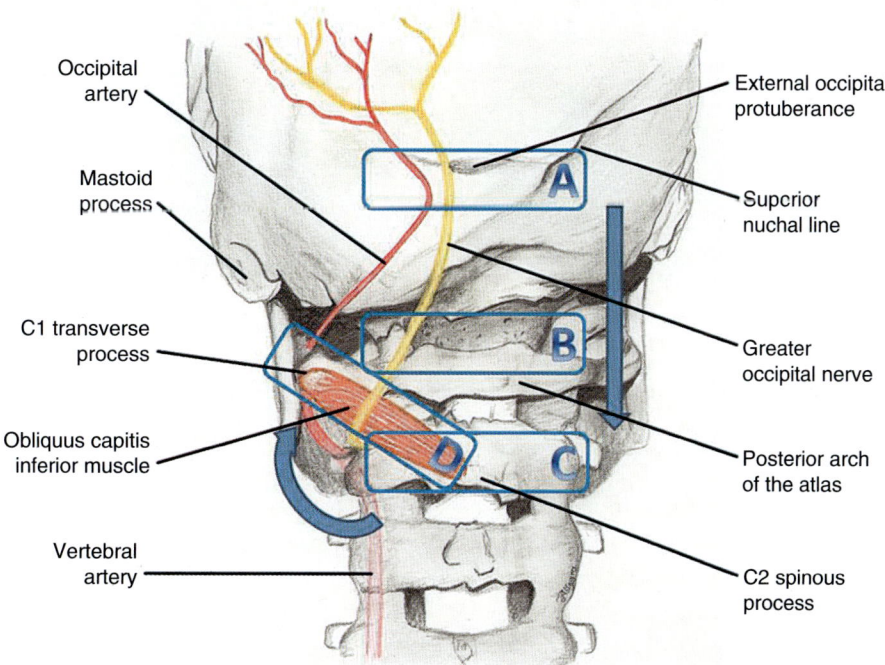

FIGURE 69.1 Drawing of the anatomy of the greater occipital nerve in the suboccipital triangle. The drawing shows the recommended scanning sequence to identify the nerve (probe positions A through D).

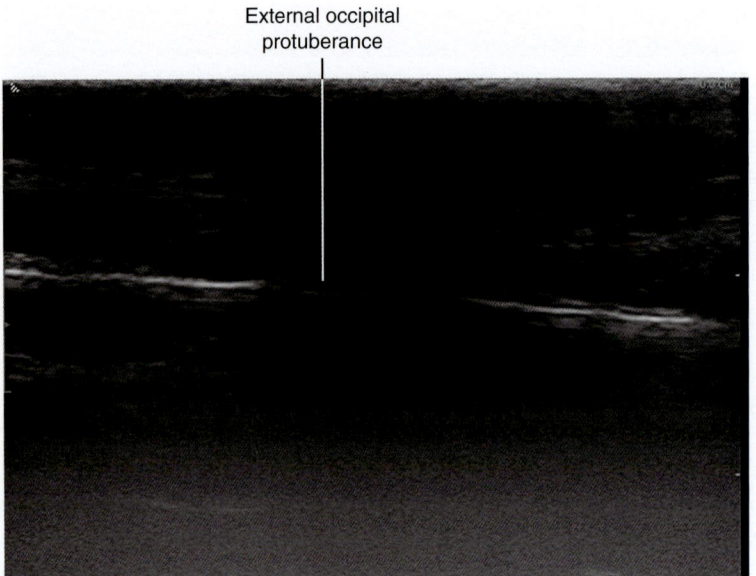

FIGURE 69.2 Sonogram showing a midline transverse view of the external occipital protuberance (probe position A in Fig. 69.1).

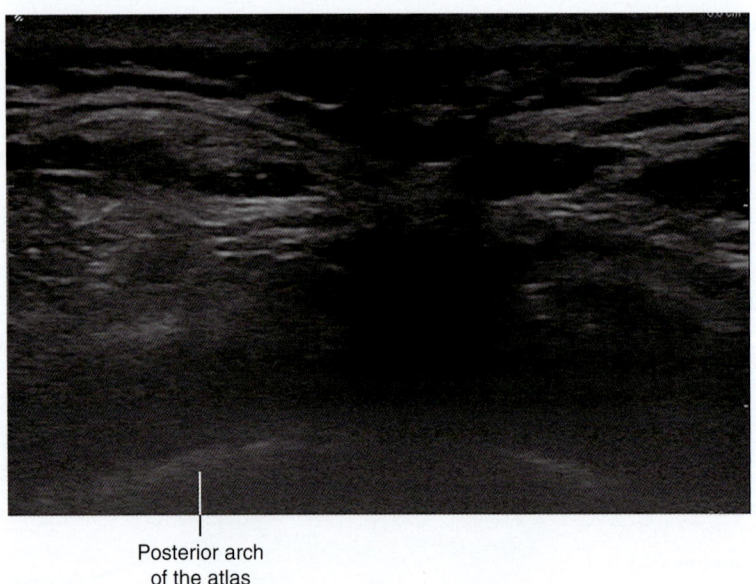

FIGURE 69.3 Sonogram showing the posterior arch of the atlas (probe position B in Fig. 69.1).

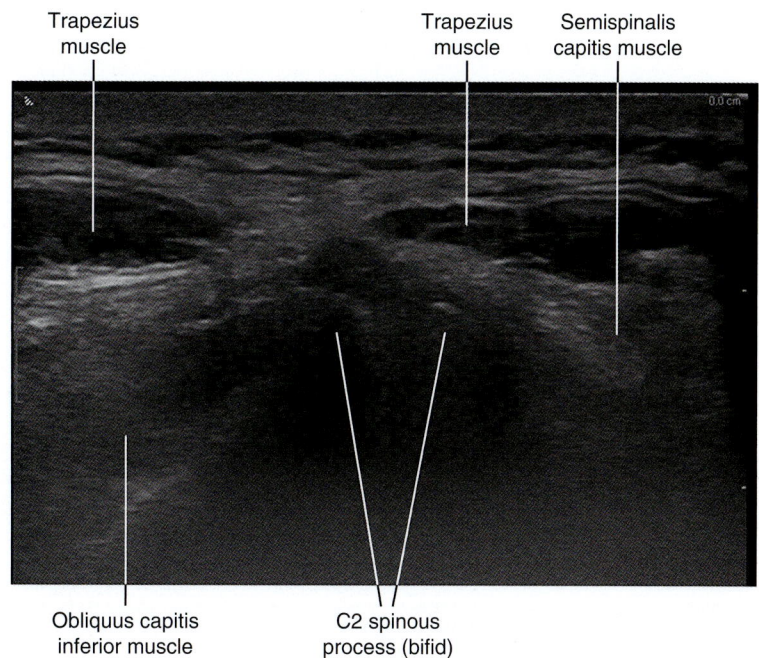

FIGURE 69.4 Sonogram showing the bifid spinous process of C2 (probe position C in Fig. 69.1).

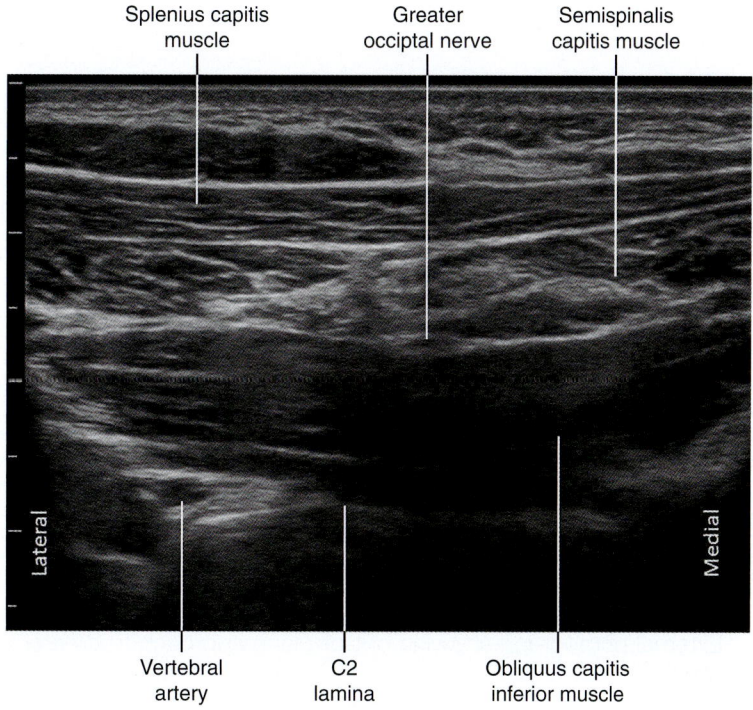

FIGURE 69.5 Sonogram showing the greater occipital nerve over the inferior oblique muscle (probe position D in Fig. 69.1). The transducer has been slid laterally and rotated to view the muscle in long axis. The vertebral artery is seen below the inferior oblique muscle.

HEAD AND NECK BLOCKS

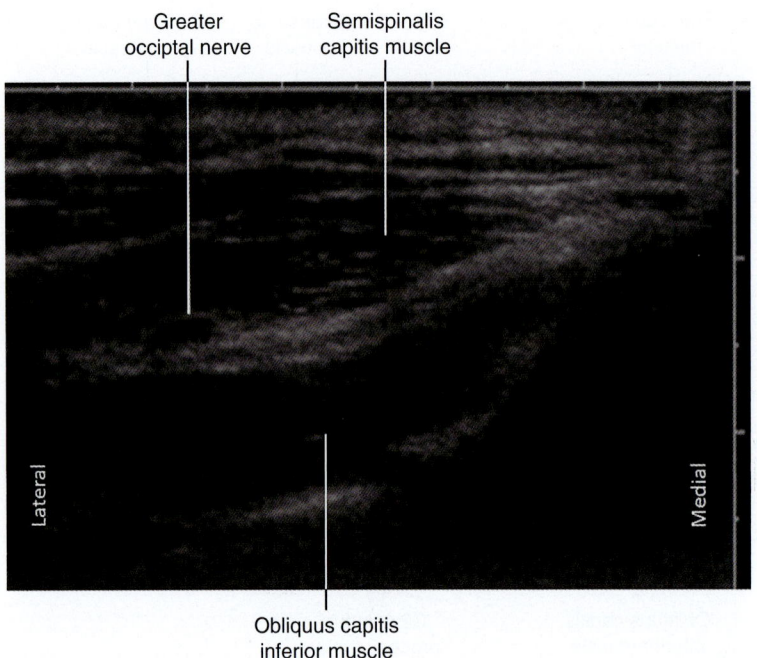

FIGURE 69.6 Sonogram after adjustment of the transducer to show the underlying lamina of C2.

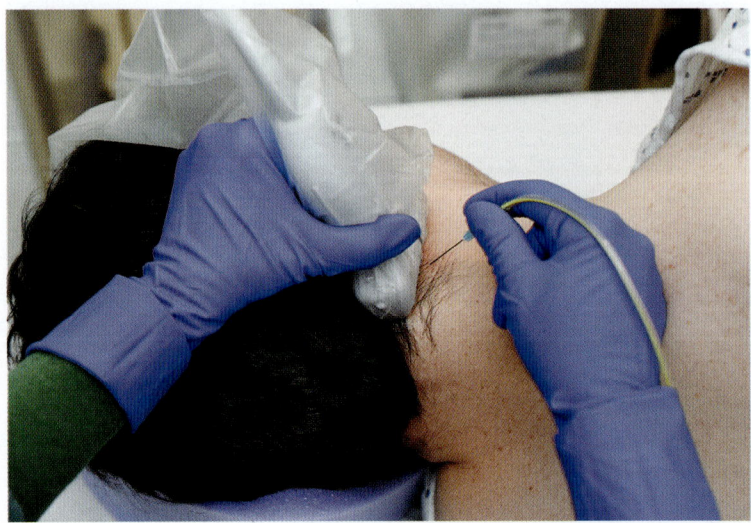

FIGURE 69.7 External photograph showing out-of-plane approach to greater occipital nerve block.

Lesser Occipital Nerve Block

CHAPTER 70

Occipital nerve blocks are useful for treatment of headaches and pain relief following cranial surgeries. Ultrasound guidance has a role in improving the efficacy of these blocks. Scalp innervation is complex and derives from many ascending nerves.

The lesser occipital nerve (LON) is a superficial branch of the cervical plexus and derives from the ventral rami of C2 and C3. The LON provides sensory innervation to the external ear and posterior occiput.[1] The LON ascends along the posterolateral border of the sternocleidomastoid (SCM) muscle behind the ear.

SUGGESTED TECHNIQUE

The patient is positioned lateral or supine with the head turned to the contralateral side.

Use a small-footprint linear transducer (hockey-stick) to image the LON.
To locate the LON, place a gel trail along the posterolateral border of the SCM, using a transverse scan and sliding the transducer in a cephalo-caudal fashion.
Follow the LON centrally to where it joins the GAN and the remainder of the cervical plexus to confirm identity. The LON and GAN are the ascending branches of the cervical plexus.
The LON emerges from underneath the posterior border of the SCM near where the spinal accessory nerve emerges.
The LON has a diameter of about 1 mm and a monofascicular appearance.[2]
The block can be performed with a 25-gauge, 38-mm needle and 1 to 2 mL local anesthetic using the in-plane technique.

Cutaneous assessment of LON block can be performed behind the ear. Also, test the territories of the adjacent nerves (great auricular nerve: on the inner rim of the posterior aspect of the external ear; spinal accessory nerve: shoulder shrug; supraclavicular nerve: skin over the clavicle).

KEY POINTS

Lesser Occipital Nerve Block	The Essentials
Anatomy	The LON is about 1 mm in diameter.
Image orientation:	The LON lies on the posterior side of the SCM.
Positioning	Lateral or supine with the head turned to the contralateral side.
Operator	Standing on the ipsilateral side of the table
Display	Across the table, on the contralateral side
Transducer	High-frequency linear, 23- to 25-mm footprint
Initial depth setting	25 mm
Needle	25 gauge, 38 mm in length
Anatomic location	Begin by scanning the posterolateral border of the SCM.
Approach	SAX view of LON, in-plane from the posterior side
	Place the needle tip underneath the LON.
	Sonographic assessment:
	Injection should track along the course of the LON (confirm with SAX slide).

Continued

KEY POINTS—CONT'D

Lesser Occipital Nerve Block	The Essentials
Anatomic variation	Accessory head of the SCM (about 20% of cases).
	LON can pierce the SCM (about 10% of cases).

LON, Lesser occipital nerve; SCM, sternocleidomastoid muscle; SAX, short axis.

Clinical Pearls

- The lesser occipital nerve is the second-largest superficial branch of the cervical plexus (the adjacent great auricular nerve is slightly larger).
- The lesser occipital nerve often divides on the surface of the sternocleidomastoid muscle at its cranial end.
- The LON ascends nearly vertically along the posterior border of the SCM. Therefore, the location of the LON crossing of the SCM border can be difficult to estimate.
- Occipital nerve blocks are relatively contraindicated in the presence of a bone defect.[3]

References

1. Pantaloni M, Sullivan P. Relevance of the lesser occipital nerve in facial rejuvenation surgery. *Plast Reconstr Surg.* 2000;105(7):2594–2599. PMID: 10845317.
2. Platzgummer H, Moritz T, Gruber GM, et al. The lesser occipital nerve visualized by high-resolution sonography—normal and initial suspect findings. *Cephalalgia.* 2015;35(9):816–824. PMID: 25414471.
3. Okuda Y, Matsumoto T, Shinohara M, Kitajima T, Kim P. Sudden unconsciousness during a lesser occipital nerve block in a patient with the occipital bone defect. *Eur J Anaesthesiol.* 2001;18(12):829–832. PMID: 11737183.

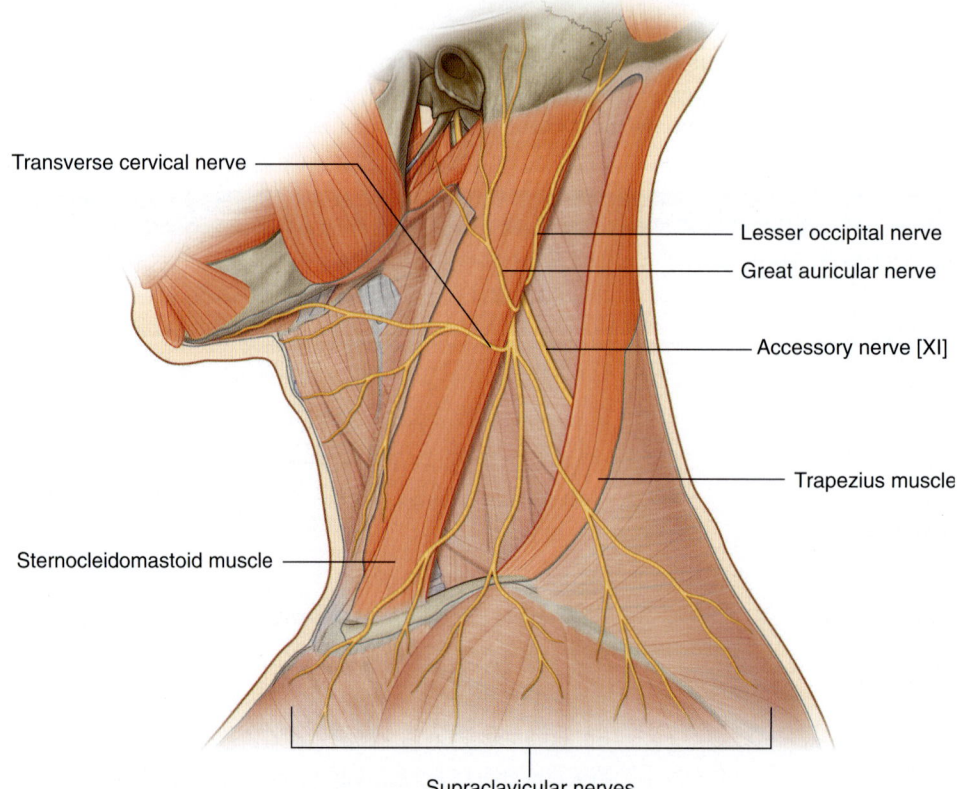

FIGURE 70.1 Course of the lesser occipital nerve. (From Drake RL, Vogl W, Mitchell AWM. *Gray's anatomy for students*. Philadelphia: Churchill Livingstone; 2004.)

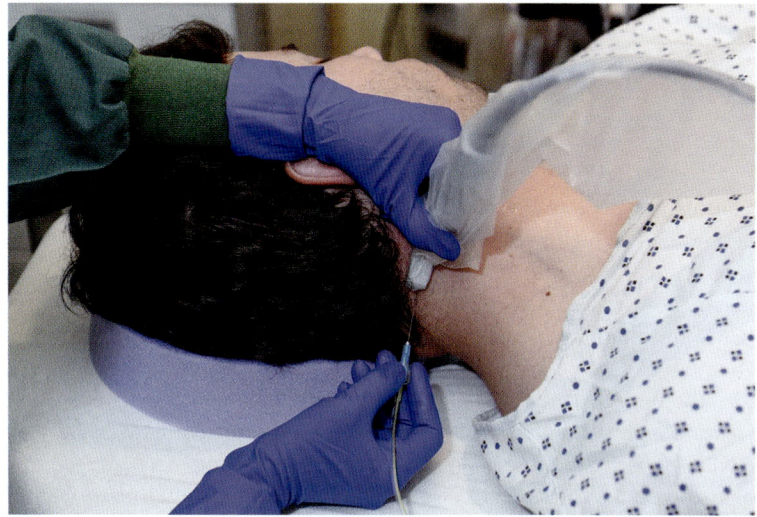

FIGURE 70.2 External photograph showing the probe position for lesser occipital nerve block at the posterolateral corner of the sternocleidomastoid muscle.

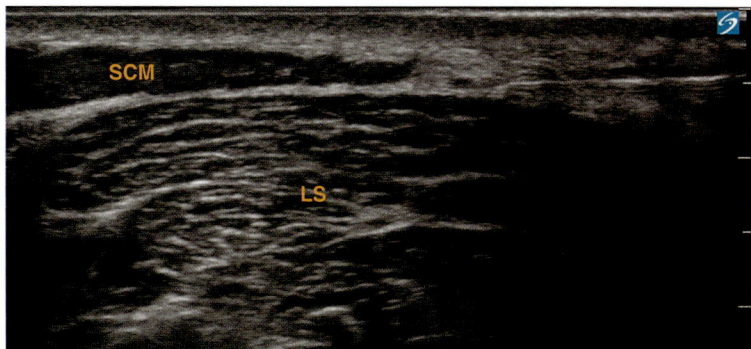

FIGURE 70.3 The lesser occipital nerve at the posterolateral corner of the sternocleidomastoid (SCM) muscle (the "dot at the corner" appearance). In this location near the transverse process of C1, the lesser occipital nerve lies over the levator scapulae (LS) muscle. A posterolateral to anteromedial in-plane approach to lesser occipital nerve block is shown, with the needle tip placed adjacent to the nerve.

Great Auricular Nerve Block

CHAPTER 71

The great auricular nerve (GAN) is the largest branch of the superficial cervical plexus (see Chapter 72, Fig. 72-1). The nerve arises mainly from the third cervical nerve (C3) with inconstant contributions from the second cervical nerve (C2). It provides cutaneous innervation to the periauricular region.[1] The GAN wraps around the posterior border of the sternocleidomastoid muscle (SCM) and then courses superiorly and anteriorly, dividing into anterior and posterior branches. Because of its superficial location, the GAN can be damaged during surgical procedures in the neck. The nerves of the superficial cervical plexus lie deep to the platysma when first emerging from the plexus, but it lies superficial to the prevertebral fascia.

The GAN lies superficial to the lateral border of the SCM and can be traced to the preauricular area or back to the superficial cervical plexus. The lesser occipital nerve has similar anatomy, except that it can be followed behind the ear.

GAN block can be used to provide anesthesia for external ear surgeries.[2,3] The average GAN diameter is 1.4 mm.[4]

SUGGESTED TECHNIQUE

The GAN has a characteristic monofascicular or bifascicular appearance on ultrasound scans where it courses over the SCM. The GAN flattens in shape slightly as it lies over the SCM. The nerve becomes difficult to image at the lateral corner of the SCM. This point is about the level of the cricoid cartilage. Isolated GAN blocks are possible, but its large size and characteristic ultrasound appearance make the GAN a convenient way of identifying the position of the remainder of the superficial cervical plexus.

Because the GAN is very superficial, an out-of-plane approach to GAN block is usually used with the nerve viewed in short axis. The GAN lies near the external jugular vein, so vascular puncture and minor bleeding are possible.

Clinical Pearls

- The GAN consists of contributions from the second and third cervical nerves. The GAN divides into anterior and posterior branches.
- The GAN often can be seen both superficial and deep to the sternocleidomastoid muscle within one plane of imaging because the nerve loops around the posterolateral border of this muscle.
- Dominance patterns of cutaneous innervation of the external ear have been examined.[5] Most patterns are either lesser occipital or great auricular dominant.

References

1. Thallaj A, Marhofer P, Moriggl B, et al. Great auricular nerve blockade using high resolution ultrasound: a volunteer study. *Anaesthesia*. 2010;65:836–840.
2. Flores S, Herring AA. Ultrasound-guided greater auricular nerve block for emergency department ear laceration and ear abscess drainage. *J Emerg Med*. 2016;50(4):651–655.
3. Ritchie MK, Wilson CA, Grose BW, Ranganathan P, Howell SM, Ellison MB. Ultrasound-guided greater auricular nerve block as sole anesthetic for ear surgery. *Clin Pract*. 2016;6(2):856.
4. Lieba-Samal D, Pivec C, Platzgummer H, et al. High-resolution ultrasound for diagnostic assessment of the great auricular nerve—normal and first pathologic findings. *Ultraschall Med*. 2015;36(4):342–347.
5. Pantaloni M, Sullivan P. Relevance of the lesser occipital nerve in facial rejuvenation surgery. *Plast Reconstr Surg*. 2000;105:2594–2599.

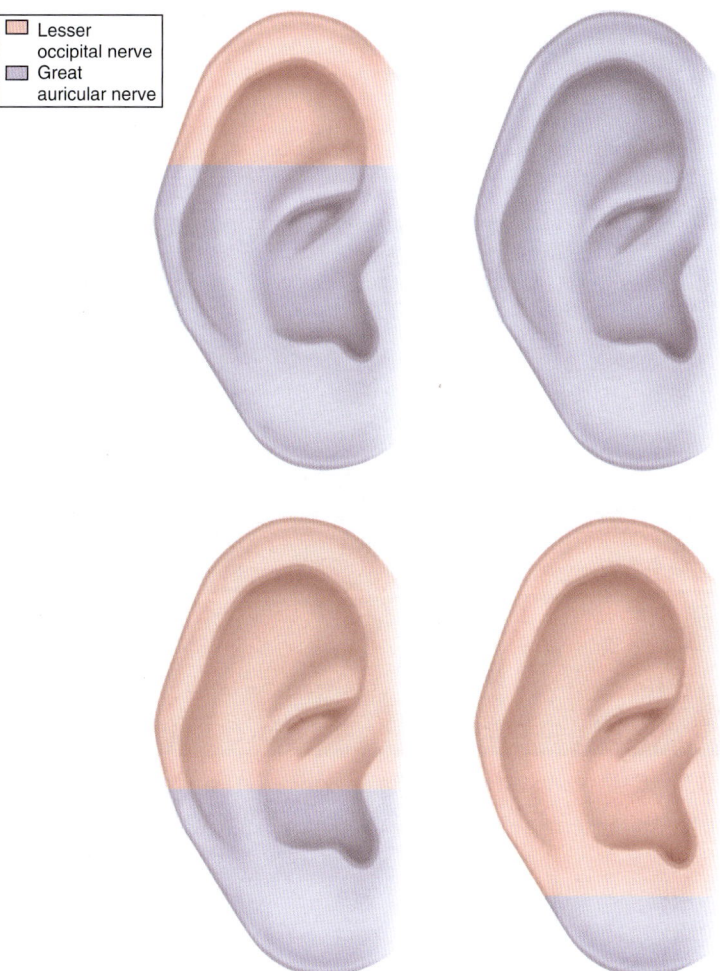

FIGURE 71.1 *Above, left,* in 11 of 19 hemifaces (58%), the lesser occipital nerve innervated the superior one-third of the ear. *Above, right,* in 3 of 19 hemifaces (16%), the great auricular nerve provided sensory supply to the entire ear. *Below, left,* in 4 of 19 hemifaces (21%), the lesser occipital nerve supplied the superior two-thirds of the ear. *Below, right,* in 1 of 19 hemifaces (5%), the lesser occipital nerve innervated the majority of the ear, and the great auricular nerve supplied the earlobe. (From Pantaloni M, Sullivan P. Relevance of the lesser occipital nerve in facial rejuvenation surgery. *Plast Reconstr Surg.* 2000;105(7):2594–2599.)

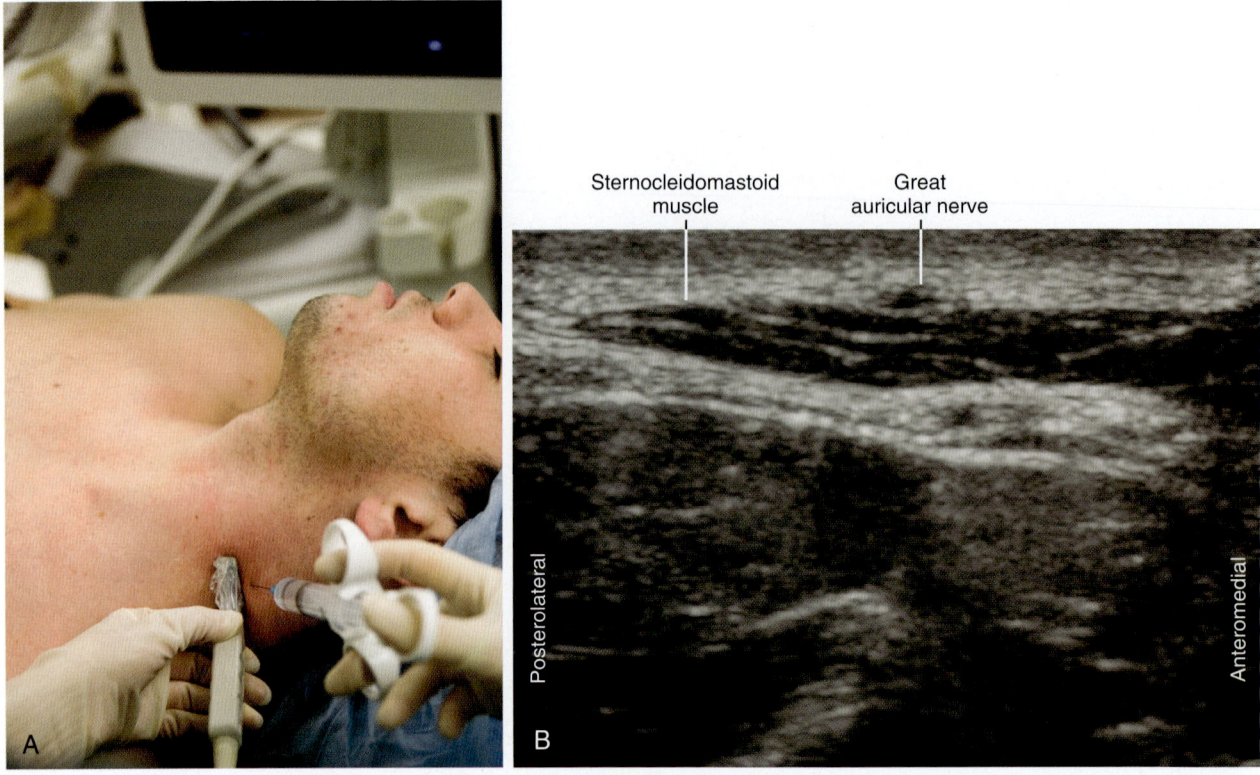

FIGURE 71.2 External photograph showing an out-of-plane approach to great auricular nerve block (A). The corresponding sonogram is shown before needle placement (B).

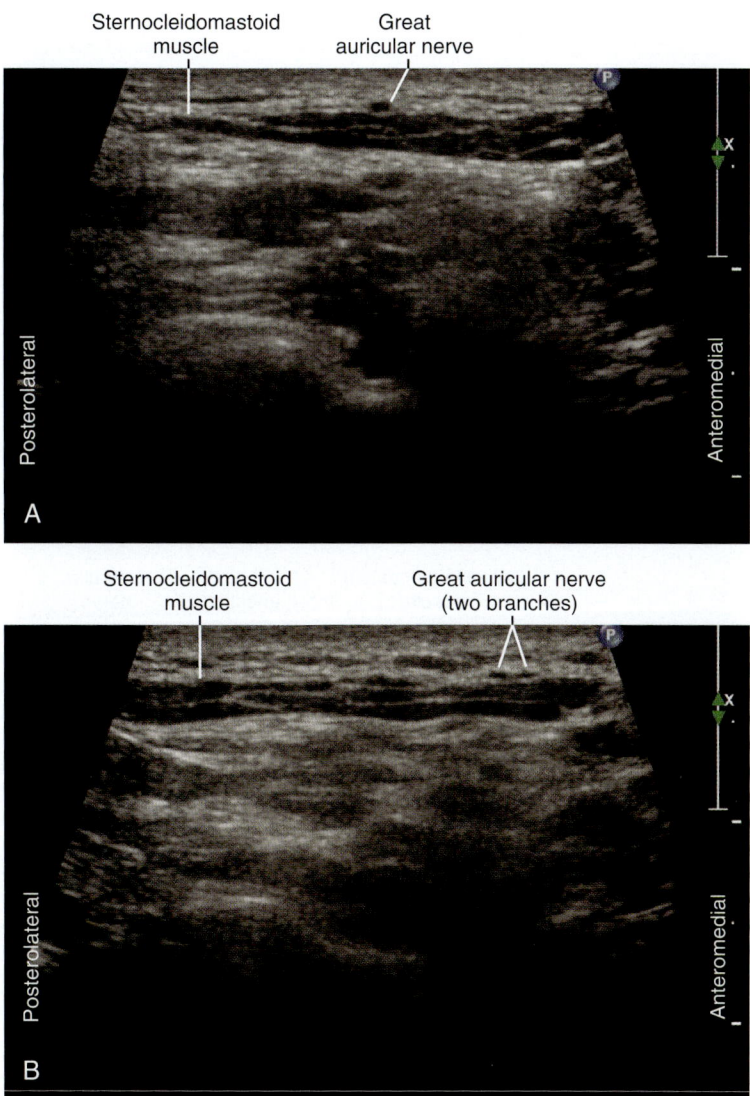

FIGURE 71.3 Short-axis view of the great auricular nerve near the posterolateral border of the sternocleidomastoid muscle (A). The great auricular nerve divides into anterior and posterior branches (B).

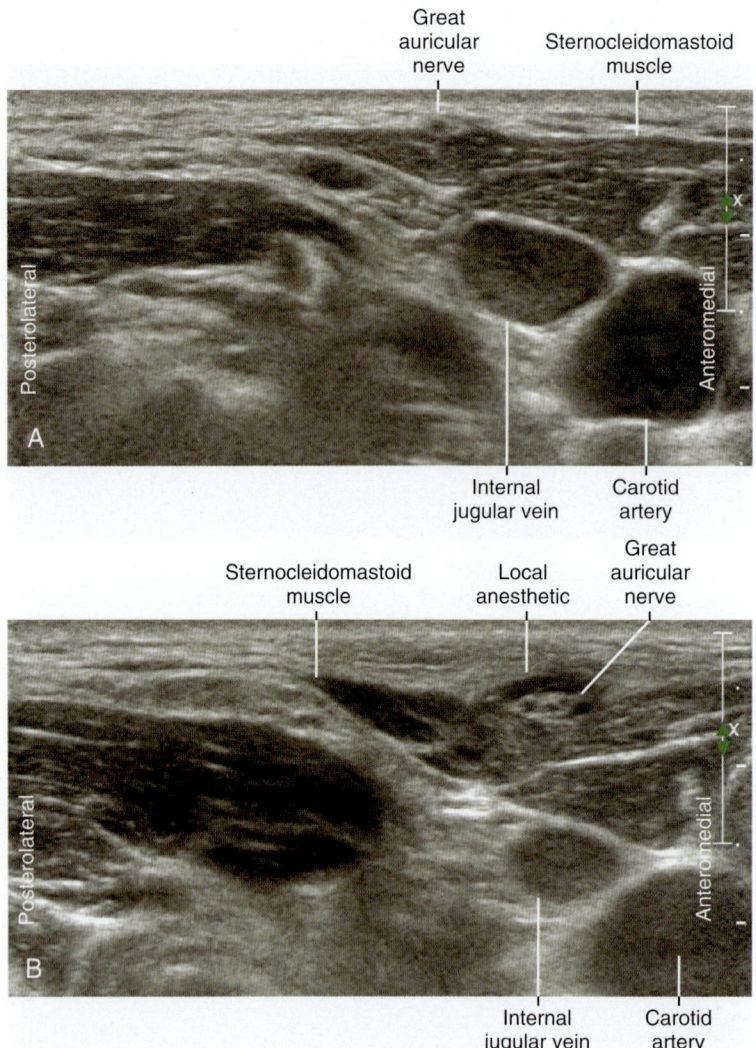

FIGURE 71.4 Short-axis view of the great auricular nerve before (A) and after (B) injection of local anesthetic. Local anesthetic is seen to distribute around the nerve.

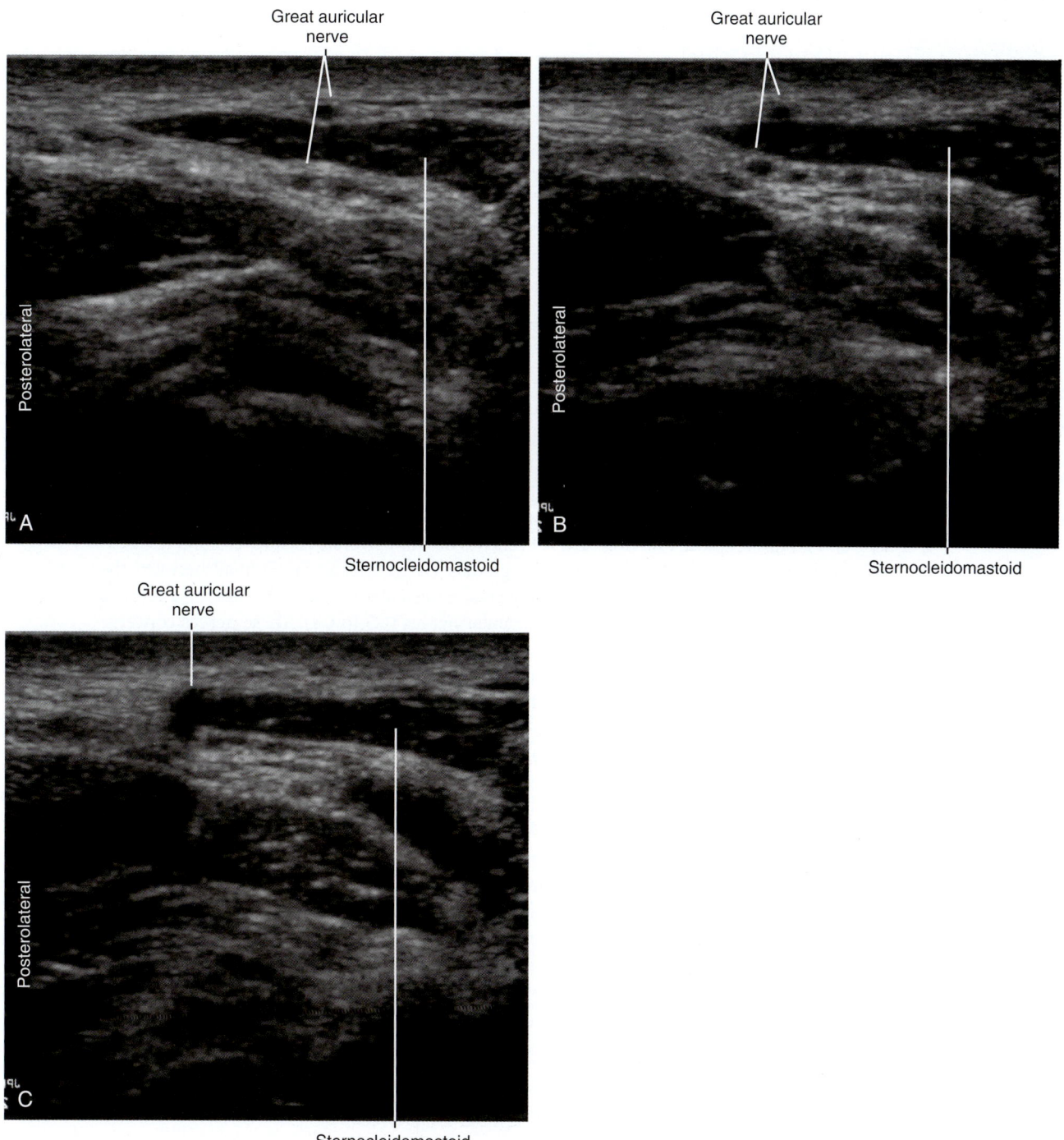

FIGURE 71.5 The great auricular nerve descends to loop around the posterolateral edge of the sternocleidomastoid muscle, and it therefore can be visible both above and below this muscle within one transverse plane of imaging (A and B, the "double dot" sign). Sliding the transducer caudally verifies that these two nerves join at the muscle border (C, the "boomerang" sign of partial long axis view of the nerve rounding the corner of the sternocleidomastoid muscle). The great auricular nerve can be blocked deep to the sternocleidomastoid muscle for more complete anesthesia.

CHAPTER 72

Cervical Plexus Block

Ronald Seidel

 See Video 72.1 on ExpertConsult.com.

INTRODUCTION

ANATOMIC BACKGROUND

The cervical plexus derives from the ventral rami of C1 to C4 and has two types of branches: muscular and cutaneous.

Muscular branches include the phrenic nerve (C4 (C3 to C5); innervation: pericardium, diaphragm), the deep cervical ansa (loop formed from C1 to C3; innervation: supra- and infrahyoid muscles), and segmental branches from C1 to C4 (innervation: rectus capitis, longus colli and longus capitis, scalene and levator scapulae muscles). These branches do not perforate the prevertebral fascia.

The superficial branches derive from the segments C2 to C4 and are formed between the prevertebral and superficial fascia. These are the greater auricular (C2 to C3), transverse cervical (C2 to C3), lesser occipital (C2), and supraclavicular nerves (C3 to C4). These nerves converge at the posterolateral border of the sternocleidomastoid muscle (SCM), perforate the superficial fascia, and innervate the skin of the neck, shoulder, and infraclavicular region (Fig. 72.1).

In addition, cranial nerves (CN) and the sympathetic trunk (ST) are involved in the innervation of the vessel walls (carotid artery: CN IX, X, ST) and neck muscles (platysma: CN VII; sternocleidomastoid and trapezius muscle: CN XI). Multiple anastomoses exist between CN and the cervical plexus.[1]

INDICATIONS AND CONTRAINDICATIONS

Common indications for cervical plexus block (CPB) include carotid endarterectomy, thyroid and parathyroid surgery, shoulder surgery, and surgery on the clavicle.

Contraindications exist when incidental block of the phrenic nerve or recurrent laryngeal nerve would lead to a potentially life-threatening situation. This applies for patients with severe obstructive lung disease and contralateral paralysis of the vocal cord or phrenic nerve. In this case, a superficial or subplatysmal injection site can be chosen.

SUGGESTED TECHNIQUE

NOMENCLATURE OF CERVICAL PLEXUS BLOCKS

In this chapter, the definition of the injection site is based on the nomenclature of Telford and Stoneham.[2] An injection superficial to the prevertebral layer of the cervical fascia (previously referred to as superficial block) has been further differentiated into intermediate (between the prevertebral and superficial layer of the cervical fascia) and superficial (subcutaneous or subplatysmal injection site) blocks. An injection deep to the prevertebral fascia is referred to as deep CPB.

ULTRASOUND GUIDANCE

Ultrasound imaging is useful for guiding deep or intermediate blocks of the cervical plexus. Sonographic landmarks can be identified, and in some cases, direct nerve imaging is possible. Optimal needle tip placement with in-plane approach can be used to target injections and potentially avoid complications.

CERVICAL PLEXUS BLOCK

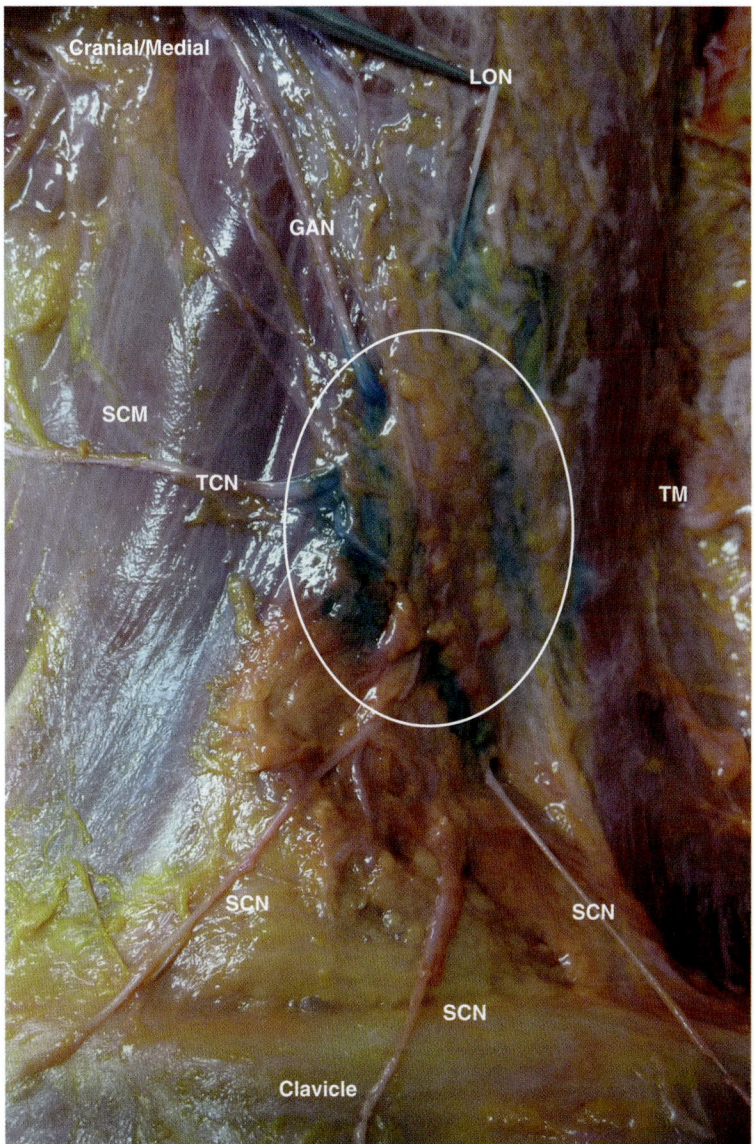

FIGURE 72.1 Cervical plexus—nervous area after intermediate cervical plexus block with methylene blue *(left side)*. *GAN*, Greater auricular nerve; *LON*, lesser occipital nerve; *SCM*, sternocleidomastoid muscle; *SCN*, supraclavicular nerves; *TCN*, transverse cervical nerve; *TM*, trapezoid muscle; white circle, subplatysmal impregnation of the nervous area with methylene blue. (The superficial lamina of the cervical fascia is impregnated by the dye.) (Modified from Seidel R, Schulze M, Zukowski K, Wree A. Ultrasound-guided intermediate cervical plexus block. Anatomical study. *Anaesthesist.* 2015;64:446.)

SONOGRAPHIC LANDMARKS

Several sonographic landmarks more precisely determine the level for CPB injections[3,4]:
1. Cervical levels can be estimated by cervical vertebral morphology on ultrasound imaging scans. The anterior tubercle of the seventh cervical transverse process is rudimentary. In contrast, the anterior tubercle of the sixth cervical transverse process (Chassaignac's tubercle) is prominent compared with its posterior tubercle (Fig. 72.2). This bony morphology can be used to identify higher cervical levels when performing CPBs. In addition, the first segment of the vertebral artery lies anterior to the seventh cervical transverse process before it enters the cervical spinal canal. The intervening space (sulcus) between the anterior and posterior tubercles becomes

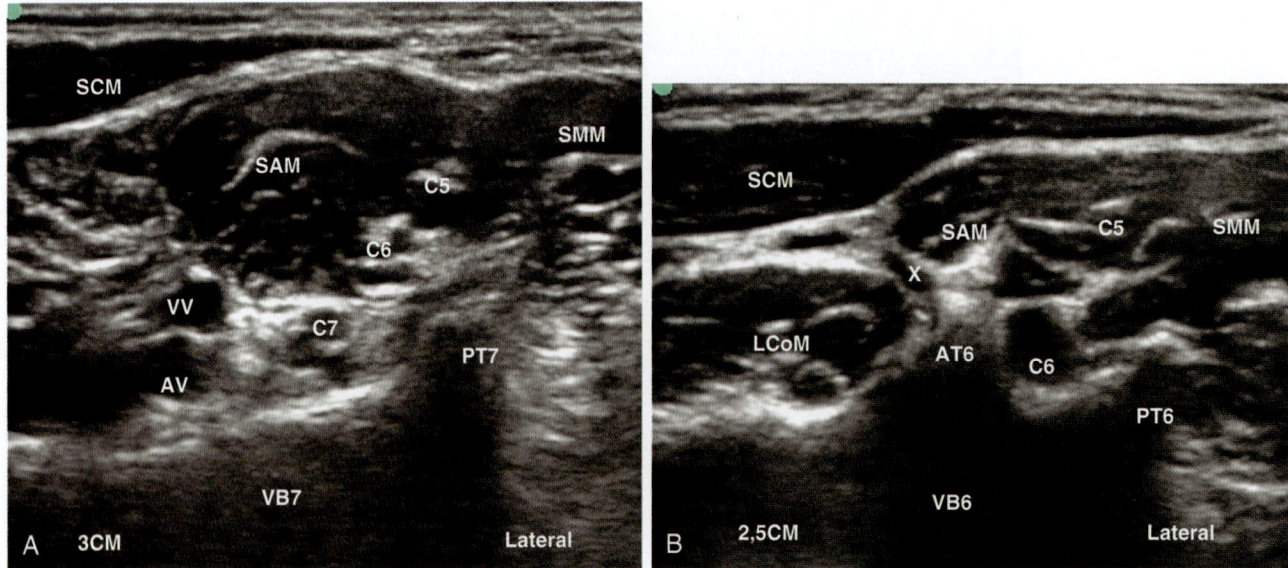

FIGURE 72.2 Internal sonographic landmarks *(right side)*. (A) Level of the seventh cervical vertebra, (B) level of the sixth cervical vertebra. *AT6*, Anterior tubercle of transverse process C6; *AV*, vertebral artery; *C5/6/7*, ventral branch of spinal nerve C5/6/7; *LCoM*, longus colli muscle; *PT6/7*, posterior tubercle of transverse process C6/7; *SAM*, scalenus anterior muscle; *SCM*, sternocleidomastoid muscle; *SMM*, scalenus medius muscle; *VB6/7*, body of vertebra C6/7; *VV*, vertebral vein.

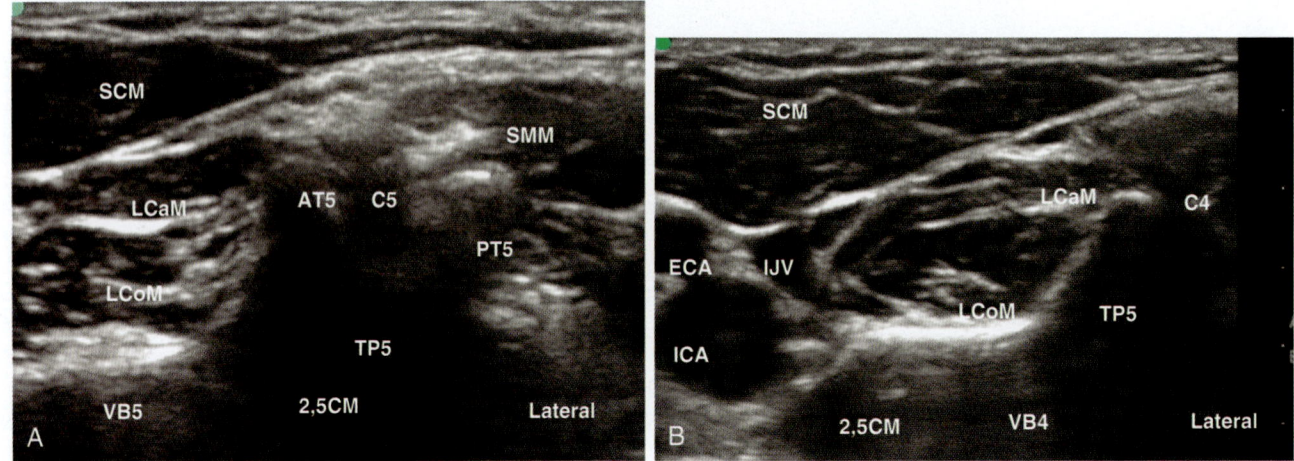

FIGURE 72.3 Internal sonographic landmarks *(right side)*. (A) Level of the fifth cervical vertebra, (B) Level of the fourth cervical vertebra. *AT5*, Anterior tubercle of transverse process C5 (TP5); *C4/5*, ventral branch of spinal nerve C4/5; *ECA*, external carotid artery; *ICA*, internal carotid artery; *IJV*, internal jugular vein; *LCaM*, longus capitis muscle; *LCoM*, longus colli muscle; *PT5*, posterior tubercle of transverse process C5 (TP5); *SCM*, sternocleidomastoid muscle; *SMM*, scalenus medius muscle; *VB4/5*, body of vertebra C4/5.

progressively smaller as one slides the transducer cephalad. This is because the exiting ventral rami are smaller at higher cervical vertebrae (Fig. 72.3).

2. At the level for CPB, the ventral rami of the brachial plexus are often difficult to identify, and the scalene muscles taper in diameter. Medial and anterior to the C4 transverse process, the longus colli and longus capitis muscles can be identified (Fig. 72.4). The longus capitis muscle inserts on the C6 anterior tubercle and is not visible at this level. Lateral and posterior to the C4 transverse process the levator scapulae muscle can be identified.
3. The superficial layer of the cervical fascia encloses the SCM and can be identified lateral to the carotid sheath. The neck muscles are enclosed by the prevertebral layer of the cervical fascia. The interfascial compartment contains the sensory branches of the cervical plexus.

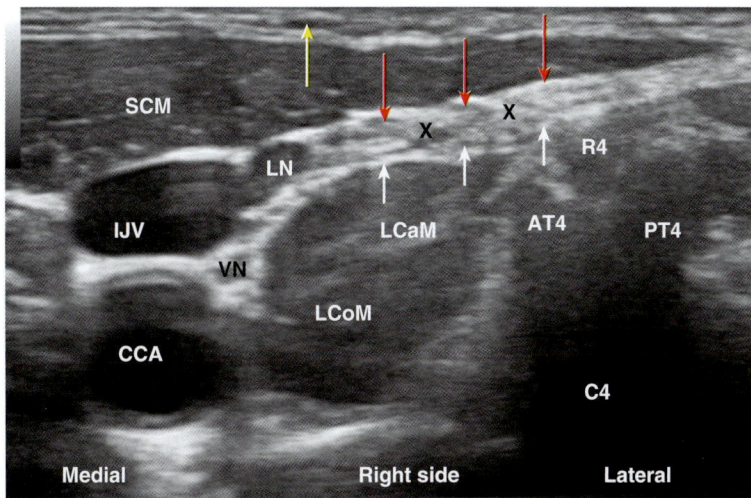

FIGURE 72.4 Sonogram at the level of the fourth cervical vertebra. *AT4*, Anterior tubercle of transverse process C4; *R4*, ventral branch of spinal nerve C4; *CCA*, common carotid artery; *IJV*, internal jugular vein; *LCaM*, longus capitis muscle; *LCoM*, longus colli muscle; *LN*, lymph node; *PT4*, posterior tubercle of transverse process C4; *red arrows*, superficial lamina of the cervical fascia; *SCM*, sternocleidomastoid muscle; *VN*, vagal nerve; *white arrows*, prevertebral lamina of the cervical fascia (prevertebral fascia); *yellow arrow*, greater auricular nerve (ascending portion); *x*, hypoechoic parts of the cervical plexus.

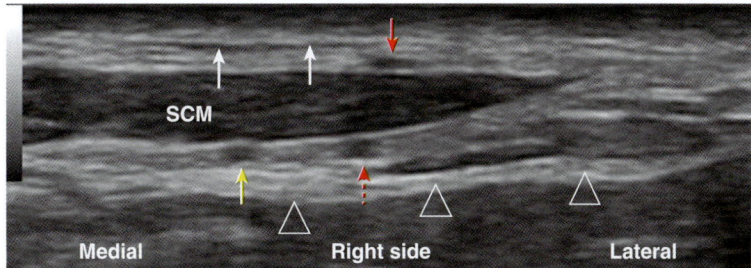

FIGURE 72.5 Greater auricular nerve *(red arrows)*: ascending branch (below the platysma *[white arrows]*) and descending branch (below the SCM). *SCM*, Sternocleidomastoid muscle; *white triangles*, prevertebral fascia; *yellow arrow*, branch of the cervical plexus or portion of the spinal accessory nerve (if entering the trapezoid muscle).

4. The greater auricular nerve (GAN) is the largest branch of the cervical plexus and is often visible where it rounds the posterolateral edge of the SCM (Fig. 72.5). Intermediate CPBs can be performed just cranially from this point to join the remainder of the cervical plexus.
5. Another sonographic landmark for CPB is the carotid bifurcation (Figs. 72.6 and 72.7). In most cases, the cranio-caudal distance between the carotid bifurcation and C4 transverse process is 1 cm or less. However, in a few cases, the carotid bifurcation is located much higher, approximately at the level of the C3 transverse process.

CHOICE OF BLOCKING TECHNIQUE

Pandit et al. demonstrated that the incidence of serious complications with deep (combined) CPBs ($n = 7558$) is significantly increased compared with intermediate or superficial blocks alone ($n = 2533$).[5] Although the complication rate for deep CPBs may be reduced using an ultrasound-guided approach, more recent studies have focused on intermediate and/or superficial blocking techniques.[6-8]

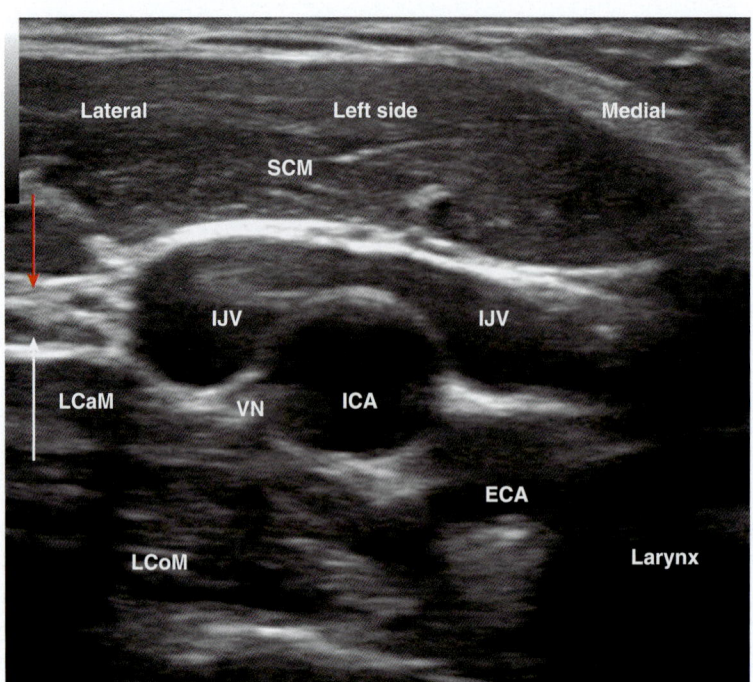

FIGURE 72.6 Carotid bifurcation *(left side)*. *ECA*, External carotid artery; *ICA*, internal carotid artery; *IJV*, internal jugular vein; *LCaM*, longus capitis muscle; *LCoM*, longus colli muscle; *red arrow*, superficial lamina of the cervical fascia; *SCM*, sternocleidomastoid muscle; *VN*, vagus nerve; *white arrow*, prevertebral lamina of the cervical fascia (prevertebral fascia).

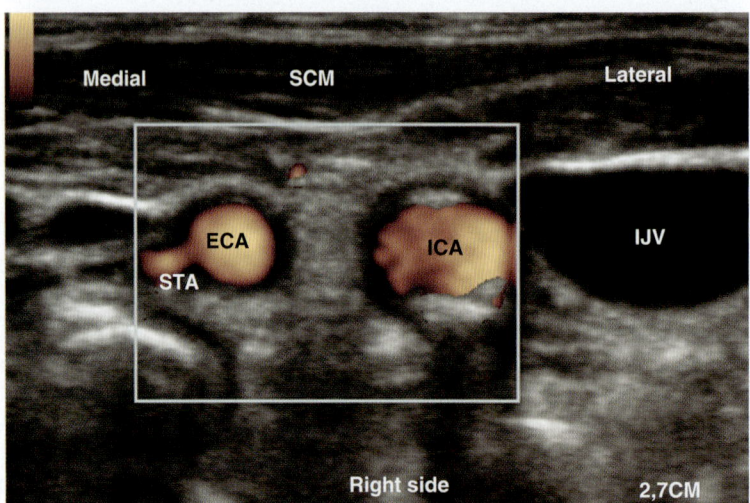

FIGURE 72.7 Carotid bifurcation *(left side)*, power Doppler mode. The external carotid artery (ECA) is identified by extracranial branches. The first branch is the superior thyroid artery *(STA)*. *ECA*, external carotid artery; *ICA*, internal carotid artery; *IJV*, internal jugular vein; *SCM*, sternocleidomastoid muscle.

The interfascial compartment (intermediate block) contains the terminal sensory branches of the cervical plexus. Anatomical studies on unembalmed cadavers showed that injected local anesthetic (LA) is evenly distributed (also in cranio-caudal direction) in this compartment, which results in a homogeneous staining of all sensory portions of the cervical plexus, provided a sufficiently large volume of LA is used.[9]

SUGGESTED TECHNIQUE (INTERMEDIATE CERVICAL PLEXUS BLOCK)

CPBs can be performed in a supine position with the head slightly turned to the opposite side and arms at the side. The head can be stabilized with a gel donut. For an in-plane approach from lateral to medial, it may be useful to raise the ipsilateral shoulder with a gel pad.

The landmarks described above determine the injection site at the level of the C4 transverse process. First, a transverse view of the carotid sheath (common carotid artery, internal jugular vein, vagus nerve) is obtained (SAX-short axis view). The transducer is then moved laterally until the tapering posterolateral edge of the SCM becomes visible. The injection should be performed with an in-plane approach, either from medial to lateral (transmuscular) or from lateral to medial (behind the lateral edge of the SCM; Fig. 72.8). A 24-gauge, 50-mm needle on extension tubing can be used to administer 10 to 20 mL of LA for the block.

DISCUSSION

CURRENT DEBATES AND LIMITATIONS

Two important questions have been raised in current debates. First, the clinical significance of the CN innervation in the neck region and the impact on block technique has not been defined. For carotid endarterectomies, recent studies have attempted to optimize the quality of anesthesia by using a combination of CPBs with an additional ultrasound-guided instillation of LA on the vessel wall (involved nerves: CN, IX, X; sympathetic trunk).[6,8] Moreover, it should be noted that the facial nerve (CN VII) innervates the platysma, which is incised during surgical preparation for carotid endarterectomy. Also, a constant anastomosis between the facial nerve (cervical branch) and the transverse cervical nerve exists (the superficial cervical ansa) (Fig. 72.9).[9] Therefore, a rationale is given for additional local infiltration of the skin incision as described in recent studies.[10] Alternatively, a selective block of the facial nerve (cervical branch) is possible (Fig. 72.10).

Second, the question arises whether the prevertebral fascia is impermeable to injected local anesthetic.[9,11] It is therefore unclear whether accidental block of the phrenic nerve (which is located deep to the prevertebral fascia) can be avoided by an intermediate cervical plexus anesthesia.

A potential cause of inadequate anesthesia may be derived from the course of the supraclavicular nerves (Fig. 72.11). These nerves are located at C4 level, deep to the prevertebral layer of the cervical fascia, and penetrate this barrier at the C5 to C6 level, 2 to 3 cm caudad to the nervous

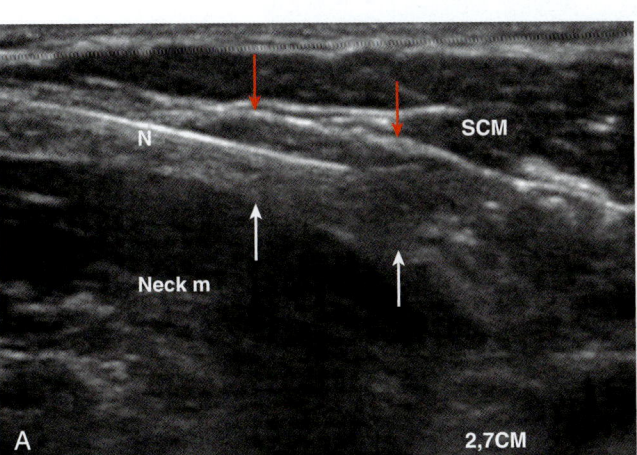 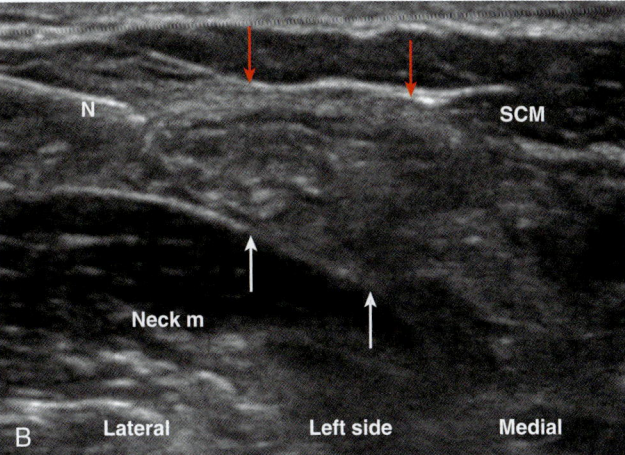

FIGURE 72.8 Intermediate cervical plexus block. In-plane approach from lateral *(left side)*. (A) Before, (B) After injection of local anesthetic. Note the thickening of the interfascial compartment. *N*, Needle within the interfascial compartment; *red arrows*, superficial lamina of the cervical fascia; *SCM*, sternocleidomastoid muscle; *white arrows*, prevertebral lamina of the cervical fascia (prevertebral fascia).

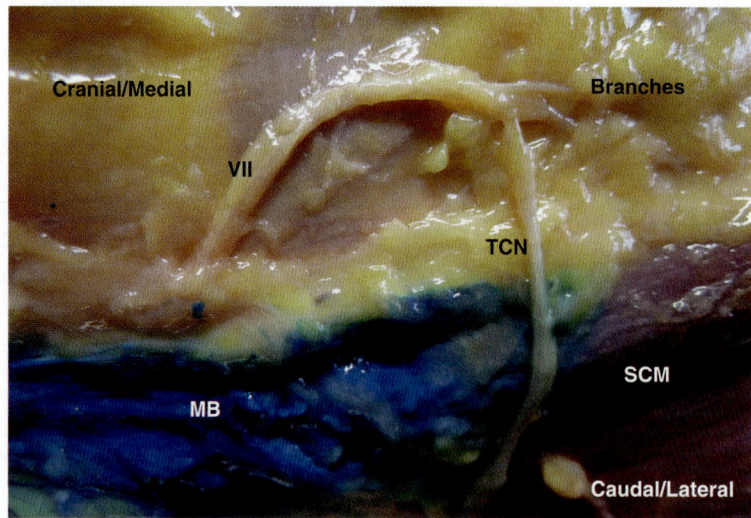

FIGURE 72.9 Superficial cervical ansa between the facial nerve (cervical branch) and the transverse cervical nerve (cervical plexus). The subplatysmal injected methylene blue *(MB)* stains the transverse cervical nerve *(TCN)* but not the facial nerve (CN VII). The submandibular injection site should be located between the ventral border of the sternocleidomastoid muscle and the submandibular gland (see Fig. 72.10). *SCM,* Sternocleidomastoid muscle. (Modified from Seidel R, Schulze M, Zukowski K, Wree A. Ultrasound-guided intermediate cervical plexus block. Anatomical study. *Anaesthesist.* 2015;64:446.)

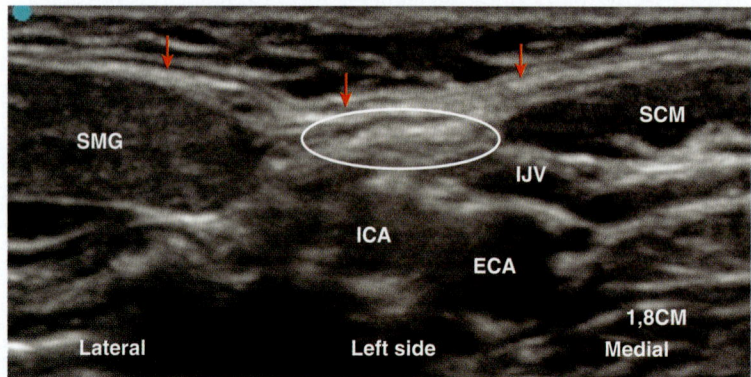

FIGURE 72.10 Selective blockade of the facial nerve (cervical branch) respectively, and the superficial cervical ansa. The injection site *(white circle)* is situated between the ventral border of the sternocleidomastoid muscle *(SCM)* and the submandibular gland *(SMG). ECA,* External carotid artery; *ICA,* internal carotid artery; *IJV,* internal jugular vein.

area. In this case, inadequate anesthesia would be expected selectively in the caudal region of the incision line (for carotid endarterectomies).

When the portions of the cervical plexus penetrate the prevertebral fascia at different levels, the necessary volume of local anesthetic needs to be determined. The interfascial compartment is a three-dimensional space. A craniocaudal distribution of local anesthetic within this space is essential for a uniform impregnation of all sensitive portions of the cervical plexus. This can be achieved with a volume of 20 mL local anesthetic. Lower volumes (5 to 10 mL) tend to lead to a differential blockade of individual portions of the cervical plexus: supraclavicular nerves (injection level C6 to C7) or greater auricular, lesser occipital and transverse cervical nerves (injection level C3 to C4).

CERVICAL PLEXUS BLOCK

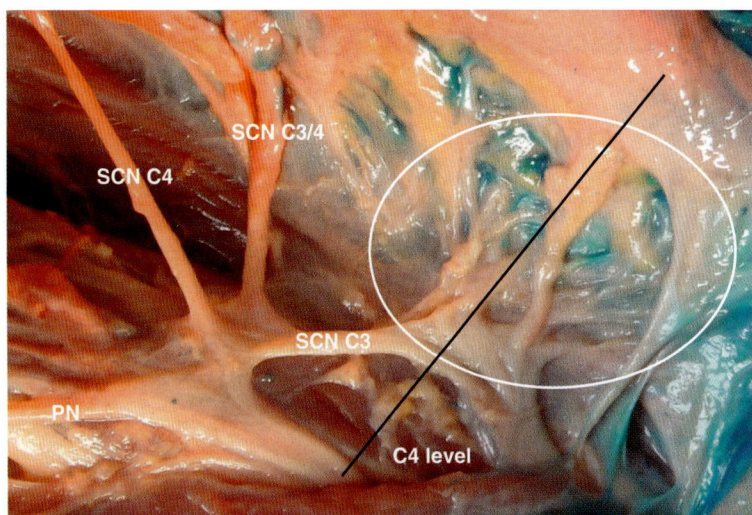

FIGURE 72.11 Course of the phrenic and supraclavicular nerves below the prevertebral fascia at the level of the transverse process C4. View from medial to lateral *(right side)* of the prevertebral fascia after intermediate cervical plexus *(white circle)* block with methylene blue. The supraclavicular nerves perforate the prevertebral fascia at the C5 to C6 level. *PN*, Phrenic nerve; *SCN*, supraclavicular nerves.

KEY POINTS

Cervical Plexus Block	Injection Site	Essential Points
Superficial	Along the posterior border of the sternocleidomastoid muscle; either superficial (landmark-guided) or subplatysmal (ultrasound-guided) injection	Avoids accidental block of the phrenic or recurrent laryngeal nerve
Intermediate	Behind the sternocleidomastoid muscle at the level of C4; between the superficial and the prevertebral lamina of the cervical fascia	Craniocaudal distribution of local anesthetic within the interfascial compartment
Deep	Below the prevertebral fascia	Block of the phrenic nerve is not avoidable

KEY POINTS

Intermediate Cervical Plexus Block	The Essentials
Anatomy	The correct puncture depth: between the superficial layer (envelops the sternocleidomastoid muscle; SCM) and the prevertebral layer of the cervical fascia; behind the SCM The correct puncture height: at the level at transverse process C4; alternatives: at the level of the carotid bifurcation (on average 1 cm more cranially) or at the point, where the greater auricular nerve loops around the posterior border of the SCM (on average 1 cm more caudally)
Patient	Supine position with arms at side, head turned to opposite side, head position supported with gel donut, perhaps ipsilateral shoulder raised with a gel pad
Operator and display	Operator standing at the side of the patient and display across the table; alternative: operator at the head of the patient and display to the ipsilateral side
Transducer	High-frequency linear transducer (>10 MHz) with 38 mm (23–50 mm) footprint; initial depth setting usually less than 30 mm

Continued

KEY POINTS—CONT'D

Intermediate Cervical Plexus Block	**The Essentials**
Needle	24–25 gauge, 38–50 mm
Imaging	SAX (Short Axis View), Step 1: represent the transverse process C7 behind the SCM (note the tapering posterolateral edge), Step 2: move the transducer cranially until the transverse process C4 appears
Approach	OOP (Out-of-Plane) when combined with an interscalene brachial plexus block; IP (In-Plane) from a medial (transmuscular) or lateral injection site

Clinical Pearls

- For some surgeries (such as shoulder surgery) an interscalene brachial plexus block can be combined with an intermediate cervical plexus block (supraclavicular nerves) from a single injection site at the level C6 to C7.
- Important sonographic landmarks include the interfascial compartment behind the sternocleidomastoid muscle (SCM; between the superficial and prevertebral layers of cervical fascia), the transverse process C4, the carotid bifurcation (on average 1 cm higher than C4), and the greater auricular nerve (loops around the lateral edge of the SCM; on average 1 cm lower than C4).
- The innervation of the neck has contributions from descending branches of cranial nerves and ascending branches that travel with sympathetic nerves. Therefore, in some cases, cervical plexus blocks do not serve as definitive anesthetics. This problem can be solved by additional doses of analgesics or by supplementary injections of local anesthetic, either by the surgeon (local infiltration as needed) or the anesthesiologist (carotid sheath, facial nerve). The key is a cooperative approach by all members of the surgical team.

References

1. Shoja MM, Oyesiku NM, Shokouhi G, et al. Anastomoses between lower cranial and upper cervical nerves: a comprehensive review with potential significance during skull base and neck operations, part II: glossopharyngeal, vagus, accessory, hypoglossal and cervical spinal nerves 1-4. *Clin Anat.* 2014;27(1):131–144.
2. Telford RJ, Stoneham MD. Correct nomenclature of superficial cervical plexus blocks. *Br J Anaesth.* 2004;92(5):775–776.
3. Choquet O, Dadure C, Cabdevila X. Ultrasound-guided deep or intermediate cervical plexus block: the target should bet the posterior cervical space. *Anesth Analg.* 2010;111(6):1563–1564.
4. Soeding P, Eizenberg N. Review article: anatomical considerations for ultrasound guidance for regional anesthesiaof the neck and upper limb. *Can J Anesth.* 2009;179(3):699–702.
5. Pandit JJ, Satya-Krishna R, Gration P. Superficial or deep cervical plexus block for carotid endarterectomy: a systematic review of complications. *Br J Anaesth.* 2007;99(2):159–169.
6. Calderon AL, Zetlaoui P, Benatir F, et al. Ultrasound-guided intermediate cervical plexus block for carotid endarterectomy using a new anterior approach: a two-centre prospective observational study. *Anaesthesia.* 2015;70(4):445–451.
7. Ramachandran SK, Picton P, Shanks A, Dorje P, Pandit JJ. Comparison of intermediate vs subcutaneous cervical plexus block for carotid endarterectomy. *Br J Anaesth.* 2011;107(2):157–163.
8. Rössel T, Kersting S, Heller AR, Koch T. Combination of high-resolution ultrasound-guided perivascular regional anesthesia of the internal carotid artery and intermediate cervical plexus block for carotid surgery. *Ultrasound Med Biol.* 2013;39(6):981–986.
9. Seidel R, Schulze M, Zukowski K, Wree A. Ultrasound-guided intermediate cervical plexus block. Anatomic study. *Anaesthesist.* 2015;64(6):446–450.
10. Martusevicius R, Swiatek F, Joergensen LG, et al. Ultrasound-guided locoregional anesthesia for carotid endarterectomy: a prospective observational study. *Eur J Endovasc Surg.* 2012;44(1):27–30.
11. Pandit JJ, Dutta D, Morris JF. Spread of injectate with superficial cervical plexus block in humans: an anatomical study. *Br J Anaesth.* 2003;91(5):733–735.

Stellate Ganglion Block
(Cervicothoracic Sympathetic Ganglion Block)

Jens Kessler

CHAPTER 73

Stellate ganglion blocks can be performed to treat sympathetically maintained pain (reflex sympathetic dystrophy, causalgia, complex regional pain syndromes). The stellate ganglion is the fusion of the inferior cervical and first thoracic sympathetic ganglia. Almost all the sympathetic innervation of the head, neck, and upper extremity travels via pathways through the stellate ganglion. The stellate ganglion is approximately 0.5 to 2.5 cm in size.[1] Despite its name, the stellate ganglion is fusiform, triangular, or globular in shape on magnetic resonance scans.[2] The stellate ganglion can have a star-shaped appearance if the fusion of the inferior cervical and first thoracic ganglion is complete. Stellate ganglion block is used to diagnose and treat chronic pain syndromes of the upper extremity and head and neck.

At the level of the first thoracic vertebral level, the stellate ganglion lies lateral and posterior to the lateral edge of the longus colli muscle. As the cervical sympathetic chain travels cephalad, it comes to lie anterior to the longus colli muscle.[3,4] This muscle lies over the anterior surface of the cervical transverse processes.

ANATOMIC STRUCTURES TO BE IDENTIFIED FOR STELLATE GANGLION BLOCK

ESOPHAGUS

The esophagus is usually a midline structure that can be deviated, most often to the left side. Tilting the chin up straightens the esophagus to move it toward the midline. The esophagus is relatively easy to identify because it has muscular walls. Any question regarding identity can be resolved by asking the patient to swallow while imaging is performed. This forces intraluminal bubbles to move and enhance their conspicuity. The esophagus is important to recognize on ultrasound scans because of the risk of mediastinitis if it is punctured. Because of its usual location, the risk of esophageal puncture is higher with left-sided stellate ganglion blocks.

INFERIOR THYROID ARTERY

The inferior thyroid artery has a tortuous course (hence its alternate name, the "serpentine" artery).[5] This artery travels over the surface of the longus colli muscle from lateral to medial.

VERTEBRAL ARTERY AND VEIN

As it ascends, the vertebral artery travels over the surface of the longus colli muscle from medial to lateral before it enters the vertebral canal. The level of entry is usually at the sixth cervical vertebra. The vertebral vein lies on the superficial aspect of the vertebral artery.

ANTERIOR AND POSTERIOR TUBERCLES

The anterior and posterior tubercles of the transverse processes of the C6 and C7 vertebrae can be identified by their morphology. The anterior tubercle of C6 is prominent (Chassaignac's tubercle), whereas the anterior tubercle of C7 is rudimentary. This helps establish the level for the block.

PHRENIC NERVE

The phrenic nerve crosses over the anterior surface of the anterior scalene muscle from lateral to medial. On ultrasound scans, the phrenic nerve appears as a small (<1 mm in diameter) monofascicular structure.[6] The phrenic nerve lies adjacent to the C5 ventral ramus at the level of the cricoid cartilage (C6). Performing stellate block caudal to this level helps avoid the phrenic nerve within the lateral to medial needle path. Similarly, the superficial cervical artery (transverse cervical artery) that also lies over the anterior scalene muscle can be avoided in this fashion.

LONGUS COLLI MUSCLE

This muscle is very hypoechoic (relatively dark) on ultrasound scans and represents the most important landmark for stellate ganglion blocks.

APPROACH AND SUGGESTED TECHNIQUE

Confirm nothing per mouth (NPO) status and place a peripheral IV prior to the procedure. Some patients may require EMLA (eutectic mixture of local anesthetics) cream over the needle insertion site and sedation for the procedure.

Stellate block is performed in supine position with arms at the side. Performing the procedure on an operating room table is optimal because it allows the operator to be close to the patient and adjust elevation of the head of the bed. The patient's head should be midline, with the chin tilted up. A blue foam headrest helps stabilize the head in this position. Preprocedural and postprocedural pain scores should be recorded. Skin temperature probes should be applied to the dorsum of the hand on the ipsilateral and contralateral sides for monitoring. The patient should be instructed to not talk, swallow, cough, or move during the procedure (use hand signals if necessary).

For the lateral-to-medial in-plane approach the needle is placed through the anterior scalene muscle on the surface of the longus colli muscle. This is usually done between C6 and C7 or between C7 and T1. Gentle pressure is held on the injection syringe until a rim of local anesthetic is seen to distribute around the lateral aspect of the longus colli muscle. There is debate regarding the correct layer for successful stellate block as being over, under, or within the fascia that invests the longus colli muscle.[7] Regardless, a rim of local anesthetic that outlines the surface of the longus colli muscle is predictive of block success. Because the site of injection is distant from the stellate ganglion (which lies closer to the level of T1), dilute local anesthetic is used for the block (4 mL has been estimated to the optimal volume for ropivacaine 0.2%). The head of the bed is elevated after injection to promote caudal and posterior distribution toward the stellate ganglion.

Many pain therapists prefer the out-of-plane approach to stellate ganglion block. If directing the needle through the thyroid gland, the bevel must be sharp and a small-size needle (e.g., 25 gauge) is recommended.

Postprocedure neurologic examination is performed to rule out somatic brachial plexus block. A temperature increase of the ipsilateral upper extremity and Horner's syndrome is expected with successful block. The sympathetic efferents to the arm are primarily found in the C8 and T1 roots.[8] It is therefore important that local anesthetic distribute to the sympathetic chain at or below those levels. Bilateral stellate ganglion blocks should be avoided or at least temporally staggered because of the risk of bilateral pneumothorax, cardiac accelerator nerve fiber block, recurrent laryngeal nerve block, and phrenic nerve block.

KEY POINTS

Stellate Ganglion Block	The Essentials
Anatomy	The CSG lies on the posterolateral aspect of LC at C7.
	The STG lies near the head of the first rib.
	The ITA, VA, ESO, and PN can lie in the needle path.
Positioning	Supine with arms at side, blue foam headrest
Operator	Standing at the side of the patient
Display	Across the table
Transducer	High-frequency linear, 38- to 50-mm footprint
Initial depth setting	35–50 mm
Needle	21 gauge, 70 mm in length

KEY POINTS—CONT'D

Stellate Ganglion Block	The Essentials
Anatomic location	Begin by imaging the C6 and C7 transverse processes.
	Perform the block between C6 and C7 or between C7 and T1.
Approach	In-plane from lateral to medial
	Aim the needle through the AS on the LC surface.
	Slowly inject over the LC surface.
Sonographic assessment	The injection should rim over the lateral surface of the LC.
Anatomic variation	Common (a distinct STG is not present in 20%)

AS, Anterior scalene muscle; *CSG*, cervical sympathetic ganglion; *ESO*, esophagus; *ITA*, inferior thyroid artery; *LC*, longus colli muscle; *PN*, phrenic nerve; *STG*, stellate ganglion; *VA*, vertebral artery.

Clinical Pearls

- Ultrasound provides valuable soft tissue information that is important for safe and effective stellate ganglion block.[9]
- The longus colli muscle lies medial to the anterior tubercles of the cervical vertebrae. The vertical fibers of this muscle extend into the chest, as low as T3.
- The borders of the longus colli muscle can be difficult to identify. The echogenic fascial plane between the longus capitis and longus collis can help identify the muscle border.
- On the left side of the neck, the esophagus more often lies in the needle path at the C7 level than at the C6 level.[10] On the right side of the neck, the esophagus is usually not present.
- The inferior thyroid artery ("serpentine" artery) ascends anterior to the longus colli muscle to supply the inferior part of the thyroid lobe and is potentially within the needle path for stellate ganglion block. The inferior thyroid artery has a tortuous course between the carotid artery and the anterior surface of the longus colli muscle (the artery runs from lateral to medial).
- The phrenic nerve lies on the surface of the anterior scalene muscle and is potentially in the needle path for stellate ganglion block.[11]
- Stellate ganglion block is considered an intermediate-risk procedure in terms of bleeding complications.[12]

References

1. Erickson SJ, Hogan QH. CT-guided injection of the stellate ganglion: description of technique and efficacy of sympathetic blockade. *Radiology*. 1993;188(3):707–709.
2. Hogan QH, Erickson SJ. MR imaging of the stellate ganglion: normal appearance. *AJR Am J Roentgenol*. 1992;158(3):655–659.
3. Ebraheim NA, Lu J, Yang H, et al. Vulnerability of the sympathetic trunk during the anterior approach to the lower cervical spine. *Spine*. 2000;25(13):1603–1606.
4. Civelek E, Karasu A, Cansever T, et al. Surgical anatomy of the cervical sympathetic trunk during anterolateral approach to cervical spine. *Eur Spine J*. 2008;17(8):991–995.
5. Narouze S. Beware of the "serpentine" inferior thyroid artery while performing stellate ganglion block. *Anesth Analg*. 2009;109(1):289–290.
6. Kessler J, Schafhalter-Zoppoth I, Gray AT. An ultrasound study of the phrenic nerve in the posterior cervical triangle: implications for the interscalene brachial plexus block. *Reg Anesth Pain Med*. 2008;33:545–550.
7. Gofeld M, Bhatia A, Abbas S, et al. Development and validation of a new technique for ultrasound-guided stellate ganglion block. *Reg Anesth Pain Med*. 2009;34(5):475–479.
8. Hogan QH, Erickson SJ, Haddox JD, et al. The spread of solutions during stellate ganglion block. *Reg Anesth*. 1992;17(2):78–83.
9. Narouze S. Ultrasound-guided stellate ganglion block: safety and efficacy. *Curr Pain Headache Rep*. 2014;18:424.

10. Siegenthaler A, Mlekusch S, Schliessbach J, et al. Ultrasound imaging to estimate risk of esophageal and vascular puncture after conventional stellate ganglion block. *Reg Anesth Pain Med.* 2012;37(2):224–227. PMID: 22157739.
11. Ojeda A, Sala-Blanch X, Moreno LA, Busquets C. Ultrasound-guided stellate ganglion block: what about the phrenic nerve? *Reg Anesth Pain Med.* 2013;38(2):170. PMID: 23423134.
12. Narouze S, Benzon HT, Provenzano DA, et al. Interventional spine and pain procedures in patients on antiplatelet and anticoagulant medications. *Reg Anesth Pain Med.* 2015;40:182–212.

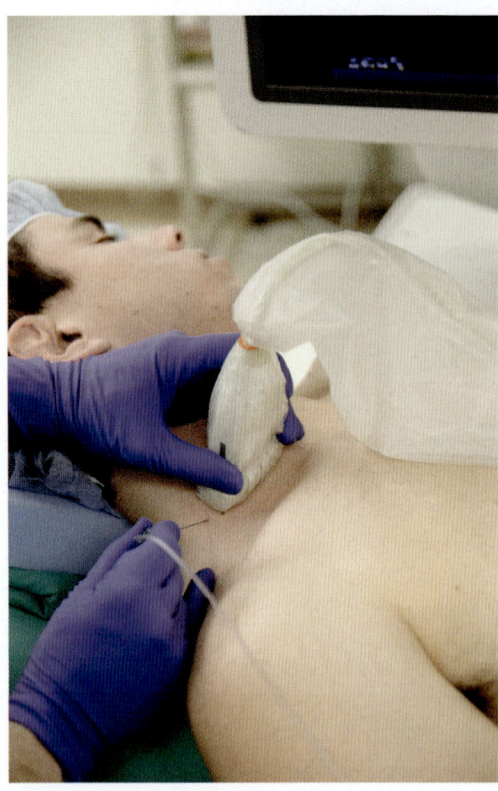

FIGURE 73.1 External photograph showing lateral in-plane approach to stellate ganglion block between the transverse processes of the sixth and seventh cervical vertebrae.

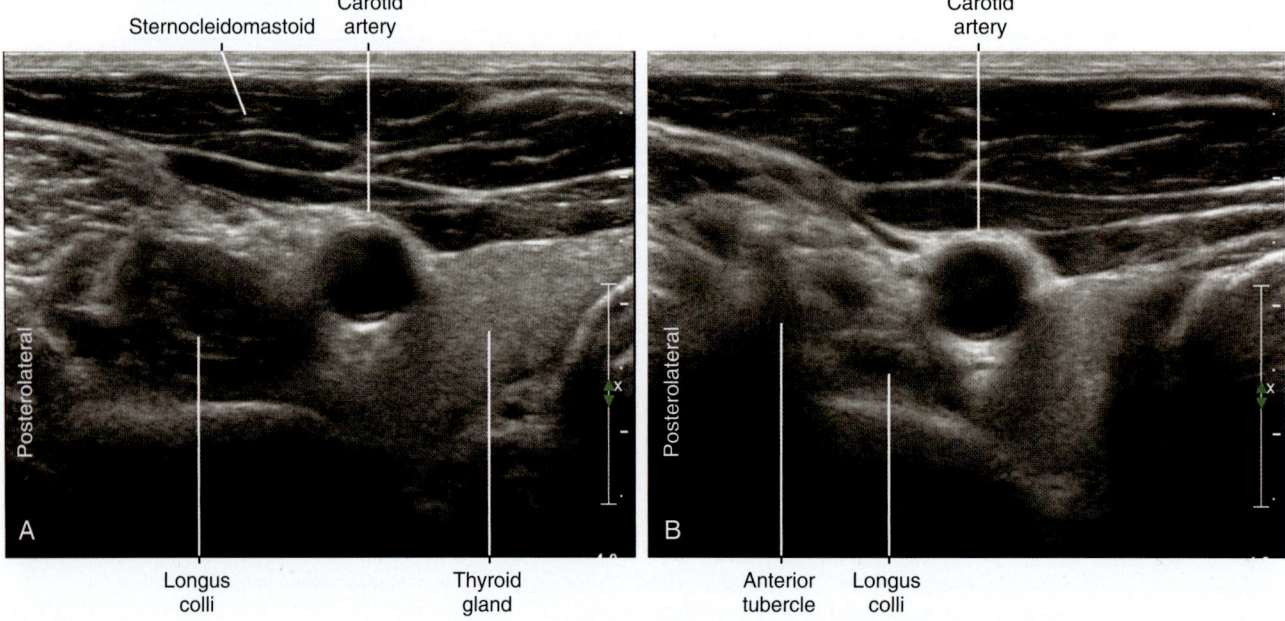

FIGURE 73.2 Transverse view of the longus colli muscle adjacent to the transverse process of sixth cervical vertebra (A). For comparison, the transverse process of the sixth cervical vertebra with a prominent anterior tubercle is shown (Chassaignac's tubercle) (B).

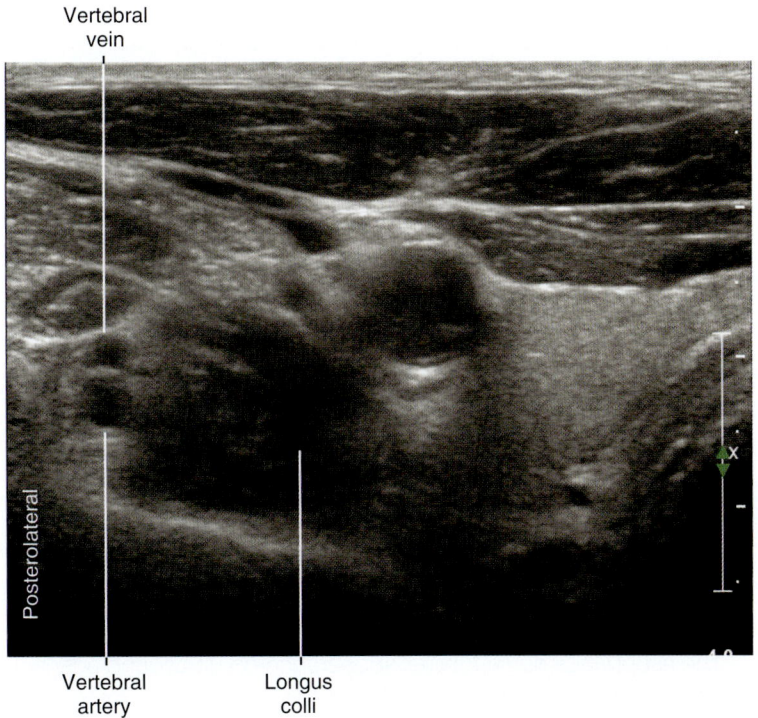

FIGURE 73.3 Transverse view of the longus colli muscle showing the position of the vertebral artery and vein. This scan was obtained adjacent to the seventh cervical vertebra.

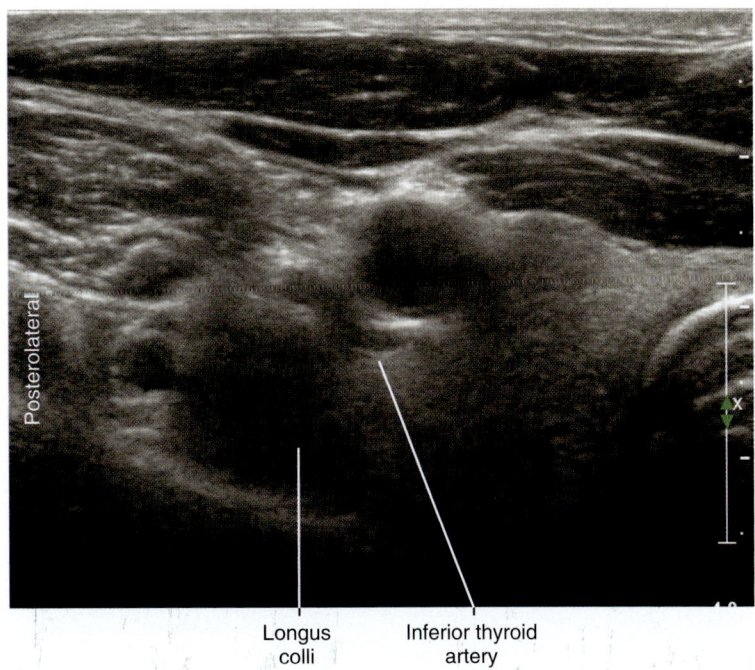

FIGURE 73.4 Long-axis view of the inferior thyroid artery. Because the artery is tortuous (the "serpentine" artery), only a limited portion of the artery is contained within the field of view (a partial long-axis view).

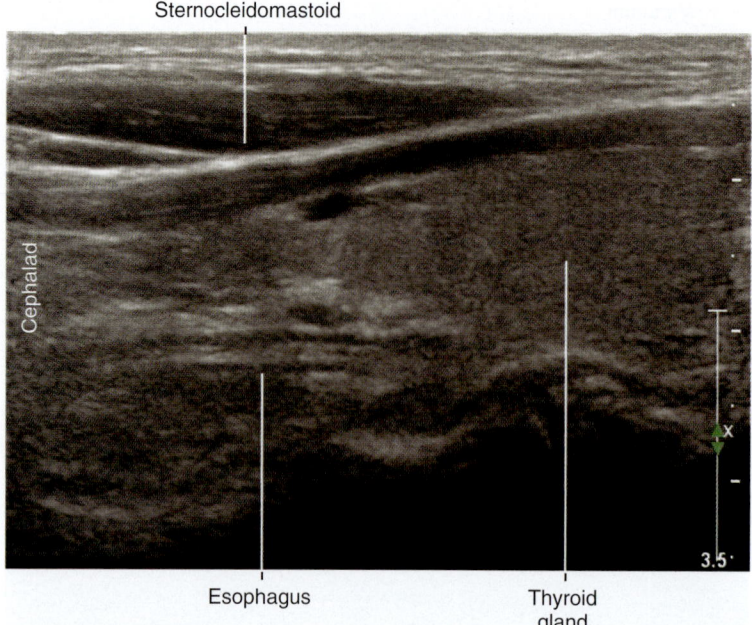

FIGURE 73.5 The esophagus has a tubular appearance on ultrasound scans. High-frequency sonography can resolve multiple layers of the muscular esophageal wall. The esophagus can often be seen posterior to the thyroid gland on the left side and can be identified by the mucosal pattern characteristic of a hollow viscus. In this example, a longitudinal view shows the esophageal lumen with hyperechoic bands.

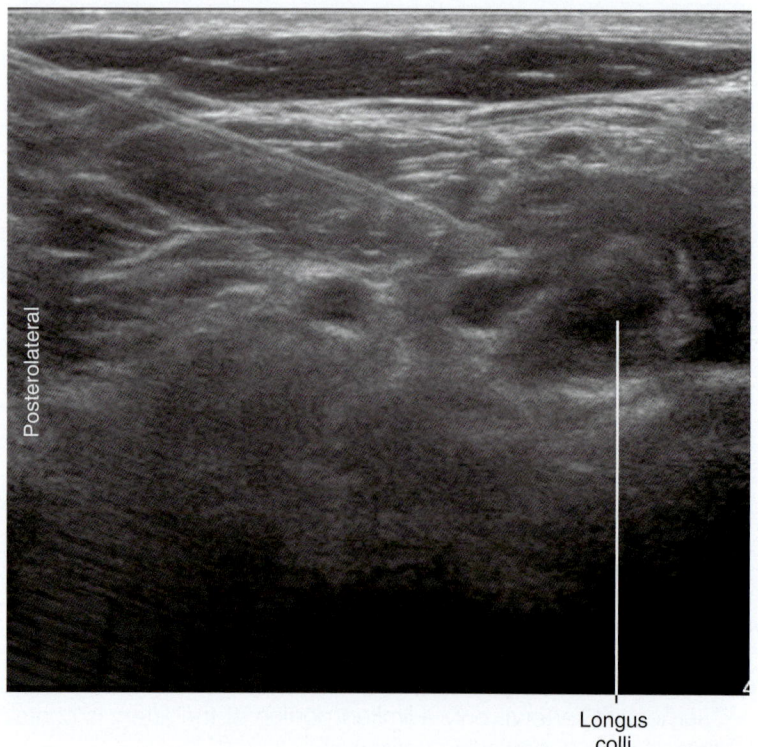

FIGURE 73.6 Lateral to medial in-plane approach to stellate ganglion block. The block needle tip has been placed in the longus colli muscle. Injection occurs as the needle is slowly withdrawn to the surface of the muscle.

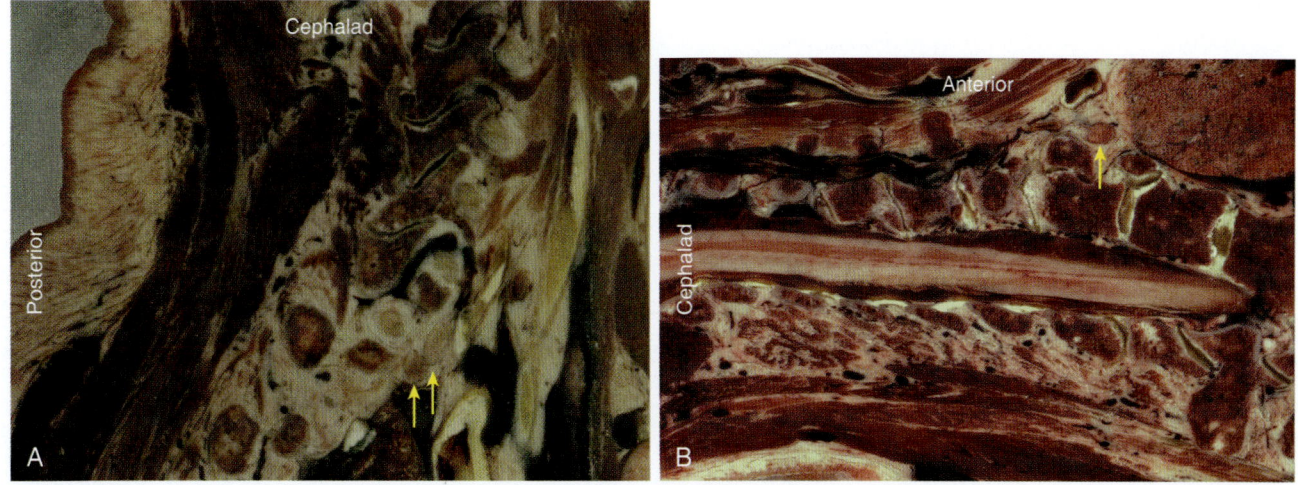

FIGURE 73.7 Anatomic sections demonstrating bi-lobed (A) and globular (B) appearances of the stellate ganglion *(yellow arrows)*. Anatomic sections are provided courtesy of Dr. Quinn Hogan.

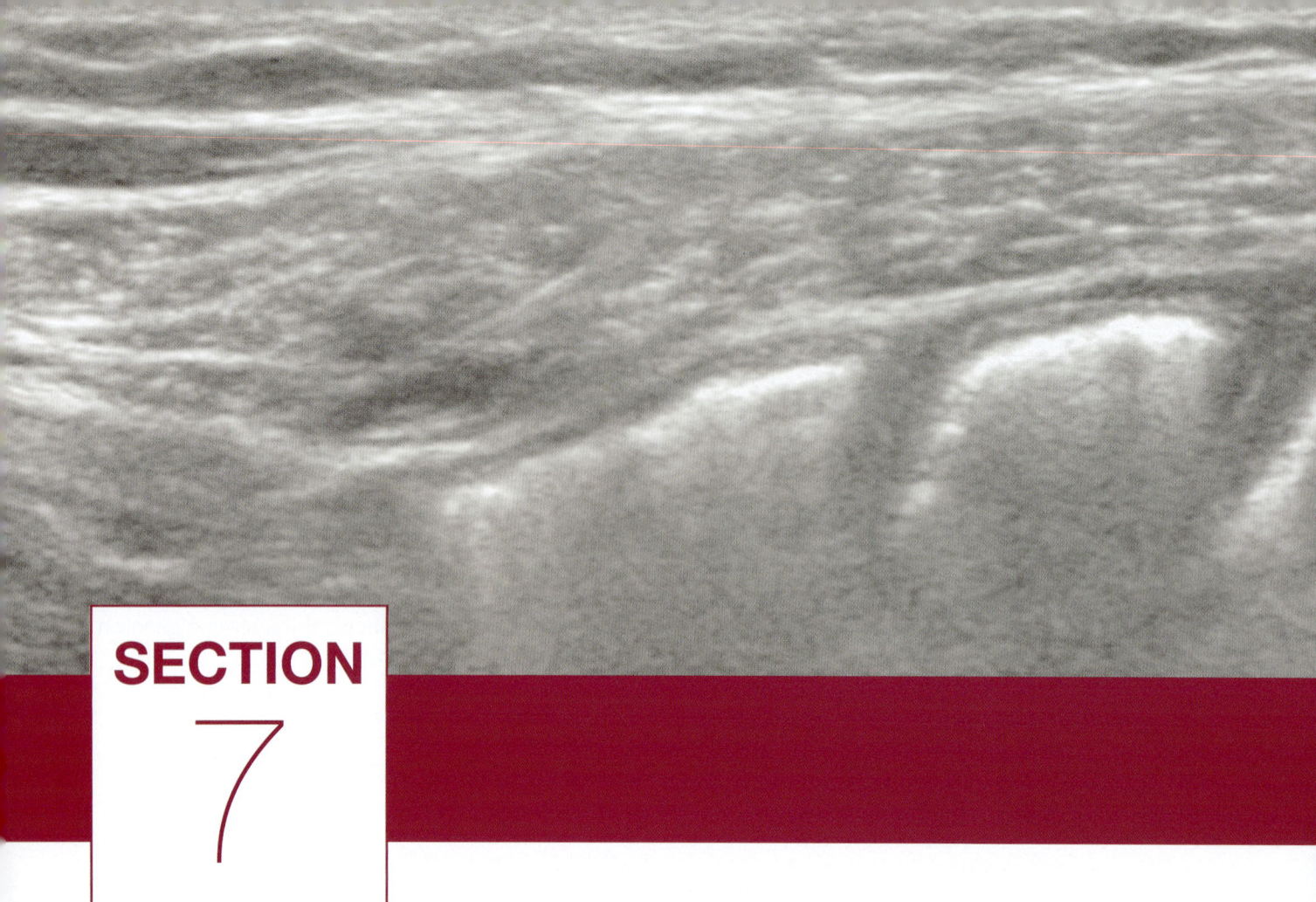

SECTION 7

Safety Issues

Safety: Practical Techniques to Prevent Complications During Ultrasound-Guided Nerve Blocks

CHAPTER 74

Michael J. Barrington | Daniel M. Wong

See Video 74.1 on ExpertConsult.com.

The goal of this chapter is to promote practical techniques that enhance safety during ultrasound-guided peripheral nerve block (PNB). Ultrasound-guided PNB can be performed with a level of precision and purpose that is not feasible with other techniques. Ultrasound imaging and guidance for PNB is unique among all the nerve localizing tools and monitors because the needle trajectory can be tracked and controlled, reducing the risk of trauma to nerves and other critical structures. However, operators find it challenging to maintain the needle in the plane of the ultrasound beam in all patients and anatomical locations. Therefore, anesthesiologists require appropriate training and education to develop this skill. As with all regional anesthesia techniques, the safety and efficacy of ultrasound-guided techniques require meticulous attention to indication, anatomy, equipment, and technique.

VASCULAR COMPLICATIONS

Inadvertent vascular puncture and injection of local anesthetic may result in local anesthetic systemic toxicity (LAST). Inadvertent vascular puncture may result in persisting bleeding or discomfort from bruising in the subcutaneous tissues or muscles. More serious cases of trauma have resulted in trauma to critical organ sites including the liver, kidney, intestinal wall, pelvis, retroperitoneum, and mediastinum.[1] Sequelae of bleeding and hematoma have included pain, neurologic complications, renal failure, postponement of surgery, surgical intervention to correct the injury, sepsis, delayed recovery, prolonged hospitalization, dyspnea, tracheostomy, and even death. Fortunately, serious hematoma and injury are rare. However, these have occurred in patients with both normal and impaired hemostasis and following both superficial and deep PNB.[2] Therefore, knowledge of the frequency and origins of the vasculature in close proximity to block locations is important so as to avoid these vessels and reduce the incidence of vascular complications. A Cochrane meta-analysis of randomized, controlled trials concluded that ultrasound guidance was associated with a reduced incidence of vascular puncture compared to nerve stimulator guidance.[3] This result is supported by observational studies.[4]

PRACTICAL SUGGESTIONS FOR REDUCING THE RISK OF VASCULAR TRAUMA

1. *Identify vessels on the sonogram along the intended needle trajectory.*
   Many PNB locations have a high level of vascularity, and vessels can be imaged using two-dimensional (2D) or color Doppler modes on the ultrasound machine. The authors recommend that practitioners routinely perform a pre-block survey sonogram to identify major and minor vessels so that a safe needle trajectory can be planned. An example presented in Fig. 74.1 is a pre-block survey sonogram obtained prior to a supraclavicular brachial plexus block. This

SAFETY ISSUES

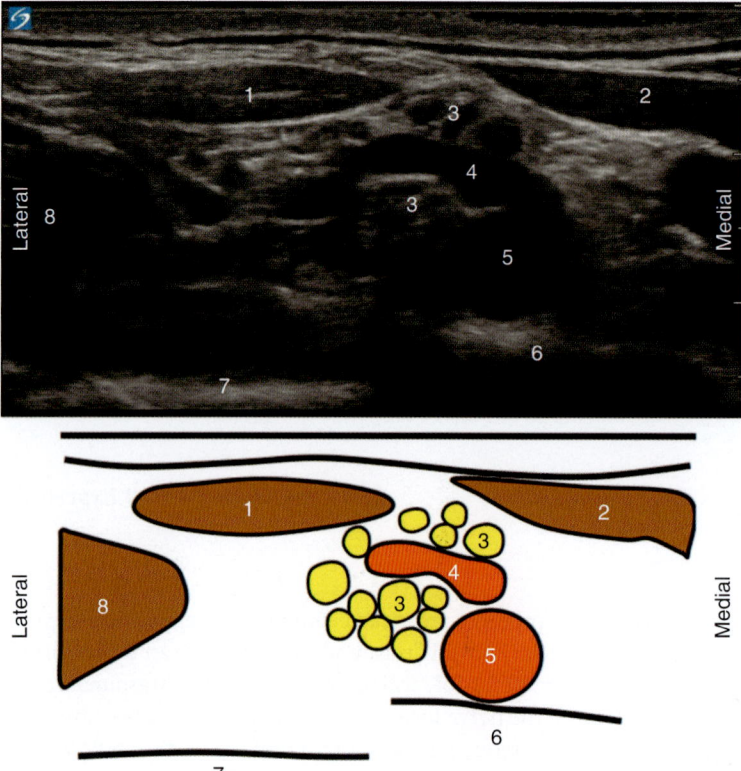

FIGURE 74.1 A pre-block survey sonogram obtained prior to a supraclavicular brachial plexus block identified a large arterial structure between the neural elements of the brachial plexus. (1) Omohyoid muscle; (2) sternocleidomastoid muscle; (3) brachial plexus; (4) dorsal scapular artery; (5) subclavian artery; (6) first rib; (7) pleura; (8) scalenius medius muscle.

pre-block sonogram identified a large arterial structure (the dorsal scapular artery) between the neural elements of the brachial plexus. It is important to note that when arterial flow is at 90 degrees to the angle of insonation, there will be no color Doppler signal. Some vessels may be difficult to identify on the sonogram related to size, circumflex course, and depth.

2. *Knowledge of common vascular branches.*
   Because the operator may not always identify vessels using ultrasound, knowledge of the location of key vasculature is of paramount importance. In this section, we provide two examples in the neck and inguinal region. The dorsal scapular, suprascapular, and superficial cervical arteries arise directly from the subclavian artery or from the thyrocervical trunk. There is substantial variation in the anatomy and nomenclature with at least four different arterial trunks described emerging directly from the subclavian artery or from the thyrocervical trunk. In a combined cadaver and clinical study, Muhly documented that arterial branches were often in close proximity to or passed between branches of the brachial plexus (Fig. 74.1).[5] In the supraclavicular region, arterial branches, usually the dorsal scapular artery, were adjacent to the plexus in 43/50 (86%) patients. In the interscalene region and arterial vessel (likely the superficial cervical artery), they were identified in 45/50 (90%) of patients. In a similar study performed by the same authors, at the level of the femoral crease, there was a 12% incidence of arterial vessels (profunda femoral, lateral circumflex femoral) located lateral to the femoral artery.[6]

3. *Plan an atraumatic needle trajectory taking into account both identified and expected vessels.*
   The anesthesiologist can implement strategies to reduce the risk of inadvertent vascular trauma (if a vessel is identified on a pre-block sonogram) including a complete change of needle trajectory, a minor change to the transducer angle so that the vessel is no longer in the planned needle trajectory, or another approach to the nerve or plexus. Using the example in Fig. 74.1, if the vessel is large, it may be sensible to choose a different approach to the brachial plexus. Using an example at the femoral block level, circumflex vessels have a medial to lateral course,

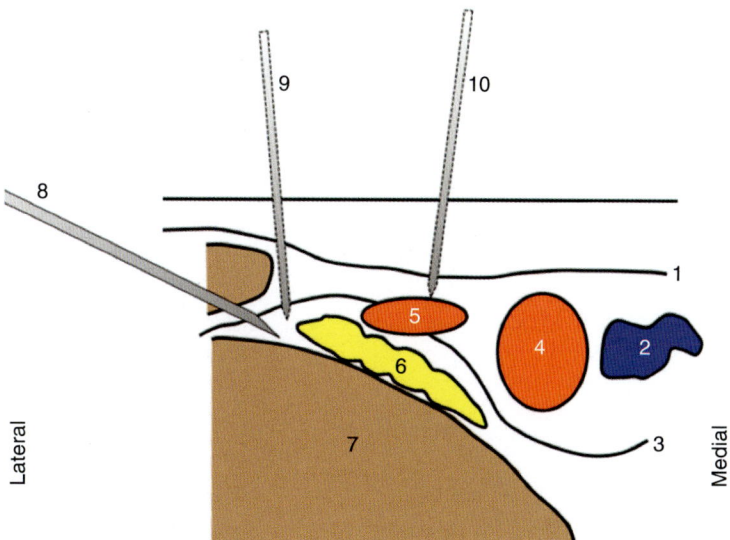

FIGURE 74.2 Examples of trajectories and relative risk of vascular injury during femoral block are illustrated. (1) Fascia lata; (2) femoral vein; (3) fascia iliaca; (4) femoral artery; (5) circumflex artery (femoral); (6) femoral nerve; (7) iliopsoas muscle; (8) lateral to medial in-plane approach; (9) out-of-plane approach; (10) out-of-plane approach too medial.

vessels may be anterior to the femoral nerve, and injury to this vessel may be less likely if an anteromedial approach is avoided and a lateral to medial approach is used. In Fig. 74.2, examples of trajectories and relative risk of vascular injury during femoral block are illustrated.

LOCAL ANESTHETIC SYSTEMIC TOXICITY

LAST is a feared complication of regional anesthesia due to its potential to result in a fatal outcome. LAST is variable in timing of onset and presentation; therefore, diagnosis can be delayed or even missed. Management of this complication has improved with the use of crisis resource algorithms, cognitive aids, checklists, and the use of intravenous lipid emulsion (ILE) therapy. ILE represents a major milestone in improving safety. Despite these advances, the most important strategy for improving patient outcomes is preventing LAST.

Recent epidemiological and registry studies have captured LAST events including presenting features and incidence. Table 74.1 summarizes the incidence of LAST, block types involved, practice setting, and severity/type of LAST.[7-17]

INCIDENCE AND RISK FACTORS FOR LAST

In 2013, a dataset from the Australian and New Zealand Registry of Regional Anaesthesia (AURORA) comprising 25,336 PNBs from 20,021 patients was analyzed. There were 22 cases of LAST (13 mild severity, 8 major, and 1 cardiac arrest) with an overall incidence of LAST of 0.87 per 1000 PNB. Analysis of this dataset using logistic regression and propensity scoring demonstrated that ultrasound guidance was associated with a 60% to 65% reduced risk of LAST.[11] Factors associated with an increased risk of LAST included site of injection (upper extremity and paravertebral block having an increased risk of LAST compared to lower extremity block), increased local anesthetic dosage, increased local anesthetic dosage per weight, and reduced patient body weight. Lidocaine was associated with an increased risk of LAST compared with ropivacaine. This result was surprising because conventional wisdom would predict that lidocaine would present a lower risk of LAST. Interestingly, lidocaine dosage was increased in ultrasound-guided techniques (4.55 [1.54 to 7.5] mg/kg) compared to nonultrasound techniques (3.38 [1.10 to 6.67] mg/kg); presented as median (10th to 90th centiles). This was in contrast to ropivacaine dosage 1.48 (0.73 to 2.71) mg/kg being reduced for ultrasound-guided techniques compared to non-ultrasound techniques 1.63 (0.74 to 2.88) mg/kg. Bupivacaine was only used in 4% of 25,336 PNB; therefore, it was not

TABLE 74.1 Local Anesthetic Systemic Toxicity: Incidence, Block Types, Practice Setting, and Severity

Author, Year	n	N	Incidence n per 1000	%	Block Type	Practice Setting	Severity and Nature of Presenting Features
Ecoffey, 2010[7]	16	29,290	0.54	0.05	Neuraxial: 10,554 Peripheral: 18,735	Pediatric	All major LAST, Seizure 1; cardiac 15 (15 occurred under GA)
Orebaugh, 2012[8]	6	14,498	0.41	0.04	Peripheral	Single-center academic	Major LAST (seizures) all with non-ultrasound technique
Sites, 2012[9]	0	12,668	–		Peripheral	Single-center academic	Events sought were seizures
Polaner, 2012[10]	0	14,917	0–2[a]		Neuraxial: 9,156 Peripheral: 5,761	Pediatric, 6 academic centers	
Barrington, 2013[11]	22	25,336	0.87	0.09	Peripheral (all)	Multi-center, mixed academic, community	Minor LAST – 13 (prodromes, agitation); major LAST – 9 (seizures 6, loss of consciousness 3, cardiac arrest 1,)
Rohrbaugh, 2013[12]	8	15,014	0.53	0.05	Interscalene		Details not provided
Gurnaney, 2014[13]	3	1954	1.53	0.2	Peripheral	Pediatric, Single-center academic	Outpatient catheters, all minor (prodromes)
Heinonen, 2015[14]	15	217,700	0.07	0.007		Nationwide center	Major LAST 15 (CV 1, seizures 14)
Liu, 2016[15]	3	80,661	0.04	0.004	Peripheral	Single-center, high-volume practice	Major LAST (seizures) – 3
Allegri, 2016[16]	10	29,545	0.3	0.03	Peripheral	Multi-center	Minor LAST – 3 (prodromes); major LAST –7 (seizures 4, CV 3)
Morwald 2017[17]	434	238,473	1.8	0.18	Peripheral	Administrative database	Surrogate outcomes

CV, Cardiovascular; *GA*, general anaesthesia; *N*, Number of events; *N*, denominator (blocks).
[a]95% confidence interval per 10,000 presented for zero events, calculated by author; one event presented as unconsciousness followed by seizure.

possible to determine if this was a potential risk factor. During the time period of the AURORA registry (2007 to 2012), epinephrine was not uniformly captured to the database; therefore, this could not be entered as a covariate in the logistic regression model. It is generally accepted that patient comorbidities and individual susceptibility to local anesthetic may increase the risk of LAST.

In 2016, the incidence of LAST reported by Liu was 0.04 per 1000 PNBs from a cohort of 80,661 PNB from the Hospital for Special Surgery.[15] This incidence is substantially lower than other reports. However, it was derived from a high-volume PNB practice that may have expertise not representative of the wide spectrum of clinical practice. A nationwide study in Finland used an electronic survey to record outcomes over a 3-year period, 2011 to 2013, where it was estimated that 211,700 PNB were performed.[14] Fifteen episodes of LAST were reported giving an overall incidence of LAST of 0.7 (95% CI, 0.4 to 1.2) per 10,000. Ultrasound guidance was used in two of three cases from the Hospital for Special Surgery and 5 of the 15 cases of LAST in the study from Finland. Ultrasound guidance does not completely prevent LAST from occurring.

Despite advances in management of LAST poor outcomes still occur. In a recent summary of 53 published case reports of LAST following patient PNB from 59 patients between 2010 and 2014, mortality was the outcome in 6 of 59 patients with LAST events.[18] From a recent cohort study that utilized a large administrative database, the authors' concluded that although the incidence of LAST is low, it remains clinically significant.[17]

PRACTICAL SUGGESTIONS FOR REDUCING THE RISK OF LAST

1. *Use lower local anesthetic dosages and volumes*
   Reducing local anesthetic dosage reduces the risk of LAST (systemic toxicity),[11] local neural toxicity, and the incidence of side effects such as a phrenic nerve block[19,20] or Horner's syndrome. Ultrasound-guided PNB techniques are associated with reduced dose requirements for PNB. Controlled clinical trials and volunteer studies have studied the minimum effective local anesthetic doses for ultrasound-guided femoral nerve block,[21] axillary brachial plexus block,[22,23] ulnar nerve block,[24] supraclavicular block,[25] sciatic nerve block,[26] and interscalene block (Table 74.2).[20,27]

2. *Monitor local anesthetic spread using ultrasound guidance and inject the total local anesthetic dosage use an incremental approach.*
   The spread of local anesthetic can be monitored using ultrasound to ensure appropriate spread. An incremental approach with intermittent aspiration should be used. If perineural spread of local anesthetic is observed, intravascular injection can be excluded. If spread of injectate is not observed in the tissues, the injectate may be out-of-plane, or intravascular injection may have occurred. If local anesthetic is injected into a vessel, it may be detected early with sonographic monitoring, thereby limiting the systemic dosage injected.

3. *Compress veins*
   During pre-block survey sonogram light pressure should be applied to the transducer so as to avoid compression of veins. However, once an appropriate needle path has been planned, avoiding such structures, compression of veins may reduce the likelihood of trauma during needle advancement. For example, compression of the large axillary vein(s) during axillary brachial plexus block allows easier navigation of the needle to the terminal nerve branches of the brachial plexus.

4. *Consider adding epinephrine*
   Addition of epinephrine reduces blood concentrations of local anesthetic following paravertebral[28] and other anatomical locations. Epinephrine when used as an adjunct to local anesthetic may allow early detection (i.e., rapid onset of tachycardia) following inadvertent vascular injection of local anesthetic.

5. *Prompting a patient for symptoms*
   For a comprehensive review of prevention of LAST, refer to the review by Mulroy.[29]

NEUROLOGICAL COMPLICATIONS ASSOCIATED WITH PERIPHERAL NERVE BLOCKADE

INCIDENCE OF PERIPHERAL NERVE INJURY DUE TO PERIPHERAL NERVE BLOCK

Nerve injury following PNB can cause long-term effects, including persisting sensory and motor deficits, neuropathic pain, and decreased quality of life. Neurological complications directly related to PNB with severe long-term sequelae occur infrequently or rarely.[30,31] The estimated incidence of long-term PNB-related nerve injury is between 2 and 4 per 10,000 blocks.[31] The incidence of PNB related injuries has remained stable despite major shifts in localizing techniques from nerve stimulator to ultrasound guidance. This highlights the importance of nontechnological factors that impact safety. This abovementioned incidence is an estimate using an epidemiology of peripheral nerve injury limited by the number of studies, their denominators, and methods used to capture and investigate potential PNB-related nerve injuries. The interaction of anesthetic, patient, and surgical factors and the challenges in diagnosis make peripheral nerve injury a very challenging topic to study. For an eloquent discussion that addresses the risk factors (host, agent, environment) and their complex interactions, refer to a recent narrative review.[32] Table 74.3 summarizes the

TABLE 74.2 Effects of Ultrasound Technology on Local Anesthetic Requirements and Respiratory Side Effects

Author, Year	Study Type	Block Type	Results
Casati, 2007[21]	RCT	Femoral	ED 95 was 22 mL (95% CI, 13–36 mL) in US group, and 41 mL (95% CI, 24–66 mL) in group NS. 42% reduction in MEAV ropivacaine 0.5%.
O'Donnell, 2009[22]	Validated up-and-down method	Axillary brachial plexus	US-guided axillary brachial plexus block may be successful with as little 1 mL lidocaine 2% per nerve.
Marhofer, 2010[23]	RCT	Axillary brachial plexus	Mepivacaine 1% 0.11 versus with 0.4 mL/mm² cross-sectional nerve area. The mean volume and success rates were 4.0/14.8 mL and 90/100% in the low/high volume groups.
Eichenberger, 2009[24]	Validated up-and-down method	Ulnar	ED 95 volume was 0.11 mL/mm² or 0.7 mL in total, volunteer study.
Duggan, 2009[25]	Validated up-and-down method	Supraclavicular brachial plexus	Minimum volume required for US-guided block in 50% and 95% of patients was 23 mL and 42 mL, respectively.
Latzke, 2010[26]	Validated up-and-down method	Sciatic	The ED 99 volume of local anesthetic for sciatic nerve block was calculated at 0.10 mL/mm² cross-sectional nerve area (range: 1.5% mepivacaine, 2.8–10.2 mL), volunteer study.
Renes, 2010[20]	Validated up-and-down design	Interscalene brachial plexus C7 level	MEAV for ultrasound-guided technique in 50 and 95% of patients was 2.9 and 3.6 mL of ropivacaine 0.75%, respectively. 100% incidence of hemidiaphragmatic paresis following 22 h of infusion of ropivacaine 0.2% 6 mL/h.
Gautier, 2011[27]	Validated up-and-down method	Interscalene brachial plexus	Surgical anesthesia for arthroscopic shoulder surgery achieved with 5 mL 0.75% ropivacaine.
Riazi, 2008[71]	RCT	Interscalene brachial plexus	US guided interscalene block: 5 mL compared to 20 mL ropivacaine 0.5%, resulted in 45 versus 100% incidence of hemidiaphragmatic paralysis.
Renes, 2009[19]	RCT	Interscalene brachial plexus C7 level	Hemidiaphragmatic paralysis: US group 2 (13%) versus NS group, 12 (93%) patients; $P < .0001$). 10 mL ropivacaine 0.75% used in both groups.
Renes, 2009[20]	RCT	Supraclavicular brachial plexus	US-guided injection of 20 mL 0.75% ropivacaine was not associated with hemidiaphragmatic paresis. Using NS-guided technique, 15 (53%) patients showed complete hemidiaphragmatic paresis.

CI, Confidence interval; *ED*, estimated dose in a proportion of patients; *MEAV*, minimum estimated anesthetic volume; *NS*, nerve stimulator; *PNB*, peripheral nerve or plexus block; *RCT*, randomized controlled trial; *RR*, risk ratio; *US*, ultrasound.

results of selected studies on PNB-related neurologic complications.[4,7,8,10,12,33–41] While acknowledging that these studies are a subset of the entire literature, they have been chosen because they represent of cross section of PNB practice. For review, refer to the summary of the American Society of Regional Anesthesia and Pain Medicine (ASRA) Practice Advisory on Neurologic Complications Associated With Regional Anesthesia and Pain Medicine.[31]

MICROANATOMY OF THE PERIPHERAL NERVE AND RELEVANCE TO NERVE INJURY

The peripheral nerve complex comprises neural elements (axons), three connective tissue layers (from inside to outside: endoneurium, perineurium, epineurium), and a supporting blood supply.

TABLE 74.3 Incidence of Neurologic Outcomes Associated With Peripheral Nerve Blockade in Selected Studies

Author, Year	PNB Type	Technique Used	N	Neurologic Outcome	Incidence, % (Time)[a]	Potential Risk Factors	Comment
Borgeat, 2001[33]	ISB	NS	521	Plexus lesion	0.2 (9 months)	Cubital and carpal tunnel syndromes	Neurologic features present in 7.9%, 3.9%, and 0.9% at 1, 3, and 6 months; serial EMGs performed
Auroy, 2002[34]	All	NS, LM	50,223	Neurologic complication[d]	0.014 (6 months)	Popliteal SNB (0.3%), paresthesia during PNB	50,223 PNB, 12 complications in total, 7 present at 6 months
Barrington, 2009[4]	All	US, NS, LM	8189	Neurologic complication[d]	0.02 (6 months)	Comorbidities: vascular disease, lumbar stenosis, radiculopathy, neuropathy	Systematic postoperative follow-up. No significant difference: US versus NS techniques
Sharma, 2010[35]	FNB	NS	729[b]	Femoral neuropathy/neuritis	0.14 (12 months)	Neuropathy: 0.7% with FNB, 0.4% with no FNB	1 patient following FNB had residual sensory symptoms at 12 months
Ecoffey, 2010[7]	UL, LL, Trunk	Not stated	20,576	Neurologic complication	0	Pediatric study	Femoral distribution hypesthesia (iliofascial block) resolved <48 h
Liu, 2010[36]	ISB, SCB	US	1169	PONS	0.4	—	No permanent injuries
Jacob, 2011[37]	LL	NS, LM	12,329[b]	PNI	0.79 (3 months)	Tourniquet time and bilateral surgery	PNI was not associated with PNB or type of anesthesia
Misamore, 2011[38]	ISB	NS	910	Neurologic complication[d]	0.8 (6 months)	Diffuse mild brachial plexopathy confirmed on EMG	Radial nerve palsy (n = 1), mild forearm/hand paresthesias (n = 5), Horner's syndrome (n = 2)
Singh, 2012[39]	ISB	US	1319	Neurological complication	0 (4 months)	Brachial plexitis (3 cases) related to underlying comorbidities	Digital numbness (0.6%), all resolved by 4 months, ulnar neuropathy (1 case) resolved
Sviggum, 2012[40]	ISB	NS, LM	1569	PNI	2.2 (3 months)	ISB did not increase the risk of PNI. GA used as primary anesthetic in 1569 patients.	Complete resolution of symptoms in 97% of patients following TSA
Orebaugh, 2012[8]	UL, LL	US, NS	14,498	Neurologic complication[d]	0.04 (6 months)	No significant difference: US versus NS techniques.	1 sensorimotor deficit persisted >1 year following FNB

Continued

TABLE 74.3 Incidence of Neurologic Outcomes Associated With Peripheral Nerve Blockade in Selected Studies—cont'd

Author, Year	PNB Type	Technique Used	N	Neurologic Outcome	Incidence, % (Time)[a]	Potential Risk Factors	Comment
Polaner, 2012[10]	All	US, NS	5221	Neurologic complication	0 (3 months)	Possible exacerbation of preoperative symptoms following LPB	Pediatric regional anesthesia, 14,917 total, 35% peripheral
Henningsen, 2013[41]	SaNB	US	97	Neurologic complication	0 (6 months)	Infrapatellar branch involved in 84% (surgical etiology).	Neurologic examination of patients following TKA
Rohrbaugh, 2013[12]	ISB	US or PNS	15,014	Neuropathy	0.03 (>6 months)	–	All sitting position, sensory neuropathy, 1 phrenic nerve injury (0.07%).

[a]Indicates elapsed postoperative time period when incidence calculated; PNB, peripheral nerve or plexus block; N, number of PNB procedures.
[b]Number of patients receiving all anesthetic types (GA and regional).
[c]Results of smaller cohort published in 2009, included in 2012 publication.
[d]PNB thought to be the cause.

Ax, Axillary brachial plexus block; *BP*, brachial plexus; *CPNB*, continuous peripheral nerve block; *EA*, epidural anesthesia; *EMG*, electromyogram; *FIB*, fascia iliaca block; *FNB*, femoral nerve block; *GA*, general anesthesia; *ICB*, infraclavicular block; *ISB*, interscalene block; *LL*, lower limb; *LM*, landmark; *MP*, mechanical paresthesia; *NS*, nerve stimulator; *PCB*, psoas compartment block; *PNB*, peripheral nerve blockade; *PNI*, new perioperative nerve injury due to any cause; *PNS*, peripheral nerve stimulator; *PONS*, postoperative neurological symptom (in distribution of PNB); *QI*, quality improvement; *SaNB*, saphenous nerve block; *SNB*, sciatic nerve block; *TA*, transarterial; *THA*, total hip arthroplasty; *TKA*, total knee arthroplasty; *TSA*, total shoulder arthroplasty; *UL*, upper limb PNB; *US*, ultrasound; *UT*, ulnar transposition.

Axons are organized into bundles called fascicles, and each fascicle is supported on the inside by a matrix of fine collagen fibers termed the endoneurium. The perineurium, wrapped around each fascicle, is the protective layer of the peripheral nerve complex providing a barrier to both physical and chemical insults to the axons. Injury or rupture of the perineurium including intrafascicular injection (deep to the perineurium) of local anesthetic disturbs the internal milieu that supports the axons and results in histological evidence of nerve injury including myelin and axonal degeneration.[42-46] The outer connective tissue layer, the epineurium gives the peripheral nerve complex its characteristic external appearance, that is, the epineurium forms the external border of the nerve.[47] However, there is also epineurial extrafascicular connective tissue within the external border of the nerve (also known as the inner or interfascicular epineurium), and this tissue can represent a substantial cross section of a peripheral nerve. The ratio of non-neural connective to neural tissue increases from proximal to distal.[48] The perineurium has mechanical characteristics that provide physical protection to its contents provides more resistance to an advancing needle than the extrafascicular connective tissue. In particular, a short-bevel (block) needle (compared to a long-bevel [hypodermic] needle) is likely to slide off the perineurium and remain in the extrafascicular tissue. Potentially, peripheral nerves characterized by tightly packed fascicles and high fascicular-to-connective tissue content, such as the proximal brachial plexus, may be at greater risk of mechanical and injection injury compared with nerves characterized by lower fascicular-to-connective tissue content.

Related to the different mechanical properties and cross-sectional area of the intraneural connective tissue, intraneural injection may be extrafascicular or result in injury to only a small proportion of axons.[49] This may explain why in the existing studies of nerve puncture and intraneural injection in humans and that there was no apparent clinical evidence of neurologic injury.[50,51] Although an extrafascicular injection is less likely to cause nerve injury, it may not be completely benign.[30,44,45] In some peripheral nerves, there are axonal communications between fascicles. Furthermore, ultrasound imaging cannot distinguish an extrafascicular from an intrafascicular injection. Therefore, the authors emphasize that all intraneural injections should be avoided, because nerve injury may occur and result in long-term neurological sequelae.

PRACTICAL SUGGESTIONS FOR REDUCING RISK OF NEUROLOGIC COMPLICATIONS INCLUDING AVOIDING INTRANEURAL TRAUMA

1. *Avoid intraneural injection: understand "intraneural" versus "extraneural"*
   Nonspecific connective tissue layers external to the epineurium separating the nerve from specialized tissues such as muscles, tendons, and vessels. Sunderland referred to this as deep fascial or paraneural connective tissue and explained that this exists to "fill the space" between and loosely connect and provide movement between the specialized tissues.[52] This provides relative mobility between the nerve and the surrounding tissues in many anatomical locations. Franco describes a *plane of cleavage* between the epineurium and the extraneural connective tissue layers or adjacent structures.[47,53] The nonspecific extraneural connective tissue layers has recently been termed the "paraneural sheath,"[54,55] or "circumneural sheath" and injecting within this "circumneural space" has been described as equivalent to injecting into the "sweet spot" around the nerve. Anatomical studies have focused on the sciatic nerve and its bifurcation,[56] but such perineural cleavage planes (between the epineurium and the extraneural connective tissue) have been described at other locations such as the brachial plexus above the clavicle where the relevant connective tissue is the prevertebral fascia.[53] In short, the epineurium of nerves have close relationships to surrounding connective tissues, identifying this boundary as important to safe practice.

   Using ultrasound guidance to inject into this plane of cleavage between the epineurium and the extraneural connective tissue layers visually results in a nerve/injectate "interface," confirming that the injection is extraneural, that is, external to the nerve. Likely, this is both a safe location to inject local anesthetic and one that results in an efficacious block. Once the needle tip is within this plane of cleavage, a low-pressure injection[57] should occur, resulting in expansion of the plane by hydrostatic pressure. This is otherwise known as hydrodissection. Hydrodissection of the tissue plane immediately external to the epineurium has an important role in ultrasound-guided PNB (Fig. 74.3).

2. *Plan a needle trajectory so as to minimize trauma to nerves and other key structures*
   The connective tissue surrounding or adjacent to a nerve may be relatively thick and difficult to breach with a short-beveled needle, and therefore an overshoot (when penetrating the

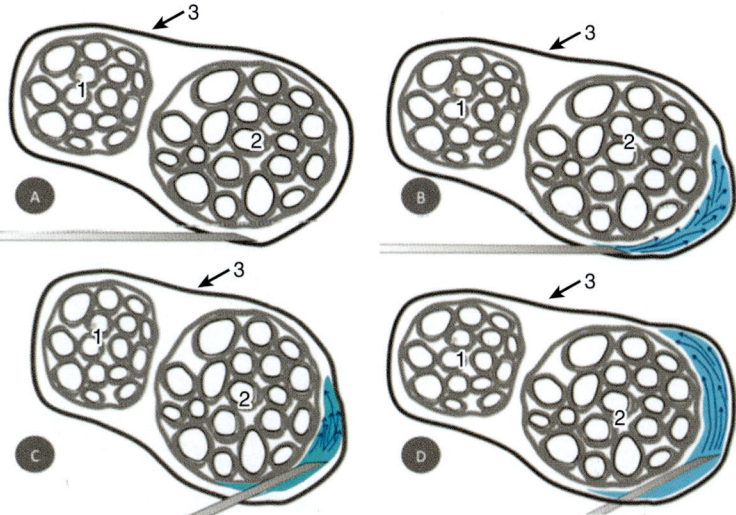

FIGURE 74.3 Demonstrating a needle trajectory that is tangential to the tibial nerve (2) to minimize the risk of trauma to nerve. Initial trajectory is to 6 o'clock on tibial nerve (A). Initial hydrodissection (B) with local anesthetic injectate of space (shaded blue with arrows) immediately adjacent to the tibial nerve, but within the connective tissue that surrounds the tibial and common peroneal (1) components of the sciatic nerve. (C and D) Demonstrate further hydrodissection and spread of local anesthetic, providing more space for needle advancement.

paraneurium or other connective tissue layer) may occur. Potentially this overshoot may cause trauma to the nerve; therefore, we recommend a tangential approach to the nerve. If the needle trajectory crosses the nerve *tangentially* and there is overshoot, the risk of trauma to the nerve is reduced (refer to Fig. 74.3A).

Beware of other nerves, because the presence of one visible nerve on the sonogram does not mean that all nerves are equally visible. For example, because of relative size and connective tissue content, the common peroneal nerve may not be imaged as well as the tibial nerve. Furthermore, in the popliteal fossa, the common peroneal component had an oblique course as it heads toward the head of the fibula. If a popliteal sciatic block is performed distal to where the two nerves have separated, a lateral to medial needle trajectory may cause trauma to the common peroneal nerve en route to the larger and often brighter (echogenic) tibial nerve (refer to Fig. 74.4).

3. *Minimize needle passes where feasible and minimize force used*
   Circumneural spread requiring more needle instrumentation close to nerves is not always required.[58,59] For example, the musculocutaneous nerve is often small and flat. In such cases, only one side needs to be targeted.[59] Other authors have advocated that only one side of the brachial plexus needs to be targeted during an interscalene nerve block.[60,61] The indication of the block, for instance, if analgesia rather than total surgical anesthesia is sought, may permit a less aggressive approach to complete perineural spread and a reduced number of needle passes. In one experimental study, significant structural injury and inflammation occurred in forced needle–nerve contact compared with nonforced needle–nerve contact.[62]

4. *Monitor the spread of local anesthetic*
   Intraneural injection may be detected visually in real time as nerve expansion.[63] However, intraneural injection is not always easy to detect with ultrasound, especially with small volumes,[64] so vigilance is always necessary. Other indicators of potential or impending nerve injury, such as high pressure or pain on injection and other patient responses, should not be ignored (refer to Section 6).

5. *Needle characteristics*
   A long-standing safety principle is to use a needle with short-bevel tip. A short-beveled (45-degree) needle is less likely to penetrate the perineurium compared with a long-bevel (15-degree) needle. In part, this is because fascicles may slide away from a short-bevel needle and it is less likely to cause fascicular damage.[65] In one cadaver experiment with deliberate impalement of the sciatic nerve, of 134 fascicles in the region of the needle trajectory, only four fascicles were

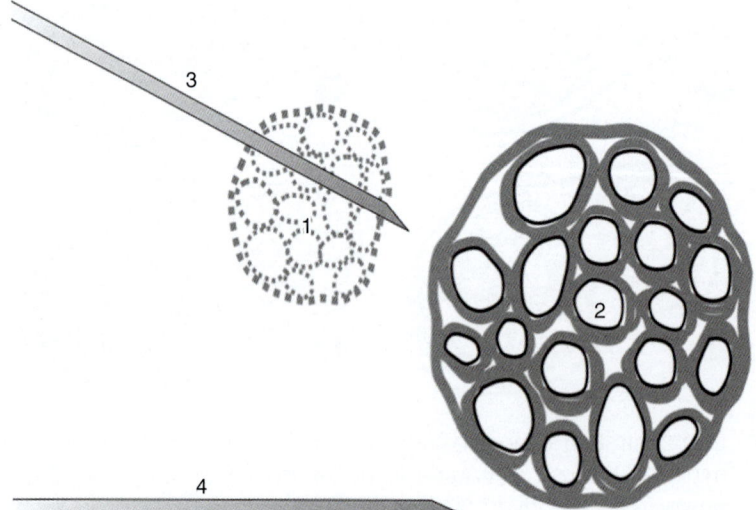

FIGURE 74.4 Demonstrates how a needle trajectory may cause injury to a nerve such as the common peroneal en route to the larger and often brighter tibial nerve. Systematic scanning is required to carefully identify the less echogenic vulnerable common peroneal nerve. (1) common peroneal nerve; (2) tibial nerve; (3) poor needle trajectory; (4) nontraumatic, tangential needle trajectory.

damaged, all involving a needle with a long-bevel (15-degrees) tip.[49] In the scenario that the perineurium is breached with a short-bevel needle, the degree of fascicular damage may be greater. Increased needle diameter is linked to increased severity of histological nerve injury.[66]

6. *Use additional nerve localizing monitors*

    Ultrasound imaging may not clearly identify the outer border of a nerve in all anatomical locations. Therefore, consider using concurrent monitors, nerve stimulator guidance, and/or injection pressure monitoring. It is recommended not to inject if an evoked motor response is present less than 0.5 mA at 0.1 ms current duration during nerve stimulation.[31] Note that an absence of motor response does not exclude needle–nerve contact; that is, there are false negatives with use of nerve stimulation.

    In experimental studies, neurologic injury and functional deficits occurred when intrafascicular injection was combined with a high-pressure injection. No neurologic injuries occurred when low-pressure injections occurred. These studies support the concept that low-pressure injections are unlikely to result in nerve injury,[43,67] and this has provided the basis for development of injection pressure monitors. It is recommended that if opening pressures are unusually high (greater than 15 psi), then the injection should be aborted.[31] Note that false positive high pressures can be recorded, and this may be due to the needle tip being against fascia.[57]

RESPIRATORY COMPLICATIONS

Phrenic nerve block and hemi-diaphragmatic paralysis are common complications of brachial plexus blocks above the clavicle. The phrenic nerve originates from the ventral ramus of the fourth cervical nerve with contributions from the third and fifth cervical nerves, but the origin of the phrenic nerve is variable. However, during its course, the phrenic nerve is located anterior to the anterior scalene muscle, deep to the prevertebral fascia. At the level of the cricoid cartilage, the phrenic nerve is as close as 2 mm[68] to the brachial plexus. During interscalene block, spread of local anesthetic under the prevertebral fascia anterior to the anterior scalene muscle to involve the phrenic nerve is likely. An alternative mechanism is cranial spread of local anesthetic to the ventral root of C4. The incidence of phrenic nerve block approaches 100% following blocks in the posterior triangle of the neck when "traditional" volumes (30 to 40 mL) of local anesthetic are used.[69] However, there is a risk of pneumothorax following procedures in the posterior triangle of the neck, thoracic paravertebral, intercostal, and pectoral blocks.[70]

PRACTICAL SUGGESTIONS FOR REDUCING RISK OF PHRENIC NERVE BLOCK AND HEMI-DIAPHRAGMATIC PARALYSIS

1. *Reduce the local anesthetic dose and use an ultrasound-guided technique*

    Reducing local anesthetic dose can reduce the risk of phrenic nerve blockade.[69] Ultrasound-guided interscalene blockade is efficacious with significantly reduced volumes of local anesthetic compared to traditional approaches (Table 74.2).[20,27,71] Ultrasound also has a role to provide a point of injection that is not immediately adjacent to the phrenic nerve. Ultrasound-guided interscalene and supraclavicular blockade are both associated with a reduced incidence of phrenic nerve blockade compared with nerve stimulator techniques.[19,71,72]

2. *Use cervical spine sonography to determine the cervical nerve level*

    Renes has demonstrated that an ultrasound-guided interscalene block at the C7 level is associated with a reduced incidence of phrenic nerve blockade.[19] Sonography can be used to identify the cervical vertebrae level by the characteristic shape of the transverse processes.[74] With the head in the neutral position or turned to the opposite side, the cervical paravertebral region can be examined in a systematic manner starting with the transducer close to the midline in the transverse plane to identify the thyroid gland. If the transducer is then slid laterally, the carotid sheath, anterior vertebral muscles, scalene muscles, brachial plexus, and the transverse processes are identified. The level of the cervical roots is identified based on the shape of the adjacent cervical transverse processes. For example, the C6 transverse process is identified by its prominent anterior tubercle and together with the posterior tubercle by a "U" shape. The oval hypoechoic structure between the tubercles is the corresponding nerve root. Transverse processes of C4 to C5 can be identified have similar "U" shapes to C6 except the anterior tubercle is less prominent. Each root leaves the intervertebral foramen and lies on its corresponding transverse process (exception, the C8 root lies at the T1 vertebrae). In this way, the cervical space morphology can be used to identify the cervical nerve level.

3. *Use suprascapular and axillary nerve blockade*
   For patients with preexisting severe pulmonary compromise, alternative techniques including combined suprascapular and axillary nerve blockade should be considered.[73]

PRACTICAL SUGGESTIONS FOR REDUCING RISK OF PNEUMOTHORAX

1. *Use ultrasound guidance to allow real-time visualization of the needle trajectory, injectate, and pleura.*
   Ultrasound guidance has a unique role in monitoring so a safe distance between the needle tip and the pleura can be maintained. It is imperative that the practitioner has attained a level of proficiency in which the needle tip can be maintained in-plane and be carefully monitored.

2. *Consider alternative approach to brachial plexus in high-risk scenarios (technical degree of difficulty or high risk patient)*
   In patients with poor access to the posterior triangle of the neck (short neck, morbid obesity, unable to position adequately) or when it is difficult to visualize the needle tip, the risks of proceeding with blocks where the pleura is in range should be weighed against the advantages of choosing alternative techniques (e.g., axillary plexus blockade for upper limb surgery may be a safer alternative in certain patients).

3. *Consider the needle trajectory and depth*
   For example, an infraclavicular block with the transducer orientated or placed too medial results in a needle trajectory closer to the pleura than necessary. With interscalene blocks, the depth to the target is often very superficial; therefore, a steep trajectory should be avoided. For supraclavicular blockade, if the pleura is difficult to visualize, it is worth imaging the position of the first rib. The first rib should highlight a depth that should not be breached.

OTHER CONSIDERATIONS

In addition to needle guidance and pleural monitoring, ultrasound has been shown to be more accurate than chest x-ray at detecting pneumothorax.[75,76] The presence of the sliding lung sign or comet tail sign are reliable indicators that pneumothorax is not present.[75,77,78] These signs are visible with 2D ultrasound, but they also are appreciated with M-mode. The hallmark sign of a pneumothorax is the absence of pleural sliding.[79]

OTHER COMPLICATIONS

1. *Myotoxicity*
   A case series of three patients who received continuous adductor canal block has been recently reported.[80] All presented with marked limb swelling and profound weakness of their quadriceps muscles in the absence of sensory deficits. Magnetic resonance imaging demonstrated increased signal intensity in the quadriceps muscles, and a diagnosis of local anesthetic-induced myositis was made. In animal experiments, local anesthetics are toxic to muscles. However, myositis is usually subclinical in humans.

2. *Deep-tissue infection*
   Necrotizing fasciitis secondary to a continuous popliteal sciatic catheter has been reported recently.[81] In-dwelling catheters and continuous catheter techniques represent an increased risk of infection compared to single-injection techniques. Strict aseptic precautions should be used in any continuous catheter technique.

> **Key Points/Clinical Pearls**
> - Vascular injury is reduced by ultrasound guidance, and we recommend a pre-block sonogram to plan a needle trajectory to minimize trauma to both major arteries and minor branches, which are often not well imaged.
> - Severe LAST still occurs in contemporary practice and can be minimized by reducing local anesthetic dosage, ultrasound guidance, and standard safety precautions.
> - Ultrasound guidance can be used to control needle trajectory and minimize needle–nerve trauma.
> - Minimize force used and the number of needle passes when instrumenting near nerves.
> - Needle tip characteristics influence the likelihood of fascicular penetration and nerve injury; consequently, short-bevel needles are recommended because they are less likely to result in fascicular injury.
> - Ultrasound guidance can be used to control local anesthetic injection and minimize spread to the phrenic nerve.
> - Ultrasound guidance can image the pleura and be used to control needle trajectory to reduce risk of pleural puncture.

References

1. Horlocker TT, Wedel DJ, Rowlingson JC, et al. Regional anesthesia in the patient receiving antithrombotic or thrombolytic therapy: American Society of Regional Anesthesia and Pain Medicine Evidence-Based Guidelines (Third Edition). *Reg Anesth Pain Med.* 2010;35:64–101.
2. Parvaiz MA, Korwar V, McArthur D, Claxton A, Dyer J, Isgar B. Large retroperitoneal haematoma: an unexpected complication of ilioinguinal nerve block for inguinal hernia repair. *Anaesthesia.* 2012;67:80–81.
3. Lewis SR, Price A, Walker KJ, McGrattan K, Smith AF. Ultrasound guidance for upper and lower limb blocks. *Cochrane Database Syst Rev.* 2015;(9):CD006459.
4. Barrington MJ, Watts SA, Gledhill SR, et al. Preliminary results of the Australasian Regional Anaesthesia Collaboration: a prospective audit of more than 7000 peripheral nerve and plexus blocks for neurologic and other complications. *Reg Anesth Pain Med.* 2009;34:534–541.
5. Muhly WT, Orebaugh SL. Sonoanatomy of the vasculature at the supraclavicular and interscalene regions relevant for brachial plexus block. *Acta Anaesthesiol Scand.* 2011;55:1247–1253.
6. Muhly WT, Orebaugh SL. Ultrasound evaluation of the anatomy of the vessels in relation to the femoral nerve at the femoral crease. *Surg Radiol Anat.* 2011;33:491–494.
7. Ecoffey C, Lacroix F, Giaufre E, Orliaguet G, Courreges P. Association des Anesthesistes Reanimateurs Pediatriques d'Expression F. Epidemiology and morbidity of regional anesthesia in children: a follow-up one-year prospective survey of the French-Language Society of Paediatric Anaesthesiologists (ADARPEF). *Paediatr Anaesth.* 2010;20:1061–1069.
8. Orebaugh SL, Kentor ML, Williams BA. Adverse outcomes associated with nerve stimulator-guided and ultrasound-guided peripheral nerve blocks by supervised trainees: update of a single-site database. *Reg Anesth Pain Med.* 2012;37:577–582.
9. Sites BD, Taenzer AH, Herrick MD, et al. Incidence of local anesthetic systemic toxicity and postoperative neurologic symptoms associated with 12,668 ultrasound-guided nerve blocks: an analysis from a prospective clinical registry. *Reg Anesth Pain Med.* 2012;37:478–482.
10. Polaner DM, Taenzer AH, Walker BJ, et al. Pediatric Regional Anesthesia Network (PRAN): a multi-institutional study of the use and incidence of complications of pediatric regional anesthesia. *Anesth Analg.* 2012;115:1353–1364.
11. Barrington MJ, Kluger R. Ultrasound guidance reduces the risk of local anesthetic systemic toxicity following peripheral nerve blockade. *Reg Anesth Pain Med.* 2013;38:289–299.
12. Rohrbaugh M, Kentor ML, Orebaugh SL, Williams B. Outcomes of shoulder surgery in the sitting position with interscalene nerve block: a single-center series. *Reg Anesth Pain Med.* 2013;38:28–33.
13. Gurnaney H, Kraemer FW, Maxwell L, Muhly WT, Schleelein L, Ganesh A. Ambulatory continuous peripheral nerve blocks in children and adolescents: a longitudinal 8-year single center study. *Anesth Analg.* 2014;118:621–627.
14. Heinonen JA, Litonius E, Pitkanen M, Rosenberg PH. Incidence of severe local anaesthetic toxicity and adoption of lipid rescue in Finnish anaesthesia departments in 2011–2013. *Acta Anaesthesiol Scand.* 2015;59:1032–1037.
15. Liu SS, Ortolan S, Sandoval MV, et al. Cardiac arrest and seizures caused by local anesthetic systemic toxicity after peripheral nerve blocks: should we still fear the reaper? *Reg Anesth Pain Med.* 2016;41:5–21.

16. Allegri M, Bugada D, Grossi P, et al. Italian Registry of Complications associated with Regional Anesthesia (RICALOR). An incidence analysis from a prospective clinical survey. *Minerva Anestesiol*. 2016;82:392–402.
17. Morwald EE, Zubizarreta N, Cozowicz C, Poeran J, Memtsoudis SG. Incidence of local anesthetic systemic toxicity in orthopedic patients receiving peripheral nerve blocks. *Reg Anesth Pain Med*. 2017;42(4):442–445.
18. Vasques F, Behr AU, Weinberg G, Ori C, Di Gregorio G. A review of local anesthetic systemic toxicity cases since publication of the american society of regional anesthesia recommendations: to whom it may concern. *Reg Anesth Pain Med*. 2015;40:698–705.
19. Renes SH, Rettig HC, Gielen MJ, Wilder-Smith OH, van Geffen GJ. Ultrasound-guided low-dose interscalene brachial plexus block reduces the incidence of hemidiaphragmatic paresis. *Reg Anesth Pain Med*. 2009;34:498–502.
20. Renes SH, van Geffen GJ, Rettig HC, Gielen MJ, Scheffer GJ. Minimum effective volume of local anesthetic for shoulder analgesia by ultrasound-guided block at root C7 with assessment of pulmonary function. *Reg Anesth Pain Med*. 2010;35:529–534.
21. Casati A, Baciarello M, Di Cianni S, et al. Effects of ultrasound guidance on the minimum effective anaesthetic volume required to block the femoral nerve. *Br J Anaesth*. 2007;98:823–827.
22. O'Donnell BD, Iohom G. An estimation of the minimum effective anesthetic volume of 2% lidocaine in ultrasound-guided axillary brachial plexus block. *Anesthesiology*. 2009;111:25–29.
23. Marhofer P, Eichenberger U, Stockli S, et al. Ultrasonographic guided axillary plexus blocks with low volumes of local anaesthetics: a crossover volunteer study. *Anaesthesia*. 2010;65:266–271.
24. Eichenberger U, Stockli S, Marhofer P, et al. Minimal local anesthetic volume for peripheral nerve block: a new ultrasound-guided, nerve dimension-based method. *Reg Anesth Pain Med*. 2009;34:242–246.
25. Duggan E, El Beheiry H, Perlas A, et al. Minimum effective volume of local anesthetic for ultrasound-guided supraclavicular brachial plexus block. *Reg Anesth Pain Med*. 2009;34:215–218.
26. Latzke D, Marhofer P, Zeitlinger M, et al. Minimal local anaesthetic volumes for sciatic nerve block: evaluation of ED 99 in volunteers. *Br J Anaesth*. 2010;104:239–244.
27. Gautier P, Vandepitte C, Ramquet C, DeCoopman M, Xu D, Hadzic A. The minimum effective anesthetic volume of 0.75% ropivacaine in ultrasound-guided interscalene brachial plexus block. *Anesth Analg*. 2011;113:951–955.
28. Karmakar MK, Ho AM, Law BK, Wong AS, Shafer SL, Gin T. Arterial and venous pharmacokinetics of ropivacaine with and without epinephrine after thoracic paravertebral block. *Anesthesiology*. 2005;103:704–711.
29. Mulroy MF, Hejtmanek MR. Prevention of local anesthetic systemic toxicity. *Reg Anesth Pain Med*. 2010;35:177–180.
30. Brull R, Hadzic A, Reina MA, Barrington MJ. Pathophysiology and etiology of nerve injury following peripheral nerve blockade. *Reg Anesth Pain Med*. 2015;40:479–490.
31. Neal JM, Barrington MJ, Brull R, et al. The Second ASRA practice advisory on neurologic complications associated with regional anesthesia and pain medicine: executive summary 2015. *Reg Anesth Pain Med*. 2015;40:401–430.
32. Sondekoppam RV, Tsui BC. Factors associated with risk of neurologic complications after peripheral nerve blocks: a systematic review. *Anesth Analg*. 2017;124:645–660.
33. Borgeat A, Ekatodramis G, Kalberer F, Benz C. Acute and nonacute complications associated with interscalene block and shoulder surgery: a prospective study. *Anesthesiology*. 2001;95:875–880.
34. Auroy Y, Benhamou D, Bargues L, et al. Major complications of regional anesthesia in France: the SOS Regional Anesthesia Hotline Service. *Anesthesiology*. 2002;97:1274–1280.
35. Sharma S, Iorio R, Specht LM, Davies-Lepie S, Healy WL. Complications of femoral nerve block for total knee arthroplasty. *Clin Orthop Relat Res*. 2010;468:135–140.
36. Liu SS, Gordon MA, Shaw PM, Wilfred S, Shetty T. Yadeau JT. A prospective clinical registry of ultrasound-guided regional anesthesia for ambulatory shoulder surgery. *Anesth Analg*. 2010;111:617–623.
37. Jacob AK, Mantilla CB, Sviggum HP, Schroeder DR, Pagnano MW, Hebl JR. Perioperative nerve injury after total knee arthroplasty: regional anesthesia risk during a 20-year cohort study. *Anesthesiology*. 2011;114:311–317.
38. Misamore G, Webb B, McMurray S, Sallay P. A prospective analysis of interscalene brachial plexus blocks performed under general anesthesia. *J Shoulder Elbow Surg*. 2011;20:308–314.
39. Singh A, Kelly C, O'Brien T, Wilson J, Warner JJ. Ultrasound-guided interscalene block anesthesia for shoulder arthroscopy: a prospective study of 1319 patients. *J Bone Joint Surg Am*. 2012;94:2040–2046.
40. Sviggum HP, Jacob AK, Mantilla CB, Schroeder DR, Sperling JW, Hebl JR. Perioperative nerve injury after total shoulder arthroplasty: assessment of risk after regional anesthesia. *Reg Anesth Pain Med*. 2012;37:490–494.
41. Henningsen MH, Jaeger P, Hilsted KL, Dahl JB. Prevalence of saphenous nerve injury after adductor-canal-blockade in patients receiving total knee arthroplasty. *Acta Anaesthesiol Scand*. 2013;57(1):112–117.
42. Gentili F, Hudson A, Kline DG, Hunter D. Peripheral nerve injection injury: an experimental study. *Neurosurgery*. 1979;4:244–253.

43. Hadzic A, Dilberovic F, Shah S, et al. Combination of intraneural injection and high injection pressure leads to fascicular injury and neurologic deficits in dogs. *Reg Anesth Pain Med.* 2004;29:417–423.
44. Hogan QH. Pathophysiology of peripheral nerve injury during regional anesthesia. *Reg Anesth Pain Med.* 2008;33:435–441.
45. Whitlock EL, Brenner MJ, Fox IK, Moradzadeh A, Hunter DA, Mackinnon SE. Ropivacaine-induced peripheral nerve injection injury in the rodent model. *Anesth Analg.* 2010;111:214–220.
46. Farber SJ, Saheb-Al-Zamani M, Zieske L, et al. Peripheral nerve injury after local anesthetic injection. *Anesth Analg.* 2013;117:731–739.
47. Franco CD. Connective tissues associated with peripheral nerves. *Reg Anesth Pain Med.* 2012;37:363–365.
48. Moayeri N, Bigeleisen PE, Groen GJ. Quantitative architecture of the brachial plexus and surrounding compartments, and their possible significance for plexus blocks. *Anesthesiology.* 2008;108:299–304.
49. Sala-Blanch X, Ribalta T, Rivas E, et al. Structural injury to the human sciatic nerve after intraneural needle insertion. *Reg Anesth Pain Med.* 2009;34:201–205.
50. Bigeleisen PE. Nerve puncture and apparent intraneural injection during ultrasound-guided axillary block does not invariably result in neurologic injury. *Anesthesiology.* 2006;105:779–783.
51. Cappelleri G, Cedrati VL, Fedele LL, et al. Effects of the intraneural and subparaneural ultrasound-guided popliteal sciatic nerve block: a prospective, randomized, double-blind clinical and electrophysiological comparison. *Reg Anesth Pain Med.* 2016;41:430–437.
52. Sunderland S. Features of nerves that protect them from injury during normal activities. In: Sunderland S, ed. *Nerve Injuries and Their Repair: A Critical Appraisal.* Edinburgh, UK: Churchill Livingstone; 1991.
53. Franco CD, Rahman A, Voronov G, Kerns JM, Beck RJ, Buckenmaier CC 3rd. Gross anatomy of the brachial plexus sheath in human cadavers. *Reg Anesth Pain Med.* 2008;33:64–69.
54. Andersen HL, Andersen SL, Tranum-Jensen J. Injection inside the paraneural sheath of the sciatic nerve: direct comparison among ultrasound imaging, macroscopic anatomy, and histologic analysis. *Reg Anesth Pain Med.* 2012;37:410–414.
55. Karmakar MK, Shariat AN, Pangthipampai P, Chen J. High-definition ultrasound imaging defines the paraneural sheath and the fascial compartments surrounding the sciatic nerve at the popliteal fossa. *Reg Anesth Pain Med.* 2013;38:447–451.
56. Perlas A, Wong P, Abdallah F, Hazrati LN, Tse C, Chan V. Ultrasound-guided popliteal block through a common paraneural sheath versus conventional injection: a prospective, randomized, double-blind study. *Reg Anesth Pain Med.* 2013;38:218–225.
57. Gadsden J, Latmore M, Levine DM, Robinson A. High opening injection pressure is associated with needle-nerve and needle-fascia contact during femoral nerve block. *Reg Anesth Pain Med.* 2016;41:50–55.
58. Sites BD, Neal JM, Chan V. Ultrasound in regional anesthesia: where should the "focus" be set? *Reg Anesth Pain Med.* 2009;34:531–533.
59. Choquet O, Morau D, Biboulet P, Capdevila X. Where should the tip of the needle be located in ultrasound-guided peripheral nerve blocks? *Curr Opin Anaesthesiol.* 2012;25:596–602.
60. Spence BC, Beach ML, Gallagher JD, Sites BD. Ultrasound-guided interscalene blocks: understanding where to inject the local anaesthetic. *Anaesthesia.* 2011;66:509–514.
61. Albrecht E, Kirkham KR, Taffe P, et al. The maximum effective needle-to-nerve distance for ultrasound-guided interscalene block: an exploratory study. *Reg Anesth Pain Med.* 2014;39:56–60.
62. Steinfeldt T, Poeschl S, Nimphius W, et al. Forced needle advancement during needle-nerve contact in a porcine model: histological outcome. *Anesth Analg.* 2011;113:417–420.
63. Lupu CM, Kiehl TR, Chan VW, El-Beheiry H, Madden M, Brull R. Nerve expansion seen on ultrasound predicts histologic but not functional nerve injury after intraneural injection in pigs. *Reg Anesth Pain Med.* 2010;35:132–139.
64. Krediet AC, Moayeri N, Bleys RL, Groen GJ. Intraneural or extraneural: diagnostic accuracy of ultrasound assessment for localizing low-volume injection. *Reg Anesth Pain Med.* 2014;39:409–413.
65. Selander D, Dhuner KG, Lundborg G. Peripheral nerve injury due to injection needles used for regional anesthesia. An experimental study of the acute effects of needle point trauma. *Acta Anaesthesiol Scand.* 1977;21:182–188.
66. Steinfeldt T, Nimphius W, Werner T, et al. Nerve injury by needle nerve perforation in regional anaesthesia: does size matter? *Br J Anaesth.* 2010;104:245–253.
67. Kapur E, Vuckovic I, Dilberovic F, et al. Neurologic and histologic outcome after intraneural injections of lidocaine in canine sciatic nerves. *Acta Anaesthesiol Scand.* 2007;51:101–107.
68. Kessler J, Schafhalter-Zoppoth I, Gray AT. An ultrasound study of the phrenic nerve in the posterior cervical triangle: implications for the interscalene brachial plexus block. *Reg Anesth Pain Med.* 2008;33:545–550.
69. Verelst P, van Zundert A. Respiratory impact of analgesic strategies for shoulder surgery. *Reg Anesth Pain Med.* 2013;38:50–53.

70. Abell DJ, Barrington MJ. Pneumothorax after ultrasound-guided supraclavicular block: presenting features, risk, and related training. *Reg Anesth Pain Med*. 2014;39:164–167.
71. Riazi S, Carmichael N, Awad I, Holtby RM, McCartney CJ. Effect of local anaesthetic volume (20 vs 5 ml) on the efficacy and respiratory consequences of ultrasound-guided interscalene brachial plexus block. *Br J Anaesth*. 2008;101:549–556.
72. Renes SH, Spoormans HH, Gielen MJ, Rettig HC, van Geffen GJ. Hemidiaphragmatic paresis can be avoided in ultrasound-guided supraclavicular brachial plexus block. *Reg Anesth Pain Med*. 2009;34:595–599.
73. Dhir S, Sondekoppam RV, Sharma R, Ganapathy S, Athwal GS. A comparison of combined suprascapular and axillary nerve blocks to interscalene nerve block for analgesia in arthroscopic shoulder surgery: an equivalence study. *Reg Anesth Pain Med*. 2016;41:564–571.
74. Martinoli C, Bianchi S, Santacroce E, Pugliese F, Graif M, Derchi LE. Brachial plexus sonography: a technique for assessing the root level. *AJR Am J Roentgenol*. 2002;179:699–702.
75. Goodman TR, Traill ZC, Phillips AJ, Berger J, Gleeson FV. Ultrasound detection of pneumothorax. *Clin Radiol*. 1999;54:736–739.
76. Wilkerson RG, Stone MB. Sensitivity of bedside ultrasound and supine anteroposterior chest radiographs for the identification of pneumothorax after blunt trauma. *Acad Emerg Med*. 2010;17:11–17.
77. Lichtenstein DA, Menu Y. A bedside ultrasound sign ruling out pneumothorax in the critically ill. Lung sliding. *Chest*. 1995;108:1345–1348.
78. Madill JJ. In-flight thoracic ultrasound detection of pneumothorax in combat. *J Emerg Med*. 2010;39:194–197.
79. Sites BD, Macfarlane AJ, Sites VR, et al. Clinical sonopathology for the regional anesthesiologist: part 2: bone, viscera, subcutaneous tissue, and foreign bodies. *Reg Anesth Pain Med*. 2010;35:281–289.
80. Neal JM, Salinas FV, Choi DS. Local anesthetic-induced myotoxicity after continuous adductor canal block. *Reg Anesth Pain Med*. 2016;41:723–727.
81. Dott D, Canlas C, Sobey C, Obremskey W, Thomson AB. Necrotizing fasciitis as a complication of a continuous sciatic nerve catheter using the lateral popliteal approach. *Reg Anesth Pain Med*. 2016;41:728–730.

Regional Anesthesia in Resource-Constrained Environments

Michael S. Lipnick | Gerald Dubowitz | Agnes Wabule

CHAPTER 75

INTRODUCTION

Regional anesthesia is a relatively low-cost and widely used technique in perioperative analgesia and anesthesia. To date, it has been primarily utilized in high-income countries (HICs) where regional anesthesia has been associated with reduced postoperative pain, reduced opioid requirements, as well as increased patient satisfaction, surgical pathway efficiency, and avoidance of general anesthesia.[1] While each of these outcomes is also relevant in low- and middle-income countries (LMICs), the role and benefits for regional anesthesia in LMICs are yet to be fully defined.

Due to significant limitations in access to analgesia and general anesthesia modalities, coupled with a disproportionately high burden of surgical diseases including trauma, the benefits of regional anesthesia may be amplified in LMICs.

Pain and surgical diseases account for more than 30% of global disease burden, which is more than that of human immunodeficiency virus (HIV), tuberculosis (TB), and malaria combined.[2] The majority of this burden exists in LMICs where critical shortages in workforce, infrastructure, and political capacity create major barriers to pain and anesthesia care.[3]

Pain alone is among the top ten causes of disability-adjusted life years (DALYs) worldwide.[4,5] Access to pain management is widely considered a basic human right, yet reliable access to analgesia does not exist for the vast majority of the world.[6-9] At present, Australia, Canada, New Zealand, the United States of America, and several European countries account for more the 90% of the world's opiate consumption, while most LMICs lack reliable access to cheap and effective medications like morphine.[10,11]

For practice settings where access to opiates is limited, exploring alternative analgesia modalities such as regional anesthesia is critical, while simultaneously working to increase access to all essential analgesic options.[12]

The barriers to regional anesthesia in resource-constrained settings are complex. In this chapter, we discuss these challenges, potential solutions, and the need for ongoing evaluation of how to best increase access to anesthesia and analgesia services worldwide.

TECHNIQUE SELECTION AND PREFERRED BLOCKS

The choice of regional anesthetic technique (e.g., ultrasound, paresthesia, or nerve stimulator) and block type (e.g., forearm or interscalene block) will be influenced by numerous factors specific to the local context. These include local disease epidemiology, provider skill level, local supply chains, as well as availability of medications and safety supplies (as discussed later in this chapter).

Safety profiles for different types of regional anesthesia vary significantly with technique, injection site, local anesthetic drug, dose, and patient weight. Each of these factors can significantly influence the risk of local anesthetic systemic toxicity (LAST). The use of ultrasound for regional anesthesia has been associated with increased safety and efficacy; however, nerve stimulator and landmark-based techniques still have a significant role.[13]

There are no guidelines or robust data to aid decision making when weighing the risks and benefits of a proposed procedure in a resource-constrained setting. Nonetheless, there are several blocks with relatively greater potential utility and more favorable safety profiles as discussed below. Many surgical procedures commonly performed with general anesthesia in HICs can be done with regional anesthesia alone, with significant potential savings in cost and time. In addition to neuraxial anesthesia, examples include field blocks for hernias, digital blocks, axillary blocks for upper extremity procedures, topical blocks for ophthalmologic procedures, penile blocks for circumcision, intravenous regional anesthesia, forearm blocks for hand surgery, ankle blocks for foot and ankle procedures, and superficial thoracic paravertebral, pectoral, and serratus anterior blocks for breast surgery or rib fractures.

While most of these blocks can be done relatively easily without ultrasound and with acceptable safety profiles, serious complications can still occur in inexperienced hands. For example, anecdotal reports of LAST fatalities during penile blocks for circumcision are still encountered regularly in some low-income countries (LICs) and are attributed to preventable causes (incorrect dosing or technique).

In general, distal blocks and the use of ultrasound are preferred when feasible in low-resource settings for a number of reasons. Distal blocks (e.g., a forearm or ankle block instead of an axillary or femoral/popliteal block for hand or foot surgery, respectively) minimize the amount of local anesthetic dose needed, thereby reducing the risk of LAST. Furthermore, due to the lower dose of local anesthetic required and the proximity to the surgical field, distal blocks also allow for intraoperative supplementation. This can help overcome limitations of using short-acting local anesthetics for longer cases and mitigate the effects of incomplete blocks due to provider skill level.

EQUIPMENT CHALLENGES

Although ultrasound has largely replaced nerve stimulation for regional anesthesia in many HICs, access to both ultrasound and nerve stimulator units in many LMICs remains limited.

In some LMICs, access to ultrasound can often be surprisingly easier than access to nerve stimulators. This is due to decreasing costs, high turnover of ultrasounds in HICs over the past 10 years, and the high utility and versatility of ultrasounds machines throughout the hospital. Nonetheless, cost is still a significant barrier, as ultrasound units can range in price from $2,000 to over $50,000, while nerve stimulators generally cost several hundred dollars. In resource-constrained settings, expensive equipment, whether donated or procured, is often locked in secure storage for fear of theft, thereby limiting its utility even when technically available on site.

An additional barrier limiting access to ultrasound and nerve stimulators in many settings is the lack of supply chain and biomedical support. When equipment fails, repairs can be costly or may not even be feasible. When deploying relatively expensive and complex technologies such as ultrasound, access to biomedical support is essential and must be part of the procurement plan. Companies that have in-country or regional technical support should be considered, and donors should adhere to World Health Organization (WHO) Equipment Donation Guidelines to avoid unintended consequences of their efforts.[14]

In the case of nerve stimulators, cost and availability of specialized, insulated needles can be prohibitive. Because improvisation using a noninsulated needle can be undertaken with many blocks, nerve stimulators still have a significant role in many resource-limited settings. Where sterile probe covers and sterile ultrasound gel are lacking (as discussed in the following), the use of nerve stimulation may provide for easier infection control over ultrasound guided regional. In addition, substitution of nerve stimulators designed for regional anesthesia with those designed for other purposes (e.g., neuromuscular blockade twitch monitoring) can be dangerous. Inability to precisely control milliamp output and dispersion can significantly increase the risk of nerve injury or block failure.

Not all ultrasounds are created equally when it comes to regional anesthesia in LMICs. Power supplies may not be compatible (110 to 240 V), and probe types may not be optimal. Where power is unreliable and battery operation is critical, special attention must be given to the wide-ranging battery performance among ultrasound units.

Although linear probes with higher frequencies are considered optimal for regional anesthesia (see Chapter 9), many blocks can surprisingly be accomplished with a wide variety of probes. Decreasing costs and replacement of older equipment by newer technology in HICs will continue to increase the prevalence of ultrasound, especially in LICs. Despite increased access to ultrasound, proficiency with nerve stimulation and landmark-based regional anesthesia techniques remains important for all anesthesiologists.

One of the most important pieces of equipment required to perform safe regional anesthesia may be a monitoring device. Monitors are perhaps more important, but they are equally as rare as ultrasounds in many LICs. Monitoring standards from HICs may not be feasible for many practice settings in LMICs. Without availability of these devices, the ability to provide safe anesthesia of any sort (including regional) may be limited. Additional safety equipment that must not be overlooked includes intravenous access supplies, vasopressors, and airway equipment to deal with emergencies.

CHALLENGES WITH CONSUMABLES

As previously mentioned, cost and supply chain shortcomings can cause major barriers to the provision of regional anesthesia, especially when it comes to consumables. The following are specific examples of these challenges as well as descriptions of potential workarounds. Some of these potentials solutions require additional investigation and refinement prior to endorsement or widespread implementation.

ULTRASOUND GEL

Ultrasound gel is traditionally a water-soluble, gas-free solution that minimizes absorption and attenuation of sound waves and is specifically marketed for use with ultrasound. Gel may come in single- or multi-use containers and sterile or nonsterile packing, with significant cost implications. While single-use, sterile packets of gel are optimal for infection control, they are not sustainable for many health facilities in LMICs due to cost and supply chain issues. In these settings, probe hygiene is critical, and "no-touch gel" techniques may be utilized. This technique involves inserting the needle through a sterile-prepped area of skin away from the unsterile probe (gel) while taking great caution not to contaminate the needle insertion site (Fig. 75.1). Because the operator is examining the ultrasound screen, contact between the probe or nonsterile ultrasound gel and the needle is common and poses an infectious risk. A narrow piece of tape can be used to provide tactile feedback when the probe is approaching the needle insertion site; however, the increased distance from the needle insertion site can increase the technical difficulty of completing the block.

Most ultrasound gel is manufactured in middle or high-income countries. This results in significant access challenges for most LICs. As a result, several substitutes have been tried including

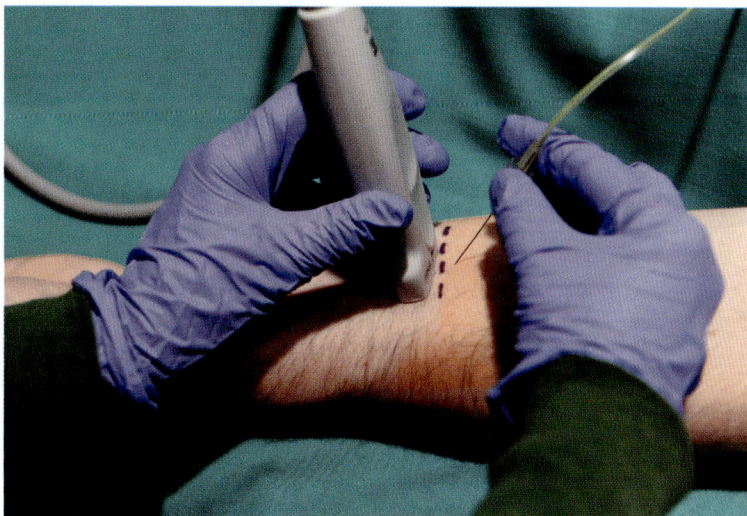

FIGURE 75.1 No-touch technique for regional anesthesia. Demonstration of no-touch technique to decrease risk of infection where sterile probe covers are not available. The technique involves inserting the needle through a sterile-prepped area of skin away from the unsterile probe (gel) while taking great caution not to contaminate the needle insertion site.

5% dextrose, betadine, oils, albumin, cassava and cornstarch-based gels, and many others with varying degrees of success.[15-18] Geographic availability, cost, and sterility can limit the utility of each of these potential alternatives.

One initiative to manufacture ultrasound gel in the Democratic Republic of the Congo from locally available cassava produced a gel alternative at a cost of approximately US$0.09 per 500 mL bottle versus the US$5.00 to >US$15.00 cost of commercial ultrasound gel.[19] Hospital staff manufactures the gel every 3 days to ensure adequate supply and sterility (Fig. 75.2).

Certain alcohol-based solutions including hand-sanitizing gels have demonstrated adequate image quality, although caution must be taken to ensure probe compatibility, as many chemicals can significantly damage probe heads.[20] Furthermore, care must be taken not to track excess alcohol-based solutions along with the needle, as this could potentially increase the risk of neural injury. Betadine may provide effective acoustic coupling, but this occurs only when wet (and thus technically not sterile). Furthermore, betadine is not always readily available and can cause skin irritation and allergies. Even when using skin-cleaning preparations for acoustic coupling, this does not obviate the need for other antimicrobial barriers and precautions.

TRANSDUCER COVERS

The previous challenges with ultrasound gel are similar to those limiting the use of transducer covers. As a result, a number of improvisations have been reported, including the use of sterile gloves, condoms, sterile adhesive dressings, or using a no-touch technique and clean probe.[21] Although the use of sterile probe covers is often recommended, little data exist to clarify actual infectious disease risks when other techniques are used for regional anesthesia. Careful probe storage (i.e., not in a cardboard box) and pre-cleaning a patient prior to placing the probe may decrease cross-contamination and nosocomial infections.[22,23]

MEDICATIONS

Inconsistent availability of drugs is a significant barrier to regional anesthesia in LICs. Although local anesthetics (lidocaine, bupivacaine, and lidocaine with epinephrine) are included on the WHO Essential Medicines List, aside from lidocaine (also known commonly as lignocaine or xylocaine), regular access to large volumes of other local anesthetics is not common in many LICs.[12] Furthermore, access to epinephrine can be challenging in many resource-limited settings outside HICs. A needs assessment survey in Uganda reported that nearly two-thirds of anesthesia providers have either no access or inconsistent access to local anesthesia for spinals.[24] Even when medications are available,

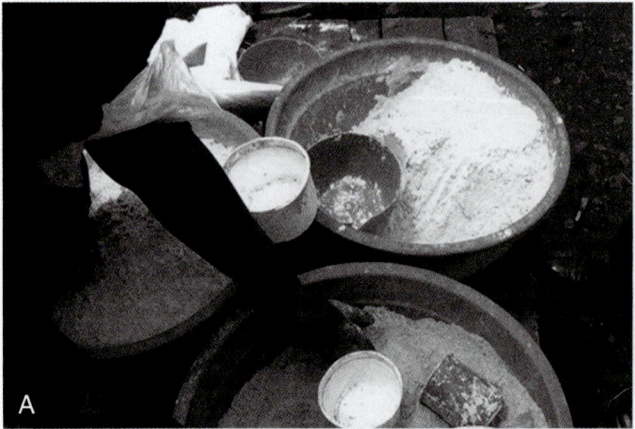
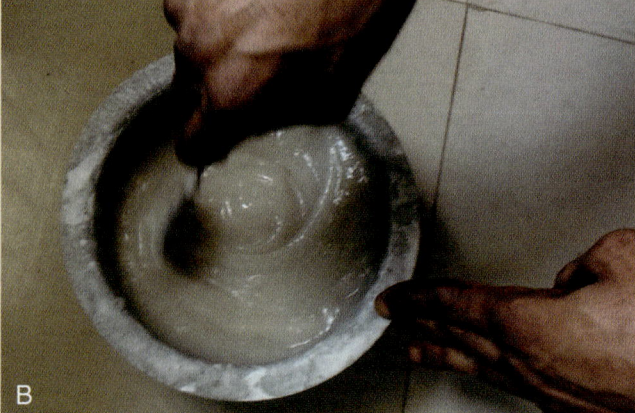

FIGURE 75.2 Manufacture of cassava-based ultrasound gel. (A) Vendors selling cassava root flour in Addis Ababa, Ethiopia. (B) Mixing cassava root flour to make ultrasound gel in Kindu, Maniema province, Democratic Republic of Congo. ([A] Reproduced with permission of Margaret Salmon under Creative Commons Attribution Licensing. Originally produced by Salmon M, Salmon C, Bissinger A, et al. Alternative ultrasound gel for a sustainable ultrasound program: application of human centered design. *PLoS One*. 2015;10(8):e0134332. [B] Courtesy of Margaret Salmon.)

concerns over quality in LICs can be significant. Concentrations reported on drug labels for many medications including local anesthetics may differ significantly from that prepared. Low-quality medications have several implications for regional anesthesia including issues of sterility, therapeutic effect, and toxicity.

Multiple uses for a single-use vial is a widespread and commonly critiqued practice in both HICs and LMICs.[25] In LMICs, where drugs are in short supply and cost savings are critical, efforts to utilize a single-use vial for multiple patients may be especially commonplace and with significantly increased risk of morbidity and mortality.[26]

The amount of local anesthetic needed to perform a single block, such as a femoral or popliteal block, may be enough for 10 spinals. For example, in East Africa, it is common practice to use multiple vials of spinal preparation bupivacaine (usually 0.5%) and dilute it to a concentration used for regional (0.25%). Limited existing data that address concerns over injecting dextrose in or around the nerve suggest neurotoxicity is unlikely.[27] In HICs, long-acting local anesthetics (bupivacaine and ropivacaine) are most commonly used for many regional blocks to afford longer operating times and provide post-op analgesia. While these goals are similar in LMICs as well, it is important to note that many procedures can be done when only short-acting local anesthetics are available.

In addition to local anesthetics, other drugs are often in short supply, including vasopressors and lipid emulsification, which can create significant challenges for providing safe regional and neuraxial anesthesia. In light of this, avoiding the use of large volume, long-acting, high-dose local anesthetics, such as 30 mL 0.5% bupivacaine for a femoral block, may be advisable. Where consistent access to standard-dose formulations is lacking, awareness of toxic dosing calculations and attention to drug labeling cannot be overemphasized. For example, last-minute substitutions of 4% or 10% lidocaine for 1% to 2% solutions may occur out of necessity, with a small margin of error for dosing miscalculations.

NEEDLES

Both echogenic needles preferred for ultrasound as well as insulated needles preferred for nerve stimulators are generally unavailable in LICs. Although several workarounds exist (discussed below), data are lacking to support superiority in safety for specialized regional needles.

The ideal needle for ultrasound-guided blocks is considered by many to be relatively long and scored to provide echogenicity while possessing a shallow bevel to facilitate tactile feedback when advancing through anatomical structures.

While there are many proprietary and relatively expensive needles designed with the previously mentioned features, almost any needle can be used for an ultrasound guided region if one recognizes the potential risks. Spinal and epidural needles have been used to provide additional length, although often, standard hypodermic needles are used. It is commonly assumed that sharper needles are more likely to injure nerves; however, this may not be true.[28] Despite the lack of clear evidence for needle type and safety (for neuronal or vascular injury), some providers in LICs attempt to mitigate these risks by manually blunting a sharp needle in the bottom of an opened, sterile glass ampule (Fig. 75.3).

Several techniques have also been reported for increasing needle echogenicity, including roughening or scoring the outer needle or inner stylet with a No. 11 surgical blade, using a guidewire, or injecting saline to help identify the needle tip[29] (Fig. 75.3).

With regard to nerve stimulator technique, non-insulated needles have been used in lieu of insulated needles, although with the increased potential risks as previously described.

TRAINING AND STAFFING

Staffing is perhaps one of the biggest challenges to providing regional anesthesia for many resource-constrained settings. Shortages in supplies affect not only provision of care but also the ability to train providers. Many hospitals in LICs have procured or received donated ultrasounds, needles, and other necessary supplies, but ultimately, local staff must be in sufficient numbers and trained to be proficient to incorporate regional techniques into the local workflow.[30] This is highly unlikely to be accomplished with a short course or in the absence of ongoing support and training.

SAFETY ISSUES

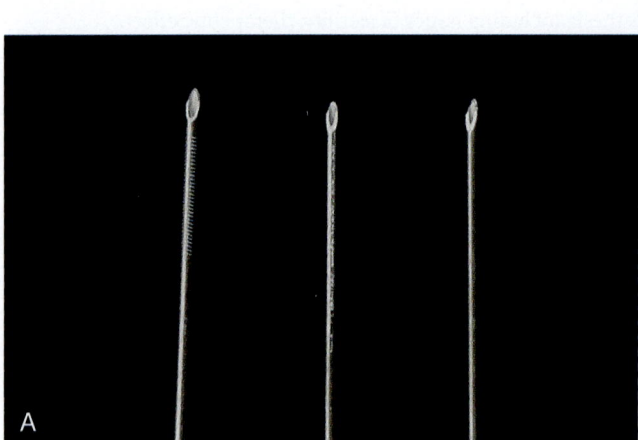 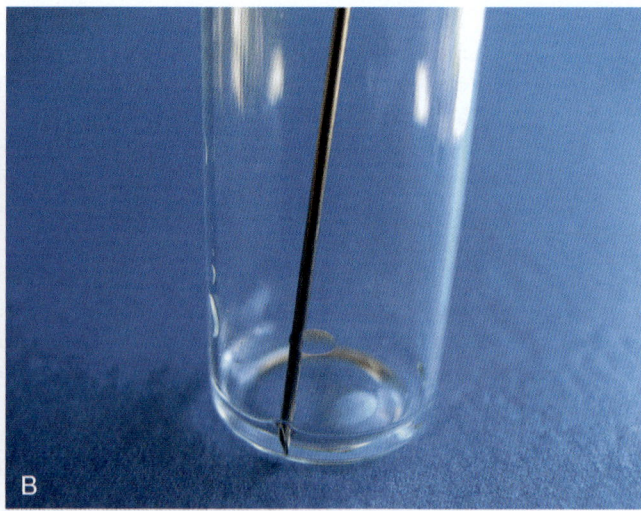

FIGURE 75.3 Comparison of various commonly found needle types. (A) *Left to right*: Echogenic, textured regional ultrasound needle; 18 g hypodermic needle that has been manually blunted and scored with a No. 11 surgical blade; 18 g hypodermic needle. (B) Demonstration of manual blunting technique for 18 g hypodermic syringe in an empty, sterile glass ampule.

Surgeon preference and comfort with regional and local techniques is another factor affecting implementation of regional anesthesia. Utilization of regional or local as the primary anesthetic for cases varies considerably in all practice settings.[31] In addition, education for non-anesthesia providers may have a role in increasing implementation of regional anesthesia. This includes properly informing patients who may not be familiar with regional anesthesia and have significant distress during a case without the commonly expected general anesthetic.

In addition to training personnel in regional techniques, practitioners must also be trained to manage complications, such as LAST with cardiovascular collapse or the loss of an airway. Training providers to comfortably perform blocks under ultrasound may be far easier than training these staff to manage an airway or convert to general anesthesia unexpectedly in an unstable patient.

Two recently published initiatives have implemented ultrasound-guided regional anesthesia at hospitals in the Democratic Republic of the Congo (DRC), Ethiopia, and the University Teaching Hospital of Kigali (CHUK) in Rwanda. In the DRC and Ethiopia, as part of a multicenter, train-the-trainers pilot study, 41 non-anesthesiologists were taught a limited number of regional anesthesia techniques (femoral, popliteal, and forearm blocks) using lidocaine 1% or 2%. During the pilot study, providers performed nearly 1000 blocks for analgesia management of digit and limb amputations, wounds, fractures, tendon rupture, fasciotomy, and gunshot wounds with high success rates and had no complications.[32]

At CHUK in Rwanda, a qualitative evaluation was recently done as part of the creation of an onsite regional anesthesia service. This evaluation concluded that lack of staff, materials, and educational resources collectively contribute to low utilization in the face of high demand by local practitioners.[33] Although regional anesthesia has the potential to increase the efficiency of operating theater utilization, the opposite is also true, especially where workflow and protocols may be lacking.

ETHICS AND SAFETY OF REGIONAL US IN LMICs

Although regional anesthesia, especially when using ultrasound, is low-risk, it is not without risk. The limited existing data on the safety of regional anesthesia are almost exclusively from HICs where training and equipment meet the highest standards. More data are needed to quantify the risks of regional and general anesthesia in both HICs and LMICs.[34]

The degree of safety that is acceptable and "bare minimum" requirements for the provision of anesthesia in resource-constrained settings is a matter of intense, ongoing debate with significant ethical and humanitarian components.[35,36]

Unanswered questions include: Who should provide or supervise regional anesthesia? How much training or supervision is adequate? Should regional anesthesia be done where there is no intralipid, pressor, or skilled provider to manage a complication? When does the potential benefit outweigh the potential risk? How best to create equipment supply chains?

Implementation of regional anesthesia in LMICs has great potential to reduce morbidity and mortality, although it requires significant resources, evaluation, and consideration beyond a workshop or the procurement of an ultrasound. Decisions regarding implementation of regional anesthesia in a resource-constrained setting, including safety and workflow, must be tailored to the local context by local experts.

References

1. Kessler J, Marhofer P, Hopkins PM, Hollmann MW. Peripheral regional anaesthesia and outcome: lessons learned from the last 10 years. *Br J Anaesth*. 2015;114:728–745.
2. Meara JG, Leather AJM, Hagander L, et al. Global Surgery 2030: evidence and solutions for achieving health, welfare, and economic development. *Lancet*. 2015;386(9993):569–624.
3. Dare AJ, Bleicher J, Lee KC, et al. Generation of national political priority for surgery: a qualitative case study of three low-income and middle-income countries. *Lancet*. 2015;385(suppl 2):S54.
4. Buchbinder R, Blyth FM, March LM, Brooks P, Woolf AD, Hoy DG. Placing the global burden of low back pain in context. *Best Pract Res Clin Rheumatol*. 2013;27:575–589.
5. GBD Data Tool|Institute for Health Metrics and Evaluation. http://ghdx.healthdata.org/gbd-results-tool. Accessed September 28, 2016.
6. Brennan F, Carr DB, Cousins M. Pain management: a fundamental human right. *Anesth Analg*. 2007;105:205–221.
7. Goldberg DS, McGee SJ. Pain as a global public health priority. *BMC Public Health*. 2011;11:770.
8. United Nations. Universal declaration of human rights; 1948. http://www.ohchr.org/EN/UDHR/Documents/UDHR_Translations/eng.pdf. Accessed September 28, 2016.
9. Seya MJ, Gelders SFAM, Achara OU, Milani B, Scholten WK. A first comparison between the consumption of and the need for opioid analgesics at country, regional, and global levels. *J Pain Palliat Care Pharmacother*. 2011;25:6–18.
10. International Narcotics Control Board. Availability of Internationally Controlled Drugs: Ensuring Adequate Access for Medical and Scientific Purposes; 2010. https://www.incb.org/documents/Publications/AnnualReports/AR2010/Supplement-AR10_availability_English.pdf. Accessed September 28, 2016.
11. Berterame S, Erthal J, Thomas J, et al. Use of and barriers to access to opioid analgesics: a worldwide, regional, and national study. *Lancet*. 2016;387:1644–1656.
12. World Health Organization. WHO Model List of Essential Medicines; 2015. http://www.who.int/selection_medicines/committees/expert/20/EML_2015_FINAL_amended_AUG2015.pdf?ua=1. Accessed August 21, 2017.
13. Barrington MJ, Kluger R. Ultrasound guidance reduces the risk of local anesthetic systemic toxicity following peripheral nerve blockade. *Reg Anesth Pain Med*. 2013;38:289–299.
14. WHO. Donation of medical equipment. WHO. http://www.who.int/medical_devices/management_use/manage_donations/en/. Accessed October 3, 2016.
15. Tsui BCH. Dextrose 5% in water as an alternative medium to gel for performing ultrasound-guided peripheral nerve blocks. *Reg Anesth Pain Med*. 2009;34:525–527.
16. Binkowski A, Riguzzi C, Price D, Fahimi J. Evaluation of a cornstarch-based ultrasound gel alternative for low-resource settings. *J Emerg Med*. 2014;47:e5–e9.
17. Gorny KR, Hangiandreou NJ, Hesley GK, Felmlee JP. Evaluation of mineral oil as an acoustic coupling medium in clinical MRgFUS. *Phys Med Biol*. 2007;52:N13–N19.
18. Luewan S, Srisupundit K, Tongsong T. A comparison of sonographic image quality between the examinations using gel and olive oil, as sound media. *J Med Assoc Thai*. 2007;90:624–627.
19. Salmon M, Salmon C, Bissinger A, et al. Alternative ultrasound gel for a sustainable ultrasound program: application of human centered design. *PLoS ONE*. 2015;10:e0134332.
20. Sutton E, Bullock WM, Khan T, Eng M, Gadsden J. Hand sanitizer as an alternative to ultrasound transmission gel. *Reg Anesth Pain Med*. 2016;41:655–656.
21. Abdullah BJ, Mohd Yusof MY, Khoo BH. Physical methods of reducing the transmission of nosocomial infections via ultrasound and probe. *Clin Radiol*. 1998;53:212–214.
22. Karadeniz YM, Kiliç D, Kara Altan S, Altinok D, Güney S. Evaluation of the role of ultrasound machines as a source of nosocomial and cross-infection. *Invest Radiol*. 2001;36:554–558.

23. Muradali D, Gold WL, Phillips A, Wilson S. Can ultrasound probes and coupling gel be a source of nosocomial infection in patients undergoing sonography? An in vivo and in vitro study. *AJR Am J Roentgenol*. 1995;164:1521–1524.
24. Hodges SC, Mijumbi C, Okello M, McCormick BA, Walker IA, Wilson IH. Anaesthesia services in developing countries: defining the problems. *Anaesthesia*. 2007;62:4–11.
25. Woodbury A, Knight K, Fry L, Margolias G, Lynde GC. A survey of anesthesiologist and anesthetist attitudes toward single-use vials in an academic medical center. *J Clin Anesth*. 2014;26:125–130.
26. Pandian JD, Sarada C, Radhakrishnan VV, Kishore A. Iatrogenic meningitis after lumbar puncture-a preventable health hazard. *J Hosp Infect*. 2004;56:119–124.
27. Sakura S, Chan VW, Ciriales R, Drasner K. The addition of 7.5% glucose does not alter the neurotoxicity of 5% lidocaine administered intrathecally in the rat. *Anesthesiology*. 1995;82:236–240.
28. Neal JM, Wedel DJ. Ultrasound guidance and peripheral nerve injury: is our vision as sharp as we think it is? *Reg Anesth Pain Med*. 2010;35:335–337.
29. McGahan JP. Laboratory assessment of ultrasonic needle and catheter visualization. *J Ultrasound Med*. 1986;5:373–377.
30. Schnittger T. Regional anaesthesia in developing countries. *Anaesthesia*. 2007;62(suppl 1):44–47.
31. Wilhelm TJ, Anemana S, Kyamanywa P, Rennie J, Post S, Freudenberg S. Anaesthesia for elective inguinal hernia repair in rural Ghana – appeal for local anaesthesia in resource-poor countries. *Trop Doct*. 2006;36:147–149.
32. Malemo KL, Salmon M, Salmon C, Mutendi MM, Reynolds T. Ultrasound guided regional anesthesia — a multicentre feasibility trial for use in low resource settings. *Can J Surg*. 2014;57:S7. http://insights.ovid.com/cmaj-canadian-medical-association/cjsu/2014/06/001/18-ultrasound-guided-regional-anesthesia/19/00002789. Accessed October 3, 2016.
33. Ho M, Livingston P, Nyandwi D, et al. Establishing a regional anesthesia service in a low-income country: factors influencing implementation; 2016. http://www.epostersonline.com/ASRAPain16/node/553. Accessed November 1, 2016.
34. Bainbridge D, Martin J, Arango M, Cheng D, Evidence-based Peri-operative Clinical Outcomes Research (EPiCOR) Group. Perioperative and anaesthetic-related mortality in developed and developing countries: a systematic review and meta-analysis. *Lancet*. 2012;380:1075–1081.
35. Gelb AW, Enright A, Merry AF, Morriss W. The bare minimum requires caution. *World J Surg*. 2016;40(11):2821–2822.
36. McQueen K, Coonan T, Ottaway A, et al. The bare minimum: the reality of global anaesthesia and patient safety. *World J Surg*. 2015;39:2153–2160.

Index

Page numbers followed by "*f*" indicate figures, "*t*" indicate tables, and "*b*" indicate boxes.

A

Abdominal wall
   lateral, ultrasound image of, 281*f*
   muscles of, 249, 255*f*
   nerves of, 267
Accessory muscle, 245
Accessory nerve (XI), 364*f*
Acoustic coupling gel, 48, 48*b*–49*b*
Acoustic enhancement, posterior, 5
   during femoral nerve block, 156, 163*f*–164*f*
Acoustic impedance, 7
Acoustic shadowing
   by bone, 5, 6*f*
   during musculocutaneous nerve block, 9*f*
Adductor canal, 169, 172*b*–173*b*
Adductor canal block, 169–173, 172*b*–173*b*
   goal of, 171
   key points, 172*t*
   quadriceps weakness of, 171–172
   suggested technique for, 170–171, 171*f*
Adductor hiatus, 169
Adhesive capsulitis, isolated SSN block in, 89
Air, ultrasound characteristics of, 7*t*
Aliasing, 19
Analgesia, caudal, inguinal hernia repair and, 259
Anatomic structures, 45–46
Anechoic fluid, injected, 42
Anesthetic injections, local, in axillary block, 105
Aneurysmal dilatation, of axillary artery, 63*f*
Angle of insonation (insertion angle), 24, 26*f*
Anisotropic, definition of, 13
Anisotropy, 13, 13*b*, 14*f*
   definition of, 13
   in femoral nerve block, 161*f*
   of muscle, 53
Ankle blocks, 204
   contraindication to, 214
   at deep peroneal nerve, 204, 208
   at superficial peroneal nerve, 214
Antebrachial cutaneous nerve, medial, 104*t*, 105, 114*f*
Anterior echo complex, 320, 320*t*
Anterior inferior iliac spine (AIIS), for fascia iliaca block, 155
Anterior intercostal nerves, 249
Anterior interosseous nerve, 132
3-Anterior quadratus lumborum (QLB3), 278, 278*t*, 283*f*
Anterior sciatic nerve block, 189, 189*b*, 190*f*–192*f*
   suggested technique for, 189
Anterior tibial artery, 208
Anterior tubercles, 381
Anterior-superior iliac spine (ASIS), 144
Aponeuroses, 249
Arteries, 60
   power Doppler imaging of, 60*f*–61*f*
   of transversus abdominis plane, 272*f*
Artifacts, 42*b*
   comet-tail, 7, 7*b*, 67–68, 67*f*
   in infraclavicular block, 93, 103*f*
   posterior acoustic enhancement, 156, 163*f*–164*f*
   posterior acoustic enhancement of, 5
   reverberation, 7, 8*f*
   sound, speed of, 3, 4*f*
   speckle, 15
ASIS. *see* Anterior-superior iliac spine
Aspiration, caudal epidural block and, 329*b*–330*b*
Atlas, posterior arch of, 359*f*–360*f*
Atraumatic needle trajectory
   for intraneural trauma reduction, 397–398, 397*f*–398*f*
   for pneumothorax reduction, 400
   for vascular trauma reduction, 390, 391*f*
Attenuation, 5, 5*b*
Audible sounds, 2
Augmentation maneuvers, distal, 64
Axilla
   brachial plexus in, 104, 104*t*, 108*f*
   musculocutaneous nerve block in, 9*f*
Axillary artery, 60*f*, 63*f*
   axillary block in, 105, 114*f*
   long axis view of, 20*f*
Axillary block, 104–106, 106*b*, 113*f*, 116*f*
   axillary artery after, 114*f*
   axillary scout view imaging in, 110*f*
   back-wall injection in, 112*f*
   clinical considerations for, with ultrasound, 104, 105*t*
   color Doppler imaging during, 20*f*
   in-plane approach to, 107*f*, 111*f*
   key points in, 106*t*
   medial antebrachial cutaneous nerve after, 114*f*
   median nerve after, 115*f*
   suggested technique for, 104–105
Axillary nerve, 104*t*
   sensory blockade of, 71
Axillary scout view imaging, in axillary block, 110*f*
Axillary vein, 64*f*–65*f*
Axons, 394–396

B

Back-wall injection, in axillary block, 112*f*
Bayonet artifacts, 4*f*
   during popliteal block, 199*f*
Beach-chair position, 75
Beam profile, 12*f*
Beam width (slice thickness), 11, 11*f*
   out-of-plane, 11, 11*f*
Bevel orientation, 24
Bifurcation, carotid, 375, 376*f*
Bilateral symmetrical anesthesia, in thoracic paravertebral block (TPVB), 291
Bilateral sympathetic blockade, in thoracic paravertebral block (TPVB), 291
Blood, ultrasound characteristics of, 7*t*
Blood vessels, intercostal, 234
Bone, 66
   acoustic shadowing by, 5, 6*f*, 66, 66*f*
   thermal index of, 66*b*
   ultrasound appearance of, 66*f*
   ultrasound characteristics of, 7*t*
Brachial cutaneous nerve, medial, 104*t*
Brachial plexus, 74, 77*f*–78*f*, 80*f*–82*f*
   anatomical variations, 74
   in axilla, 104, 104*t*, 108*f*
   cervical ventral rami of, imaging of, 49*f*
   dorsal scapular nerve and, 87, 88*f*
   infraclavicular block in, 93, 97*f*, 101*f*
   pass-over, 75, 83*f*
   pass-through, 75, 83*f*
   peripheral blocks of, 125
   supraclavicular nerves, 71, 72*f*–73*f*
Bulk modulus, 3
Bupivacaine, in thoracic paravertebral block (TPVB), 290

C

C1, transverse process of, 359*f*
C2
   lamina of, 362*f*
   spinous process of, 359*f*, 361*f*
Cadaveric dissection, in thoracic paravertebral block (TPVB), 290–291
Carotid artery, 370*f*
Carotid bifurcation, 375, 376*f*
Cassava-based ultrasound gel, 408, 408*f*
"Cat ears", 319–320
Catheter, 34
   peripheral nerve
     in popliteal fossa, 38*f*
     short-axis in-plane approach to, 34
     ultrasound imaging of, 40*f*
   placement of, 34
     in thoracic paravertebral block (TPVB), 292–293

Catheter (*Continued*)
  popliteal placement, 37*f*
    peripheral nerve, 38*f*
Catheter-over-needle (CON) technique, 35
Catheter-through-needle (CTN) technique, 35
Caudal analgesia, inguinal hernia repair and, 259
Caudal epidural block, 328–331, 329*b*–330*b*
  longitudinal in-plane approach to, 331*f*, 334*f*
  normal adult values for, 328*t*
  pediatric, 335*f*
  suggested technique for, 329
  transverse out-of-plane approach to, 334*f*
Cephalic vein, axillary block in, 105
Cervical nerve, transverse, 364*f*
Cervical plexus, 372, 373*f*
  muscular branches of, 372
  superficial branches of, 372
Cervical plexus block, 372–380, 380*b*
  anatomic background in, 372
  blocking technique, 375–376
  contraindications to, 372
  current debates on, 377–378
  deep, 375, 379*t*
  indications for, 372
  in-plane approach to, 73*f*
  intermediate, 376–377, 377*f*, 379*t*–380*t*
  limitations of, 377–378, 378*f*
  nomenclature of, 372
  sonographic landmarks in, 373–375, 374*f*–375*f*
  suggested technique to, 372–377
  superficial, 379*t*
  supraclavicular, 73*f*
  ultrasound guidance for, 372
Cervical ribs, 74
Cervical spine sonography, for phrenic nerve block, 399–400
Cervical triangle, posterior, sonoanatomy of, 74
Cervical ventral ramus
  of brachial plexus, 49*f*
  fourth, phrenic nerve and, 84
  seventh, 74, 76*b*
Chassaignac's tubercle, 373–374, 384*f*
Children, pudendal nerve block in, 316–317, 317*b*
  discussion and comments for, 316
  suggested technique for, 316, 317*f*–318*f*
Circumflex artery, 259
Circumneural sheath, 397–399
CMAPs. *see* Compound motor action potentials
Color Doppler imaging, 19, 20*f*
Comet tail sign, 400

Comet-tail artifacts, 7, 7*b*, 8*f*
  imaging of, 67, 67*f*
  in peritoneal imaging, 68
  during rectus sheath block, 8*f*
Common peroneal nerve, 193, 196*f*
Compact transducer, for interscalene block, 75
Compound imaging, spatial, 15–16, 16*b*, 17*f*–18*f*
Compound motor action potentials (CMAPs), 174
Compression, 2
Connective tissue, 48
  muscle and, 54*b*
Continuous catheter transversus abdominis plane blocks, 268–269
Continuous femoral nerve block, advancement of peripheral nerve catheter for, 40*f*
Contraction, of muscle, 53
Cord topography, in infraclavicular block, 93
Cricoid, arch of, 355*f*
Cricoid cartilage, 356*f*
Cricopharyngeus muscle, 349*f*
Cricothyroid ligament, 355*f*
Cricothyroid membrane, 356*f*
  identification of, 353
Cricothyroid muscle, 349*f*
Curved arrays, 21, 21*f*
Curvilinear arrays, 21
Cutaneous nerve
  medial antebrachial, 104*t*, 105, 114*f*
  medial brachial, 104*t*
Cutaneous nerve block, posterior femoral, 200–202, 202*f*–203*f*
  distal, 201, 201*b*, 201*t*
  neurologic assessment for, 200
  proximal, 200
  suggested technique for, 200

D

"Dark stripe sign", 94
DCIA. *see* Deep circumflex iliac artery
Decibels (dB), 5*b*
Deep cervical artery, 76*b*, 78*f*
Deep cervical plexus block, 375, 379*t*
Deep circumflex iliac artery (DCIA), 150, 151*b*, 259
Deep peroneal nerve, 204, 208
  ultrasound guidance for, 208, 211*f*
Deep peroneal nerve block, 208–209, 209*b*, 210*f*–213*f*
  key points, 209*t*
  suggested technique for, 208
Deep radial nerve, 126
Density, 3
Dermis, 47
"Devil's horns" appearance, of cricoid cartilage and cricothyroid membrane, 356*f*

Distal augmentation maneuvers, 64
Distal SSN block, 89
Doppler imaging, 19, 19*b*
  color, 19, 20*f*
  power, 19, 19*b*
  of supraorbital artery, 341*f*
  variance, 19
Dorsal scapular artery, 76*b*, 78*f*, 87, 87*b*
  inferior trunk and, 75
Dorsal scapular nerve, 87
  imaging of, 87*f*–88*f*
Double-layer sign, 249, 254*f*
Doughnut sign, 32
Dynamic motion, of muscle, 53

E

Echogenic modifications, 25
Echogenic needles, 409, 410*f*
Echolucent, 2
Elbow, median nerve block proximal to, 132
Endoneurium, 394–396
Endothoracic fascia, 286, 289*f*
Epidermis, 47
Epidural block, caudal, 328–331, 329*b*–330*b*
  longitudinal in-plane approach to, 331*f*, 334*f*
  normal adult values for, 328*t*
  pediatric, 335*f*
  suggested technique for, 329
  transverse out-of-plane approach to, 334*f*
Epidural needles, 409
Epidural space
  depth of, 322*t*
  localization, in thoracic paravertebral block (TPVB), 291
  posterior, 326*f*
    AP width of, 321*t*
    depth of, 321*t*
  sacral, 329
Epidural spread, in thoracic paravertebral block (TPVB), 290–291
Epigastric arteries, 249, 255*f*
  TAP blocks and, 268
Epimysium, 53
Epinephrine
  for LAST, 393
  in thoracic paravertebral block (TPVB), 290
Epineurium, 394–396
Equals sign, 320, 320*t*
Erector spinae muscle, 280*f*, 282*f*
Esophagus, 381, 386*f*
External occipital protuberance, 359*f*–360*f*
Extrapleural paravertebral compartment, 286
Extrinsic muscles, forearm blocks in, 125

F

Facial muscles, motor block of, due to supraorbital nerve block, 338
Facial nerve, blockade of, cervical branch, 377, 378f
Fascia iliaca block, 150–151, 151b, 153f–155f
   in-plane approach to, 150, 152f–153f
   positioning for, 152f
   proximal, 150, 152f, 155f
   suggested technique for, 150–151
Fascicles, 394–396
Fascicular echotexture, 48, 49f–50f, 52f, 56
FCU. see Flexor carpi ulnaris
Femoral artery, 60f, 62f, 156, 161f, 163f, 166f
Femoral artery plaque, 167f
Femoral cutaneous nerve block, posterior, 200–202, 202f–203f
   distal, 201, 201b, 201t
   neurologic assessment for, 200
   proximal, 200
   suggested technique for, 200
Femoral nerve, 156
   course of, 159f
   imaging of, 59f
   in inguinal region, 156, 160f–162f
   long-axis view of, 163f
   morphologies of, 162f
   short-axis view of, 156, 161f–166f
Femoral nerve block, 156–158, 157b–158b
   approaches to, 160f
   continuous, advancement of peripheral nerve catheter for, 40f
   imaging of, 69, 69f
   in inguinal region, 160f
   in-plane approach to, 156–157, 160f, 164f
   key points, 157t
   out-of-plane approach to, 156–157, 160f
   posterior acoustic enhancement artifact with, 156, 163f–164f
   suggested technique for, 156–157
   transducer location for, 157b–158b
   verification of, 163f, 166f
Femoral vein, 62f
Fibrillar echotexture, 56–57, 59f
Fibroadipose connective tissue, 53
Fixed predetermined distance, of needle, in thoracic paravertebral block (TPVB), 292
Flexor carpi ulnaris (FCU), 138
   tendon, 56
Flexor digitorum longus, 232f
Flexor pollicis longus (FPL) tendon, imaging of, 58f
"Flying bat", 319–320
Foot, innervation of, 204
Forearm
   median nerve in, 132, 134f, 136f
   ulnar nerve block in, 140f–141f

Forearm blocks, 125
Frozen shoulder syndrome, isolated SSN block in, 89

G

GON. see Greater occipital nerve
Great auricular nerve, 364f, 366, 367f, 369f–371f
Great auricular nerve block, 366, 366b
   out-of-plane approach to, 368f
   suggested technique to, 366
Greater auricular nerve, 373f, 375, 375f
Greater occipital nerve (GON), 357, 359f, 361f
Greater occipital nerve block, 357–359, 358b–359b
   discussion and comments on, 358
   key points on, 358t
   out-of-plane approach to, 362f
   suggested technique for, 357
Gut sliding, 68

H

Hand-on-needle approaches, 30f
Hand-on-needle hub technique, 29
   for interscalene block, 75
Hand-on-syringe technique, 29, 30f
Hand-sanitizing gels, 408
Head and neck blocks
   greater occipital nerve block, 357–359, 358b–359b
      discussion and comments on, 358
      key points on, 358t
      out-of-plane approach to, 362f
      suggested technique for, 357
   mental nerve block, 342–343, 343b, 344f, 346f
      key points on, 343t
      suggested technique for, 342
   superior laryngeal nerve block, 347–348, 347b–348b, 350f
      suggested technique for, 347
   supraorbital nerve block, 336–339, 338b–339b
      comments on, 338
      incomplete, 338
      in-plane approach to, 340f
      key points on, 338t
      suggested technique for, 337
   transtracheal block, 353–355, 354b
      key points on, 354t
      out-of-plane approach to, 356f
      suggested technique for, 353–354
Hematoma, due to supraorbital nerve block, 338
Hemi-diaphragmatic paralysis, reducing risk of, 399–400
Hemothorax, 235
Hernia, inguinal, 259
Hiccups, intractable, phrenic nerve imaging, 84

High-resolution ultrasound, 46
   for lateral femoral cutaneous nerve, 144
   for persistent median artery, 132
Hockey stick transducers, 21f
Honeycomb echotexture, 48, 51f
Hunter canal, 169
Hustead needle tips, 25b
Hydrodissection, 397–399, 397f
Hyoid bone, 347, 350f–351f, 355f
Hyperechoic reverberation artifacts, 7b
Hypodermic needles, 410f
Hypoechoic muscle, 53, 55f

I

Iliohypogastric nerve, 259
   course of, 259
   in quadratus lumborum (QL) muscle, 277
Iliohypogastric nerve block, 259–262, 261b, 262f–266f
   benefits of, 259
   key points for, 260t–261t
   suggested techniques for, 259–260
Ilioinguinal nerve, 259
   course of, 259
Ilioinguinal nerve block, 259–262, 261b, 262f–266f
   benefits of, 259
   key points for, 260t–261t
   suggested techniques for, 259–260
Ilioinguinal transversus abdominis plane block, 268, 274f
Iliopsoas tendon, 156, 157b–158b, 166f
   imaging of, 59f
Inadvertent vascular puncture, 389
Increased through-transmission, 5
Inferior pharyngeal constrictor muscle, 349f
Inferior thyroid artery, 381, 385f
Inferior trunk, interscalene block and, 75
Infraclavicular block, 93–96, 96b, 97f, 99f, 101f
   advantage of, 93–94, 93t
   artifacts during, 93, 103f
   comments in, 94–95
   disadvantage of, 93, 93t
   in-plane approach to, 94, 97f–98f
   intraneural injection during, 102f
   key points in, 95t
   sonographic assessment of, 94, 95t, 98f
   suggested technique in, 94
   transducer for, 94, 100f
"Infraclavicular" configuration, 93
Inguinal hernia, 259
Inguinal lymph nodes, 69, 167f
Injected anechoic fluid, 42
Injections
   intraneural, to infraclavicular block, 98f
   sonographic signs of success, 32, 33f
   test, 25

In-plane approach, 28t, 29, 30f
  to axillary block, 107f, 111f
  to infraclavicular block, 94, 97f–98f
  to musculocutaneous nerve block, 119f
  needle redirection during, 29
  to radial nerve block, 126, 128f–129f
Insertion angle (angle of insonation), 24, 26f
Intercostal approach, to thoracic paravertebral space, ultrasound-guided thoracic paravertebral block in, 293, 311–313, 312f–313f
Intercostal arteries, 234
Intercostal nerve block, 233–236, 235b, 237f–238f
  positioning for, 234, 236f
  suggested technique for, 234–235
Intercostal nerves, 234, 249
  anterior, 249
  in thoracic paravertebral space (TPVS), 286
Intercostal vessels, in thoracic paravertebral space (TPVS), 286
Intercostobrachial nerve, 104t, 105
Intercostobrachial nerve block, 105
Intermediate cervical plexus block, 376–377, 377f, 379t–380t
Internal intercostal membrane, 286
Internal intercostal muscle, 286
Internal jugular vein, 370f
Internal mammary vessels, 244
Interscalene block, 71b, 74–76
  dorsal scapular nerve and, 87
  imaging of, 50f, 77f–78f, 80f–82f
  lateral to medial approach to, 75, 76b, 80f, 82f
  medial to lateral approach to, 75, 76b, 80f–81f
  phrenic nerve and, 84
  probe position, 79f
  suggested technique for, 75
  ultrasound-guided, 399–400
Interscalene plexus, 80f
Interspaces, lumbar
  distance of, 321t
  imaging of, 326f–327f
  length of, 321t
  level estimation of, 322
Intertransverse ligament, 286
Intractable hiccups, phrenic nerve imaging, 84
Intraneural injection
  during femoral nerve block, 168f
  to infraclavicular block, 98f
  peripheral nerve injury and, 396–399
Intraneural trauma, reducing risk of, 397–399, 397f–398f
Investing fascia, 53

Ipsilateral Horner syndrome, after thoracic paravertebral block (TPVB), 286–289
Ipsilateral lumbar spinal nerves, in thoracic paravertebral space (TPVS), 289, 291
Ipsilateral segmental thoracic anesthesia, thoracic paravertebral block (TPVB) and, 290
iSlice display, of thoracic paravertebral region
  sagittal, 306f
  transverse, 308f
Isolated SSN block, 89
Isotropic (term), 13

L

Lamina, inclination of, 321t
Landmark based techniques, in thoracic paravertebral block (TPVB), 289–292
Laparoscopic surgery, transversus abdominis plane blocks in, 270
Large bifascicular nerve, in thigh, 147f
Large-bore needles, 25b
Laryngeal nerve, superior, 347, 347b–348b, 349f
  external branch of, 347, 347b–348b, 349f
  internal branch of, 347, 347b–348b, 349f
Laryngeal nerve block, superior, 347–348, 347b–348b, 350f
  suggested technique for, 347
Larynx, nerves of, 349f
LAST. see Local anesthetic systemic toxicity
Lateral abdominal wall, ultrasound image of, 281f
Lateral circumflex femoral artery, 60f, 163f
Lateral decubitus position, thoracic paravertebral block (TPVB) in, 291
Lateral femoral cutaneous nerve (LFCN), 144, 145b
  anatomic variations of, 144, 149f
  course of, 144
  imaging of, 144, 147f
  pass-through, 144, 149f
Lateral femoral cutaneous nerve block, 53t, 145b, 147f–148f
  in-plane approach, 144, 146f, 148f
  key points, 145t
  suggested technique for, 144–145
Lateral position, for quadratus lumborum blocks, 279
1-Lateral quadratus lumborum (QLB1), 277, 278t, 283f–284f
Lateral transversus abdominis plane block, 269–270, 275f
Latissimus dorsi muscle, 280f, 285f

Leg, saphenous nerve block in, 205–206, 206b, 207f
  key points, 205t–206t
  suggested technique for, 205
Lesser occipital nerve (LON), 358, 364b, 364f, 367f, 373f
Lesser occipital nerve block, 363–364, 363t–364t, 364b, 365f
LFCN. see Lateral femoral cutaneous nerve
Ligaments, 56–57
  as sonographic landmarks, 57, 57t
Linear array test tool imaging, 15–16, 17f
Linear arrays, 21, 21f
Local anesthetic, 33f
  in adductor canal, 169, 171, 171f
  after musculocutaneous nerve block, 117, 122f
  in axillary block, 105
  in femoral nerve, 156, 164f–166f, 168f
  in lateral femoral cutaneous nerve, 144, 148f–149f
  in obturator nerve, 174, 177f–178f
  regional anesthesia and, 408–409
Local anesthetic systemic toxicity (LAST), 389, 391–393
  block types involved with, 392t
  effects of ultrasound technology on, 394t
  incidence of, 391–393, 392t
  reducing risk of, 393, 394t
  risk factors for, 391–393
LON. see Lesser occipital nerve
Long-axis in-plane approach, to continuous peripheral nerve blocks, 34
Long-axis view, 29
  of femoral artery, 62f
  of fibrillar echotexture, 59f
  flexor pollicis longus tendon in, 58f
  of muscle, 54b
  of peripheral nerves, 48b–49b, 52f
Longitudinal wave, 2
Longus colli muscle, 382, 384f–385f
Loss-of-resistance techniques, 250
  in thoracic paravertebral block (TPVB), 291–292
Low-income countries (LICs), regional anesthesia in, 405–412
  challenges with consumables, 407–409
  equipment challenges to, 406–407
  ethics and safety of, 410–411
  preferred blocks for, 405–406
  staffing for, 409–410
  technique selection for, 405–406
  training for, 409–410
Lumbar epidural catheter placement, offline, suggested technique for, 320–322

INDEX

Lumbar interspaces
  distance of, 321t
  imaging of, 326f-327f
  length of, 321t
  level estimation of, 322
Lumbar plexus block, 150
Lung sliding, 67
Lymph nodes, 69, 69b
  inguinal, 69, 167f
  ultrasound appearance of, 69f

M

Mastoid process, 359f
Matrix arrays, four-dimensional imaging with, 42
Mechanical waves, 2
Medial antebrachial cutaneous nerve, 104t, 105, 114f
Medial brachial cutaneous nerve, 104t
Median artery, persistent, 132, 137f
Median nerve, 104t, 105, 115f, 132, 133b
  anisotropy of, 14f
  imaging of, 51f
  musculocutaneous and, fusion of, 117, 123f
  in short axis, 31f
Median nerve block, 132-133, 134f-136f
  key points, 133b, 133t
  neurologic assessment of, 132
  suggested technique for, 132, 137f
Medications, regional anesthesia and, 408-409
Mental foramen, 342, 345f-346f
Mental nerve, 342
Mental nerve block, 342-343, 343b, 344f, 346f
  key points on, 343t
  suggested technique for, 342
Meralgia paresthetica, 144
M-mode center line, 28
Monofascicular echotexture, 49f-50f
Monofascicular ventral rami, 74
Motion, of muscle, 53
Motor block, of opponens pollicis, 132
Muscle, 53-54
  echogenicity, 53t
  hypoechoic, 53, 55f
Musculocutaneous nerve, 104t, 117
  cutaneous branch of, 117, 124f
  division of, 120f
  imaging of, 44f
  pass-over, 117, 124f
Musculocutaneous nerve block, 117-118
  acoustic shadowing during, 9f
  image sequence of, 121f
  in-plane approach to, 119f
  key points in, 118t
  local anesthetic after, 117, 122f
  suggested technique in, 117

Musculocutaneous-median nerve fusion, 117, 123f
Musculoskeletal imaging, 46
Musculotendinous junctions, 57b
Myositis, 400

N

Neck, anterior view of, 355f
Necrotizing fasciitis, 400
Needle gauge, 24
Needle imaging, 24-26
Needle motion, 25
Needle tip visibility, 24
  factors that influence, 24, 24t
  influence of angle of insonation on, 26f
  influence of bevel orientation on, 25t, 27f
Needle tips, Hustead, 25b
Needles, 34
  echogenic modifications, 25
  large-bore, 25b
  peripheral nerve block and, 34
  redirection during in-plane technique, 29
  for regional anesthesia, 409, 410f
  for regional block, 24, 25b, 27f
  side-port, 25b
Nerve(s)
  of abdominal wall, 267
  anisotropy of, 13
  characteristics of, 56, 56t
  genitofemoral, 259
  iliohypogastric, 259
    course of, 259
  ilioinguinal, 259
    course of, 259
  imaging of, 42, 43f
  intercostal, 249
    anterior, 249
  of larynx, 349f
  musculocutaneous, imaging of, 44f
  peripheral, 48-49
  superficial, 48b-49b
  thoracoabdominal, 252f
Nerve block
  anterior sciatic, 189, 189b, 190f-192f
    suggested technique for, 189
  axillary, 104-106, 106b, 113f, 116f
    axillary artery after, 114f
    axillary scout view imaging in, 110f
    back-wall injection in, 112f
    clinical considerations for, with ultrasound, 104, 105t
    in-plane approach to, 107f, 111f
    key points in, 106t
    medial antebrachial cutaneous nerve after, 114f
    median nerve after, 115f
    suggested technique for, 104-105

Nerve block (*Continued*)
  deep peroneal, 208-209, 209b, 210f-213f
    key points, 209t
    suggested technique for, 208
  femoral, 156-158, 157b-158b
    approaches to, 160f
    in inguinal region, 160f
    in-plane approach to, 156-157, 160f, 164f
    key points, 157t
    out-of-plane approach to, 156-157, 160f
    posterior acoustic enhancement artifact with, 156, 163f-164f
    suggested technique for, 156-157
    transducer location for, 157b-158b
    verification of, 163f, 166f
  great auricular, 366, 366b
    out-of-plane approach to, 368f
    suggested technique to, 366
  intercostobrachial, 105
  lateral femoral cutaneous, 145b, 147f-148f
    in-plane approach, 144, 146f, 148f
    key points, 145t
    suggested technique for, 144-145
  lesser occipital, 363-364, 363t-364t, 364b, 365f
  median, 132-133, 134f-136f
    key points, 133b, 133t
    neurologic assessment of, 132
    suggested technique for, 132, 137f
  mental, 342-343, 343b, 344f, 346f
    key points on, 343t
    suggested technique for, 342
  musculocutaneous, 117-118
    image sequence of, 121f
    in-plane approach to, 119f
    key points in, 118t
    local anesthetic after, 117, 122f
    suggested technique in, 117
  obturator, 174-175, 175b, 176f-178f
    key points, 175t
    suggested technique for, 174
  peripheral
    continuous, long-axis in-plane approach to, 34
    sonographic assessment of, 39f
    ultrasound-guided continuous, 34-36, 35b, 37f
  posterior femoral cutaneous, 200-202, 202f-203f
    distal, 201, 201b, 201t
    neurologic assessment for, 200
    proximal, 200
    suggested technique for, 200
  pudendal, in children, 316-317, 317b
    discussion and comments for, 316

Nerve block (*Continued*)
    suggested technique for, 316, 317f–318f
    radial, 126–127, 127b, 131f
        in-plane approach to, 126
        key points in, 127t
        neurologic assessment of, 127
        suggested technique in, 126
        superficial, 128f–129f
    saphenous, in leg, 205–206, 206b, 207f
        key points, 205t–206t
        in mid-leg, 207f
        suggested technique for, 205
    sciatic, 179–181, 180b–181b, 182f–188f
        fascia iliaca block before, 151b
        in gluteal region, 188f
        key points, 180t
        position for, 179
        proximal, 179, 184f
        in subgluteal region, 179, 183f
        suggested technique, 179–180
    superficial peroneal, 214–216, 216f–220f
        key points, 215b, 215t
        suggested technique, 214
    superior laryngeal, 347–348, 347b–348b, 350f
        suggested technique for, 347
    supraorbital, 336–339, 338b–339b
        comments on, 338
        incomplete, 338
        in-plane approach to, 340f
        key points on, 338t
        suggested technique for, 337
    suprascapular, 89–90, 90b, 91f–92f
        clinical assessment of, 90
        selectivity of, 90
        suggested technique for, 89–90
    ulnar, 138–139, 139b, 140f–142f
        key points, 138t–139t
        neurologic assessment of, 138
        suggested technique for, 138
    ultrasound-guided, 125, 388–404, 401b
Nerve fiber, 48
Nerve fusion, musculocutaneous-median, 117, 123f
Nerve stimulation, in thoracic paravertebral space (TPVS), 290
Nerve to the vastus medialis (NVM), 169, 171, 172b–173b
Neuraxial block, 319–324, 323b
    anatomic structures seen in, 320, 320t
    comments on, 322
    longitudinal paramedian view of, 319, 323b, 326f–327f
    measurements useful for guiding, 321t
    offline approaches to, 319, 324f–325f
    outcomes on, 323
    suggested technique for, 320–322
    transducer position for, 324f–325f
    transverse midline view of, 319–320, 324f

Neuraxis, high-resolution ultrasound imaging of, 322–323
Neurologic assessment, of radial nerve block, 127
Neurovascular bundle, 227
No touch technique, for regional anesthesia, 407, 407f
Nomenclature, for transducer manipulation, 22
NVM. *see* Nerve to the vastus medialis

O
Obesity, neuraxial block and, 322
Oblique subcostal line, 267–268, 274f
Obliquus capitis inferior muscle (OCIM), 357, 359f
Obturator nerve, 174
    accessory, 175b
    divisions of, 174, 176f–178f
    imaging of, 176f–178f
Obturator nerve block, 174–175, 175b, 176f–178f
    key points, 175t
    suggested technique for, 174
Occipital artery, 359f
Occipital nerve
    greater, 357, 359f, 361f
    lesser, 358, 364b, 364f
Occipital nerve block, 363
    greater, 357–359, 358b–359b
        discussion and comments on, 358
        key points on, 358t
        out-of-plane approach to, 362f
        suggested technique for, 357
    lesser, 363–364, 363f–364f, 364b, 365f
OCIM. *see* Obliquus capitis inferior muscle
Offline markings, 28
Offline techniques, 28
Omohyoid muscle, 90
    interscalene block and, 75
Online guidance, 28
Opponens pollicis, motor block of, 132
Optimal spectral Doppler angle, 19
Osseous structures, transverse scan of, 300f
Out-of-plane approach, 28–29, 28t, 30f
Out-of-plane beam width (slice thickness), 11, 11f

P
Palmar cutaneous nerve, 132
Paramedian sagittal oblique scan, of thoracic paravertebral region, 305f, 307f
Paramedian sagittal scan with in-plane needle insertion, ultrasound-guided thoracic paravertebral block in, 309–311, 310f–311f
Paramedian sagittal sonogram, of thoracic paravertebral region, 304f

Paramedian transverse scan, of thoracic paravertebral region, 297f–300f, 302f
Paramedian transverse sonogram, of thoracic paravertebral region, 303f
Paraneural sheath, 397–399
Paravertebral block (PVB), 259
Parenchymal lung disease, 7b
Pass-over brachial plexus, 75, 83f
Pass-over musculocutaneous nerve, 117, 124f
Pass-through brachial plexus, 75, 83f
Pectoral nerve block (Pecs block), 239–240, 240b, 241f–243f
    key points in, 239t–240t
    neurologic assessment of, 239
    relation with other blocks, 239
    suggested technique for, 239
Pectoral nerves, 239
    course of, 241f
Pectoralis minor muscle, imaging of, 54f
Pediatric caudal epidural block, 335f
Pediatric patients, neuraxial scans of, 66b
Pennate muscle, 53, 54b
Perimysium, 53
Perineurium, 394–396
Peripheral nerve block
    continuous, long-axis in-plane approach to, 34
    neurological complications associated with, 393–399
    peripheral nerve injury due to, 393–394, 395t–396t
    sonographic assessment of, 39f
    ultrasound-guided, 389
    ultrasound-guided continuous, 34–36, 35b
        equipment of, 37f
Peripheral nerve catheter
    in popliteal fossa, 38f
    short-axis in-plane approach to, 34
    ultrasound imaging of, 40f
Peripheral nerve injury
    due to peripheral nerve block, 393–394, 395t–396t
    microanatomy of peripheral nerve and, 394–396
Peripheral nerves, 32, 48–49
    arteries and, 60
    long-axis view, 48b–49b, 52f
    microanatomy of, 394–396
    veins and, 64
Peritoneum, 68, 68f
Peroneal nerve, imaging of, 51f
Peroneal nerve block
    deep, 208–209, 209b, 210f–213f
        key points, 209t
        suggested technique for, 208
    superficial, 214–216, 216f–220f
        key points, 215b, 215t
        suggested technique, 214
Persistent median artery, 132, 137f

Pharmacokinetics, transversus abdominis plane blocks and, 269
Pharyngeal constrictor muscle, inferior, 349f
Phrenic nerve, 84, 379f, 381, 399
  course of, 85f
  imaging of, 84, 84f–86f
  interscalene block and, 75
Phrenic nerve block, 399
  reducing risk of, 399–400
Piriformis muscle, 53
Plane of cleavage, 397–399
Plaque, femoral artery, 167f
Pleura, 67
Pleural line, 7b
Pneumothorax, 7b
  after intercostal nerve block, 235
  reducing risk of, 400
Popliteal block, 193–195, 194b–195b, 196f–198f
  Bayonet artifact during, 199f
  key points, 194t
  suggested technique for, 193–195
Popliteal catheter placement, 37f
Popliteal fossa
  bifurcation of the sciatic nerve in, 193t
  imaging of, 193
  peripheral nerve catheter in, 38f
  sciatic nerve block in, 33f, 194
  sonographic anatomy of, 198f
Posterior acoustic enhancement, 5
  during femoral nerve block, 156, 163f–164f
Posterior echo complex, 320, 320t, 326f
Posterior epidural space, 326f
  AP width of, 321t
  depth of, 321t
Posterior femoral cutaneous nerve block, 200–202, 202f–203f
  distal, 201, 201b, 201t
  neurologic assessment for, 200
  proximal, 200
  suggested technique for, 200
2-Posterior quadratus lumborum (QLB2 block), 277, 278t, 283f–284f
Posterior tibial artery, 227
Posterior tubercles, 381
Power Doppler imaging, 19, 19b
Pre-block survey sonogram
  for reducing LAST, 393
  for reducing vascular trauma, 389–390, 390f
Prevertebral fascia, brachial plexus, 73f
Profunda brachii artery, 109f
Prone position
  for quadratus lumborum blocks, 279
  thoracic paravertebral block (TPVB) in, 291
Proximal fascia iliaca block, 150, 152f, 155f
Proximal sciatic nerve block, 179, 189

Psoas major muscle, in thoracic paravertebral space (TPVS), 289
Psoas muscle, 277, 281f–282f
Pudendal nerve, 316
Pudendal nerve block, in children, 316–317, 317b
  discussion and comments for, 316
  suggested technique for, 316, 317f–318f
PVB. see Paravertebral block

Q
QLB1. see 1-Lateral quadratus lumborum
QLB2 block. see 2-Posterior quadratus lumborum
QLB3. see 3-Anterior quadratus lumborum
Quadratus lumborum blocks, 53t, 277–280, 279b, 284f
  clinical anatomy/sonoanatomy in, 277
  main features of, 278t
  nomenclature and points of injection of, 277–278, 283f
  patient positioning and equipment selection for, 278–279
Quadratus lumborum (QL) muscle, 259, 267, 277, 280f–282f, 285f

R
Radial nerve, 104t, 126
  deep, 126
  in distal arm, 131f
  snake-eyes appearance of, 126, 130f
  superficial, 126
Radial nerve block, 126–127, 127b, 131f
  in-plane approach to, 126
  key points in, 127t
  neurologic assessment of, 127
  suggested technique in, 126
  superficial, 128f–129f
Radiopaque contrast medium, in thoracic paravertebral space (TPVS), 290
Rarefaction, 2
Receiver gain, 25
Rectus abdominis, 249, 256f
Rectus sheath block, 68f, 249–251, 251b, 253f–255f, 257f–258f
  comet-tail artifacts during, 8f
  goal of, 249
  indication for, 249
  key points in, 250t
  suggested technique for, 249–251
Recurrent laryngeal nerve, right, 349f
Red blood cells, veins and, 64
Reflection, 7–8
Regional anesthesia, in resource-constrained environments, 405–412
  challenges with consumables, 407–409
  equipment challenges to, 406–407
  ethics and safety of, 410–411
  preferred blocks for, 405–406
  staffing for, 409–410

Regional anesthesia, in resource-constrained environments (Continued)
  technique selection for, 405–406
  training for, 409–410
Regional block
  for hip fracture pathways, 151b
  in-plane approach to, 28t, 29
  needles used for, 24, 25b, 27f
  out-of-plane approach to, 28–29
  ultrasound transducers for, 21f
Renal fascia, 280f
Reverberation artifacts, 7, 8f
Ribs, cervical, 74
Right recurrent laryngeal nerve, 349f
Running the groove, for interscalene block, 75

S
Sacral cornua, 329, 332f–333f, 335f
Sacrococcygeal ligament, 329, 332f
Sagittal scan, of thoracic paravertebral region, 299–307, 303f–307f
Sagittal sonograms, of thoracic paravertebral region, 305f
Saphenous nerve (SN), 64, 169, 172b–173b, 205
Saphenous nerve block, 62f
  in leg, 205–206, 206b, 207f
  key points, 205t–206t
  in mid-leg, 207f
  suggested technique for, 205
Saphenous vein, 64
Sartorius muscle, 62f
Saw sign, 319
Scalene muscle
  anomalies, 74
  middle, dorsal scapular nerve and, 87, 88f
Scan lines, spatial compound imaging of, 18f
Scapular nerve, dorsal, 87
Sciatic nerve, 189, 190f–192f
  anatomic variations of, 179
  bifurcation, in popliteal fossa, 193t
  course of, 182f, 187f
  imaging of, 51f
  morphologies of, 186f
Sciatic nerve block, 179–181, 180b–181b, 182f–188f
  anterior, 189, 189b, 190f–192f
  suggested technique for, 189
  fascia iliaca block before, 151b
  in gluteal region, 188f
  key points, 180t
  popliteal, 193
  in popliteal fossa, 33f
  position for, 179
  proximal, 179, 184f
  in subgluteal region, 179, 183f
  suggested technique, 179–180

SCTL. *see* Superior costotransverse ligament
Sector transducer, 21f
"Seesaw" sign, 194b–195b
Segmental contralateral anesthesia, in thoracic paravertebral block (TPVB), 291
Semi-sitting position, 75
Sensory anesthesia, in thoracic paravertebral block (TPVB), 290–291
Sensory block, of median nerve, 132
"Serpentine" artery, 381, 385f
Short-axis in-plane approach, to peripheral nerve catheter, 34
Short-axis sliding, 48, 48b–49b
Short-axis view, 28–29
    of axillary artery, 60f, 63f
    of fibrillar echotexture, 59f
    flexor pollicis longus tendon in, 58f
Side-port needles, 25b
Singultus, phrenic nerve imaging, 84
Sitting position
    for quadratus lumborum blocks, 279
    thoracic paravertebral block (TPVB) in, 291
    transverse ultrasound scan of thoracic prevertebral region in, 294f
Skin, normal, 47
Skin markings, neuraxial block and, 322
Slice thickness, beam width, 11, 11f
Sliding lung sign, 400
Small nerve imaging, 16b
Small saphenous vein, 64, 65f
Smooth metal, 15–16
Snake-eyes appearance, of radial nerve, 126, 130f
Soft tissue
    thermal index of, 66b
    ultrasound characteristics of, 7t
SON. *see* Supraorbital nerve
Sonoanatomy
    relevant for thoracic paravertebral block (TPVB), 293–313
        basic considerations in, 293–294
        thoracic paravertebral region. *see* Thoracic paravertebral region
    three dimensional, of thoracic paravertebral region, 307–309, 308f
Sonogram
    of fascia iliaca block, 154f
    of medial thigh, 176f
    of median nerve block, 135f
Sonographic assessment, of infraclavicular block, 94, 95t, 98f
Sonographic signs, of successful injections, 32, 33f
Sound, speed of, 2–3

Sound artifacts, speed of, 3, 4f
Sound velocity, 3
Spatial compound imaging, 15–16, 16b, 17f–18f
    advantages and disadvantages of, 15t
    needle tip visibility in, 25
Speckle, 15
Specular reflections, 7
Speed of sound artifacts, 3, 4f
Spinal needles, 409
Spinal nerves, in thoracic paravertebral space (TPVS), 286
Spinous process, 323b, 324f, 327f
SSN. *see* Suprascapular nerve
Steel, stainless, 7t
Steep in-plane approach, to median nerve, 132
Stellate ganglion, 381, 387f
Stellate ganglion block, 381–384, 382t–383t, 383b
    anatomic structures in, 381–382
    approach and suggested technique to, 382
    lateral-to-medial in-plane approach to, 382, 384f, 386f
    out-of-plane approach to, 382
Sternalis muscle, 245
Sternocleidomastoid muscle, 73f, 364f, 371f, 373f
    brachial plexus and, 74, 77f
Steroid suspensions, 10f
Subarachnoid space, 325f, 329
    AP width of, 321t
Subcostal nerve, 234
    in quadratus lumborum (QL) muscle, 277
Subcostal transversus abdominis plane block, 267–268, 268b, 276f
Subcutaneous tissue, 47, 47f
    veins and, 64, 65f
Subendothoracic paravertebral compartment, 286
Subsartorial canal, 169
Subserous fascia, 286
Superficial cervical ansa, 378f
Superficial cervical artery, 61f, 79f
    phrenic nerve imaging and, 85f
Superficial nerves, 48b–49b
Superficial peroneal nerve, 214
Superficial peroneal nerve block, 214–216, 216f–220f
    key points, 215b, 215t
    suggested technique, 214
Superficial radial nerve, 126
Superficial radial nerve block, 128f–129f
Superficial ulnar artery, 138, 139b, 142f
    imaging of, 141f
Superior costotransverse ligament (SCTL), 286, 287f
Superior laryngeal artery, 347, 352f

Superior laryngeal nerve, 347, 347b–348b, 349f
    external branch of, 347, 347b–348b, 349f
    internal branch of, 347, 347b–348b, 349f
Superior laryngeal nerve block, 347–348, 347b–348b, 350f
    suggested technique for, 347
Superior nuchal line, 359f
Supine position, for quadratus lumborum blocks, 279
"Supraclavicular" configuration, 93
Supraclavicular nerve block, 41f, 71–76, 72f–73f, 78f
    catheter placement for, 41f
    suggested technique for, 71
Supraclavicular nerves, 71, 72f, 373f, 377–378, 379f
Suprainguinal injection, under fascia iliaca, 151b
Supraorbital artery, Doppler image of, 341f
Supraorbital nerve (SON), 337
    branching pattern of, 339f
Supraorbital nerve block, 336–339, 338b–339b
    comments on, 338
    incomplete, 338
    in-plane approach to, 340f
    key points on, 338t
    suggested technique for, 337
Suprascapular nerve (SSN), 89, 91f–92f
Suprascapular nerve block, 89–90, 90b, 91f–92f
    clinical assessment of, 90
    selectivity of, 90
    suggested technique for, 89–90
Suprascapular notch, 89
Sural nerve, 65f
Sural nerve block, 221–222, 223f–226f
    key points, 221t–222t, 222b
    suggested technique for, 221
Swelling, due to supraorbital nerve block, 338

T
"TACA" technique, 354b
TAP. *see* Transversus abdominis plane
Techniques, 28–30
Tendons, 56–57
    anisotropy of, 13
    characteristics of, 56, 56t
    in muscle, 53
Test injections, 25
Test tool image, 17f
TF. *see* Transversalis fascia
TGC. *see* Time gain compensation
Thermal index of bone, 66b
Thermal index of soft tissue, 66b

INDEX

Thigh
    large bifascicular nerve in, 147f
    lateral incisions of, lateral femoral cutaneous nerve block for, 144, 146f
    right, surface anatomy of, 170f
Third occipital nerve (TON), 358
Thoracic paravertebral anesthesia, 290
Thoracic paravertebral block (TPVB), 286-315
    anatomical landmark based techniques in, 291-292
    gross anatomy in, 286, 287f-289f
    mechanism of, 289-291
    sonoanatomy relevant for, 293-313
        basic considerations in, 293-294
        thoracic paravertebral region. *see* Thoracic paravertebral region
    ultrasound-guided, 292-293
        techniques of, 309-313
Thoracic paravertebral region
    anatomy of, 288f
    sagittal scan of, 299-307, 303f-307f
    three dimensional sonoanatomy of, 307-309, 308f
    transverse scan of, 294-299, 294f-303f
Thoracic paravertebral space (TPVS), 286
    caudal boundary of, 289
    communications of, 286-289
    intercostal approach to, ultrasound-guided thoracic paravertebral block in, 293, 311-313, 312f-313f
    sagittal anatomy of, 287f
    transverse anatomy of, 287f
Thoracic spine, 327f
    cross sectional cadaver anatomic section of, 301f
    magnetic resonance imaging (MRI) of, 302f
    midline transverse scan of, 297f
    transverse computed tomography of, 301f
    transverse scan of, in thoracic paravertebral region, 296f, 299f
Thoracoabdominal nerves, 252f
    quadratus lumborum blocks in, 277
Thoracolumbar fascia (TLF), 277, 280f
Three dimensional sonoanatomy, of thoracic paravertebral region, 307-309, 308f
Three-dimensional ultrasound, 42-43, 42b, 43f-44f
    potential advantage of, 42
    of thoracic paravertebral region, 308f
    multiplanar, 295f, 306f
Through-transmission, increased, 5
Thyroid gland
    isthmus of, 355f
    left lobe of, 355f
    right lobe of, 355f
Thyroid notch, 355f
Thyroid prominence, 355f

Tibial nerve, 193, 196f, 198f, 227
    course of, 227
    imaging of, 51f
    medial calcaneal branch of, 227
    ultrasound appearance of, 227, 229f-230f, 232f
Tibial nerve block, 227-228, 228b, 229f-232f
    key points, 227t-228t
    suggested technique for, 227
Time gain compensation (TGC), 5
Tissue
    subcutaneous, 47, 47f
    thermal index of soft tissue, 66b
TKA. *see* Total knee arthroplasty
TLF. *see* Thoracolumbar fascia
TMQL block, 278
TON. *see* Third occipital nerve
Total knee arthroplasty (TKA), 169, 172b-173b
TPVB. *see* Thoracic paravertebral block
TPVS. *see* Thoracic paravertebral space
Transducer covers, 408
Transducer manipulation, 22, 23f
Transducer position
    for dorsal scapular nerve imaging, 87b
    for phrenic nerve imaging, 84f
Transducers
    conceptual illustration of, 18f
    for infraclavicular block, 94, 100f
    modern, 21
    ultrasound, 21
Transmuscular QBL, 278, 278t, 284f
Transtracheal block, 353-355, 354b
    key points on, 354t
    out-of-plane approach to, 356f
    suggested technique for, 353-354
Transversalis fascia (TF), 249, 259, 277
Transverse cervical nerve, 364f, 373f
Transverse process, of thoracic vertebra, 286, 287f
    ligaments attach to, 288f
    size, shape, and orientation of, 298f
Transverse scan
    with short-axis needle insertion, ultrasound-guided thoracic paravertebral block in, 309, 310f
    of thoracic paravertebral region, 294-299, 294f-303f
Transverse sonogram, of thoracic paravertebral region, 295f
Transversus abdominis muscle, imaging of, 55f
Transversus abdominis plane (TAP)
    arteries in, 272f
    block zones in, 272f
    muscles in, 271f
Transversus abdominis plane blocks, 53t, 259, 267-270, 267b, 271f-276f
    anatomic background of, 267
    continuous catheter, 268-269

Transversus abdominis plane blocks (*Continued*)
    discussion and comments on, 269-270
    dual, 269-270
    ilioinguinal, 268, 274f
    indications and contraindications for, 267
    in laparoscopic surgery, 270
    lateral, 269-270, 275f
    pharmacokinetics and, 269
    subcostal, 267-268, 268b, 276f
    suggested techniques for, 267-269
Transversus muscle, 255f
Transversus thoracis muscle, 244
Transversus thoracis muscular plane block, 244-246, 246b, 247f-248f
    anatomic considerations for, 244-245
    anatomic variation and, 245
    key points in, 245t
    suggested technique for, 244-245
Trapezius muscle, 364f
Trapezoid muscle, 373f
Trunk blocks
    caudal epidural block, 328-331, 329b-330b
        longitudinal in-plane approach to, 331f, 334f
        normal adult values for, 328t
        pediatric, 335f
        suggested technique for, 329
        transverse out-of-plane approach to, 334f
    neuraxial block, 319-324, 323b
        anatomic structures seen in, 320, 320t
        comments on, 322
        longitudinal paramedian view of, 319, 323b, 326f-327f
        measurements useful for guiding, 321t
        offline approaches to, 319, 324f-325f
        outcomes on, 323
        suggested technique for, 320-322
        transducer position for, 324f-325f
        transverse midline view of, 319-320, 324f
    pudendal nerve block, in children, 316-317, 317b
        discussion and comments for, 316
        suggested technique for, 316, 317f-318f

U

Ulna, acoustic shadowing by, 6f
Ulnar artery, superficial, 138, 139b, 142f
    imaging of, 141f
Ulnar nerve, 104t, 138, 139b
Ulnar nerve block, 138-139, 139b, 140f-142f
    key points, 138t-139t
    neurologic assessment of, 138
    suggested technique for, 138

Ultrasound, 1–2, 46
  approaches and techniques for, 28–30
  axillary block with, 104, 105t
  characteristics of biologic tissue, 7t
  of median nerve, 132
  for meralgia paresthetica, 144
  in musculocutaneous nerve block, 117
  three-dimensional, 42–43, 42b, 43f–44f
    potential advantage of, 42
Ultrasound gel, 407–408, 408f
Ultrasound probe, for quadratus lumborum blocks, 278–279
Ultrasound systems, beam width (slice thickness) and, 11
Ultrasound transducer, in paramedian sagittal scan, of thoracic paravertebral region, 303f
Ultrasound-guided continuous peripheral nerve block, 34–36, 35b
  equipment of, 37f
  suggested technique of, 34
Ultrasound-guided fascia iliaca block, 152f–153f
Ultrasound-guided nerve blocks, 125, 388–404, 401b
  deep tissue infection in, 400
  local anesthetic systemic toxicity in, 389, 391–393
    block types involved with, 392t
    effects of ultrasound technology on, 394t
    incidence of, 391–393, 392t
    reducing risk of, 393, 394t
    risk factors for, 391–393
  myotoxicity in, 400
  neurological complications in, 393–399
    microanatomy of peripheral nerve and, 394–396
    peripheral nerve injury in, 393–394, 395t–396t
    reducing risk of, 397–399, 397f–398f
  respiratory complications in, 399
  vascular complications in, 389–390
    reducing risk of, 389–390, 390f–391f
Ultrasound-guided thoracic paravertebral block, 292–293
  in-plane technique for, 293
  techniques of, 309–313
    intercostal approach to thoracic paravertebral space, 311–313, 312f–313f
Ultrasound-guided thoracic paravertebral block (*Continued*)
    paramedian sagittal scan with in-plane needle insertion, 309–311, 310f–311f
    transverse scan with short-axis needle insertion, 309, 310f
U-shaped distribution, of infraclavicular block, 94

V

VAM. *see* Vastoadductor membrane
Variance Doppler imaging, 19
Vascular trauma, reducing risk of, 389–390, 390f–391f
Vastoadductor membrane (VAM), 169
Veins, 64
Ventral rami, 74
Vertebral artery, 359f, 361f, 381
Vertebral vein, 381

W

Water, ultrasound characteristics of, 7t
"White walls sign", 94
Wrist, median nerve block with, 132